AAOS
AMERICAN ACADEMY OF ORTHOPAEDIC SURGEONS

Nancy Caroline's
Emergency
Care in the Streets
Author: Bob Elling, MPA, EMT-P

Student Workbook CUSTOM EDITION

JONES & BARTLETT
LEARNING

World Headquarters
Jones & Bartlett Learning
5 Wall Street
Burlington, MA 01803
978-443-5000
info@jblearning.com
www.jblearning.com

American Academy of Orthopaedic Surgeons
Chief Education Officer: Ellen C. Moore
Director, Department of Publications: Hans J. Koelsch, PhD
Senior Manager, Book Program: Lisa Claxton Moore
Senior Editor, Publications: Steven Kellert

AAOS Board of Directors, 2017–2018
President: William J. Maloney, MD
First Vice President: David A. Halsey, MD
Second Vice President: Kristy L. Weber, MD
Treasurer: M. Bradford Henley, MD, MBA
Past President: Gerald R. Williams, Jr., MD
Chair Board of Councilors: Daniel K. Guy, MD
Chair-Elect Board of Councilors: Basil R. Besh, MD
Secretary Board of Councilors: Robert M. Orfaly, MD
Chair Board of Specialty Societies: Lisa K. Cannada, MD
Chair-Elect Board of Specialty Societies: Amy L. Ladd, MD
Secretary Board of Specialty Societies: Dirk H. Alander, MD
Lay Member: James J. Balaschak
Members-At-Large:
  Robert H. Brophy, MD
  Jacob M. Buchowski, MD, MS
  Brian J. Galinat, MD, MBA
  Ronald A. Navarro, MD
CEO (Ex-Officio): Thomas E. Arend, Jr., Esq., CAE

Jones & Bartlett Learning books and products are available through most bookstores and online booksellers. To contact Jones & Bartlett Learning directly, call 800-832-0034, fax 978-443-8000, or visit our website, www.jblearning.com.

16330-8

Production Credits
General Manager and Executive Publisher: Kimberly Brophy
VP, Product Development: Christine Emerton
Senior Acquisitions Editor: Tiffany Sliter
Senior Editor: Carol B. Guerrero
Editorial Assistant: Jessica Sturtevant
Editorial Assistant: Ashley Procum
Vendor Manager: Nora Menzi
VP, Sales, Public Safety Group: Matthew Maniscalco
Director of Marketing Operations: Brian Rooney

VP, Manufacturing and Inventory Control: Therese Connell
Composition and Project Management: S4Carlisle Publishing Services
Cover Design: Kristin E. Parker
Rights & Media Specialist: Robert Boder
Media Development Editor: Troy Liston
(Title Page, Part Opener, Chapter Opener): © Jones & Bartlett Learning.
  Courtesy of MIEMSS. Background: © Photos.com/Getty
Printing and Binding: Edwards Brothers Malloy
Cover Printing: Edwards Brothers Malloy

6048

Printed in the United States of America
21 20 19 18 17   10 9 8 7 6 5 4 3 2 1

6. When developing a prevention program, the type of objective that declares that all mobile homes will be provided with a

smoke alarm and CO monitor is known as a(n) _____ _____.

7. Specific, nonjudgmental advice given on a scene to a patient who is receptive to the message is called a(n) _____

_____.

Identify

In the following case study, list the pertinent negatives that can lead to injury.

Mrs. M is so tired. She is 6 months pregnant with Katie's new brother. She works a night shift and takes care of curious 3-year-old Katie during the day. Their day starts with a bath for Katie. Mrs. M takes her out, dries her off, and gets her dressed but forgets to pull the plug in the tub because the phone is ringing. Katie runs off to get some breakfast in the kitchen, where she finds a pot of hot water for oatmeal boiling on the stove. Meanwhile, Mrs. M is still on the phone with her overbearing mother. Because Katie can't find anything to eat, she decides to go outside and play on the trampoline. Mr. M didn't get the safety net up last night when he put it together. Mrs. M finally gets off the phone with her mother and has a hard time finding Katie. Later on in the day, Mrs. M sneaks a nap while Katie is playing on the floor. Katie decides she wants to play that she is sewing like her mommy and finds the knitting needles and scissors in mommy's bag beside the chair. Luckily, Katie decides to play barber shop instead of doctor on her mommy. When Mrs. M wakes up, she is horrified to find lots of her own hair on the chair. Mrs. M. decides it would be better to take Katie to day care in the mornings while she catches up on her sleep!

1. Pertinent negatives

a. _____

b. _____

c. _____

d. _____

Ambulance Calls

The following case scenarios provide an opportunity to explore the concerns associated with patient management and paramedic care. Read each scenario, and then answer each question.

2. Mary and Jake are on duty when the tones go off for a man down. As they respond to the call, they radio dispatch for more information. Dispatch tells them that this is a lifeline call, and they are unable to get any response when they call the residence. Not knowing what they will encounter, Mary and Jake radio for law enforcement backup. When they arrive at the residence and first knock on the door, they can hear shouts for help from inside the house. A police officer shows up to help, and they determine that all doors and windows are locked, and there is no way into the house. The officer determines the basement window is the best one to break. Because Mary is the smallest person there, she is chosen to crawl through the basement window. She enters the house and finds an elderly man on the bathroom floor. After checking on the patient, she goes to unlock the front door. Mary and Jake determine that the man fell when trying to get from the toilet back to his wheelchair. He has no injuries and doesn't want to go to the hospital. He just needs a hand getting up. After calling a neighbor to come stay with the gentleman until his caregiver gets home, they load up and head back.

a. Why is it a good idea that Mary and Jake call for an officer before they get to the scene?

_____

_____

b. Which equipment should Mary have taken with her when she entered the home through the basement window?

_____

_____

_____ **4.** Which of the following patients could benefit from a "teachable moment"?
  A. An 18-year-old not wearing his seat belt who received cuts and bruises as a result of a motor vehicle crash
  B. A 3-year-old drowning patient
  C. An elderly person suffering from dementia
  D. A 45-year-old woman with a dog bite

_____ **5.** Which of the following is NOT a primary injury prevention measure?
  A. Wearing your seat belt
  B. Using safe lifting techniques
  C. Smoking only a pack a day
  D. Wearing gloves at the scene of a crash

_____ **6.** When developing a prevention program, what is the second step of the five steps discussed in the text?
  A. Plan and test interventions.
  B. Conduct a community assessment.
  C. Set goals and objectives.
  D. Define the problem.

_____ **7.** According to the Centers for Disease Control and Prevention (CDC), more than _____ children and teenagers are evaluated in the emergency department (ED) for _____.
  A. 0.5 million; home injuries
  B. 1.5 million; motor vehicle injuries
  C. 2.6 million; sports-related injuries
  D. 5 million; abuse-related injuries

_____ **8.** What is the primary focus for an EMS provider when dealing with prevention?
  A. Primary injury prevention
  B. Secondary injury prevention
  C. Illness prevention
  D. Intervention research

_____ **9.** Which of the following is NOT a reason EMS should be involved in the prevention field?
  A. EMS providers reflect the composition of the community.
  B. EMS providers are high-profile role models.
  C. EMS personnel are contacted by auto makers for safety recommendations.
  D. EMS providers are welcomed by school systems.

_____ **10.** What is the leading killer among those aged 1 to 19 in the United States?
  A. Heart disease and congenital defects of the heart
  B. Diabetes
  C. Influenza and pneumonia
  D. Injury

Fill in the Blank

Read each item carefully, and then complete the statement by filling in the missing word(s).

1. A(n) _____ is a specific prevention measure that increases safety and positive health outcomes.

2. Assault, suicide, and intentional overdose are defined as _____ injuries.

3. The four Es of prevention are _____, _____, _____/_____, and _____ _____.

4. A toy manufacturer no longer sews buttons on the teddy bears for eyes; instead, it paints on the eyes with nontoxic paint. An automatic protection for our children such as this is known as _____ _____.

5. The top five causes of death in 2014 were _____, _____, _____, _____, and _____.

Contents

Section 8: **Shock and Resuscitation** — 437

Section 9: **Special Patient Populations** — 463

Section 10: **Operations** — 539

Section 11: **Career Development** — 609

Appendices — 615

EMS Systems

© Jones & Bartlett Learning.

Try seeing it from the patient's point of view.

Matching

Match each of the definitions in the left column to the appropriate term in the right column.

_____ **1.** Outlined measures that may be difficult to obtain in a research project.

A. Systematic sampling

_____ **2.** A research format that uses a hypothesis to prove one finding from another.

B. Reciprocity

_____ **3.** A computer-generated list of subjects or groups for research.

C. Parameters

_____ **4.** A type of study in which the subjects are advised of all aspects of the study.

D. Inferential

_____ **5.** A process in which a person, an institution, or a program is evaluated and recognized as meeting certain predetermined standards to provide safe and ethical care.

E. Evidence-based practice

_____ **6.** The process of granting licensure or certification to a provider from another state or agency.

F. Unblinded study

_____ **7.** Time parameters set during a research project.

G. Certification

_____ **8.** The process used by medical magazines, journals, and other publications to ensure the quality and validity of an article before publishing it; it involves sending the article to subject matter experts for review of the content and research methods.

H. Peer review

_____ **9.** The use of practices that have been proven to be effective in improving patient outcomes.

I. Online (direct) medical control

_____ **10.** Medical direction given in real time to an EMS service or provider.

J. Alternative time sampling

Multiple Choice

Read each item carefully, and then select the best response.

_____ **1.** In which year did the National Academy of Science and the National Research Council release the white paper entitled "Accidental Death and Disability: The Neglected Disease of Modern Society"?

A. 1965

B. 1967

C. 1968

D. 1969

_____ **2.** Which of the following was NOT an emergency medical services (EMS) system element during the 1980s and 1990s?

A. Resource management

B. Public information and education

C. Decrease in number of providers

D. Medical direction

_____ **3.** What does EMR stand for?

    A. Emergency medical reaction

    B. Emergency medical receiver

    C. Emergency management response

    D. Emergency medical responder

_____ **4.** Which of the following may involve radio or electronic communications during patient care?

    A. Off-line medical control

    B. Online medical control

    C. Protocols

    D. Standing orders

_____ **5.** Which type of research is considered a basic observation only, may involve interviews with subjects, and specifies that no alterations occur?

    A. Experimental

    B. Descriptive

    C. Cross-sectional

    D. Qualitative

_____ **6.** Attributes of professionalism, as a paramedic, include all of the following, EXCEPT:

    A. communication.

    B. patient advocacy.

    C. empathy.

    D. reciprocity.

_____ **7.** Which of the following is considered a high-risk activity from a continuous quality improvement point of view?

    A. Taking vital signs

    B. Intravenous therapy

    C. Handing off patients

    D. Basic airway management

_____ **8.** Who is considered the father of paramedicine?

    A. Dr. David Boyd

    B. Dr. Eugene Nagel

    C. Dr. Jean Larrey

    D. Dr. Peter Safar

_____ **9.** Who is usually the first EMS professional with whom the public deals?

    A. EMT

    B. Law enforcement officer

    C. Dispatcher

    D. Paramedic

_____ **10.** Which level of EMS was changed to Advanced EMT in the most recent National EMS Education Standards?

    A. EMR

    B. EMT

    C. EMT-Intermediate

    D. Paramedic

_____ **11.** Which of the following is NOT considered a traditional EMS employment career for paramedics?

    A. Fire-based EMS

    B. Third-service EMS

    C. Emergency department technicians

    D. Private EMS agency

_____ **12.** In a community where the municipality operates the EMS agency, and it is not part of a public safety entity, this is referred to as:

    A. hospital-based EMS.

    B. a hybrid system.

    C. fire-based EMS.

    D. third-service EMS.

_____ **13.** When a paramedic is employed to work with a physician or other primary care provider to provide specific services to the physician's patients, this is referred to as:

    A. a municipal EMS system.

    B. a hybrid system.

    C. hospital-based EMS.

    D. a private EMS agency.

Fill in the Blank

Read each item carefully, and then complete the statement by filling in the missing word(s).

1. In the late 1950s and early 1960s, the _____ _____ _____ _____ were staffed by specially trained physicians.

2. The _____ receives and enters all information on the call, interprets the information, and relays it to the appropriate resources.

3. When a state grants certification (or licensure) to a provider from another state, it is known as _____.

4. The paramedic who can demonstrate to the patient, the patient's family members, and other health care providers the ability to identify and understand their feelings is showing _____.

5. During scene management, ensuring your own safety and the safety of your crew is your _____ _____.

6. The tool often used to continually evaluate your care is called _____ _____ _____.

7. _____ research is based on a clearly defined problem or question and gathers information as events occur in real time.

Ambulance Calls

The following case scenarios provide an opportunity to explore the concerns associated with patient management and paramedic care. Read each scenario, and then answer each question.

1. You are exiting a theater after watching a movie, when suddenly the woman in front of you falls down on the carpeted floor, landing on her knees and hands. She apparently has tripped in the dark on the steps. As you try to help her to a seated position, you find that she is not responding to you as she should. She says she feels very faint, so you lower her back to the ground. She then loses consciousness, and you lower her all the way to a supine position and make sure that her airway is open and that she is breathing. You ask your spouse to call 9-1-1 on her cell phone and to find management to bring up the theater lights and get the nearest automated external defibrillator (AED). Your patient is a 60-year-old woman who wakes up and says she is fine and doesn't want anyone making a fuss over her. She just wants to go home.

    a. Which information should you give your spouse to tell the dispatcher?

_____

_____

_____

b. What are some reasons this patient should go to the hospital to get checked out?

_____

_____

_____

2. Wow, what an evening at the theater! After your patient has left in an ambulance, you head out the door to go home. Just as you are getting into your vehicle, you hear a woman scream. It seems she has been hit by a small pickup truck that was backing up to get a good parking spot. You hurry over to find a 40-year-old woman who is conscious and alert. She is sprawled out on the ground. She is screaming about her left leg, which is where the bumper of the pickup impacted her. She was knocked to the pavement. The driver of the pickup stopped when he heard the impact and then pulled forward, which caused no more injury to the woman. She has an obvious deformity at midthigh on the left leg. An emergency medical technician (EMT) comes running to help because several people have already called 9-1-1. Because you are first on scene and the more highly trained responder, you take charge of this patient.

a. What is the first thing you should do on this scene?

_____

_____

_____

b. Which steps should you take in treating this patient before the ambulance arrives?

_____

_____

_____

True/False

If you believe the statement to be more true than false, write the letter "T" in the space provided. If you believe the statement to be more false than true, write the letter "F."

_____ **1.** The *first* documented ambulance service was started in 1869 in New York City out of Bellevue Hospital.

_____ **2.** "The White Paper" provided authority and financial support for the development of basic and advanced life support services.

_____ **3.** An emergency medical dispatcher can give simple medical instructions to the caller.

_____ **4.** The primary and backbone level of employment in the traditional EMS system is the EMR.

_____ **5.** In EMS, paramedics constitute the greatest number of trained and certified individuals in the field.

_____ **6.** The first priority at the scene is assessment of the patient.

_____ **7.** Peer review is used as a means of continuous quality improvement.

_____ **8.** Retrospective research uses available data from medical records or patient care reports (PCRs).

_____ **9.** Only the emergency vehicle operator is responsible for restocking the unit after a call.

_____ **10.** Injury prevention in the home is a topic the paramedic should be comfortable discussing with patients and bystanders.

Short Answer

Complete this section with short written answers using the space provided.

1. Pretend you are a fly on the wall during this scene: A team of paramedics arrives on scene for a routine geriatric call. The woman fell and has a broken hip. Her daughter found her and called 9-1-1. List the professional attributes the paramedics should demonstrate on this and every call.

   a. _____

   b. _____

   c. _____

   d. _____

   e. _____

   f. _____

   g. _____

   h. _____

   i. _____

   j. _____

   k. _____

2. Paramedics follow an important sequence of procedures for every emergency call. List the eight procedures.

   a. _____

   b. _____

   c. _____

   d. _____

   e. _____

   f. _____

   g. _____

   h. _____

3. No paramedic service in the United States can perform advanced life support procedures without medical direction. What is medical direction, and why is it necessary?

   _____

   _____

   _____

4. Medical control consists of several different parts. Give an example of each of the following:

   a. Online medical control:_____

   b. Protocols:_____

   c. Standing orders: _____

Although some states do require even off-duty EMS providers to stop at the scene of an accident, this law can vary from state to state. Make sure you know the laws in your area.

© Jones & Bartlett Learning.

Workforce Safety and Wellness

Matching

Part I

Stress is a major part of a paramedic's job. Indicate which of the following two types of stress you are more likely to experience in the following scenarios.

A. Eustress   B. Distress

_____ **1.** You are running a 10-km road race with your best friend. You have been training to beat her, and she is about 15 steps in front of you.

_____ **2.** You respond to a rollover collision and find out that the unrestrained driver of the vehicle is your 17-year-old daughter.

_____ **3.** You are assigned to work with Billy Bob for the next month. Billy Bob is not your favorite person and is always criticizing every move you make.

_____ **4.** You are taking your National Registry Paramedic exam next week, and you are studying in hopes of passing the test with an excellent grade the first time you take it.

_____ **5.** You find out the ambulance service that you work for is merging with a larger service. There is talk that your position will be eliminated.

_____ **6.** You are climbing Pikes Peak, and you are about to make the summit (your lifelong dream), but you don't feel that you have enough energy left to climb the last 500 feet.

_____ **7.** Your spouse has just left a letter explaining to you that he/she is divorcing you and that he/she has already cleaned out the bank accounts.

Part II

Match each psychological defense mechanism with the situation in which it is most likely to be used.

A. Projection   **B.** Denial   **C.** Regression

_____ **1.** Your patient is ignoring the symptoms he has been having over the past few days.

_____ **2.** Your school-aged patient is upset by her injuries and seems to be acting like a toddler.

_____ **3.** Your patient seems to be blaming his symptoms on the bad behaviors of his family members.

Part III

Match each of the definitions in the left column to the appropriate term in the right column.

_____ 1. A fear reaction in which a person's judgment seems to disappear entirely; it is particularly dangerous because it may precipitate mass panic among others.

A. Defense mechanism

_____ 2. Pathogenic microorganisms that are present in human blood and can cause disease in humans; they include, but are not limited to, hepatitis B virus and human immunodeficiency virus.

B. Transmission

_____ 3. Any disease that can be spread from person to person or from animal to person.

C. Denial

_____ 4. An event that overwhelms a person's ability to cope with the experience, either at the scene or later.

D. Blind panic

_____ 5. Psychological ways to relieve stress; they are usually automatic or subconscious (eg, denial, regression, projection, and displacement).

E. Standard precautions

_____ 6. An early response to a serious medical emergency in which the severity of the emergency is diminished or minimized.

F. Bloodborne pathogens

_____ 7. Exposure to, or transmission of, a communicable disease from one person to another by physical contact.

G. Direct contact

_____ 8. A disease that is caused by the growth and spread of small harmful organisms within the body or one that is capable of being transmitted with or without direct contact.

H. Communicable disease

_____ 9. Protective measures that have traditionally been developed by the Centers for Disease Control and Prevention for use in dealing with objects, blood, body fluids, or other potential exposure risks of communicable disease.

I. Infectious disease

_____ 10. The way in which an infectious agent is spread: contact, airborne, foodborne, or by vectors.

J. Critical incident

Multiple Choice

Read each item carefully, and then select the best response.

_____ 1. You respond to a 12-year-old boy who has been hit by a car. He is alert but has a deformity of his lower left leg. The boy "baby talks" as he is answering your questions. This is a form of:

    A. denial.

    B. projection.

    C. regression.

    D. displacement.

_____ 2. You respond to a multiple-casualty incident (MCI) involving a collision of a charter bus of senior citizens and a car with four teenagers. At the scene, you find one teen with no obvious injuries. You have to tell him numerous times to sit on the side of the road and stay away from the moving traffic. His judgment seems impaired, and he may be experiencing:

    A. conversion hysteria.

    B. projection.

    C. depression.

    D. blind panic.

_____ 3. Which of the following would NOT be a symptom of impending paramedic burnout?

    A. Increased interest in hobbies

    B. Chronic fatigue and irritability

    C. Cynical, negative attitude

    D. Decreasing ability to concentrate

_____ **4.** As a result of your partner's careless behavior, you have been stuck by a needle that was used to start an IV on your patient. Which of the following should be done immediately?

    A. Get a medical evaluation from the emergency department physician.

    B. Document the negligence of your partner.

    C. Wash the area of the exposure with soap and water.

    D. Get a booster shot for all of your immunizations.

_____ **5.** According to the Centers for Disease Control and Prevention, when should you wear an N95 or N100 respirator?

    A. Between patient contacts

    B. When working with a patient who has tuberculosis

    C. When touching mucous membranes

    D. When dealing with blood or body fluids

_____ **6.** You are on your first "code." As you arrive on scene, you feel stressed. Which of the following management techniques would NOT help you during this call?

    A. Focusing on the immediate situation

    B. Controlled deep breathing

    C. Progressive relaxation

    D. Regression

_____ **7.** You are on the scene of a major car crash. Your patient is an elderly man who has now accepted the fact that he is really hurt and could be in the hospital for a long time. Which of the following reactions might the patient experience?

    A. Depression

    B. Fear

    C. Anger

    D. All of the above

_____ **8.** At a vehicle collision, you believe that you have everyone accounted for and managed. Suddenly you hear a baby crying and realize there is a child whom you have not found yet. Your heart begins to race; this is an example of a(n):

    A. delayed reaction.

    B. alert response.

    C. defense mechanism.

    D. fight-or-flight response.

_____ **9.** After being told she might be having a heart attack, a 66-year-old female patient hits the paramedic in anger and tells him that he doesn't know what he is talking about. Which defense mechanism is associated with this kind of reaction?

    A. Displacement

    B. Projection

    C. Alarm reaction

    D. Denial

_____ **10.** A paramedic who has been on duty for 6 months of double shifts (without a personal day) begins to show signs of physical and emotional breakdown. He is cynical and doesn't seem to be able to sleep. These are signs of:

    A. eustress.

    B. burnout.

    C. anxiety.

    D. alert response.

Fill in the Blank

Read each item carefully, and then complete the statement by filling in the missing word(s).

1. The following paragraphs describe behaviors of different individuals under stress. For each description, fill in the defense mechanism that the individual is apparently using.

    a. Your partner has been irritable and ill-tempered ever since he arrived at work today. You are doing your best to keep a low profile and not annoy him further, but nonetheless he snaps at you, "You sure are in a lousy mood today." Your partner is showing the mechanism of defense known as _____.

    b. You are called by a very distraught woman to treat her husband, who has been having chest pain. When you reach the patient's house, he says, "I can't understand why my wife called for an ambulance; I'm just having a little indigestion, that's all." His face is gray, and he is sweating profusely. He is using the psychological defense mechanism known as _____.

    c. A 22-year-old woman is extricated from a wrecked automobile in which her boyfriend remains trapped. She says she has lost all sensation in her hands and feet. She does not appear terribly upset about that fact, and you cannot find any signs of injury on her body. She is using the psychological defense mechanism known as _____.

    d. At the scene of a car crash, you are trying to extricate an entrapped front-seat passenger who is seriously injured. The driver, who has not suffered any apparent injury, is giving you a hard time. "Be careful, will you! Don't drop her! Watch what you're doing, you damn idiot!" He is very aggressive toward you, but you realize that his behavior is simply a(n) _____ of the anger he feels toward himself for having caused the injury to his passenger.

2. Being a paramedic is a stressful job. For some, the stresses are too much, and burnout can occur. The time to start thinking about burnout—and how to prevent it—is now, during your training. Develop strategies that will keep burnout from happening to you by listing some of the steps you plan to take to keep from burning out as a paramedic.

    a. _____

    b. _____

    c. _____

    d. _____

    e. _____

    f. _____

    g. _____

    h. _____

Identify

In the following case study, list the six pertinent negatives with regard to the well-being of your partner, Tommy Jones. Also, identify two stress reactions of the patient.

It is midnight, and Tommy Jones is still awake, watching a horror movie on TV and drinking his last soda out of the six-pack that he brought to work today. You are both on a 24-hour shift, and he has just been lying around the TV room when he was not out on calls. He skipped his workout today so that he could watch his favorite soap opera. He is bummed out that he is out of cigarettes and is searching the kitchen for yet another bag of popcorn when the tones go off, indicating another call.

As you head from the bunk room to the ambulance, Tommy is yelling that it is all your fault there is another call. "If you hadn't gone to bed, we wouldn't have had another call tonight," he grumbles.

You arrive at the scene to find a 72-year-old woman who has fallen and fractured her hip. As you begin your treatment, the patient begins to blame you for all of her problems. As you load her into the ambulance, the patient reaches out and pinches your arm as hard as she can.

After you deliver your patient to the hospital, Tommy stops to grab another pack of smokes and a bean burrito. As you pull into the bay, Tommy tells you to restock because he wants to watch the end of the movie. As he heads into the TV room, he tells you that his stomach is killing him and that he might be your next patient.

1. Pertinent negatives

a. _____

b. _____

c. _____

d. _____

e. _____

f. _____

2. Stress reactions

a. _____

b. _____

Ambulance Calls

The following case scenarios provide an opportunity to explore the concerns associated with patient management and paramedic care. Read each scenario, and then answer each question.

1. Your unit responds to a call for a 3-month-old boy who is not breathing. When you enter the house, you find a mother holding the boy, who is not breathing and is very pale. You and your partner, John, begin working the code. You start the steps of cardiopulmonary resuscitation (CPR), with compressions, while gathering as much information as possible about what has happened. As you arrive at the hospital with the infant, you know in your heart that the child is dead. The code team works further on the child, and finally, the doctor calls for the time of death. John storms out of the room and out to the ambulance to begin cleanup. John begins to yell about the fact that the child died and how if he hadn't missed the first IV on the child, he might still be alive. You finish your patient care report (PCR) and then head back to the station. At the station, John refuses to talk about the call and says he wants to be alone. He ends up sitting at the table just staring off into space for the rest of the afternoon. At the next shift, John is very negative and flies off the handle at everyone that day. After the shift is over, John heads for the local bar instead of going home to his wife and his 2-month-old son. Two weeks later, John is put on mandatory leave for his mental well-being.

a. Explain how this one incident could have triggered John's decline.

_____

_____

_____

b. What are some steps that every paramedic can take to reduce stress on the job?

_____

_____

2. A call comes in for a motor vehicle crash involving a small car and a pickup truck. It was a head-on collision, with both vehicles going 60 mi/h. Your patient is a 56-year-old man. He was not wearing his seat belt when the crash occurred. He has multiple breaks of both arms and legs. He has a large cut on his forehead that is bleeding profusely. You begin your trauma assessment on him after doing a rapid extrication with a long backboard. In the back of the ambulance, you begin treatment by applying oxygen and starting two large-bore IVs en route to the hospital. The patient is alert and is able to respond to you correctly. His blood pressure is 78/40 mm Hg, and respirations are 32 breaths/min and shallow. His skin is cool and clammy, and you have no pulses in the wrists or the feet. The cardiac monitor is showing sinus tachycardia with multifocal premature ventricular complexes (PVCs) that are becoming very frequent. You don't hear good lung sounds, and you prepare for needle decompression of the right chest. You know that this patient is approaching death and will more than likely turn into a trauma code.

a. Your patient looks up at you and asks, "Am I going to die?" How do you respond to him?

_____

_____

_____

b. What are the five stages that you might witness in this patient, and how will the patient act during these stages?

(1)_____

(2)_____

(3)_____

(4)_____

(5)_____

True/False

If you believe the statement to be more true than false, write the letter "T" in the space provided. If you believe the statement to be more false than true, write the letter "F."

_____   **1.** The USDA 2015 dietary guidelines contain five different food groups.

_____   **2.** You should avoid caffeine and keep a regular sleep schedule.

_____   **3.** When lifting, you should use your back, so you don't injure your knees.

_____   **4.** Indirect contact involves the spread of infection between the patient with an infection to another person through a contaminated inanimate object.

_____   **5.** You should sanitize your stethoscope with alcohol or disinfectant wipes.

_____   **6.** Anger is a defense mechanism.

_____   **7.** Blind panic is present when a patient converts anxiety to a bodily dysfunction, such as a paralyzed extremity.

_____   **8.** Burnout is a consequence of chronic, unrelieved stress.

_____   **9.** The stages of the grieving process, in order, are denial, anger, bargaining, depression, and acceptance.

_____   **10.** Gloves are absolutely essential on every emergency medical services (EMS) call.

_____   **11.** Gloves are the only personal protective equipment (PPE) needed when suctioning a patient.

_____   **12.** A mask worn by you can protect the patient from your germs.

_____   **13.** Your maximum heart rate during exercise should be 320 minus your age.

_____   **14.** The redirecting of one's emotions from the original source to the paramedic is known as displacement.

Short Answer

Complete this section with short written answers using the space provided.

1. When faced with a perceived threat, the body reacts with a fight-or-flight response. From your own experience, list four signs or symptoms of the fight-or-flight response.

   a. _____

   b. _____

   c. _____

   d. _____

2. At times, you are the person who will be dealing with a grieving family. List the six guidelines for helping the family begin the process of coping with their loss.

   a. _____

   b. _____

   c. _____

   d. _____

   e. _____

   f. _____

3. In general, people who have any of five types of reactions to mass casualties should be removed from the scene. These five types of reactions are:

   a. _____

   b. _____

   c. _____

   d. _____

   e. _____

Problem Solving

Calculate the maximum heart rate and target heart rate for a person with a resting heart rate of 76 beats/min and an age of 46 years.

1. a. Resting heart rate _____

   b. 220 – _____ (age in years) = _____ (Maximum heart rate)

   c. _____ (Maximum heart rate) – _____ (Resting heart rate) = _____ × 0.7 = _____ (round up)

   d. _____ (Total) + _____ (Resting heart rate) = _____ (Target heart rate)

c. During this call, Mary and Jake can apply the teachable moment. What are some things they can teach their patient?

_____

_____

3. Courtney and Larry have been called by the local elementary school to do a program for the third and fourth grades. They decide to educate the children on how and why to call 9-1-1. They arrive with a video of a dispatcher taking a "call" from a child. They show all the steps of how and when to call, what the dispatcher will say, and how the ambulance will respond to them. The video shows a child calling 9-1-1 after she finds her grandpa "asleep" on the floor and is unable to wake him up. Three days later during their shift, Courtney and Larry get a call for a woman who won't wake up. The dispatcher has the woman's 8-year-old son on the phone. When they arrive, they find a woman who won't wake up on the couch and a very upset little boy. With a few good questions, they determine the mother has diabetes. After getting a reading of 66 on the glucometer, they start an IV and give her D_{50}. The woman wakes up, and after eating a peanut butter and jelly sandwich, her glucose level stabilizes. Courtney and Larry stay a little longer to make sure everything is going well and wait for her neighbor to arrive. After receiving approval from medical control, they allow the patient to sign off and not be transported. During this time, they find out the boy, Ryan, was at their demonstration a few days ago.

a. When Larry and Courtney created an implementation plan for their program, they developed their objective with the SMART plan. What does the SMART plan stand for?

S _____

M _____

A _____

R _____

T _____

b. How did their program help Ryan decide to get help for his mother?

_____

_____

True/False

If you believe the statement to be more true than false, write the letter "T" in the space provided. If you believe the statement to be more false than true, write the letter "F."

_____   **1.** Primary prevention is defined as reducing the effects of an injury that has already happened.

_____   **2.** Unintentional injuries are the leading cause of death for people between 1 and 19 years of age.

_____   **3.** The three factors used in making a Haddon injury matrix are the host, the event, and the post-event.

_____   **4.** The process of collecting, analyzing, and interpreting injury data is called injury surveillance.

_____   **5.** A risk factor for an intentional injury would be not wearing your seat belt.

_____   **6.** In creating an implementation plan, you need a realistic time line to complete your project.

_____   **7.** Two of the five steps in developing a prevention plan are conducting a community assessment and setting goals and objectives.

_____   **8.** When using SMART to meet your objectives, the R in this acronym stands for risk.

_____   **9.** Funding for a prevention program can include donations from local media, grants, and sponsorships from different organizations.

_____   **10.** Every EMS call includes a teachable moment.

Short Answer

Complete this section with short written answers using the space provided.

1. Define primary injury prevention and secondary injury prevention, and give an example of each.

Primary injury prevention: _____

Secondary injury prevention: _____

2. Give three examples of why EMS providers should be active in the prevention field.

a. _____

b. _____

c. _____

3. List the four Es of prevention, and explain each one.

a. _____

b. _____

c. _____

d. _____

4. A public health model will help to identify a problem and how to approach the problem. Use this approach to list the three key factors involved in the problem of children and swimming-pool drowning deaths.

a. _____

b. _____

c. _____

Fill in the Table

Fill in the missing parts of the table.

The Five Steps to Developing a Prevention Program
1. _____
2. _____
3. Set goals and objectives.
4. _____
5. _____

Medical, Legal, and Ethical Issues

As a paramedic you will frequently encounter situations for which there is no right or wrong answer—and for which no amount of studying can prepare you. Use your best judgment, consult with supervisors if possible, and ask yourself, "What is best for the patient?"

Matching

Part I

Match the following sentences with the correct situation. For questions 1 to 6, indicate whether:

   A. You may treat the patient without obtaining the patient's expressed consent.

   B. You may NOT treat the patient without obtaining the patient's expressed consent.

_____   **1.** A 10-year-old child is struck by a car. He is bleeding profusely. His parents cannot be located.

_____   **2.** A 48-year-old man is injured in a motor vehicle crash in which his car was demolished. He has bruises on his forehead. He seems confused. He says, "I'm all right. Let me alone. I just called for an Uber car."

_____   **3.** A 56-year-old woman has chest pain. Her husband phoned for an ambulance. The patient says, "It's nothing, just my gastroesophageal reflux disease." She refuses to be examined or treated.

_____   **4.** A 26-year-old woman is pulled from the beach surf in cardiac arrest.

_____   **5.** A 23-year-old man is injured in a barroom altercation. He is bleeding profusely from his nose and mouth. He smells strongly of alcohol. He is very belligerent and shouts at you, "Leave me alone, you creeps. If you come any closer, I'll knock your teeth in."

_____   **6.** An 82-year-old woman has fainted at home. Her son found her on the floor and called for an ambulance. She is conscious when you arrive. She says to you, "You are all very sweet, but one can't live forever, you know, and I don't fancy hospitals."

For questions 7 to 10, match the following words to the correct situation.

   A. Slander

   B. Defamation

   C. Battery

   D. Assault

_____   **7.** The reporting paramedic wrote on his patient care report (PCR) that Mr. Paul was obviously drunk. The paramedic made that statement because he has a long-running feud with Mr. Paul and thought this was a great way to pay him back.

_____   **8.** Mrs. O'Malley told the emergency medical technician (EMT) not to touch her. She did not want any help. The EMT went ahead and tried to grab Mrs. O'Malley and put her on the cot.

_____   **9.** Mitch is taking a patient into the hospital. The patient asks about the doctor on staff. Mitch tells the patient, "Sorry, buddy, but I wouldn't want that witch doctor treating me. Good luck, partner."

_____   **10.** Ryan is in the back of the ambulance with his patient, Jake, who is 16 years old and has just rolled his car. Jake is really wound up and wants out of the ambulance. Ryan tells Jake that if he doesn't calm down, he is going to strap him down and give him a shot.

Match each of the following items to the appropriate situation.

E = Ethical   **M** = Moral   **UE** = Unethical practice

_____ **11.** The patient's religion determines that no matter how sick the person is, the person will not seek medical attention.

_____ **12.** The physician believes that Mother is terminal, but he wants to try at least one more medication to see if it can help her.

_____ **13.** My patient has overdosed on crack cocaine, so he is not worth working on.

_____ **14.** Even though my patient, who was drinking and driving, has just killed a family of four in a car crash, I will do my best to provide medical attention to him.

_____ **15.** A 40-year-old woman has tried to commit suicide by overdosing; if she wants to die, let's give her that wish by working this as a "slow code."

_____ **16.** The patient does not want any pain medication because he feels that those medications are considered "drugs."

_____ **17.** This patient obviously doesn't have the money for this emergency department (ED) visit; let's wait until all of the other patients have been taken care of before we work on this welfare case.

_____ **18.** Mark intentionally left out the fact that he gave five times the normal epinephrine dose on the PCR.

_____ **19.** After helping the mother give birth to a premature stillborn child, the paramedic blessed the infant because the mother requested that the child be blessed.

_____ **20.** The paramedic gave the apparently "drunk" 18-year-old patient Lasix on the long transport to the hospital. He wanted to teach the patient a lesson. He thought that if the patient wet himself, it would be funny.

Part II

Match each of the definitions in the left column to the appropriate term in the right column.

_____ **1.** Unauthorized act committed outside the scope of medical practice defined by law.

A. Abandonment

_____ **2.** A person who is younger than the legal age (generally 18 years) in a given state but is legally considered an adult because of other circumstances.

B. Advance directive

_____ **3.** Legal protection from penalties that could normally be incurred under the law.

C. Borrowed servant doctrine

_____ **4.** A right to a fair procedure for a legal action against a person or agency; has two components: notice and opportunity to be heard.

D. Common law

_____ **5.** Act(s) committed by a plaintiff that contribute(s) to adverse outcomes.

E. Contributory negligence

_____ **6.** A principle that absolves an institution of liability when one of its members acts beyond his or her scope of certification or training by following someone else's orders.

F. Defamation

_____ **7.** Termination of medical care for the patient without giving the patient sufficient opportunity to find another suitable health care professional to take over his or her medical treatment.

G. Due process

_____ **8.** A decision that has been made by a judge through a court case based on his or her interpretation of the statutes and constitutions; it can be overturned either by another court with a higher authority or the issuing court at a later time; also called case law.

H. Emancipated minor

_____ **9.** A written document or oral statement that expresses the wants, needs, and desires of a patient in reference to future medical care; examples include living wills, do not resuscitate (DNR) orders, and organ donation orders.

I. Immunity

_____ **10.** Intentionally making a false statement, through written or verbal communication that injures a person's good name or reputation.

J. Malfeasance

Multiple Choice

Read each item carefully, and then select the best response.

_____ **1.** You have responded to a fender bender, where your patient is conscious and alert. The patient is able to answer all questions correctly and declines treatment. Your overzealous partner starts to put a cervical collar on the patient. What could he be charged with?

   A. Assault

   B. Battery

   C. False imprisonment

   D. Libel

_____ **2.** You are on a volunteer squad in a small town. At the grocery store, your neighbor starts asking you what happened the night before. You proceed to tell her that the local dentist was hitting his wife, and you had to take her up to the hospital for a broken jaw. Along the way, you let slide a few of your own opinions about the dentist. Soon the story is all over town. The dentist is upset and contacts a lawyer to initiate a lawsuit against you. What will you be charged with?

   A. Defamation

   B. Libel

   C. Slander

   D. Assault

_____ **3.** What does the Health Insurance Portability and Accountability Act (HIPAA) guarantee the patient?

   A. The hospital cannot transfer a mother in labor.

   B. The paramedic can treat the patient without consent if she or he believes the patient has a life-threatening problem.

   C. The paramedic meets minimum qualifications.

   D. The patient's medical information will remain confidential at all times.

_____ **4.** Which of the following is NOT needed to prove the negligence of the paramedic?

   A. The paramedic treated an unconscious patient.

   B. The paramedic had a legal duty to act.

   C. The paramedic breached his or her duty to act.

   D. The patient was harmed by the paramedic.

_____ **5.** You arrive at the ED with a patient complaining of "chest pain" as your pager goes off for the next call of the night. In your hurry to get out of the hospital, you hand off your patient to the ward clerk, knowing that a registered nurse (RN) will be coming soon to take over. You are guilty of:

   A. proximate cause.

   B. ordinary negligence.

   C. gross negligence.

   D. abandonment.

_____ **6.** You are called to the local elementary school for a child who has fallen from the top of the slide. The child is not making any sense and is vomiting. The school is unable to reach her parents. Under which type of consent can you treat and transport this child?

   A. Informed

   B. Implied

   C. Expressed

   D. Involuntary

_____ **7.** You respond to a man down. You find a homeless person in an alley. Which of the following findings would allow you to take the man to the hospital under implied consent?

   A. He has not eaten for at least 6 hours.

   B. He does not appear clean.

   C. His oxygen level is 82%.

   D. His blood glucose level is normal.

_____ **8.** After transferring care of the homeless man in the preceding question to the nurse, which of the following does NOT belong in your PCR?

    A. The patient was unkempt and stunk badly.

    B. The patient had an oxygen level of 92%.

    C. The patient has not had anything to eat.

    D. The patient's blood glucose was 100 mg/dL.

_____ **9.** Which of the following patients must be reported?

    A. A 16-year-old girl who refuses to eat

    B. A new mother who is feeling very depressed

    C. A 10-year-old boy who was bitten by a dog

    D. A 25-year-old man who was binge drinking

_____ **10.** How are most civil cases resolved?

    A. A settlement process

    B. A trial by a judge

    C. A trial by jury

    D. None of the above

_____ **11.** What is the paramedic's best protection in court?

    A. A voice recording of every call

    B. A complete and accurate PCR

    C. Rewriting the PCR at a later date or time

    D. Video cameras in the back of the units

_____ **12.** In which of the following situations would you work "the code"?

    A. A woman who was found in rigor mortis in her bathroom

    B. A patient who was decapitated in a car wreck

    C. A 6-year-old child who was trapped under ice for 20 minutes

    D. A 56-year-old man who had a tractor crush his chest area and has been trapped for 40 minutes

_____ **13.** What is the person (or procedure) called when one adult has the legal authority to make the health care decisions for another?

    A. Power of attorney

    B. Parents

    C. Surrogate decision maker

    D. None of the above

_____ **14.** Which of the following is NOT an advance directive?

    A. The doctor's recommendations

    B. A DNR order

    C. A living will

    D. A health care power of attorney

_____ **15.** In the National Association of Emergency Medical Technicians (NAEMT) _Code of Ethics for Emergency Medical Technicians_, which of the following is NOT a fundamental responsibility?

    A. Alleviating suffering

    B. Promoting health

    C. Conserving life

    D. Providing moral support

Fill in the Blank

Read each item carefully, and then complete the statement by filling in the missing word(s).

1. Failure to obtain consent before providing medical treatment might give rise to charges of technical assault and battery. What are the requirements for obtaining consent to treat in the following scenarios?

    a. From a conscious, mentally competent adult, consent must be _____.

    b. To treat a child, consent must be obtained from the _____ _____ or _____ _____.

2. The patient is claiming that he was harmed by the paramedic's actions. In a lawsuit, the patient will be the _____, and the paramedic will be the _____.

3. The paramedic is permitted by the medical director to carry out certain treatments. This is known as the paramedic's

    _____ _____ _____.

4. A document that expresses the patient's wants, needs, and desires in relation to the patient's future medical care is

    known as a(n) _____ _____.

5. A minor who has been _____ is a minor younger than legal age but is treated as an adult because of marriage,

    pregnancy, or active military service.

6. Another significant _____ and _____ problem that has occurred in emergency medical services (EMS) is the

    _____ of training and certification records.

Identify

In the following case study, list the chief complaint, vital signs, and pertinent negatives.

You are called to the local sports bar for a man not feeling well. When you arrive, you are confronted by a 30-year-old man who is acting very strangely. He is yelling that he doesn't need anyone's help and just to leave him alone. All he wants is a sandwich and a beer. The patient refuses any type of help and correctly answers all of your questions. Once again, he says he wants to be left alone. Without consent and with a cranky patient, you don't feel that you can treat this patient. As you are ready to leave, the man falls off the barstool and is unconscious. You begin treatment by opening his airway and checking for breathing. He is breathing 20 breaths/min with an oxygen saturation level of 97%. The patient moans but makes no other noises. Your partner notices a medical ID bracelet stating the man has diabetes. You take a blood glucose reading and find it to be 42 mg/dL. Your partner applies oxygen by a non-rebreathing mask and starts an IV on the patient. Vital signs for this patient are as follows: blood pressure is 132/70 mm Hg, pulse is 96 beats/min, lung sounds are clear bilaterally, skin is cool, and pupils are a bit sluggish. You give 25 g of D_{50} by IV. The patient begins to wake up very quickly and asks what is going on. He tells you he had taken his sugar reading earlier and realized he needed to eat, so he stopped for food. He is now competent and does not want to be transported to the ED. After making sure that his vital signs are within normal ranges and that his blood glucose level has come up to a reading of 118 mg/dL, you discontinue the IV. Your partner writes up a report, and once again you check all of the patient's vital signs, finding them normal. The patient again refuses transport after you have determined that he is competent. With approval from medical control, you have the patient sign off, and you return to your unit, back in service for the next call.

1. Chief complaint: _____

    _____

    _____

2. Vital signs: _____

    _____

    _____

3. Pertinent negatives: _____

_____

_____

Ambulance Calls

The following case scenarios provide an opportunity to explore the concerns associated with patient management and paramedic care. Read each scenario, and then answer each question.

1. Six emergency calls are described in the following list. Circle the letter beside those calls in which it is permissible for a paramedic to give treatment without obtaining expressed consent from the patient. In those cases in which you may *not* treat the patient without expressed consent, describe which action you would take.

   a. A 10-year-old boy has fallen at school and sprained his right ankle. The school authorities have so far been unable to reach the boy's parents.

   _____

   _____

   b. A 45-year-old woman is found in cardiac arrest.

   _____

   _____

   c. A 21-year-old man called for an ambulance after his 19-year-old girlfriend swallowed a large number of sleeping pills. She is awake and refuses treatment. She says, "Go away and let me die."

   _____

   _____

   d. A 20-year-old man has taken PCP (a psychedelic drug that often induces violent behavior) and has tried to gouge out his eyes. He is bleeding profusely from the face and screaming, "Don't come near me."

   _____

   _____

   e. A 14-year-old boy was knocked from his bicycle and hit by a truck. He is unconscious and bleeding. Both legs appear fractured. Bystanders do not know the boy or his parents.

   _____

   _____

   f. A 48-year-old man has crushing chest pain. His wife called for the ambulance. The man says he doesn't need an ambulance; he just has indigestion. His face is gray, and he is sweating profusely.

   _____

   _____

2. You are called to the scene of a crash in which a pedestrian has been struck by a car. The driver of the car says the pedestrian staggered out into the street in front of him. The pedestrian is now sitting on the curb. He has an obvious bruise on his head. He is unkempt and smells strongly of alcohol. He tells you that he doesn't want to go to the hospital. You suspect that the patient might not be competent to make that decision. List three things you can check to assess his mental competence.

   a. _____

   b. _____

   c. _____

True/False

If you believe the statement to be more true than false, write the letter "T" in the space provided. If you believe the statement to be more false than true, write the letter "F."

_____ 1. You can be sued for slander when you write a false statement on your PCR.

_____ 2. The discovery period during a lawsuit can take anywhere from a few months to more than 2 years.

_____ 3. You should contact medical control in the case of a physician's orders on a scene if the orders do not fit the emergency situation.

_____ 4. HIPAA protects the patient's right to confidentiality.

_____ 5. Good Samaritan laws are designed to protect all paramedics from lawsuits.

_____ 6. To prove negligence on the part of the paramedic, the plaintiff must prove legal duty, breach of duty, failure to act, and harm.

_____ 7. A DNR order is not considered an advance directive.

_____ 8. You must gain informed consent from every competent adult before beginning treatment.

_____ 9. You must have parental consent even for an emancipated minor.

_____ 10. The paramedic's best defense in a lawsuit is his or her written report on the patient.

_____ 11. Ethics is a code of conduct that is defined by society and religion along with a person's conscience.

_____ 12. The *Code of Ethics for Emergency Medical Technicians* states that EMTs should adhere to standards of personal ethics that reflect credit upon the profession.

_____ 13. You should always place the welfare of your patient ahead of any personal considerations, except for your own safety.

_____ 14. Patient autonomy is the power of attorney making medical decisions for the patient.

_____ 15. A DNR order can be printed on a medical ID bracelet.

_____ 16. Advance directives are usually created once the patient can no longer make the decisions for his or her own health care.

_____ 17. A person who makes health care decisions for another or carries the power of attorney is called a surrogate decision maker.

_____ 18. Your general focus during resuscitation should be to provide at least 30 minutes of your best efforts.

_____ 19. If you witness misconduct by another EMS provider, you should report that person immediately to the chain of command.

_____ 20. You should always work on a baby with sudden infant death syndrome (SIDS), even if the baby is in rigor mortis.

Short Answer

Complete this section with short written answers using the space provided.

1. Every state in the United States defines certain cases as "coroner's cases"—that is, cases of death that you are obliged to report to law enforcement authorities. Although regulations vary somewhat from state to state, certain categories of cases are nearly universally regarded as coroner's cases. List three such categories.

a. _____

b. _____

c. _____

2. Good Samaritan legislation was written to prevent lawsuits from being brought against people who try to assist at an emergency scene. Explain why the Good Samaritan laws would not be a good defense for a paramedic who has a lawsuit brought against him or her.

_____

_____

_____

3. If legal action is taken against a paramedic, the charge most likely to be brought is that of professional negligence (malpractice). To prove that the paramedic was negligent, the plaintiff must demonstrate four things. List the four elements required to prove negligence.

a. _____

b. _____

c. _____

d. _____

4. List four types of cases that paramedics or other health care professionals in your state are required to report to the appropriate authorities.

a. _____

b. _____

c. _____

d. _____

5. (a) What is MOLST?
(b) Is it used in your state?

a. _____

b. _____

6. Ethics refers to the rules of right and wrong that we live by. Medical ethics refers to rules of right and wrong that guide the behavior of health care professionals. State in one or two sentences what you regard as the guiding principle of your work as a paramedic.

_____

_____

_____

7. How would you handle a paramedic who continually makes racist remarks about your patients?

_____

_____

_____

8. Explain the things you would look for in a DNR order when you arrive on scene and find the patient in cardiac arrest.

_____

_____

_____

Communications

© Jones & Bartlett Learning.

Look rookie, only your mother would be willing to order a pizza for you—and don't talk with your mouth full.

Matching

Part I

Indicate whether each of the following questions from a patient interview is an open-ended question or a closed-ended question.

O = open-ended question

C = closed-ended question

_____ **1.** What happened today?

_____ **2.** Do you remember the collision?

_____ **3.** What does your blood pressure usually run?

_____ **4.** Are you pregnant?

_____ **5.** Have you been sick in the last few weeks?

_____ **6.** Do you have asthma?

_____ **7.** Which medications do you take daily?

_____ **8.** What does the pain feel like to you?

_____ **9.** Do you wear contact lenses?

_____ **10.** How much do you weigh?

Part II

Match each of the definitions in the left column to the appropriate term in the right column.

_____ **1.** The number of cycles (oscillations) per second of a radio signal.

_____ **2.** Radio system using paired frequencies to permit the use of remote repeaters or simultaneous transmission and reception.

_____ **3.** The location to which 9-1-1 calls are routed, which may or may not serve as the dispatch center.

_____ **4.** Remote radio transceiver that receives radio signals and rebroadcasts them at a higher power, extending the range of a radio communications system.

_____ **5.** Public safety communications systems that are compatible across all local, tribal, state, and federal agencies.

_____ **6.** Computer-based system permitting real-time two-way audio, video, and data communication between the paramedic and the medical control physician.

_____ **7.** Simultaneous transmission of multiple data streams, most often voice and electrocardiogram signals.

A. Base station

B. Biotelemetry

C. Computer-assisted dispatch (CAD)

D. Crew resource management (CRM)

E. Cultural competence

F. Digital radio

G. Duplex

_____ **8.** Computerized sharing of radio frequencies by multiple units, agencies, or systems.

_____ **9.** A radio at a fixed location consisting of a transmitter, receiver, and antenna.

_____ **10.** Linked dispatch center computer consoles and vehicle-mounted mobile data terminals.

_____ **11.** The transmission of information via radio waves using native digital data or analog (voice) signals that have been converted to a digital signal and compressed.

_____ **12.** An understanding of the predominant cultures that exist in the geographic area in which the paramedic provides patient care.

_____ **13.** Transmission of physiologic data, such as electrocardiogram, from the patient to a distant point of reception (commonly referred to in emergency medical services as telemetry).

_____ **14.** An operational practice designed to enhance communication and teamwork, thereby reducing preventable errors.

H. Frequency

I. Interoperability

J. Multiplex

K. Public safety answering point (PSAP)

L. Repeater

M. Telemedicine

N. Trunked radio system

Part III

The following statements come from a patient's case history. Arrange them in the correct order for a paramedic radio transmission to medical command.

1. **A.** Pulse is 50 beats/min and regular, respirations are 36 breaths/min and deep, blood pressure (BP) is 180/126 mm Hg, and SpO_2 is 94%.
   B. The patient has a history of hypertension.
   C. The deep tendon reflexes are hyperactive.
   D. Her daughter says the patient complained of a severe headache before she collapsed.
   E. The patient was still responsive on our arrival, but she rapidly became unresponsive.
   F. The patient is a 60-year-old woman who collapsed in the bathroom while sitting on the toilet.
   G. We are administering supplemental oxygen at 4 L/min by nasal cannula.
   H. The patient's medications include nitroglycerin and Aldomet (methyldopa).
   I. Her left pupil is larger than the right and does not react to light.
   J. Her daughter states, "She was well until 9:00 a.m. this morning."
   K. Her neck is somewhat stiff.
   L. She was hospitalized 6 years ago for an acute myocardial infarction (AMI).

(1)_____   (5)_____   (9)_____

(2)_____   (6)_____   (10)_____

(3)_____   (7)_____   (11)_____

(4)_____   (8)_____   (12)_____

Multiple Choice

Read each item carefully, and then select the best response.

_____ **1.** Which of the following best describes the use of slang terms?
   A. Helpful when communicating with the hospital because of patient confidentiality
   B. Breaks up the stress of the job by interjecting "dark humor"
   C. Unprofessional and disrespectful
   D. Helpful when communicating with other paramedics

_____ **2.** Emergency medical services (EMS) systems require a large number of personnel to work and communicate together. All of the following are part of this communication EXCEPT:
   A. an emergency medical dispatcher (EMD).
   B. a citizen notifier.
   C. computer-aided dispatch (CAD).
   D. online medical control with base station physician.

3. Federal oversight of emergency medical communication is accomplished by the:
  A. State Emergency Management Organization.
  B. Department of Homeland Security.
  C. Federal Emergency Management Agency (FEMA).
  D. Federal Communications Commission (FCC).

4. What is the mode of two-way radio transmission that allows users to talk and listen simultaneously by using two separate radio frequencies at once?
  A. Multiplex
  B. Stereo
  C. Duplex
  D. Simplex

5. Which of the following is a method of transmitting information to communicate with a patient?
  A. Verbal
  B. Nonverbal
  C. Electronic
  D. All of the above

6. What is the best way to develop rapport with a patient?
  A. Have genuine concern for the patient.
  B. Always call the patient by a pet name.
  C. Hug the patient.
  D. Always use medical terminology.

7. Which of the following would suggest a mental impairment when first addressing the patient?
  A. The patient responds with a coherent speech pattern.
  B. The patient does not turn and look at you when you speak.
  C. The patient waits a second before answering your question.
  D. The patient has a meaningful response to your greeting.

8. When dealing with a fearful patient, which of the following will NOT be useful?
  A. Showing concern for the patient
  B. Standing with your arms crossed
  C. Acting like a professional
  D. Telling the patient about his electrocardiogram (ECG) rhythm

9. Which of the following strategies will help you get a useful response from the patient?
  A. Asking questions with specific medical terms
  B. Talking constantly with the patient
  C. Being quiet and letting the patient talk
  D. Speaking calmly and clearly

10. If you do not understand what the patient is trying to say to you, you should:
  A. just nod and say, "I understand."
  B. let the patient continue until you do catch something you understand.
  C. ask the patient to explain in more detail.
  D. ask the patient a closed-ended question.

11. What is the best way to demonstrate to the patient that you are honest?
  A. Using frequent and direct eye contact
  B. Patting the patient on the arm
  C. Kneeling on the floor in front of the patient
  D. Always having a smile on your face

_____ **12.** When assessing a patient's memory, which of the following is NOT a useful tool?

    A. Asking the patient his or her name

    B. Asking the patient what he or she had for breakfast the day before

    C. Asking the patient where she or he is

    D. Asking the patient what happened to her or him

_____ **13.** Which of the following cultures considers direct eye contact to be rude?

    A. Islamic

    B. French

    C. Brazilian

    D. Asian

_____ **14.** When treating a patient from another culture, what is a good rule of thumb?

    A. Always use hand gestures to make your points.

    B. Never use hand gestures when communicating.

    C. Always use medical terms in your conversation with the patient.

    D. Use pet names for the patient because it makes the patient feel that you like him or her.

Fill in the Blank

You have just been appointed the communications director for your regional EMS system, and you have been asked to draw up plans for an EMS communications system. To do so, you have to figure out who needs to communicate with whom in such a system and what is the best technical means (pager, radio, landline, or cellular phone) to achieve each link in the communications chain. Complete the following statements.

1. The _____ needs to be able to talk with _____. The best technical means of establishing that link is

    _____.

2. The _____ needs to be able to talk with _____. The best technical means of establishing that link is _____.

3. The _____ needs to be able to talk with _____. The best technical means of establishing that link is

    _____.

4. The _____ needs to be able to talk with _____. The best technical means of establishing that link is

    _____.

5. The _____ needs to be able to talk with _____. The best technical means of establishing that link is

    _____.

6. The act of transmitting information to another person is called _____.

7. When dealing with a crisis, your challenge is to remain _____.

8. A(n) _____ _____ _____ is a question that does not have a yes or no answer.

9. When using touch to assure a patient, you should touch a(n) _____ part of the patient's body.

10. If the patient is hostile and you are unable to diffuse the patient's anger, you should call the _____.

11. When treating a child, _____ are useful tools for bridging the emotional gap with the child.

12. The best way for you to recognize cross-cultural differences and understand how they may affect interactions with the

    diverse population you serve is to learn more about _____ _____.

Identify

After reading the following case history, provide the indicated assessment information.

The patient is a 52-year-old man who called for an ambulance because of chest pain. The pain was "squeezing" in character, was a 6 out of 10 in severity, radiated to the left shoulder and jaw, and had been present for 2 hours. The pain was accompanied by increasing difficulty in breathing, relieved somewhat by sitting upright. The patient denied nausea, vomiting, sweating, or palpitations. He is known to be a cardiac patient and takes nitroglycerin at home; he took two nitroglycerin doses today, without relief. He denies any history of hypertension or diabetes. He has been treated for a peptic ulcer in the past.

On physical examination, the patient was sitting bolt upright; he appeared alert and apprehensive and was in moderate respiratory distress, breathing shallowly at 30 breaths/min. Pulse was 130 beats/min, weak and regular; BP was 200/90 mm Hg; and SpO_2 was 94%. His neck veins were distended to the angle of the jaw at 45°. Wet crackles were heard at both lung bases, and auscultation of the heart revealed a gallop rhythm. The abdomen was not distended. There was 1+ presacral and ankle edema.

The patient was given supplemental oxygen by non-rebreathing mask at 12 L/min, a 12-lead ECG, and an IV of normal saline, then transported to the regional cardiac center in semi-Fowler position. His vital signs remained stable throughout transport.

1. Chief complaint:

   _____

   _____

2. History of the present illness:

   _____

   _____

3. Other medical history:

   _____

   _____

4. General appearance:

   _____

   _____

5. Vital signs:

   _____

   _____

6. Physical exam:

   _____

   _____

7. Treatment given:

   _____

   _____

8. Pertinent negatives:

   _____

   _____

Ambulance Calls

Part I

The following case scenarios provide an opportunity to explore the concerns associated with patient management and paramedic care. Read each scenario, and then answer each question.

1. Following is a transcript of a transmission between a paramedic unit in the field and a local hospital. **The transmission does *not* follow the guidelines for good radio communications.** Read through the transmission, and then list all the errors in it that you can find.

    Ambulance: Medic 12 to County Hospital.
    Hospital: Who's calling County Hospital?
    Ambulance: This is Medic 12.
    Hospital: Go ahead, Medic 12.
    Ambulance: Be advised that we are en route to your location with Maggie Jones, a lady well endowed with adipose tissue who's complaining of SOB.
    Hospital: Could you please 10-9 that chief complaint?
    Ambulance: What's the matter, are you deaf or something? S. O. B. S as in silly, O as in old, B as in bag. Stand by for the ECG. [Pause.]
    Ambulance: Medic 12 to County Hospital. Did you get the strip?
    Hospital: Yes.
    Ambulance: Say again.
    Hospital: Yes, we received the strip. The doctor wants to know how old the patient is.
    Ambulance: She's 58.
    Hospital: And does she have any medical history?
    Ambulance: Yeah, she's a cardiac patient and takes digitalis, atenolol, potassium chloride, chlorothiazide, and a whole bunch of other stuff.
    Hospital: Did you get any vitals?
    Ambulance: That's affirmative. The blood pressure is 180/120 mm Hg, the pulse is 44 beats/min, and the respirations are. . .let's see. . .here it is. . .the respirations are 30 breaths/min.
    Hospital: Doctor's orders are to give 1 mg of atropine IV.
    Ambulance: That's a 10-4. Will do.
    Hospital: What's your ETA?
    Ambulance: About 10 minutes.
    Hospital: We'll see you then.
    Ambulance: Roger. Pop a few doughnuts into the microwave for us, will you?
    What's wrong with this transmission?

    a. _____

    b. _____

    c. _____

    d. _____

    e. _____

    f. _____

    g. _____

    h. _____

2. You are covering for the dispatcher during his lunch break. ("Don't worry about a thing," you tell him as he heads out the door. "This job's a piece of cake.") The dispatcher has no sooner departed than the telephone rings. You answer on the first ring, and a caller blurts out, "There's been a terrible crash. Oh my God, it's terrible, it's terrible," and he starts sobbing. List the questions you will ask this caller, and indicate at which point you will dispatch an ambulance.

_____

_____

_____

Part II

The following case scenarios provide an opportunity to explore the concerns associated with patient management and paramedic care. Read each scenario, and then answer each question.

1. You are called to the scene of a bad motor vehicle crash in which a semitrailer plowed head-on into a passenger car. The driver of the car is pinned inside his vehicle, very seriously injured. You manage to gain access to the patient and start tending to him while you await help in what will be a lengthy extrication procedure. The patient is still conscious, and he asks you, "Am I going to die?" There is, in fact, a high probability that he will die. Describe how you would reply to this patient's question.

_____

_____

_____

2. You are called to a suburban neighborhood where a 32-year-old female patient with diabetes is having some problems with her glucose levels. Your assessment determines that you need to start an IV and give the patient D_{50}. How would you explain to your patient what you are about to do?

_____

_____

_____

3. You are dispatched to a call for chest pain. The scene is a large farm in the rural Midwest. Upon your arrival, a man in a pickup truck meets you at the front gate. He waves for you to follow him. He leads you to a large area on the farm where many camper-trailers are parked. As you get out of your ambulance, the driver of the truck approaches you. He introduces himself as the owner of the farm and tells you that the grandmother of his harvest foreman is experiencing chest pain. He also explains that the foreman and his family are migrant farm workers who speak mostly Spanish.

As you enter a camper, a worried Hispanic gentleman meets you, and the farmer introduces you as "el paramedico." The man extends his hand to you to shake it and says, "Gracias, gracias, señor," and gestures for you follow him. You are led to a cramped bedroom, where an elderly Hispanic woman is lying on a bed, propped up with several blankets. There are several Catholic icons on the wall, as well as a statue of the Virgin Mary at the bedside. The woman has a string of beads in her hand. You notice several small candles burning on a dresser next to the bed. The man gestures toward her and says, "Mi abuela." The woman presents with pale complexion, diaphoresis, obvious dyspnea, and a facial grimace that you associate with severe pain. You have an emergency medical technician (EMT) partner and an EMT student intern riding with you, so you direct your partner to start setting up the ECG monitor and the student to take vital signs. The excited student says, "Yo," and starts to work. Knowing the patient needs oxygen, you bend over and blow out the candles, not wanting the hazard of open flame around the oxygen. This action really seems to upset the woman, who lets out a little cry. You don't speak any Spanish, so you kneel beside the bed and very slowly ask, "What... is... your... name?" The woman looks in confusion to her grandson, who says "nombre." The woman tells you, very proudly, "Mi nombre es Señora Talia Elizabet Cordoba de Castille." You feel around your uniform for your pen to write it down and realize you left it in the ambulance. You find the red pen you have been using to correct the students' reports and begin to write down her name. The woman lets out a hysterical shriek and tries to back away from you on the bed. There is suddenly much excited confusion in the room, and the grandson is trying desperately to calm his grandmother.

The woman is very agitated, and the ECG monitor shows you a sinus tachycardia with several premature ventricular complexes (PVCs). You tell the EMT student to run and get the cot. He responds with another "yo" and makes the "rock on" sign with his left hand. The woman's eyes get wide, and she shrieks again, and this time she faints. The grandson cries out, "Abuela!" and then tearfully asks you to perform last rites. You inform the grandson that his grandmother is not dead but needs to be transported immediately. You really don't like the way this call is progressing and just want to get back in the ambulance.

In the preceding scenario, you not only have a language barrier but a religious one as well. Hispanic families are very close-knit, and older Hispanics are generally very religious, especially those who have come from the "old country." The majority practice Roman Catholicism and may also be very superstitious. Old World beliefs in the forces of good and evil may be very prevalent, and traditional religious practices may also be interspersed with additional spiritual beliefs. Some of these may include Candomble, which is a mixture of Roman Catholicism and African Voodoo, practiced predominately in the Pan-Caribbean regions and South America; Santeria, which is popular in Cuba, the Caribbean, and South America; espiritismo, which is practiced predominately in Puerto Rico and Central America; and curanderismo, which is found in Mexico and the American Southwest and still exists in "Old Spain."

In some of these traditions, the color yellow is associated with death, the color red with witchcraft, and white with resisting evil spells. Thus, writing a person's name in red ink may be perceived as an attempt to "cast a spell" and gain power over the individual.

Hispanic people generally use two surnames. The first surname listed is from the father, and the second surname listed is from the mother. When speaking to someone, use his or her father's surname. A married woman may attach her husband's surname to the end of hers with a *de*. A widow may indicate her widowed status by including *-vda* ("widow of") in her name as well. Hispanics are very proud of their family names, and a good name is often more important than wealth or status. They also expect to be treated with dignity and respect (familiar theme, no?) and will reciprocate the same. It is very important in the paramedic–patient relationship to treat the Hispanic patient with polite formality and address him or her by title (Mr., Mrs., Señor, Señora). Once rapport is established, the paramedic can gain valuable inroads in the trust factor by politely asking about family members or loved ones. Hispanics, especially older Hispanics, base clinical trust on *individual* perception, not an institutional one.

a. What should you have asked the farmer before you entered the residence?

_____

_____

_____

b. Upon seeing all the religious symbols in the room, what should you have done before blowing out the candles?

_____

_____

_____

c. Why did the student intern upset the woman?

_____

_____

_____

d. Why is a translator so important at this scene?

_____

_____

_____

True/False

If you believe the statement to be more true than false, write the letter "T" in the space provided. If you believe the statement to be more false than true, write the letter "F."

_____   **1.** EMS may use very high frequency (VHF), ultra high frequency (UHF), and "trunking systems."

_____   **2.** aramedics skilled in dysrhythmia recognition do not rely heavily on ECG telemetry.

_____   **3.** An EMS base station consisting of a transmitter, receiver, and antenna is usually mounted in the front console of an ambulance for emergency communications.

_____   **4.** To have clarity of transmission, there must be a sender, a clear message, a receiver, and a feedback loop.

_____   **5.** Most EMS agencies use radio codes to comply with Health Insurance Portability and Accountability Act (HIPAA) requirements for transmitting patient information over the radio.

_____   **6.** Sometimes it might be more practical to step out of the patient exam room or to speak in a softer tone to provide the history and transfer information to the receiving medical practitioner.

_____   **7.** An EMD is nothing more than a "call taker" who relays the initial dispatch information.

_____   **8.** The description of "feeling what the patient is feeling" is used to describe empathy.

_____   **9.** Saying to the patient, "Please feel welcome to tell me about that" is referred to as facilitation.

_____   **10.** People in a crisis could not care less about your nonverbal communications.

_____   **11.** It is okay to use pet names like "dolly" or "chief" with your patients.

_____   **12.** One of the most important treatments you can provide is reassurance.

_____   **13.** When caring for patients with alcoholism or behavioral problems, you will need to use patience and persistence.

_____   **14.** A paramedic who frowns or smirks during a patient interview is demonstrating empathy.

_____   **15.** You show respect to other cultures when you make an effort to learn their language.

Short Answer

Complete this section with short written answers using the space provided.

1. You are planning a radio system for your ambulance service, which consists of six vehicles serving an area of 150 square miles. List the components you will need, and state the function of each component.

Component	Function

2. To the paramedic who is knee-deep in mud while trying to extricate a patient involved in a motor vehicle crash, the dispatcher's job looks pretty easy. In fact, the job is not easy at all. List four tasks the dispatcher has to perform to ensure that the EMS system operates as it should.

a. _____

b. _____

c. _____

d. _____

3. According to the dictionary, communication is a process by which information is exchanged. In EMS, information must go back and forth in several different channels. Suppose you had to design the communications network for *your* EMS system. Who needs to be connected to whom? Draw a diagram to show those connections, or describe which parties should be in contact with one another.

4. Create a radio report from the ambulance to the emergency department (ED) for the following patient scenario. Be sure to include all findings, the care provided, and the status of improvement of the patient.

    You are en route to the hospital with a conscious, alert 58-year-old man who appears to be having an AMI. The estimated time of arrival (ETA) is about 20 minutes. With the patient's consent, you have mutually decided that the most appropriate facility to treat him is one that has a 24-hour interventional cardiac catheter lab.

    The patient's chief complaint is substernal chest pressure that was radiating down his left arm. It began after he started shoveling snow. He describes the pain initially to be 10 on a 10-point scale, with 10 being the worst pain he ever felt. He also states feeling nauseated and appears to be anxious and sweaty.

    His previous medical history includes hypertension and hypercholesterolemia. The patient states that he believes that his father had a heart attack when he was in his 40s. The patient is allergic to Novocain (procaine; causes nausea). He takes 81 mg of aspirin daily PO. He also takes atorvastatin (Lipitor). The patient ate lunch 3 hours ago and was directed to self-administer 162 mg of aspirin by the EMD.

    The patient's exam includes bilateral crackles in the bases, pulse of 110 beats/min, BP of 146/82 mm Hg, and SpO_2 of 94%. He is on high-flow supplemental oxygen via non-rebreathing mask. The 12-lead ECG indicates a sinus tachycardia and elevations in V_3 and V_4.

    The patient has been treated with morphine, oxygen, nitroglycerin, and self-administered aspirin.

_____

_____

_____

_____

_____

_____

_____

_____

_____

_____

_____

_____

_____

_____

_____

_____

_____

_____

_____

_____

_____

Fill in the Table

Fill in the table with the International Radiotelephony Phonetic Alphabet.

A		J		S	
B		K		T	
C		L		U	
D		M		V	
E		N		W	
F		O		X	
G		P		Y	
H		Q		Z	
I		R			

Documentation

My neck hurts. It feels really stiff and hard to move.

Translation—point tenderness at C4 and C5 and limited range of motion with left-side rotation.

© Jones & Bartlett Learning.

Matching

Part I

It does little good to take a careful history and conduct a thorough physical examination if you cannot communicate your findings to others. To do so, you need to know how to organize those findings in such a way that other medical professionals will be able to read your patient care report (PCR) and get a good understanding of your assessment findings and management of the patient.

Label each of the following statements to indicate which part of the PCR pertains to each item.

_____ **1.** There was no pedal edema (edema of the ankles).

_____ **2.** The patient is allergic to penicillin.

_____ **3.** The pain came on while he was watching television.

_____ **4.** The blood pressure was 190/110 mm Hg.

_____ **5.** He was administered supplemental oxygen by non-rebreathing mask at 12 L/min.

_____ **6.** The patient is a 51-year-old man with chest pain.

_____ **7.** The chest was clear.

_____ **8.** His skin was pale, cold, and sweaty (diaphoretic).

_____ **9.** The patient was transported in semi-Fowler position.

_____ **10.** Nothing seemed to make the pain better or worse.

_____ **11.** The pulse was 52 beats/min and full, with an occasional premature beat.

_____ **12.** The neck veins were not distended.

_____ **13.** There was no cyanosis of the lips.

_____ **14.** The patient takes alumina/magnesia (Maalox) and cimetidine (Tagamet) regularly.

_____ **15.** He also felt nauseated.

_____ **16.** His abdomen was soft and nontender.

_____ **17.** His respirations were 20 breaths/min and unlabored.

_____ **18.** He was sitting in a chair and appeared to be frightened.

_____ **19.** He is under the care of Dr. Tums for an ulcer.

_____ **20.** He was alert and oriented to person, place, and day.

_____ **21.** He denies any shortness of breath.

_____ **22.** An 18-gauge IV was started with normal saline at TKO rate.

_____ **23.** The pain radiates down his left arm.

_____ **24.** The blood pressure came down to 170/90 mm Hg during transport.

A. Chief complaint

B. Part of the history of the present illness

C. Part of the patient's other medical history

D. Part of the description of the patient's general appearance

E. Part of the vital signs

F. Part of the physical examination

G. Part of the management

H. Part of the patient's condition during transport

_____ **25.** He describes the pain as squeezing.

_____ **26.** Breath sounds were clear bilaterally.

27. Rearrange the preceding 26 statements into the order in which they should be presented.

(1)_____   (10)_____   (19)_____

(2)_____   (11)_____   (20)_____

(3)_____   (12)_____   (21)_____

(4)_____   (13)_____   (22)_____

(5)_____   (14)_____   (23)_____

(6)_____   (15)_____   (24)_____

(7)_____   (16)_____   (25)_____

(8)_____   (17)_____   (26)_____

(9)_____   (18)_____

Part II

Now try the same exercise with a patient who has been injured. Keeping in mind what you will need to document on your PCR, label each of the following statements to indicate which part of the PCR pertains to each item.

_____ **1.** The right leg was severely angulated at the midfemur.

_____ **2.** The pulse was 92 beats/min, weak, and regular.

_____ **3.** Bystanders state, "The car that hit him was traveling very fast."

_____ **4.** His medical ID bracelet says he is a diabetic.

_____ **5.** There is a bruise on the left forehead.

_____ **6.** His skin is pale, cool, and moist.

_____ **7.** He was secured to a scoop stretcher.

_____ **8.** The patient is a middle-aged man who was struck by a car while crossing the street.

_____ **9.** Respirations were 30 breaths/min, deep, and noisy; blood pressure was 160/100 mm Hg.

_____ **10.** The patient was unresponsive and did not withdraw from painful stimuli.

_____ **11.** An OPA was inserted, and supplementary oxygen was given by non-rebreathing mask at 12 L/min.

_____ **12.** He apparently staggered into the street without looking, as if he were drunk.

_____ **13.** Chest wall was stable, and breath sounds were equal bilaterally.

_____ **14.** We put the right leg in a traction splint.

_____ **15.** The pupils were equal, midposition, and reactive to light.

_____ **16.** There was no change in his condition during transport.

_____ **17.** There was no blood or fluid draining from his nose or ears.

_____ **18.** His abdomen was soft.

_____ **19.** The dorsalis pedis pulses were equal.

A. Chief complaint

B. Part of the history of the present illness

C. Part of the patient's other medical history

D. Part of the description of the patient's general appearance

E. Part of the vital signs

F. Part of the physical examination

G. Part of the management condition during transport

H. Part of the patient's condition during transport

20. Rearrange the preceding 19 statements in the correct order for presentation.

(1)_____   (8)_____   (14)_____

(2)_____   (9)_____   (15)_____

(3)_____   (10)_____   (16)_____

(4)_____   (11)_____   (17)_____

(5)_____   (12)_____   (18)_____

(6)_____   (13)_____   (19)_____

(7)_____

Part III

Sometimes you will be given information or obtain it in a sequence that needs to be rearranged into the standardized flow of information in which all health care professionals process a case. The following statements come from a patient's case history. Arrange them in the correct order for documentation on the PCR.

1. **A.** Pulse is 50 beats/min and regular, respirations are 36 breaths/min and deep, blood pressure is 180/126 mm Hg, and SpO_2 is 94%.
    B. The patient has a history of hypertension.
    C. The deep tendon reflexes are hyperactive.
    D. Her daughter says the patient complained of a severe headache before she collapsed.
    E. The patient was still conscious when we arrived, but she rapidly lost consciousness.
    F. The patient is a 60-year-old woman who collapsed in the bathroom while sitting on the toilet.
    G. We are administering supplemental oxygen at 12 L/min by non-rebreathing mask.
    H. The patient's medications include nitroglycerin and methyldopa (Aldomet).
    I. Her left pupil is larger than the right and does not react to light.
    J. Daughter states, "She was well until this morning."
    K. Her neck is somewhat stiff.
    L. She was hospitalized 6 years ago for an AMI.

(1)_____   (5)_____   (9)_____

(2)_____   (6)_____   (10)_____

(3)_____   (7)_____   (11)_____

(4)_____   (8)_____   (12)_____

Multiple Choice

Read each item carefully, and then select the best response.

_____ 1. Which of the following would NOT be an example of a significant finding that indicates medical necessity for ambulance transport?
    A. Patient is transported in an emergency mode per standard operating procedure (SOP).
    B. Patient needs to be chemically and physically restrained.
    C. Patient has no other means of transport for his doctor's appointment.
    D. Patient has uncontrollable hemorrhage.

_____ **2.** Patient data include the basic patient information collected on a PCR, which documents such information as the chief complaint and the:

A. call location.

B. assessment findings.

C. arrival time at the hospital.

D. disposition hospital.

_____ **3.** A thorough patient refusal should involve documentation on the PCR of each of the following, EXCEPT:

A. your opinion that the patient is a system abuser.

B. the willingness of EMS to return.

C. evidence that the patient is able to make rational, informed decisions.

D. discussion with medical control according to protocols.

_____ **4.** In most states, the paramedic is required to provide a supplemental report, aside from the PCR, in the case of a:

A. patient injured in a car crash.

B. cardiac arrest patient.

C. child who was abused.

D. burn patient.

_____ **5.** Each of the following is a method used to organize the narrative section of the PCR, EXCEPT:

A. body systems/parts approach.

B. AVPU.

C. CHARTE method.

D. SOAP method.

_____ **6.** Proper documentation is an essential job function of a paramedic. Today, in the majority of the jurisdictions in the United States, this formal _written_ report is referred to as a:

A. trip sheet.

B. patient care report.

C. call sheet.

D. contact file.

_____ **7.** PCRs may be used as all of the following, EXCEPT:

A. a patient description for the media.

B. legal documents.

C. quality assurance reviews.

D. billing documents.

_____ **8.** Different EMS systems might use a variety of report-writing formats. Which of the following is an example of a report-writing format?

A. HEARSAY

B. TALK

C. SOAP

D. SAMPLE

_____ **9.** Patients may have the ability and right to refuse medical care. Which of the following patients would have an appropriate case for refusing care?

A. A 10-year-old boy who was injured in a skateboard crash

B. A 28-year-old woman who fell off a barstool and struck her head

C. A 19-year-old woman who is conscious and alert

D. A 70-year-old man who called for assistance and was found shivering in an unheated house

_____ **10.** When a paramedic discovers that he or she has made a documentation error on a paper PCR, it is okay for the paramedic to take which of the following actions?

A. Erase or "white out" the mistake.

B. Destroy the original report, and rewrite the report without the error.

C. Draw a single line through the error, initial it, and insert the correct information next to it.

D. Have the paramedic's partner write an addendum.

Fill in the Blank

How to Write a Narrative

Paramedics write a narrative on almost every call. Next to each topic in the following list, fill in the items you should include for each.

1. Standard precautions: _____

2. Scene safety: _____

3. MOI/NOI: _____

4. Number of patients: _____

5. Additional resources: _____

6. Cervical spine: _____

7. Initial general impression: _____

8. LOC: _____

9. Chief complaint: _____

10. Life threats: _____ _____

11. ABCDE: _____ _____

12. Oxygen: _____ _____

13. Primary survey, patient history, secondary assessment, or reassessment: _____ _____

    _____

14. SAMPLE/OPQRST: _____ _____

15. Vital signs: _____ _____

16. Medical direction: _____ _____

17. Management of secondary injuries/treat for shock: _____ _____

Identify

After reading the following case history, provide the indicated information for a PCR.

The patient is a 53-year-old woman who called 9-1-1 because she was having chest pain. She described the pain as a pressure in the center of the chest, with numbness of her left arm, which was present for 30 minutes. The pain was accompanied by difficulty in breathing with no relief. The patient denied vomiting but has some nausea and has been sweating profusely. She is known to have angina and takes nitroglycerin at home; she took one nitroglycerin dose today, without relief. She denies any history of hypertension or diabetes. She has been treated for asthma in the past.

On physical examination, the patient was sitting bolt upright; she appeared alert and apprehensive and was in moderate respiratory distress, breathing shallowly at 26 breaths/min. Pulse was 136 beats/min, weak and regular; blood pressure was 180/82 mm Hg; and SpO_2 was 95%. Her neck veins were distended to the angle of the jaw at 45°. Rales were heard at both lung bases, and auscultation of the heart revealed a gallop rhythm. The abdomen was not distended. There was no pedal edema.

The patient was given supplemental oxygen by non-rebreathing mask at 12 L/min, and a 12-lead ECG was acquired and transmitted because there was evidence of an ST segment elevation myocardial infarction (STEMI). She was transported to St.

Joseph's Hospital cath lab in semi-Fowler position. An IV of normal saline at to keep open (TKO) was started, and she was given 5 mg morphine, 324 mg acetylsalicylic acid (ASA), and nitroglycerin. Her vital signs remained stable throughout transport.

1. Chief complaint:

_____

_____

2. History of the present illness:

_____

_____

3. Other medical history:

_____

_____

4. General appearance:

_____

_____

5. Vital signs:

_____

_____

6. Physical exam:

_____

_____

7. Management:

_____

_____

8. Pertinent negatives:

_____

_____

True/False

If you believe the statement to be more true than false, write the letter "T" in the space provided. If you believe the statement to be more false than true, write the letter "F."

_____   **1.** Times used to document actions on a PCR generally use Greenwich Mean Time (GMT).

_____   **2.** To document time accurately, paramedics should "synchronize" their watches with the public safety access point (PSAP).

_____   **3.** Accurate documentation depends on all information being provided, including times, narrative, and check boxes.

_____   **4.** A false statement written about a patient could be considered libel.

_____   **5.** It is not acceptable practice to "document findings to meet medical necessity standards" to help bring in revenue.

_____ **6.** To ensure that data can be shared on a national level, electronic documentation systems need not be National Emergency Medical Services Information System (NEMSIS) compliant.

_____ **7.** The military time for 1 hour after noon is 1300 hours.

_____ **8.** In a suspected child abuse case, it is best to document your objective findings and allow the legal system to investigate and make the ultimate determination of abuse or neglect.

_____ **9.** Your PCR may be used in legal proceedings against you or someone else and is the only record of the care you provided and why.

_____ **10.** Falsifying information on the PCR may result in suspension and/or revocation of your certification/license.

Short Answer

Complete this section with short written answers using the space provided.

1. A PCR must also contain other information besides that found in a traditional medical history. List at least one other item of information that needs to be recorded on a PCR, and explain why that information is important.

   a. Information that should be recorded:

   _____

   _____

   _____

   b. Why that information is important:

   _____

   _____

   _____

2. Give two reasons why you should make certain that your PCR is as accurate and complete as possible.

   a.

   _____

   _____

   _____

   b.

   _____

   _____

   _____

3. Give specifics to document for each of the following topics:

   a. Number of patients:

   _____

   _____

   _____

b. Standard precautions:

_____

_____

_____

c. MOI/NOI:

_____

_____

_____

d. Oxygen:

_____

_____

_____

Complete the Patient Care Report

This feature will be found in a number of the chapters of this workbook. Read the incident scenario, and then complete the following PCR.

You and your partner are posted at the corner of 2nd Avenue and 14th Street, completing the paperwork for a recent diabetic call, when the dispatcher calls your unit. "Medic 185," the dispatcher says immediately.

"Medcom 185," you respond.

"Medic 185, Charlie response to 3-5-5 East 16th Street for a male with severe bleeding. Show your time of dispatch at sixteen fifty-three."

You copy the assignment and slowly roll out into traffic after activating the lights and siren, proceeding to the address, which is about six blocks away.

Five minutes later, you pull up outside a well-kept apartment house with a parking spot right in front of the building and are met by a woman frantically waving her arms.

"Please hurry!" She shouts as you open your door. "My husband was working with an electric saw in the basement and has a really deep cut on his leg. He's bleeding really bad!"

You and your partner grab your bags and walk down a flight of stairs into the basement area, where there is a woodshop. The man, whom you estimate to weigh about 170 pounds, is sitting on a pile of wood, pale and shaking, holding an old, bloody T-shirt against his lower left leg. A huge circle of blood is soaking into the wood pile under him.

"Sir, we're from the ambulance service, and we're here to help you," you say, kneeling next to the man. "Can you tell me what happened?"

As the 42-year-old man describes how the saw glanced off of a knot in the shelving he was cutting, sending it deep into the flesh of his leg, you remove the T-shirt from the wound—observing a jagged laceration approximately 9 cm long—and replace it with a wide trauma dressing. Your partner then places a non-rebreathing mask on the patient with the supplemental oxygen set to 15 L/min and begins assessing vital signs.

At 1704 hours, your partner reports the patient's vital signs as follows: systolic blood pressure (BP), 136; diastolic BP, 86; pulse, 128, strong and regular; respirations, 16, with good tidal volume; pale, cool, and diaphoretic skin; and pulse oximetry, 94%.

About 5 minutes after obtaining vital signs, you have stopped the bleeding using a pressure bandage and are loading the patient into the ambulance, keeping him covered with a blanket and in the supine position.

His wife tells you that he is allergic to amoxicillin and that he has been taking a cholesterol medication called Crestor ever since he suffered a transient ischemic attack in the spring of last year. You thank her for the information and climb into the patient compartment while your partner jumps into the driver's seat. Within a minute, you are en route to the emergency department (ED) and taking the patient's vital signs again.

This time they are as follows: systolic BP, 122; diastolic BP, 76; pulse, 136, weak and regular; respirations, 20 and shallow but with adequate tidal volume; skin still pale, cool, and diaphoretic; and pulse oximetry, 94%.

At 1715, you arrive at the ambulance bay of the Beth Israel Medical Center, quickly move the patient inside, and transfer his care to the ED staff. After giving a full report to the receiving nurse and properly cleaning and preparing the ambulance, you and your partner go back available at 1735.

EMS Patient Care Report (PCR)

Date:	Incident No.:	Nature of Call:	Location:

Dispatched:	En Route:	At Scene:	Transport:	At Hospital:	In Service:

Patient Information

Age:	Allergies:
Sex:	Medications:
Weight (in kg [lb]):	Past Medical History:
	Chief Complaint:

Vital Signs

Time:	BP:	Pulse:	Respirations:	SpO$_2$:
Time:	BP:	Pulse:	Respirations:	SpO$_2$:
Time:	BP:	Pulse:	Respirations:	SpO$_2$:

EMS Treatment
(circle all that apply)

Oxygen @ _____ L/min via (circle one): NC NRM Bag-mask device	Assisted Ventilation	Airway Adjunct	CPR
Defibrillation	Bleeding Control	Bandaging	Splinting	Other:

Narrative

Medical Terminology

CHAPTER

Medical Terminology

7

Beware the leading question!

© Jones & Bartlett Learning.

Matching

Part I

Match each of the definitions in the left column to the appropriate term in the right column.

_____	**1.** The straightening of a joint.	**A.** Abduction
_____	**2.** The posterior surface of the body, including the back of the hand.	**B.** Adduction
_____	**3.** Farther inside the body and away from the skin.	**C.** Anatomic position
_____	**4.** An imaginary plane in which the body is cut into front and back portions.	**D.** Anterior
_____	**5.** A word containing more than one word root.	**E.** Anteroposterior axis
_____	**6.** A word root followed by a vowel.	**F.** Antonyms
_____	**7.** Rotating an extremity at its joint away from the midline.	**G.** Apex
_____	**8.** The name of a disease, device, procedure, or drug that is based on the person who invented, discovered, or first described it.	**H.** Bilateral
_____	**9.** Farther from the trunk and nearer to the free end of the extremity.	**I.** Combining form
_____	**10.** The product of slicing an object cross-wise, perpendicular to its long axis.	**J.** Combining vowel
_____	**11.** On the opposite side of the body.	**K.** Compound word
_____	**12.** The vowel used to combine two word roots or a word root and a prefix or suffix.	**L.** Contralateral
_____	**13.** In anatomy, a body part or condition that appears on both sides of the midline.	**M.** Coronal plane
_____	**14.** Pairs of word roots, prefixes, or suffixes that have opposite meanings.	**N.** Cross section
_____	**15.** The front surface of the body; the side facing you in the anatomic position.	**O.** Deep
_____	**16.** Movement of a limb toward the midline.	**P.** Distal
_____	**17.** The pointed extremity of a conical structure.	**Q.** Dorsal
_____	**18.** The axis that runs perpendicular to the coronal plane.	**R.** Eponym
_____	**19.** The position of reference, in which the patient stands facing you, arms at the side, with the palms of the hands facing forward.	**S.** Extension
_____	**20.** Movement of a limb away from the midline.	**T.** External rotation

Part II

Match each of the definitions in the left column to the appropriate term in the right column.

_____	**1.** Turning the palms downward.	**A.** Flexion
_____	**2.** In anatomy, the back surface of the body; the side away from you in the standard anatomic position.	**B.** Fowler position
_____	**3.** The forward-facing part of the hand in the anatomic position.	**C.** Homonyms
_____	**4.** Lying flat, face down.	**D.** Horizontal axis

_____ **5.** Part of a term that appears before a word root, changing the meaning of the term.

_____ **6.** The sole or bottom surface of the foot.

_____ **7.** An imaginary vertical line drawn from the middle of the forehead through the nose and the umbilicus to the floor.

_____ **8.** The view of an object cut along its long axis.

_____ **9.** In anatomy, parts of the body that lie farther from the midline.

_____ **10.** Rotating the anterior surface of an extremity toward the midline.

_____ **11.** Maximum flexion or flexion beyond the normal range of motion.

_____ **12.** The axis that runs perpendicular to the sagittal plane; also called the mediolateral axis.

_____ **13.** A sitting position, with the head elevated at a 90° angle.

_____ **14.** The bending of a joint.

_____ **15.** Words that sound alike but are spelled differently and have different meanings.

_____ **16.** Maximum extension or extension beyond the normal range of motion.

_____ **17.** Below or closer to the feet.

_____ **18.** On the same side of the body.

_____ **19.** The axis that runs perpendicular to the transverse plane.

_____ **20.** Closer to the midline.

E. Hyperextension
F. Hyperflexion
G. Inferior
H. Internal rotation
I. Ipsilateral
J. Lateral
K. Longitudinal axis
L. Longitudinal section

M. Medial
N. Midsagittal plane
O. Palmar
P. Plantar
Q. Posterior
R. Prefix
S. Pronation
T. Prone

Multiple Choice

Read each item carefully, and then select the best response.

_____ **1.** Most medical terms have origins in the _____ or _____ language.
   A. French; Italian
   B. English; Roman
   C. Greek; Latin
   D. German; Russian

_____ **2.** The language of medicine includes many eponyms and terms that have resulted from advances and discoveries. Which of the following is NOT considered an eponym?
   A. McBurney point
   B. Dysphagia
   C. Apgar score
   D. Levine sign

_____ **3.** The portion of a medical term that appears before the root word is called the:
   A. combining vowel.
   B. suffix.
   C. prefix.
   D. antonym.

_____ **4.** When comparing the terms or parts of terms listed here, which are NOT synonyms?
   A. pulmon/o and pneum/o
   B. dextro and sinister/o
   C. nephr/o and ren/o
   D. angi/o and vas/o

_____ **5.** Each of the following is considered a common numerical prefix, EXCEPT:
   A. deca-.
   B. octo-.
   C. quad-.
   D. cardio-.

_____ 6. Which common numerical prefix would be found in the word used to describe a congenital anomaly involving four anatomic abnormalities of the heart?

    A. bi-

    B. tetra-

    C. quint-

    D. multi-

_____ 7. The root words used in medicine often describe a color. Which root is used for the color green?

    A. alb-

    B. polio/o

    C. chlor/o

    D. cirrh/o

_____ 8. The imaginary plane that would divide the body into right and left sides is called the:

    A. coronal plane.

    B. sagittal plane.

    C. transverse plane.

    D. frontal plane.

_____ 9. Terminology associated with the body region of the stomach would use the term:

    A. buccal.

    B. axillary.

    C. cutaneous.

    D. gastric.

_____ 10. Which of the following terms means "pertaining to the skin"?

    A. Gluteal

    B. Inguinal

    C. Cutaneous

    D. Lumbar

_____ 11. Which of the following terms means "pertaining to the armpit"?

    A. Brachial

    B. Axillary

    C. Hepatic

    D. Cranial

_____ 12. Which of the following terms means "pertaining to the sole of the foot or the palm of the hand"?

    A. Volar

    B. Sacral

    C. Perineal

    D. Renal

_____ 13. The common directional term used to describe the area closest to the point of attachment is:

    A. posterior.

    B. distal.

    C. lateral.

    D. proximal.

_____ 14. The common directional term used to describe the area closest to the head is:

    A. superficial.

    B. superior.

    C. inferior.

    D. ventral.

_____ **15.** To avoid potentially dangerous mistakes, the paramedic should always write down medication doses:
  A. by spelling out the full trade name.
  B. without trailing zeros and naked decimals.
  C. twice for clarity.
  D. All of the above

Fill in the Blank

Read each item carefully, and then complete the statement by filling in the missing word(s).

1. The _____ around the heart is called the _____.

2. The term _____ refers to _____ or through the vagina.

3. The term _____ refers to below or at the _____ of the thorax.

4. During pregnancy, when the embryo develops outside the _____, it is called a(n) _____ pregnancy.

5. A(n) _____ who is pregnant for the _____ time is called a primigravida.

6. A woman who has had _____ pregnancies resulting in _____ live births is called a quintipara.

7. The inflammation of an organ, such as _____ of the liver, causes yellow-orange pigmentation of the _____.

8. The _____ blood cell that contains hemoglobin to carry _____ is called a(n) _____.

9. The _____ passing horizontally through the body at the waist, creating top and bottom portions, is referred to as the _____ plane.

10. The _____ in the _____ is referred to as the deltoid.

True/False

If you believe the statement to be more true than false, write the letter "T" in the space provided. If you believe the statement to be more false than true, write the letter "F."

_____ **1.** *Abdominal* means "pertaining to the abdomen."

_____ **2.** *Brachial* means "pertaining to the upper arm."

_____ **3.** *Cranial* means "pertaining to the superior segment."

_____ **4.** The term meaning "pertaining to the buttocks" is *buccal*.

_____ **5.** *Inguinal* means "pertaining to the depressions in the abdominal wall near the thighs."

_____ **6.** *Lumbar* means "pertaining to the loin."

_____ **7.** *Plantar* means "relating to the palm of the hand."

_____ **8.** The inferior, posterior region of the head is called the occipital.

_____ **9.** Males do not have an umbilical region.

_____ **10.** The vessel in the posterior knee is the popliteal.

_____ **11.** The range of motion is the full range over which a joint can move.

_____ **12.** In the anatomic position, all extremities are in extension.

_____ **13.** The abduction of an extremity moves it toward the midline.

_____ **14.** *Internal rotation* means turning the anterior portion of an extremity away from the midline.

_____ **15.** The term *ipsilateral* refers to the same side of the body.

THE HUMAN BODY AND HUMAN SYSTEMS

Anatomy and Physiology

You have to consume something besides caffeine, fat, and sugar. How else can you pass the recertification exam?

Nutritional deficiencies have been shown to result in depression of bone marrow function and reduction in white blood cell development.

© Jones & Bartlett Learning.

Matching

Part I

Match each of the definitions in the left column to the appropriate term in the right column.

_____ **1.** A pathologic condition resulting from the accumulation of acids in the body (blood pH less than 7.35).

_____ **2.** Any molecule that can give up a hydrogen ion, thereby increasing the concentration of hydrogen ions in a water solution.

_____ **3.** The socket formed by the coxal (hip) bone into which the ball-shaped femoral head fits snugly.

_____ **4.** A neurotransmitter released at synapses within the autonomic nervous system and by motor neurons to stimulate skeletal muscle contraction.

_____ **5.** The commonly used blood classification system, based on the antigens present or absent in the blood.

_____ **6.** The muscles not normally used during quiet breathing; examples include the sternocleidomastoid muscles of the neck, the chest pectoralis major muscles, and the abdominal muscles.

_____ **7.** The ability of the lens of the eye to change its shape to focus on a close object.

_____ **8.** The building of larger substances from smaller substances, such as the building of proteins from amino acids.

_____ **9.** The air sacs of the lungs in which the exchange of oxygen and carbon dioxide takes place; also, the bony sockets for the teeth that reside in the mandible and maxilla.

_____ **10.** The tip of the shoulder and the site of attachment for the clavicle and various shoulder muscles.

_____ **11.** The sequence of changes in the membrane potential that occurs when an excitable cell (neuron or muscle) is stimulated.

_____ **12.** The outer layer of the adrenal gland; it produces hormones that are important in regulating the water and salt balance of the body.

_____ **13.** The temporary or permanent reduction of sensitivity to a particular stimulus.

_____ **14.** A method used to move compounds across a cell membrane to create or maintain an imbalance of charges, usually against a concentration gradient and requiring the expenditure of energy.

_____ **15.** Variant forms of a gene, which can be identical or slightly different in a sequence of deoxyribonucleic acid.

A. ABO system

B. Accessory muscles

C. Accommodation

D. Acetabulum

E. Acetylcholine

F. Acid

G. Acidosis

H. Acromion process

I. Action potential

J. Active transport

K. Adaptation

L. Adrenal cortex

M. Adrenergic

N. Aerobic metabolism

O. Afterload

_____ **16.** A pathologic condition resulting from the accumulation of bases in the body (blood pH greater than 7.45).

_____ **17.** The pressure in the aorta against which the left ventricle must pump blood.

_____ **18.** A hormone responsible for the reabsorption of sodium and water from the kidney tubules.

_____ **19.** Metabolism that can proceed only in the presence of oxygen.

_____ **20.** Having the characteristics of the sympathetic division of the autonomic nervous system.

P. Aldosterone

Q. Alkalosis

R. Alleles

S. Alveoli

T. Anabolism

Part II

Match each of the definitions in the left column to the appropriate term in the right column.

_____ **1.** Nerve endings that are stimulated by pressure changes, including increased arterial blood pressure; they are located in the aortic arch and carotid sinuses.

_____ **2.** White blood cells that contain histamine granules and other substances that are released during inflammatory and allergic responses.

_____ **3.** Long, slender extension of a neuron (nerve cell) that conducts electrical impulses away from the nerve cell body to adjacent cells.

_____ **4.** The chromosomes that do not carry the genes that determine sex.

_____ **5.** Imaginary line joining the positive and negative electrodes of a lead; also the second cervical vertebra.

_____ **6.** The portion of the skeleton made up of the skull, thoracic cage, and vertebral column.

_____ **7.** The area of the brain between the spinal cord and cerebrum that contains the midbrain, pons, and medulla; it controls functions that are necessary for life, such as breathing.

_____ **8.** Soft tissue that fills the inside of bones and is the site of production of red blood cells, platelets, and most white blood cells.

_____ **9.** A layer of tightly adhered cells that protects the brain and spinal cord from exposure to medications, toxins, and infectious particles.

_____ **10.** The ability of cardiac pacemaker cells to initiate an electrical impulse spontaneously without being stimulated by another source (such as a nerve).

_____ **11.** A group of cells that conduct an electrical impulse through the heart; located in the floor of the right atrium immediately behind the tricuspid valve and near the opening of the coronary sinus.

_____ **12.** A molecule that blocks the ability of a given chemical to bind to its receptor, preventing a biologic response.

_____ **13.** A prominence of the sternum that indicates the point where the second rib joins the sternum; also called the sternal angle or manubriosternal junction.

_____ **14.** Watery fluid filling the anterior eye cavity; the quantity determines the intraocular pressure, which is critical to sight.

_____ **15.** The portion of the skeletal system made up of the upper extremities, shoulder girdle, pelvic girdle, and lower extremities.

_____ **16.** The semilunar valve that regulates blood flow from the left ventricle to the aorta.

_____ **17.** The principal artery leaving the left side of the heart and carrying freshly oxygenated blood to the body; the largest artery in the body.

_____ **18.** The first cervical vertebra (C1), which provides support for the head.

_____ **19.** A condition where parts of the image are out of focus and others are in focus; caused by irregularities in the shape of the eye lens.

_____ **20.** Six paired cartilages stacked on top of each other in the larynx.

A. Angle of Louis

B. Antagonist

C. Aorta

D. Aortic valve

E. Appendicular skeleton

F. Aqueous humor

G. Arytenoid cartilages

H. Astigmatism

I. Atlas

J. Atrioventricular node

K. Automaticity

L. Autosomes

M. Axial skeleton

N. Axis

O. Axon

P. Baroreceptors

Q. Basophils

R. Blood-brain barrier

S. Bone marrow

T. Brainstem

Part III

Match each of the definitions in the left column to the appropriate term in the right column.

_____ 1. A thin, flap-like structure that allows air to pass into the trachea but prevents food and liquid from entering.

A. Depolarization

_____ 2. A leukocyte that may play a role following infection in various areas in the body.

B. Dermatome

_____ 3. Substances designed to speed up the rate of specific biochemical reactions.

C. Diaphragm

_____ 4. The layer of the serous pericardium that lies closely against the heart; also called the visceral pericardium.

D. Diaphysis

_____ 5. Glands that have no ducts and secrete chemicals directly into tissue fluid or blood.

E. Diastole

_____ 6. Salt or acid substances that become ionic conductors when dissolved in a solvent (such as water); chemicals dissolved in the blood.

F. Diencephalon

_____ 7. The outermost of the three meninges that enclose the brain and spinal cord; the toughest meningeal layer.

G. Diffusion

_____ 8. The thin membrane lining the inside of the heart.

H. Dura mater

_____ 9. Glands that secrete chemicals into ducts that open onto a surface for elimination.

I. Electrolytes

_____ 10. The passive part of the breathing process, in which the diaphragm and the intercostal muscles relax, forcing air out of the lungs.

J. Endocardium

_____ 11. The ability of cardiac muscle cells to respond to an electrical, chemical, or mechanical stimulus.

K. Endocrine glands

_____ 12. A branch of the internal auditory canal that connects the middle ear to the oropharynx.

L. Enzymes

_____ 13. A hormone released from the ovaries that stimulates the uterine lining during the menstrual cycle.

M. Eosinophil

_____ 14. The rapid movement of electrolytes across a cell membrane in response to an action potential, which changes the overall charge of the cell; the main catalyst for muscle contractions and neural transmissions.

N. Epicardium

_____ 15. The area of the skin supplied by a specific sensory spinal nerve.

O. Epiglottis

_____ 16. The portion of the brain between the brainstem and the cerebrum; contains the epithalamus, thalamus, hypothalamus, and subthalamus.

P. Estrogen

_____ 17. The process of particles moving from an area of higher concentration to an area of lower concentration along a concentration gradient until equilibrium is achieved.

Q. Eustachian tube

_____ 18. The shaft of a long bone.

R. Excitability

_____ 19. The large skeletal muscle that plays a major role in breathing and separates the chest cavity from the abdominal cavity.

S. Exhalation

_____ 20. The phase of the cardiac cycle in which the atria and ventricles relax between contractions and blood enters these chambers.

T. Exocrine glands

Part IV

Match the following types of epithelial tissue with their function and/or location in the human body.

_____ 1. Simple squamous

A. Distensibility, protection of the inner urinary bladder lining

_____ 2. Simple cuboidal

B. Protection of the outer layer of the skin

_____ 3. Simple columnar

C. Protection of gland ducts, pancreas, and salivary glands

_____ 4. Pseudostratified columnar

D. Absorption and secretion in the kidney tubule linings

_____ 5. Stratified squamous

E. Protection and secretion in part of male urethra and parts of pharynx

_____ 6. Stratified cuboidal

F. Secretion in the endocrine, salivary, and sweat glands

_____ 7. Stratified columnar

G. Movement of mucus, protection and secretion in respiratory passage linings

_____ 8. Transitional

H. Diffusion, filtration, osmosis, covering of surfaces in air sacs of lungs and blood vessels

_____ 9. Glandular

I. Absorption, protection, and secretion in the intestine, stomach, and uterine lining

Multiple Choice

Read each item carefully, and then select the best response.

_____ 1. All of the cells in the body, with the exception of the _____, have between a hundred and a few thousand organelles called _____, which are the powerhouses of the cell.

   A. white blood cells; lysosomes
   B. red blood cells; Golgi apparatus
   C. white blood cells; endoplasmic reticulum
   D. red blood cells; mitochondria

_____ 2. The movement of a solvent from an area of low solute concentration to one of high concentration through a selectively permeable membrane is called:

   A. facilitated diffusion.
   B. osmosis.
   C. active transport.
   D. differentiation.

_____ 3. There are 230 joints in the human body. The most complex joints, which allow free movement and are surrounded by an outer layer of ligaments forming a capsule, are called the:

   A. fibrous joints.
   B. cartilaginous joints.
   C. synovial joints.
   D. immovable joints.

_____ 4. The kidneys are found in which body cavity?

   A. Thoracic
   B. Abdominal
   C. Retroperitoneal
   D. Pelvic

_____ 5. The proximal end of the humerus articulates with the:

   A. clavicle.
   B. glenoid fossa.
   C. scapula.
   D. acromion process.

_____ 6. The neurotransmitter that stimulates skeletal muscle to contract is called:

   A. sarcoplasmic reticulum.
   B. myosin.
   C. actin.
   D. acetylcholine.

_____ 7. The muscle group located in the anterior femur is called the:

   A. gastrocnemius.
   B. rectus abdominis.
   C. quadriceps.
   D. triceps.

_____ 8. The muscle group that points the toes away from the head is called the:

   A. gastrocnemius.
   B. rectus abdominis.
   C. tibialis anterior.
   D. pectoralis.

_____ 9. The heart valve that separates the left atrium from the left ventricle is called the _____ valve and is a _____ valve.

    A. semilunar; tricuspid

    B. pulmonic; bicuspid

    C. mitral; bicuspid

    D. aortic; tricuspid

_____ 10. What percentage of the blood is made up of plasma?

    A. 0.9%

    B. 25%

    C. 45%

    D. 55%

_____ 11. Of the following vessels, which is designed to withstand the highest pressures of any vessel in the body?

    A. Common carotid artery

    B. Ascending aorta

    C. Brachial artery

    D. Inferior vena cava

_____ 12. The specialized portion of the venous system that drains blood from the stomach, intestines, and spleen is called the:

    A. hepatic portal system.

    B. lymphatic system.

    C. abdominal aortic aneurism.

    D. renal residual circulation.

_____ 13. What percentage of the plasma is water?

    A. 26%

    B. 48%

    C. 72%

    D. 92%

_____ 14. Which of the following substances found in the plasma of the blood is NOT considered a protein?

    A. Albumin

    B. Sodium bicarbonate

    C. Globulin

    D. Fibrinogen

_____ 15. The occipital lobe of the brain is responsible for:

    A. hearing, smell, and language.

    B. vision and storage of visual memories.

    C. basic emotions and basic reflexes, such as chewing.

    D. judgment and predicting the consequences of actions.

_____ 16. Which portion of the brain is responsible for emotions, temperature control, and interface with the endocrine system?

    A. Occipital lobe

    B. Temporal lobe

    C. Prefrontal area

    D. Diencephalon

_____ 17. The fifth cranial nerve is called the:

    A. optic nerve.

    B. oculomotor nerve.

    C. vagus nerve.

    D. trigeminal nerve.

_____ **18.** The ninth cranial nerve is called the:
    A. oculomotor nerve.
    B. glossopharyngeal nerve.
    C. facial nerve.
    D. abducens nerve.

_____ **19.** The cranial nerve that is responsible for the sense of hearing and balance is the _____ cranial nerve.
    A. 3rd
    B. 8th
    C. 9th
    D. 10th

_____ **20.** When a patient has _____, the eyes may be oriented correctly, but one fails to send adequate signals to the vision center, causing a loss of depth perception and poor-quality images.
    A. strabismus
    B. amblyopia
    C. macular degeneration
    D. a blind spot

Fill in the Blank

Read each item carefully, and then complete the statement by filling in the missing word(s).

1. The _____ is a large, solid organ that takes up most of the area immediately beneath the diaphragm. The _____ is an outpouching from the bile ducts that serves as a reservoir and concentrating organ for _____ produced in the liver.

2. The _____ _____ is the major hollow organ of the abdomen whose cells produce enzymes and mucus to aid in digestion. The _____ _____ consists of the cecum, the _____, and the rectum.

3. The _____ system is made up of various glands located throughout the body. These glands release _____ such as insulin into the bloodstream. The major _____ glands include the pituitary, thyroid, and adrenal glands. The major _____ glands include the sweat glands, which secrete outside the body.

4. Let's review the pituitary gland hormones. The _____ hormone increases the size and division rate of body cells. The _____-stimulating hormone controls the thyroid gland hormone secretion. The sex cell hormone that aids in the release of female egg cells is called the _____ hormone. The hormone _____ is designed to contract the uterine wall muscles as well as _____ milk–secreting gland muscles.

5. Let's review the functions of the female reproductive organs. The female reproductive organ that produces oocytes and sex hormones is(are) the _____. The _____ _____ transport secondary oocytes in the direction of the uterus so that fertilization can occur normally. The muscular organ in which implantation, _____ formation, and fetal development occur is the uterus. The uterine secretions are transported to the outside of the female's body by the _____. The _____ _____ protects and encloses the female's external reproductive organs, and the _____ _____ protects the openings of the vagina and the urethra, which are contained in the _____.

Labeling

1. Bones of the skull
Label the names of the bones in the cranium.

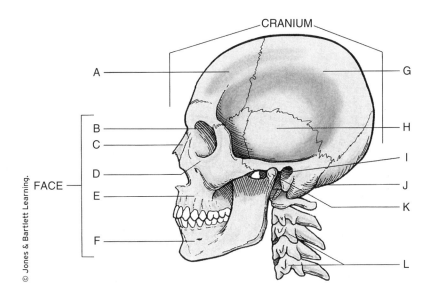

A. _____

B. _____

C. _____

D. _____

E. _____

F. _____

G. _____

H. _____

I. _____

J. _____

K. _____

L. _____

2. Lower extremity
Label the names of the principal parts of the lower extremity.

A. _____

B. _____

C. _____

D. _____

E. _____

F. _____

G. _____

H. _____

I. _____

J. _____

K. _____

3. Respiratory system
Label the names of the structures in the respiratory system.

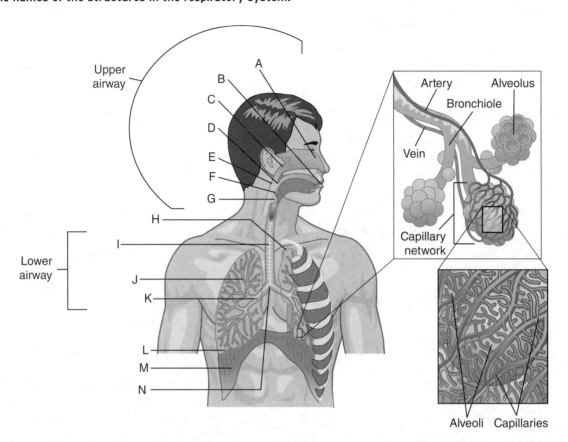

A. _____

B. _____

C. _____

D. _____

E. _____

F. _____

G. _____

H. _____

I. _____

J. _____

K. _____

L. _____

M. _____

N. _____

True/False

If you believe the statement to be more true than false, write the letter "T" in the space provided. If you believe the statement to be more false than true, write the letter "F."

_____   **1.** Parasympathetic stimulation can cause constriction of the pupil.

_____   **2.** Sympathetic stimulation can cause secretion of the hormone adrenalin.

_____   **3.** Parasympathetic stimulation can cause increased urination.

_____   **4.** Sympathetic stimulation causes increased emptying of the colon.

_____   **5.** Parasympathetic stimulation speeds up the heart.

_____   **6.** Sympathetic stimulation constricts the bronchioles.

_____   **7.** Parasympathetic stimulation increases the secretion of saliva.

_____   **8.** Sympathetic stimulation stops the secretion of the parotid gland.

_____   **9.** Parasympathetic stimulation increases the motility of the small intestines.

_____   **10.** The sympathetic division of the autonomic nervous system is responsible for the "rest and digest" reaction.

_____   **11.** The distal end of the radius articulates the irregularly shaped carpal bones of the wrist.

_____   **12.** The carpometacarpal joint of the thumb is a gliding joint.

_____   **13.** A plexus is an area where the spinal nerves come together and transmit their impulses to areas of the body through a common nerve.

_____   **14.** Four types of proteins make up myofilaments.

_____   **15.** The limbic system is responsible for fluid elimination in the body.

Pathophysiology

Two days until the recertification exam?

Excessive output can rapidly upset homeostasis; for example, severe perspiration, no matter what the reason, can cause excessive water loss and dehydration.

© Jones & Bartlett Learning.

Matching

Part I

Match each of the definitions in the left column to the appropriate term in the right column.

_____	**1.** Antibodies directed against the person's own proteins.	**A.** Acidosis
_____	**2.** The production of antibodies or T cells that work against the tissues of a person's body, producing autoimmune disease or a hypersensitivity reaction.	**B.** Acquired immunity
_____	**3.** A pattern of inheritance that involves genes that are located on autosomes or the nonsex chromosomes. Inheritance of only one copy of a particular form of a gene is needed to show the trait.	**C.** Activation
_____	**4.** A pattern of inheritance that involves genes located on autosomes or the nonsex chromosomes. Inheritance of two copies of a particular form of a gene is needed to show the trait.	**D.** Adhesion
_____	**5.** A severe hypersensitivity reaction that involves bronchoconstriction and cardiovascular collapse.	**E.** Alcoholic ketoacidosis
_____	**6.** The growth of new blood vessels.	**F.** Alkalosis
_____	**7.** A protein secreted by certain immune cells that bind antigens to make them more visible to the immune system.	**G.** Allergen
_____	**8.** A foreign substance recognized by the immune system.	**H.** Allergy
_____	**9.** Normal, genetically programmed cell death.	**I.** Anaphylactic shock
_____	**10.** A chronic inflammatory lower airway condition resulting in intermittent wheezing and excess mucus production.	**J.** Angiogenesis
_____	**11.** A decrease in cell size due to a loss of subcellular components.	**K.** Antibody
_____	**12.** An allergic tendency.	**L.** Antigen
_____	**13.** An increase in extracellular H$^+$ ions; a blood pH of less than 7.35.	**M.** Apoptosis
_____	**14.** The metabolic acidotic state that manifests because of the inadequate nutritional habits associated with chronic alcohol abuse. The liver and body experience inadequate fuel reserves of glycogen and, therefore, have to switch to fatty acid metabolism.	**N.** Asthma
_____	**15.** The attachment of polymorphonuclear neutrophils to endothelial cells, mediated by selectins and integrins.	**O.** Atopic
_____	**16.** Mediators of inflammation trigger the appearance of molecules known as selectins and integrins on the surfaces of endothelial cells and polymorphonuclear neutrophils, respectively.	**P.** Atrophy

_____ **17.** The immunity that occurs when the body is exposed to a foreign substance or disease and produces antibodies to the invader.

_____ **18.** A decrease is extracellular H^+ ions; a blood pH greater than 7.45.

_____ **19.** Any substance that causes a hypersensitivity reaction.

_____ **20.** A hypersensitivity reaction to the presence of an agent (allergen) that is intrinsically harmless.

Q. Autoantibodies

R. Autoimmunity

S. Autosomal dominant

T. Autosomal recessive

Part II

Match each of the definitions in the left column to the appropriate term in the right column.

_____ **1.** A group of plasma proteins whose function is to do one of three things: attract leukocytes to sites of inflammation, activate leukocytes, and directly destroy cells.

A. Carpopedal spasm

_____ **2.** The system that forms blood clots in the body and facilitates repairs to the vascular tree.

B. Cell-mediated immunity

_____ **3.** The movement of additional white blood cells to an area of inflammation in response to the release of chemical mediators, such as neutrophils, injured tissue, and monocytes.

C. Central shock

_____ **4.** Components of the activated complement system that attract leukocytes from the circulation to help fight infections.

D. Chemotaxins

_____ **5.** A type of shock caused by central pump failure, including cardiogenic shock and obstructive shock.

E. Chemotaxis

_____ **6.** An inherited disease in which the body absorbs more iron than it needs and stores it in the liver, kidneys, and pancreas.

F. Coagulation system

_____ **7.** A type of T lymphocyte that is involved in cell-mediated and antibody-mediated immune responses. It secretes cytokines that stimulate the B cells and other T cells.

G. Complement system

_____ **8.** A substance that normally does not stimulate an immune response but can be combined with an antigen and at a later point initiate an antibody response.

H. Cytokines

_____ **9.** A reaction of bacteria to a Gram stain in which the bacteria retain the dark purple stain; these types of bacteria have thick cell walls composed of many layers.

I. Distributive shock

_____ **10.** A whitish, filamentous protein formed by the action of thrombin on fibrinogen; the protein that polymerizes (bonds) to form the fibrous component of a blood clot.

J. Dysplasia

_____ **11.** Swelling caused by excessive fluid trapped in the body tissues.

K. Edema

_____ **12.** An alteration in the size, shape, and organization of cells.

L. Fibrin

_____ **13.** The type of shock caused by widespread dilation of the resistance vessels (small arterioles), the capacitance vessels (small venules), or both.

M. Fibrinolysis cascade

_____ **14.** The products of cells that affect the function of other cells.

N. Free radicals

_____ **15.** A reaction of bacteria to a Gram stain in which the bacteria do not retain the dark purple stain; these types of bacteria have cell walls that consist largely of lipids and have pathogenic qualities that make them especially problematic for humans.

O. General adaptation syndrome

_____ **16.** A three-stage description of the body's short- and long-term reactions to stress.

P. Gram-negative

_____ **17.** A molecule that is missing one electron in its outer shell.

Q. Gram-positive

_____ **18.** The breakdown of fibrin in blood clots and the prevention of the polymerization of fibrin into new clots.

R. Hapten

_____ **19.** A contorted position of the hand or foot in which the fingers or toes flex in a claw-like manner; may result from hyperventilation or hypocalcemia.

S. Helper T cells

_____ **20.** The immune process by which T-cell lymphocytes recognize antigens and then secrete cytokines (specifically lymphokines) that attract other cells or stimulate the production of cytotoxic cells that kill the infected cells.

T. Hemochromatosis

Part III

Match each of the definitions in the left column to the appropriate term in the right column.

_____ **1.** An abnormal condition in which some part of the body's immune system is inadequate, and consequently, resistance to infectious disease is decreased.

A. Hyponatremia

_____ **2.** The body system that includes all of the structures and processes designated to mount a defense against foreign substances and disease-causing agents.

B. Hypoperfusion

_____ **3.** The body's defense reaction to any substance that is recognized as foreign.

C. Hypophosphatemia

_____ **4.** A condition that occurs when the circulating blood volume is inadequate to deliver adequate oxygen and nutrients to the body.

D. Hypothalamic-pituitary-adrenal axis

_____ **5.** A major part of the neuroendocrine system that controls reactions to stress. It is the mechanism for a set of interactions among glands, hormones, and parts of the midbrain that mediate the general adaptation syndrome.

E. Hypovolemic shock

_____ **6.** An elevated white blood cell count, often due to inflammation.

F. Immune response

_____ **7.** Anaerobic cellular respiration due to hypoperfusion of tissues and organs.

G. Immune system

_____ **8.** A group of polypeptides that mediate inflammatory responses by stimulating visceral smooth muscle and relaxing vascular smooth muscle to produce vasodilation.

H. Immunodeficiency

_____ **9.** Acidic by-products of fat metabolism.

I. Immunogen

_____ **10.** An acidotic state created by the production of ketones via fat metabolism.

J. Immunoglobulins

_____ **11.** The formation of antibodies or T cells that are directed against antigens or another person's cells.

K. Incidence

_____ **12.** A serum sodium level that is less than or equal to 135 mEq/L.

L. Inflammatory response

_____ **13.** A condition that occurs when the level of tissue perfusion decreases below that needed to maintain normal cellular functions.

M. Interferon

_____ **14.** A decreased serum phosphate level.

N. Interleukins

_____ **15.** An antigen that is capable of generating an immune response.

O. Isoimmunity

_____ **16.** Antibodies secreted by the B cells.

P. Ketoacidosis

_____ **17.** The number of new cases of a disease in a population.

Q. Ketones

_____ **18.** Chemical substances that attract white blood cells to the sites of injury and bacterial invasions.

R. Kinin system

_____ **19.** A protein produced by cells in response to viral invasion that is released into the bloodstream or intercellular fluid to induce healthy cells to manufacture an enzyme that counters the infection.

S. Lactic acidosis

_____ **20.** A reaction by tissues of the body to irritation or injury, characterized by pain, swelling, redness, and heat.

T. Leukocytosis

Multiple Choice

Read each item carefully, and then select the best response.

_____ 1. When a patient hyperventilates and has carpopedal spasm, this reaction is a result of a developing:
   A. metabolic acidosis.
   B. respiratory alkalosis.
   C. metabolic alkalosis.
   D. respiratory acidosis.

_____ 2. An increase in the size of cells caused by the synthesis of more subcellular components, which in turn leads to an increase in tissue and organ size, is called:
   A. hypertrophy.
   B. hyperplasia.
   C. dysplasia.
   D. metaplasia.

_____ 3. Long-duration exercise in the heat, causing excessive sweating, may lead to life-threatening deficits in:
   A. phosphate.
   B. calcium.
   C. sodium.
   D. magnesium.

_____ 4. When examining rates of disease, which of the following terms refers to the number of cases in a particular population?
   A. Incidence
   B. Prevalence
   C. Distribution
   D. Tendency

_____ 5. Normal serum level of potassium should be:
   A. 1.3 to 2.1 mEq/L.
   B. 3.5 to 5.0 mEq/L.
   C. 8.2 to 10.2 mg/dL.
   D. 136 to 142 mEq/L.

_____ 6. Which of the following is caused by autosomal dominant inheritance (where a person needs to inherit only one copy of the particular form of the gene to show the trait)?
   A. Sickle cell anemia
   B. Attached earlobe
   C. Tay-Sachs disease
   D. Freckles

_____ 7. Individuals who suffer from long QT syndrome are at risk for all of the following, EXCEPT:
   A. ventricular dysrhythmias.
   B. palpitations.
   C. torsades de pointes.
   D. atrial fibrillation.

_____ 8. Chronic obstructive pulmonary disease (COPD) gradually destroys lung tissue and inhibits oxygen and carbon dioxide exchange, eventually resulting in:
   A. respiratory alkalosis.
   B. respiratory acidosis.
   C. metabolic alkalosis.
   D. metabolic acidosis.

9. Central shock consists of which two types of shock?
   A. Hypovolemic and distributive
   B. Cardiogenic and distributive
   C. Cardiogenic and obstructive
   D. Hypovolemic and obstructive

10. Normal cell death is referred to as:
   A. necrosis.
   B. gangrene.
   C. apoptosis.
   D. liquefaction.

11. Which of the following is NOT considered a neuromuscular disease?
   A. Multiple sclerosis
   B. Muscular dystrophy
   C. Huntington disease
   D. Gout

12. The disease-causing ability of a microorganism is referred to as:
   A. toxicity.
   B. inflammation.
   C. virulence.
   D. pyrogen.

13. Of the following, which is NOT an example of a cause of metabolic acidosis?
   A. Gastrointestinal losses
   B. Excessive water intake
   C. Lactic acidosis
   D. Aspirin overdose

14. The major intracellular cation that is crucial to many cell functions is:
   A. potassium.
   B. calcium.
   C. phosphate.
   D. sodium.

15. The total body water found in an infant is approximately_____of the infant's total weight.
   A. 50%
   B. 60%
   C. 70%
   D. 80%

Fill in the Blank
Read each item carefully, and then complete the statement by filling in the missing word(s).

1. Perfusion is defined as the delivery of _____ and _____ and _____ of wastes from cells, organs, and _____ by the _____ system.

2. Cardiogenic _____ occurs when the _____ cannot circulate enough _____ to maintain adequate peripheral _____ delivery.

3. Obstructive _____ occurs when blood _____ becomes _____ in the heart or great vessels.

4. Two types of _____ shock—_____ and endogenous—are possible, depending on where _____ loss occurs.

5. Anaphylactic shock occurs when histamine and other _____ proteins are _____ on exposure to a(n) _____.

6. _____ is an elevated potassium level.

7. The molecules that modulate the changes in pH are called _____.

8. Normal cell death is called _____.

9. _____ _____ _____ _____ is a progressive condition usually characterized by concurrent failure of several organs, such as the lungs, liver, and kidneys.

10. _____ are lipopolysaccharides that are part of the cell walls of gram-negative bacteria. They cause inflammation, fever, and chills.

Labeling

1. Type I allergic reaction
Fill in the missing words that describe a type I allergic reaction.

A. _____

B. _____

C. _____

D. _____

E. _____

F. _____

G. _____

H. _____

I. _____

J. _____

Sensitization stage

Antigen

Antigen (A) enters the body

(B) cells synthesize and release large amounts of IgE antibodies

IgE (C) bind to (D) located in many body tissues

IgE antibodies

Mast cell with IgE antibodies attached

Histamine-containing granules

Secondary responses

More of same allergen enters body

Antigen

Allergen combines with (E) on mast cells, triggering release of histamine from mast cell

Histamine and other chemicals

(F) stimulates (G) of blood vessels, causing fluid to leak out; stimulates release of copious amounts of (H), and causes (I) of (J) muscle in bronchioles

Fluid pours out of capillaries

Mucus is copiously released

Small respiratory passages (bronchioles) constrict

Identify

After reading the following case study, list the chief complaint, vital signs, and pertinent patient history.

You respond to a call to an assisted living manor for a 78-year-old man who is having difficulty breathing. Upon arrival, you find the patient sitting forward in a dining room chair with his "elbows out." He is looking rather distressed. You walk up to his table, introduce yourself, and ask what's wrong. The patient responds, with what appears to be great difficulty, "I... can't... breathe." Your partner starts to obtain vital signs as you place the patient on a non-rebreathing mask.

You obtain the history from the patient and the staff of the facility. The symptoms started about 30 minutes ago, with shortness of breath and coughing. The night nurse's aide tells you the patient said he was chilled, was sweaty, and felt warm. His temperature was taken before your arrival and was recorded on the chart as 102.5°F. The medical record states he has COPD, with a 40-year history of smoking two packs of cigarettes per day. Your partner tells you that respirations are 28 breaths/min and shallow, the pulse is 90 beats/min with occasional irregular beats, blood pressure (BP) is 160/90 mm Hg, and oxygen saturation is 90%.

You and your partner decide to place the patient on continuous positive airway pressure (CPAP) to assist his breathing. Just before you place the mask, the patient starts to cough and brings up blood-tinged sputum. You prepare the patient and transport. He is hospitalized for a week with a diagnosis of pneumonia before being placed in a nursing home.

1. Chief complaint:

2. Vital signs:

3. Pertinent patient history:

4. What was your presumptive diagnosis?

Ambulance Calls

The following case scenarios provide an opportunity to explore the concerns associated with patient management and paramedic care. Read each scenario, and then answer each question.

1. While on a call for a patient with chest pain, you are taking the SAMPLE history, and the patient tells you he is taking an angiotensin-converting enzyme (ACE) inhibitor for hypertension. Your partner has placed the patient on the electrocardiogram (ECG) monitor and informs you that there is a peaked T wave and a wide QRS complex with tachycardia.

a. What do you suspect is the life-threatening emergency that is being identified on the ECG?

b. Which drug should be considered as the first-line medication for this condition?

2. Approximately 500,000 people living in the United States are believed to have Crohn disease. When a person has an acute episode, he or she may call emergency medical services (EMS).

a. Crohn disease is a disorder of which body system?

_____

_____

b. Which symptoms would you expect a patient with Crohn disease to have?

_____

_____

3. It is not uncommon to encounter an elderly patient who has Alzheimer disease as an underlying problem. What are some of the factors that might affect your ability to get a good SAMPLE history and provide care for a patient with Alzheimer disease?

_____

_____

_____

True/False

If you believe the statement to be more true than false, write the letter "T" in the space provided. If you believe the statement to be more false than true, write the letter "F."

_____ **1.** Plasma cells are white blood cells (WBCs) that develop from B cells.

_____ **2.** Helper B cells phagocytize bacteria.

_____ **3.** Acquired immunity is also called native immunity.

_____ **4.** The primary immune response takes place during the first exposure to an antibody.

_____ **5.** Cell-mediated immunity is characterized by the formation of a population of lymphocytes that can destroy foreign material.

_____ **6.** With autosomal recessive inheritance, a person must inherit only one copy of a particular form of a gene to show that trait.

_____ **7.** Distributive shock occurs when blood flow becomes blocked in the great vessels.

_____ **8.** Acquired immunity is a highly specific, inducible, discriminatory, and unforgetting method by which armies of cells respond to an immune stimulant.

_____ **9.** Type 1 diabetes is considered an autoimmune disease.

_____ **10.** The immune system includes all structures and processes associated with the body's defense against foreign substances and disease-causing agents.

_____ **11.** Myasthenia gravis is a chronic systemic disease that affects the body's lymphatic system.

_____ **12.** When hemoglobin is broken down, the iron in this molecule is recycled.

_____ **13.** Iron is transported in blood by transferrin.

_____ **14.** The disease sickle cell anemia causes pancreatic failure and mucus buildup in the lungs.

_____ **15.** Small masses of uric acid or calcium salts that form in the urinary system are called kidney stones.

Short Answer

Complete this section with short written answers using the space provided.

1. Allergens that can cause hypersensitivity reactions include:

   a. _____

   b. _____

   c. _____

   d. _____

   e. _____

   f. _____

2. Cellular injury can result from various causes. List five causes.

   a. _____

   b. _____

   c. _____

   d. _____

   e. _____

3. List seven common respiratory diseases that may be caused by environmental pollutants, viruses, or bacteria.

   a. _____

   b. _____

   c. _____

   d. _____

   e. _____

   f. _____

   g. _____

4. List four conditions for which you should always consider syncope to be caused by a life-threatening dysrhythmia until proved otherwise.

   a. _____

   b. _____

   c. _____

   d. _____

5. The goal of the cellular component of the acute inflammatory response is for the inflammatory cells (polymorphonuclear neutrophils) to arrive at the site in the tissue where they are needed. The process involves two major stages: intravascular phase and extravascular phase. During the later phase, leukocytes travel to the inflammation site and kill organisms. Name the five events in this sequence.

a. _____

b. _____

c. _____

d. _____

e. _____

6. What are the three stages of the general adaptation syndrome?

a. _____

b. _____

c. _____

Fill in the Table

Fill in the missing parts of the table on shock.

Signs and Symptoms of Compensated and Decompensated Hypoperfusion	
Compensated	**Decompensated**
Agitation, anxiety, restlessness	Altered mental status (verbal to unresponsive)
Sense of impending doom	_____
_____	_____
Clammy (cool, moist) skin	Thready or absent peripheral pulses
_____	Ashen, mottled, or cyanotic skin
Shortness of breath	_____
_____	_____
Delayed capillary refill time in infants and children	Impending cardiac arrest
_____	
Normal BP	

Prior to administering nitroglycerin, always ask the patient if he has used erectile dysfunction medication.

Life Span Development

Matching

Part I

Match each of the definitions in the left column to the appropriate term in the right column.

_____ **1.** People who are 1 month to 1 year of age.

_____ **2.** People who are 61 years of age or older.

_____ **3.** The average amount of years a person can be expected to live.

_____ **4.** People who are 41 to 60 years of age.

_____ **5.** The cessation of menstruation, which begins in a woman's late 40s or early 50s and marks the end of the reproductive years.

_____ **6.** A female's first menstrual period.

_____ **7.** A parenting style that balances parental authority with the child's freedom by setting and enforcing rules but also allowing the child to have some freedom.

_____ **8.** Trauma resulting from increased pressure—for example, from too much pressure in the lungs.

_____ **9.** The formation of a close, personal relationship.

_____ **10.** Increased carbon dioxide levels in the bloodstream.

_____ **11.** Structures located on either end of an infant's bone that aid in lengthening bones as the child grows.

_____ **12.** Areas where the infant's skull has not fused together; usually disappear at approximately 18 months of age; also called soft spots.

_____ **13.** People who are 13 to 17 years of age.

_____ **14.** A swelling or enlargement of part of a blood vessel, resulting from weakening of the vessel wall.

_____ **15.** A bond between an infant and the parent/caregiver in which the infant is repeatedly rejected and develops an isolated lifestyle that does not depend on the support and care of others.

_____ **16.** The second phase of an infant's response to a situational crisis; characterized by monotonous wailing.

_____ **17.** A type of reasoning in which a child looks for approval from peers and society.

_____ **18.** People who are 18 to 40 years of age.

_____ **19.** A parenting style that demands absolute obedience.

_____ **20.** A disorder in which cholesterol and calcium build up inside the walls of the blood vessels, forming plaque, which eventually leads to partial or complete blockage of blood flow.

A. Adolescents

B. Aneurysm

C. Anxious avoidant attachment

D. Atherosclerosis

E. Authoritarian

F. Authoritative

G. Barotrauma

H. Bonding

I. Conventional reasoning

J. Despair phase

K. Early adults

L. Fontanelles

M. Growth plates

N. Hypercapnia

O. Infants

P. Late adults

Q. Life expectancy

R. Menarche

S. Menopause

T. Middle adults

Part II

Match each of the definitions in the left column to the appropriate term in the right column.

_____   **1.** An instructional technique that builds on what has already been learned.

_____   **2.** People who are 6 to 12 years of age.

_____   **3.** A bond between an infant and the parent/caregiver in which the infant understands that parents/caregivers will be responsive to his or her needs and provide care when help is needed.

_____   **4.** A person's perception of himself or herself.

_____   **5.** A parenting style in which the parent does not impose many rules, if any, on the child; two subcategories include indifferent and indulgent.

_____   **6.** A type of reasoning in which a child bases decisions on his or her conscience.

_____   **7.** A type of reasoning in which a child acts almost purely to avoid punishment and to get what he or she wants.

_____   **8.** People who are 3 to 5 years of age.

_____   **9.** In the context of infant behavior, the final phase of an infant's response to a situational crisis; characterized by apathy and boredom.

_____   **10.** A phrase that refers to a stage of development from birth to approximately 18 months of age, during which infants gain the trust of their parents and/or caregivers if their world is planned, organized, and routine.

_____   **11.** People who are 1 to 3 years of age.

_____   **12.** The theory that a person's mental function declines in the last 5 years of life.

_____   **13.** An infant reflex that occurs when something is placed in the infant's palm; the infant grasps the object.

_____   **14.** The basic filtering units of the kidneys.

_____   **15.** An infant reflex in which, when caught off guard, the infant opens his or her arms wide.

_____   **16.** An infant reflex that occurs when something touches an infant's cheek, and the infant instinctively turns his or her head toward the touch.

_____   **17.** An infant's initial response to a situational crisis; characterized by loud crying.

_____   **18.** A crisis caused by a specific set of circumstances.

_____   **19.** How a person feels about himself or herself and how he or she fits in with peers.

_____   **20.** An infant reflex in which the infant starts sucking when his or her lips are stroked.

A. Moro reflex

B. Nephrons

C. Palmar grasp

D. Permissive

E. Postconventional reasoning

F. Preconventional reasoning

G. Preschoolers

H. Protest phase

I. Rooting reflex

J. Scaffolding

K. School-age children

L. Secure attachment

M. Self-concept

N. Self-esteem

O. Situational crisis

P. Sucking reflex

Q. Terminal drop hypothesis

R. Toddlers

S. Trust and mistrust

T. Withdrawal

Multiple Choice

Read each item carefully, and then select the best response.

_____   **1.** When a newborn's cheek is touched, he or she turns toward the touch. This is called the _____ reflex.

    A. Moro

    B. palmar

    C. sucking

    D. rooting

_____ **2.** The tidal volume of an infant starts at _____ mL/kg.
  A. 4 to 6
  B. 6 to 8
  C. 8 to 12
  D. 12 to 14

_____ **3.** Which of the infant's fontanelles can be used as a possible indicator of dehydration if sunken?
  A. Posterior
  B. Mastoid
  C. Sphenoidal
  D. Anterior

_____ **4.** At approximately what age does an infant start to become afraid of strangers?
  A. 2 months
  B. 7 months
  C. 9 months
  D. 1 year

_____ **5.** The filtration function of the kidneys declines by _____ between 20 and 90 years of age.
  A. less than 25%
  B. about 25%
  C. about 50%
  D. about 75%

_____ **6.** Bleeding can empty into voids in the older adult brain, resulting in which type of hemorrhage?
  A. Meningeal
  B. Epidural
  C. Ventricular
  D. Subdural

_____ **7.** In the 5 years preceding death, mental function is presumed to decline, a theory referred to as the:
  A. terminal drop hypothesis.
  B. organic dementia hypothesis.
  C. geriatric shrinkage syndrome.
  D. end-of-life physiopsych decline.

_____ **8.** In late adults, the vital capacity of the lungs decreases, and residual volume increases. The effect can produce which of the following conditions?
  A. Hypercapnia
  B. Hypocarbia
  C. Hypoxia
  D. Hyperoxygenation

_____ **9.** Which one of the following is NOT a usual response of the cardiovascular system in late adults?
  A. Decrease in heart rate
  B. Cardiac output that matches demand
  C. Increase in systolic blood pressure
  D. Partial blockage of blood flow

_____ **10.** School-age children learn various types of reasoning in their development. Which of the following is a type of reasoning they learn?
  A. Cognitive
  B. Distributive
  C. Conventional
  D. Affective

Fill in the Blank

Read each item carefully, and then complete the statement by filling in the missing word(s).

1. A full-term infant usually weighs approximately _____ pounds at birth. After birth, infants usually lose

   _____% to _____% of their birth weight due to the loss of _____ in the first week.

2. A(n) _____ _____ occurs when an object is placed in the infant's palm.

3. An infant's _____ allow the head to be molded when the newborn passes through the birth canal.

4. _____ _____, located on either end of the infant's bones, aid in the lengthening of a child's bones.

5. _____, or the formation of a close, personal relationship, is usually based on a secure attachment.

6. _____ and _____ refer to a stage of development from birth to about 18 months of age. Most infants desire

   that their world be planned, organized, and routine

7. Atherosclerosis can contribute to the development of a(n) _____, or weakening and bulging of a blood vessel wall.

8. In late adults, blood flow in the _____ (membranes that connect organs to the abdominal wall) may drop by as

   much as 50%.

9. In the 5 years preceding death, mental function is presumed to decline. This is a theory referred to as the _____

   _____ _____.

10. In late adults, the size of the airway (_____), and the surface area of the alveoli (_____).

Labeling

Label the four fontanelles of the infant's head.

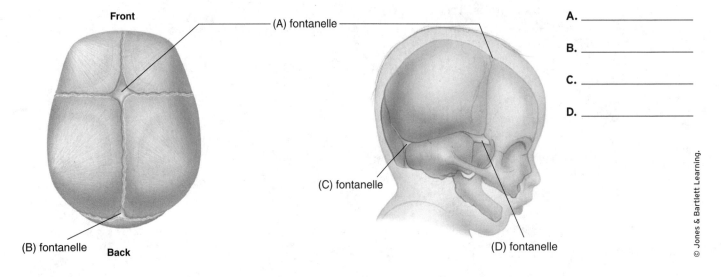

Front

(A) fontanelle

(B) fontanelle   Back

(C) fontanelle

(D) fontanelle

A. _____

B. _____

C. _____

D. _____

© Jones & Bartlett Learning.

Identify

Read the following case study, and then list the chief complaint, vital signs, and SAMPLE history.

A call to an assisted living facility brings you to a 75-year-old woman who tripped on a chair and fell while walking from the living room to the kitchen. When you enter the apartment, the patient tells you she fell and has a great deal of pain in her hip. You gently palpate the injured area, and the patient yells. You take a set of vital signs and find a pulse of 90 beats/min and thready, respirations of 24 breaths/min and shallow, and blood pressure of 100/70 mm Hg. The SAMPLE history identifies an externally rotated foot and discoloration of the hip on the same side. The patient reports no allergies and is on several medications for congestive heart failure. She had a heart attack last year, and she has a two-pack-a-day history of smoking for more than 30 years but stopped smoking about 5 years ago. She ate breakfast 3 hours ago. You place the patient on an electrocardiogram (ECG) monitor, establish an IV, and package her for transport.

1. Chief complaint:

_____

_____

2. Vital signs:

_____

_____

3. SAMPLE history:

_____

_____

Ambulance Calls

The following case scenarios provide an opportunity to explore the concerns associated with patient management and paramedic care. Read each scenario, and then answer each question.

1. Your unit is dispatched to a call for an infant with a seizure. The response time is 5 minutes, and when you enter the residence, you find a distraught mother who is very anxious. The seizure seems to have stopped, but you understand the importance of an immediate primary survey (the MS–ABC Priority Plan). You immediately notice that the child has good color except for a little cyanosis of the fingers. The child is actively breathing, and the rate is adequate. Your partner starts to administer blow-by oxygen, and you examine the child quickly from head to toe to make sure there is no external bleeding or signs of trauma. The child is starting to respond and become more active. You prepare for transport and decide the child is stable and alert enough that the neurologic status can be assessed. Which reflexes would you check, and how would you test them? What are considered to be the appropriate responses from the infant? Fill in the following table.

Reflex	How to Test	Appropriate Response

2. A call to an assisted living facility finds a 75-year-old woman sitting with her partner and complaining of general body weakness. You approach the patient but have trouble communicating with her, and while doing the SAMPLE history, you have trouble getting necessary information from her. You decide that when asking about her past medical history, you should ask about individual body systems because this might help to identify the current problem.

a. What are some of the communication issues you might have encountered while taking the history of this patient?

_____

_____

_____

_____

b. What are some possible concerns you are thinking of while attempting to obtain the past medical history?

_____

_____

_____

_____

3. You receive a call to the residence of a 16-year-old girl with a chief complaint of abdominal pain. The girl is lying on the couch in the living room; her mother and a girlfriend are also in the room. Your partner is a man who is taking the lead on the assessment and SAMPLE history. While doing the SAMPLE history, he asks the patient if there is a possibility she is pregnant. She immediately and emphatically answers no. He then decides that he should palpate the abdomen and immediately proceeds to do so, with little explanation. The patient seems embarrassed. You realize that you need to package the patient and transport.

   a. Which consideration should your partner have taken into account before questioning this patient about the possibility of pregnancy?

_____

_____

_____

_____

   b. Is there a more appropriate way to handle the physical exam of the abdomen?

_____

_____

_____

_____

True/False

If you believe the statement to be more true than false, write the letter "T" in the space provided. If you believe the statement to be more false than true, write the letter "F."

_____ **1.** An infant's ventilations that are too forceful can result in barotrauma.

_____ **2.** The rooting reflex occurs when an infant's lips are stroked.

_____ **3.** If the posterior fontanelle is sunken, the infant is most likely dehydrated.

_____ **4.** Anxious avoidant attachment is observed in infants who are repeatedly rejected.

_____ **5.** A toddler is at the critical age in human development to learn various types of reasoning.

_____ **6.** Cardiac function declines with age consequent to anatomic and physiologic changes largely related to atherosclerosis.

_____ **7.** In late adults, the vital capacity of the lungs decreases, and stagnant air remains in the alveoli and hampers gas exchange, which can produce hypercapnia.

_____ **8.** In late adults, there is a surge of increased mental functioning in the last few years of life.

_____ **9.** Age-related shrinkage creates a void between the brain and outermost layer of the meninges.

_____ **10.** The number of nephrons in the kidneys increases between the ages of 30 and 80.

Short Answer

Complete this section with short written answers using the space provided.

1. Infants are born with certain reflexes and responses that can assist you in the neurologic assessment of an infant. Name four of these reflexes.

    a. _____

    b. _____

    c. _____

    d. _____

2. Cardiac function declines with age largely as a result of atherosclerosis. This disorder, which commonly affects coronary vessels, results from the formation of plaque. Which two substances are responsible for the buildup of plaque?

    a. _____

    b. _____

3. Loss of which mechanisms in the respiratory system of the late adult makes aspiration and obstruction more likely?

    a. _____

    b. _____

    c. _____

    d. _____

    e. _____

4. Late adults have sensory changes that can affect mobility and safety. Which sensory changes occur in this age group?

    a. _____

    b. _____

    c. _____

    d. _____

    e. _____

    f. _____

    g. _____

5. Colds often develop in toddlers and preschool-age children and may manifest as which types of infections?

    a. _____

    b. _____

6. Playing games is the way that toddlers learn. What can a child of this age learn from play?

    a. _____

    b. _____

    c. _____

7. In the late elderly, the vital capacity of the lungs decreases. Name three factors that contribute to this decline.

d. _____

e. _____

f. _____

Fill in the Table

Fill in the missing parts of the tables.

1. Subtle changes occur during adolescence; one change is the development of secondary sexual characteristics. Fill in the table with these characteristics.

Male Characteristics	Female Characteristics

2. Fill in the table with the appropriate noticeable characteristics for various ages in the infant's development.

Psychosocial Characteristics at Various Ages

Age (in months)	Noticeable Characteristics
2	Recognizes familiar faces; (A) _____
3	Brings objects to the mouth; (B) _____
4	Reaches out to people; drools
5	Sleeps through the night; (C) _____
6	Teething begins; (D) _____
7	Afraid of strangers; (E) _____
8	Responds to "no"; sits upright alone; plays peek-a-boo
9	Pulls himself or herself up; (F) _____
10	Responds to his or her name; crawls efficiently
11	(G) _____; _____
12	Knows his or her name; can walk

Patient Assessment

Being good at patient assessment is a lot
like being a good detective

© Jones & Bartlett Learning.

Matching

Part I

Match each of the definitions in the left column to the appropriate term in the right column.

_____ **1.** An acute confusional state characterized by global impairment of thinking, perception, judgment, and memory.

_____ **2.** Double vision.

_____ **3.** Localized bruising or collection of blood within or under the skin.

_____ **4.** A crackling, grating, or grinding sound often heard when fragments of broken bones rub together.

_____ **5.** An abnormal whooshing sound heard over the heart that indicates turbulent blood flow around a cardiac valve.

_____ **6.** A blotchy pattern on the skin; a typical finding in states of severe protracted hypoperfusion and shock.

_____ **7.** Outward curve of the thoracic spine.

_____ **8.** Wet rattling, bubbling, or crackling lung sounds indicative of fluid in the small airways; also known as rales.

_____ **9.** Ear wax.

_____ **10.** Unequal pupils with a difference greater than 1 mm.

_____ **11.** A language impairment that affects the production or understanding of speech and the ability to read or write.

_____ **12.** The entry of fluids or solids into the trachea, bronchi, and lungs; the act of drawing material in or out by suction.

_____ **13.** Abnormal accumulation of fluid in the peritoneal cavity; typically signals liver failure.

_____ **14.** Sounds related to blood pressure measurement that are heard by stethoscope.

_____ **15.** Looking at the patient, either in general or at a specific area (ie, a patient's overall appearance from the doorway versus looking specifically at the chest wall for abnormalities/deformities).

_____ **16.** Related to a side effect or complication of medications or other medical treatment.

_____ **17.** Contraction of the abdominal muscles indicating peritoneal irritation.

_____ **18.** Sideways curvature of the spine.

_____ **19.** Involuntary motor responses to specific sensory stimuli, such as a tap on the knee or stroking the eyelash.

A. Anisocoria

B. Aphasia

C. Ascites

D. Aspiration

E. Battle sign

F. Beck triad

G. Bronchial sounds

H. Bruit

I. Cerumen

J. Crackles

K. Crepitus

L. Delirium

M. Diplopia

N. Ecchymosis

O. Guarding

P. Iatrogenic

Q. Inspection

R. Korotkoff sounds

S. Kyphosis

_____ **20.** The perception of the position and movement of the body or limbs.

T. Mottling

_____ **21.** Physical touching for the purpose of obtaining information (ie, to detect tenderness).

U. Murmur

_____ **22.** An abnormal whooshing sound of turbulent blood flow moving through a narrowed artery; usually heard in the carotid arteries.

V. Palpation

_____ **23.** Hollow, tubular, lower-pitched sounds heard over the trachea.

W. Proprioception

_____ **24.** The combination of a narrowed pulse pressure, muffled heart tones, and jugular venous distention (JVD) associated with cardiac tamponade; usually caused by penetrating chest trauma.

X. Reflexes

_____ **25.** Bruising over the mastoid process, which may indicate a basilar skull fracture; also known as retroauricular ecchymosis or raccoon eyes.

Y. Scoliosis

Part II

During your EMT course, you learned many assessment findings. In the paramedic program, you will broaden your knowledge of assessment findings and learn their diagnostic significance so that you can come to a presumptive diagnosis. Using the knowledge you already have at this point, try to match each of the signs listed to the right with the phrase that best describes its possible diagnostic significance or presumptive diagnosis. (Note: More than one sign may have the same diagnostic significance.)

_____ **1.** Narcotics overdose

A. Ecchymosis (discoloration) around the eyes

_____ **2.** Cardiac arrest

B. Fruity (acetone) odor to the breath

_____ **3.** Heart failure

C. Stridor on inspiration

_____ **4.** Skull fracture

D. Pitting edema of both ankles

_____ **5.** Stroke

E. Paralysis of upward gaze

_____ **6.** Hypoxemia

F. Muffled heart sounds

_____ **7.** Respiratory distress

G. Battle sign (discoloration of mastoid area)

_____ **8.** Shock

H. Patient lies very still; cries out when stretcher is jarred

_____ **9.** Diabetic ketoacidosis

I. Pinpoint pupils

_____ **10.** Spinal cord injury

J. Cyanosis of the lips

_____ **11.** Increased right ventricular pressure

K. Capillary refill takes 5 seconds

_____ **12.** Laryngeal edema

L. Restlessness

_____ **13.** Pelvic fracture

M. Absent pulse

_____ **14.** Fluid/blood in the pericardium

N. Retraction of the suprasternal muscles

_____ **15.** Intra-abdominal bleeding

O. Jugular veins distended to 10 cm when the patient is sitting

_____ **16.** Peritonitis

P. Crackling sensation in the skin over the chest

_____ **17.** Fracture of the orbit (eye socket in the skull)

Q. Distended, bruised abdomen in trauma victim

_____ **18.** Pneumothorax

R. Pain on compression of the iliac crests

S. Priapism

T. No movement or sensation in the right arm or leg

U. S_3 gallop (heart sound)

V. Clear fluid draining from the ear

Part III

For each of the following patients, indicate whether their signs and/or symptoms classify them as sick or not sick.

S—Sick (life-threatening)   NS—Not sick

_____ **1.** 18-month-old boy who is limp and dusky blue in the face

_____ **2.** 54-year-old woman with diffuse abdominal pain

_____ **3.** 43-year-old man with confusion, sweating, and left arm pain

_____ **4.** 22-year-old woman with rapid breathing and tingling in arms and feet

_____   **5.** 4-year-old girl who is crying and has pain in her ear

_____   **6.** 75-year-old man who is unable to speak or answer questions

_____   **7.** 66-year-old woman who is unresponsive and breathing deeply and rapidly

_____   **8.** 36-year-old woman who is depressed and does not want to talk

Multiple Choice

Read each item carefully, and then select the best response.

_____   **1.** When responding to a call, a paramedic's demeanor and appearance should be all of the following, EXCEPT:
- **A.** clean.
- **B.** overbearing.
- **C.** positive.
- **D.** efficient.

_____   **2.** Which of the following statements/questions would be considered a facilitation communication technique?
- **A.** That's all the information I need.
- **B.** You don't have to tell me if you don't want to.
- **C.** Can you think of anything else about his medical history?
- **D.** Can you narrow down his history to just the past few months?

_____   **3.** Which communication technique is NOT helpful in a stressful situation?
- **A.** Confrontation
- **B.** Facilitation
- **C.** Empathetic response
- **D.** Clarification

_____   **4.** What should the thinking paramedic do when faced with a possible physical abuse situation?
- **A.** Document.
- **B.** Gather evidence in a paper bag.
- **C.** Accuse the abuser to try to get the real story.
- **D.** Call for law enforcement before leaving the scene.

_____   **5.** When a patient has a period of silence during a call, it should make you:
- **A.** begin to ask more questions.
- **B.** realize that the patient may not trust you, prompting you to respect the silence.
- **C.** look for a reason the patient is not talking, such as a change in condition.
- **D.** look for a weapon on the patient.

_____   **6.** Your patient will not quit talking! Which of the following is NOT a reason for chattiness?
- **A.** The patient is on methamphetamine.
- **B.** The patient is very nervous.
- **C.** The patient has had several cups of coffee.
- **D.** All of the above can lead to chattiness.

_____   **7.** You are dealing with a very angry young man who is being arrested for driving while intoxicated (DWI). He has a broken leg and arm, and you are transporting him to the hospital. What is the best way to treat this situation?
- **A.** Make sure you strap him down tight to the backboard so that he cannot get away.
- **B.** Tell him that if he does not calm down, you will give him a medication to calm him down.
- **C.** Treat him as you would any patient, and keep your anger and comments to yourself.
- **D.** Yell back at him, and let him know that you are the boss and will not tolerate this in the back of your squad.

_____   **8.** Which of the following statements describes behavior that is NOT correct when interacting with a blind person?
- **A.** Always put things back exactly where you picked them up from.
- **B.** Speak very, very slowly and clearly.
- **C.** Announce your identity and reason for being there.
- **D.** Let the person know where you are and where you are going at all times during transport.

9. Which of the following signs and symptoms is NOT a sign of depression?

  A. Feeling of high energy

  B. Irritability

  C. Eating disruptions

  D. Pain with no source

10. What is a good thing to remember when asking for history from family members?

  A. They will always know the patient's history.

  B. They will be aware of drug or alcohol use.

  C. You are not at liberty to share the patient's condition with them.

  D. You will be able to give them an update on the patient once they reach the hospital.

11. While assessing a trauma patient, you press down lightly on the abdomen. This technique is called:

  A. inspection.

  B. percussion.

  C. auscultation.

  D. palpation.

12. Which of the following statements is NOT true regarding the use of a pulse oximeter?

  A. It measures only the percentage of hemoglobin saturation.

  B. It can help determine the patient's heart rhythm.

  C. A cold person can have a false reading.

  D. A hypotensive patient can have a false reading.

13. What is essential in getting an accurate blood pressure reading?

  A. Using the right cuff size

  B. Not having any clothing on the arm

  C. Having the arm perfectly straight

  D. The age of the patient

14. When assessing a patient's mental status, "P" on the AVPU scale stands for which of the following?

  A. Pupil size

  B. Pallor of the skin

  C. Painful stimuli

  D. Presence

15. Clubbing of the fingertips is possibly caused by which of the following conditions?

  A. Bacterial endocarditis

  B. Systemic illness

  C. Chronic respiratory disease

  D. Cirrhosis of the liver

16. An elderly woman who was walking across the living room reports that she felt and heard a "pop" in her hip, and then she fell to the floor. You think that there is a possibility she has a broken hip. Which process has happened to create this injury?

  A. Pathologic fracture

  B. Physiologic fracture

  C. Psychogenic fracture

  D. Psychical fracture

17. In assessing a patient's spine, you find an exaggerated inward curve of the lumbar area. This is known as:

  A. kyphosis.

  B. lordosis.

  C. the Cullen sign.

  D. dislocation of the lumbar spine.

_____ **18.** You are auscultating a patient's carotid arteries and hear a "whooshing." You are hearing bruit, which indicates:

    A. a heart murmur.

    B. turbulent blood flow around a cardiac valve.

    C. turbulent blood flow in the carotid arteries.

    D. reduced blood flow around a cardiac valve.

_____ **19.** When checking the cranial nerve IV, you will be checking for which of the following?

    A. Hearing and balance

    B. Smell

    C. Visual acuity

    D. Eye movements

_____ **20.** You are assessing a patient and notice cyanotic patches on the lower extremities. This finding is known as _____, and it is seen in severe states of shock and hypoperfusion.

    A. tenting

    B. turgor

    C. mottling

    D. crepitus

_____ **21.** The scene size-up component of the patient assessment includes all of the following, EXCEPT:

    A. focused assessment.

    B. mechanism of injury (MOI).

    C. requesting additional resources.

    D. scene safety.

_____ **22.** During the primary survey, the paramedic must:

    A. treat medical and trauma patients differently.

    B. determine the SAMPLE history.

    C. identify priority patients.

    D. obtain baseline vital signs.

_____ **23.** Which of the following standard precautions may be appropriate during the scene size-up and examination of a patient found lying on the kitchen floor for about a week?

    A. Gloves

    B. Gowns

    C. N95 masks

    D. All of the above

_____ **24.** When on a scene where people act aggressively or appear to be threatening, it is best for the paramedic to:

    A. consider retreating to the ambulance until the scene is secure.

    B. explain that you are there to help and do not intend any harm to the patient.

    C. explain that you are not law enforcement.

    D. begin acting authoritarian and aggressive toward the instigators.

_____ **25.** The most time-sensitive and important aspect of the patient assessment, where life threats are detected and quickly treated, is considered the:

    A. primary survey.

    B. focused assessment.

    C. secondary assessment.

    D. general impression.

_____ **26.** Which of the following is considered a "priority patient"?

    A. A pregnant patient involved in a low-speed motor vehicle crash without any complications

    B. A large multiple-casualty incident with a patient in cardiac arrest

    C. A patient who does not pass the "look test," giving a poor general impression

    D. A bystander who witnessed the event and is traumatized by what he saw

27. Evaluating an unresponsive medical patient requires you, the paramedic, to rely on which of the following?
  A. A head-to-toe physical exam
  B. The presence of a medical identification tag
  C. The bystander or family information
  D. All of the above

28. The rapid trauma exam is generally completed:
  A. on all patients entrapped in a vehicle.
  B. on any patient who does not have a readily identifiable medical problem.
  C. before all life threats have been identified and treated.
  D. prior to conducting a secondary assessment on the patient.

29. Which of the following patients typically requires a head-to-toe exam?
  A. A man with a minor laceration obtained while cutting vegetables in the kitchen.
  B. An athlete who was kicked in the shin while playing soccer.
  C. An intoxicated bar patron who fell off a stool and struck his head.
  D. A baseball catcher struck in the face while wearing his protective mask.

30. When assessing a patient's airway status, it is often helpful to do which of the following?
  A. Think from the simple to the complex.
  B. Intubate the patient quickly to manage the airway definitively.
  C. Alter your assessment based on the patient's age.
  D. Always open an unconscious patient's airway with a head tilt–chin lift maneuver.

Labeling

Label the following diagram with the missing terms.

1. Nine regions of the abdomen

A. _____

B. _____

C. _____

D. _____

E. _____

F. _____

G. _____

H. _____

I. _____

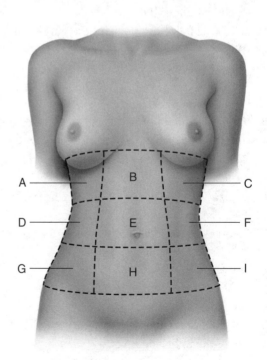

Fill in the Blank

Read each item carefully, and then complete the statement by filling in the missing word(s).

1. You will make your _____ _____ based on the patient's chief complaint, vital signs, and history.

2. The first step in making an approach to a patient is to _____ _____.

3. Once you have established the patient's chief complaint, you will want to check into the history of the _____ _____.

4. When using a translator to help interview your patient, be aware that medical terms and _____ often do not translate well.

5. You respond to a patient who is deaf. When communicating with the patient, you should orient yourself to be in _____-_____-_____ position with him or her.

6. _____ is described as one step further than sympathy.

7. When talking with a patient, you pause to consider something significant that you have just been told before proceeding. This technique is known as _____.

8. The federal law abbreviated as_____ governs the disclosure of patient information.

9. Always review transfer information before transferring a patient to a new facility so that you know the patient's _____ _____.

10. During your history taking, ensure the questions you ask are _____-appropriate and _____-appropriate.

Ambulance Calls

The following case scenarios provide an opportunity to explore the concerns associated with patient management and paramedic care. Read each scenario, and then answer each question.

1. You are called to the crash scene pictured here.

a. List four potential sources of information about what happened to the patient or about his medical background.

(1)_____

(2)_____

(3)_____

(4)_____

b. List five pieces of information you can derive simply from observing the scene.

(1)_____

(2)_____

(3)_____

(4)_____

(5)_____

c. List four reasons why it is necessary to take a history from the driver of the car.

(1)_____

(2)_____

(3)_____

(4)_____

d. Before you start taking the history, however, you need to take some preliminary steps. List them.

(1)_____

(2)_____

(3)_____

(4)_____

(5)_____

True/False

If you believe the statement to be more true than false, write the letter "T" in the space provided. If you believe the statement to be more false than true, write the letter "F."

_____   **1.** Being able to think and perform well under pressure is a big part of being a good paramedic.

_____   **2.** Patients will always be honest when it comes to their sexual history.

_____   **3.** You will always be able to tell who is a heavy user of alcohol.

_____   **4.** Patients sometimes need a few seconds to gather their thoughts and answer your questions.

_____   **5.** Law enforcement should be called for *every* hostile patient.

_____   **6.** You should check blood glucose on every patient who has an altered mental status.

_____   **7.** Patients may suffer trauma because of a medical problem or their current health status.

_____   **8.** You should be able to make your field diagnosis based on the patient's chief complaint.

_____   **9.** Using "pet names" with a patient will put the person at ease.

_____   **10.** The clarification communication technique is used when trying to clear up a vague history.

_____   **11.** Children do not become dehydrated as fast as adults do.

_____   **12.** Delirium is associated with an acute, sudden change in mental status.

_____   **13.** Aphasia is difficulty speaking, which is common in patients who have experienced cardiovascular disease or a stroke.

_____   **14.** The Babinski reflex is a normal finding in an older adult.

_____   **15.** When assessing a limb for signs of venous obstruction or insufficiency, you should check for edema and mild erythema.

_____   **16.** You should always assess a pulse in three different places on the foot.

_____   **17.** To assess a shoulder dislocation, you should be in front of the patient and looking down at both shoulders.

_____   **18.** Female and male genitalia should be assessed in a limited and discreet fashion.

_____   **19.** Right-sided heart failure is a common cause of JVD.

_____   **20.** You must have a stethoscope for evaluating blood pressure (BP).

Short Answer

Complete this section with short written answers using the space provided.

1. A male patient's chief complaint is "pain in my gut."

   a. List six questions you would ask in eliciting the history of the present illness.

     (1) _____

     (2) _____

     (3) _____

     (4) _____

     (5) _____

     (6) _____

   b. List four questions you would ask about his other medical history.

     (1) _____

     (2) _____

     (3) _____

     (4) _____

2. Taking the history of a patient requires excellent communications skills. List five communications techniques used by the paramedic in the field.

   a. _____

   b. _____

   c. _____

d. _____

e. _____

3. You are called to the scene of a multiple-vehicle crash on the interstate highway. As you approach the scene, you begin making your size-up. List four questions you need to answer in making your size-up of the collision scene.

a. _____

b. _____

c. _____

d. _____

4. Patient assessment consists largely of detective work—searching for and interpreting clues to form a picture of the patient's problem. At the scene of an incident or, for that matter, in the patient's home, there may be several sources of information about the patient. List four potential sources of information about the patient and what has happened to him or her.

a. _____

b. _____

c. _____

d. _____

Fill in the Blank

Fill in the missing parts of the tables.

1. When testing the cranial nerves, a number of simple maneuvers can be employed to determine the presence and degree of disability. Fill in the following table to indicate what to test for disability in the cranial nerves.

Tests for Disability in Cranial Nerves	
Cranial Nerve	**Test**
I	
II	
III	
IV	
V	
VI	
VII	
VIII	
IX, X	
XI	
XII	

2. In the secondary assessment physical exam of a patient with multisystem trauma, you must look for very specific clues to specific injuries. Fill in the following table to indicate what you will be looking for in particular as you examine each part of the body.

Body Region	What I Will Be Looking for in Particular
Head	
Neck	
Chest	
Abdomen	
Extremities	
Back/buttocks	

Critical Thinking and Clinical Decision Making

Matching

Part I

For each of the following scenarios, decide if you would follow protocols or use independent decisions.

A. Follow protocols   B. Use independent decisions

_____ **1.** An 86-year-old woman with facial droop and slurred speech

_____ **2.** A 14-year-old boy, unconscious, who is trapped in a drain pipe

_____ **3.** A diabetic woman with low blood glucose

_____ **4.** A 57-year-old man with "classic ischemic" chest pain

_____ **5.** A crop-duster crash with a conscious pilot who is yelling for help

_____ **6.** A school where a person has shot several students

_____ **7.** An allergic reaction to a bee sting in a 12-year-old girl

_____ **8.** A motor vehicle crash where the car is smoking and appears to be on fire

_____ **9.** A 20-year-old basketball player in cardiac arrest during a game

_____ **10.** A man who is stuck inside a grain elevator and is being pulled under the grain

Part II

Match each of the definitions in the left column to the appropriate term in the right column.

_____ **1.** Vague or unclear aspects of medicine.   **A.** Affect

_____ **2.** Blindly following a protocol or algorithm without thinking about what is being done and whether it is working.   **B.** Comorbidity

_____ **3.** The patient's emotional state as reflected in the patient's physical behavior.   **C.** Concept formation

_____ **4.** The existence of two or more chronic diseases or conditions in a patient.   **D.** Cookbook medicine

_____ **5.** Focusing on or considering only one aspect of a situation without first taking into account all possibilities.   **E.** Medical ambiguity

_____ **6.** Pattern of understanding based on the initially obtained information; the first stage of the critical thinking process n prehospital care.   **F.** Tunnel vision

Multiple Choice

Read each item carefully, and then select the best response.

_____ **1.** _____ is processing the information presented by the patient you are treating.

    A. Gathering

    B. Evaluating

    C. Synthesizing

    D. Thinking

_____ **2.** Which of the following items is NOT included in the concept-formation process?

    A. Smell

    B. Sample history

    C. Hearing

    D. Seeing

_____ **3.** What is the second stage of critical thinking?

    A. Application of principle

    B. Reflection in action

    C. Concept formation

    D. Data interpretation

_____ **4.** What does _reflection in action_ mean?

    A. A call review of the run you just completed

    B. Checking your interventions as you apply them to your patient

    C. Stopping before you apply the intervention to make sure you are doing the right thing

    D. Checking the protocols prior to doing anything

_____ **5.** Which of the following is NOT one of the "Six Rs" discussed in the chapter?

    A. Read the scene.

    B. Read the protocols.

    C. Read the patient.

    D. React.

_____ **6.** You respond to a patient's home for a report of chest pain. You are determining the chief complaint and taking the baseline vital signs. In which of the "Six Rs" are you working right now?

    A. Reading the scene

    B. Reacting

    C. Reevaluating

    D. Reading the patient

_____ **7.** When responding to a critical patient, why is it best to use a mental checklist?

    A. So that you do not forget to take vital signs

    B. So that you always follow your protocols

    C. To facilitate better thinking on the scene

    D. So that you will never be sued

_____ **8.** Which of the following is NOT used in synthesizing the patient's information?

    A. Patient history

    B. Patient allergies

    C. Current complaints

    D. Previous diseases

_____ **9.** Which of the following adult patients would be considered to have a serious condition?

    A. Acute presentation of a first-time event

    B. Acute presentation of a chronic event

    C. Patient with small lacerations

    D. Partial-thickness burns to an extremity, with less than 5% of body surface area (BSA) burned

_____ **10.** What is the "third cornerstone" of effective paramedic practice?
   A. Development and implementation of a patient care plan
   B. Having the ability to think and work under pressure
   C. Having the ability to use judgment and make independent decisions
   D. Having the ability to gather, evaluate, and synthesize information

Fill in the Blank

Read each item carefully, and then complete the statement by filling in the missing word(s).

1. By taking a SAMPLE history and baseline vital signs, you are _____ information about the patient that will be used to assess and evaluate the patient and help form your treatment plan.

2. Your care plan for your patient is almost always defined by your _____.

3. Your final cornerstone of practicing as a paramedic is to _____ and _____ under pressure.

4. The process of gathering information by smell, sight, hearing, and touch is known as _____ _____.

5. Patients with major multisystem trauma, acute chronic conditions, and devastating single-system trauma would be examples of patients with critical_____ _____.

6. Once you have assessed the patient and begin treatment, you are using a(n) _____ _____.

7. Some of the primary elements involved in _____ the scene are evaluating the overall safety of the situation, the environmental conditions, the immediate surroundings, access and egress issues, and the MOI.

8. When dealing with a critical patient, you take vital signs three or more times. The readings allow you to assess _____.

Identify

After reading the following case study, list the chief complaint, vital signs, and any pertinent negatives.

It is 1600 hours, and you have been called to a residence for a woman who is not feeling well. When you arrive, you find a 56-year-old woman with a general feeling of malaise. You begin talking with her to gather some information while your partner takes baseline vital signs. During your SAMPLE history, you find out that she has diabetes. Your partner tests her blood glucose level, and it is 110 mg/dL. The patient states that she is very careful because of her illness. Her blood pressure (BP) is 160/100 mm Hg, and her pulse is 92 beats/min and regular, with normal sinus rhythm showing on the ECG monitor, but she is showing a little ST-segment depression. You ask her if she has ever had a heart attack, and she says no. Her SpO2 is 97% on room air, all lung fields are clear, and she is breathing at 18 breaths/min. The patient's skin is warm and dry, and her pupils are PERRLA (Pupils Equal, Round, and Reactive to Light and Accommodation). She says she has been feeling this way for a few days and is so tired that she hasn't been able to do anything. She was afraid something major might be wrong with her, so she decided to give 9-1-1 a call. You tell the woman that she might have had a cardiac event and that you want to take her in. You apply oxygen by non-rebreathing mask at 15 L/min, start an IV at a to-keep-open (TKO) drip, and give her some nitroglycerin paste to bring down the BP en route. You take a 12-lead electrocardiogram (ECG) en route and transport her to the local emergency department (ED). The nitroglycerin brings the BP down to 120/70 mm Hg. All other vital signs stay the same. Later, you learn she has had a small myocardial infarction (MI), but because of her diabetes, she never had the classic signs.

1. Chief complaint:

   _____

   _____

   _____

2. Vital signs:

_____

_____

_____

3. Pertinent negatives:

_____

_____

_____

Ambulance Calls

The following case scenario provides an opportunity to explore the concerns associated with patient management and paramedic care. Read the scenario, and then answer each question.

1. You are on a rural squad, with no regional trauma center nearby. You are dispatched to an elementary school for a child who has fallen out of a tree. The school is reporting that the child is still on the ground outside on the playground. When you arrive, you find a 9-year-old girl sitting up. You ask your partner to take cervical spine precautions while you start your primary survey. The teacher says she was approximately 15 feet up when she fell. You note a large broken branch about 7 feet off the ground, and the teacher says that the child hit that branch on the way down on her left side and then landed on her head on the hard dirt. The child is unable to tell you her name and is confused about where she is and the day of the week. After finding no obvious life threats during the primary survey, you proceed with a rapid trauma exam because of the significant mechanism of injury (MOI). You decide she is a critical patient because of the MOI and call for Life Flight to take her to the regional trauma center. Your partner applies an extrication collar, and you carefully place her on a long backboard. You apply supplemental oxygen by nonrebreathing mask at 15 L/min. Your partner takes baseline vital signs that reveal a BP of 130/80 mm Hg, pulse of 52 beats/min, and respirations at 6 breaths/min. Lung sounds are clear. The patient responds only to painful stimuli at this point, and her SpO_2 is 88%. Her pupils are unequal, with the left pupil much larger than the right. The patient begins to gag and vomit. You suction all secretions, place an oropharyngeal airway, and start to assist her ventilations with the bag-mask device. Your partner gets an IV started as the helicopter is landing. The patient no longer has a gag reflex, so the flight medics insert an advanced airway. The Life Flight crew loads her and takes off, heading for the regional trauma center. Later, you learn that the girl died in the operating room (OR) as a result of massive head injury.

a. What is your first clue that this patient should be treated as a critical patient?

_____

_____

_____

b. Under which type of consent can you transport this child without her parents' permission?

_____

_____

_____

c. What do your baseline vital signs suggest for this patient?

_____

_____

_____

d. What is your first concern with the patient, and how can you manage that concern?

_____

_____

_____

2. You are traveling to Grandma's house for what you anticipate will be a wonderful Thanksgiving dinner. Traffic slows and comes to a stop. Knowing what you do about traffic and collisions, you pull out your primary survey kit and head up the road. A minivan loaded with people has crossed left of the center line and hit a car with another family in it. There are people everywhere—some trying to help patients from the vehicles and others just standing around. The 9-1-1 system has already been called, but you can't hear any sirens yet because you are about 20 miles from any town. You realize there are critical patients trapped in the van, and the Jaws of Life will be needed to extricate those patients.

a. How do you identify yourself and gain control of this scene?

_____

_____

_____

b. Which type of equipment will you need at this scene?

_____

_____

_____

c. Will you begin any type of treatment before help arrives?

_____

_____

_____

True/False

If you believe the statement to be more true than false, write the letter "T" in the space provided. If you believe the statement to be more false than true, write the letter "F."

_____ **1.** The first cornerstone of your practice is having the ability to gather, evaluate, and synthesize information on the scene.

_____ **2.** Once you have evaluated the information you obtained from the scene, the patient, or a bystander and have determined which information is valid or invalid, you need to process—or synthesize—this information.

_____ **3.** Protocols, standing orders, and patient care algorithms will address every patient for the paramedic and give a clear, defined path to treatment.

_____ **4.** The patient who presents with an acute presentation of a new medical condition is considered a patient with a critical life threat.

_____ **5.** The second stage of critical thinking is concept formation.

_____ **6.** Reflection in action is the process of reassessing the patient.

_____ **7.** When you identify a patient with medical ambiguity, it means that you have pinpointed the cause of the patient's medical problem.

_____ **8.** When reading the scene, you are looking for information that is available only at the scene.

Short Answer

Complete this section with short written answers using the space provided.

1. Discuss the use of the "Six Rs" when responding to a routine call.

   a. Read the scene:

   _____

   _____

   _____

   b. Read the patient:

   _____

   _____

   _____

   c. React:

   _____

   _____

   _____

   d. Reevaluate:

   _____

   _____

   _____

   e. Revise the plan:

   _____

   _____

   _____

   f. Review your performance:

   _____

   _____

   _____

2. When using the cornerstone principles of critical thinking, discuss the differences in gathering information, evaluating information, and synthesizing.

_____

_____

_____

_____

_____

_____

_____

PHARMACOLOGY

Are you allergic to any drugs?

According to my PDA, we should be giving the patient morphine.

Morphine.

Do not administer a medication to which the patient has an allergy!

© Jones & Bartlett Learning.

Principles of Pharmacology

Matching

Part I

Listed here are medications that are considered controlled substances. Write the schedule, I to V, for the example given.

_____ **1.** Hydrocodone (Vicodin)

_____ **2.** Narcotic cough medicines

_____ **3.** Heroin

_____ **4.** Fentanyl (Sublimaze)

_____ **5.** Diazepam (Valium)

_____ **6.** Lorazepam (Ativan)

_____ **7.** High abuse potential and no recognized medical purpose

_____ **8.** High abuse potential and legitimate medical purpose

_____ **9.** Cocaine

_____ **10.** Codeine

Part II

Match each of the definitions in the left column to the appropriate term in the right column.

_____ **1.** Medications that bind with heavy metals in the body and create a compound that can be eliminated; used in cases of ingestion or poisoning.

A. Absolute refractory period

_____ **2.** Widening of the bronchial tubes.

B. Absorption

_____ **3.** Narrowing of the bronchial tubes.

C. Acetylcholinesterase

_____ **4.** A process with four possible effects on a medication absorbed into the body: (1) an inactive substance can become active, capable of producing desired or unwanted clinical effects; (2) an active medication can be changed into another active medication; (3) an active medication can be completely or partially inactivated; or (4) a medication can be transformed into a substance (active or inactive) that is easier for the body to eliminate.

D. Active metabolite

_____ **5.** A term used to describe paralytic agents that act at the neuromuscular junction by binding with nicotinic receptors on muscles, causing fasciculations and preventing additional activation by acetylcholine.

E. Active transport

_____ **6.** Medications that temporarily bind with cellular receptor sites, displacing agonist chemicals.

F. Adverse effect

_____ **7.** The grouping to which a medication belongs. Medications are grouped according to their characteristics, traits, or primary components.

_____ **8.** A term used to describe the fibers in the parasympathetic nervous system that release a chemical called acetylcholine.

_____ **9.** The percentage of the unchanged medication that reaches systemic circulation.

_____ **10.** The state in which cardiac cells are at rest, waiting for the generation of a spontaneous impulse from within.

_____ **11.** The medications used to kill or suppress the growth of microorganisms.

_____ **12.** The medications used to treat fungal infections.

_____ **13.** The early phase of cardiac repolarization, in which the heart muscle cannot be stimulated to depolarize; also known as the effective refractory period.

_____ **14.** The process by which the molecules of a substance are moved from the site of entry or administration into the systemic circulation.

_____ **15.** An enzyme that breaks down acetylcholine.

_____ **16.** A medication that has undergone biotransformation and is able to alter a cellular process or body function.

_____ **17.** The medications used to fight infection by killing the microorganisms or preventing their multiplication to allow the body's immune system to overcome them.

_____ **18.** The group of medications that prevent endogenous or exogenous agonist chemicals from reaching cell receptor sites and initiating or altering a particular cellular activity.

_____ **19.** A medication that causes the inability to feel sensation.

_____ **20.** An extreme systemic form of an allergic reaction involving two or more body systems.

_____ **21.** The process of molecules binding with carrier proteins when energy is used to move the molecules against a concentration gradient.

_____ **22.** Abnormal or harmful effect to an organism caused by exposure to a chemical; it is indicated by some result, such as death, a change in food or water consumption, altered body and organ weights, altered enzyme levels, or visible illness.

_____ **23.** The ability of a medication to bind with a particular receptor site.

_____ **24.** The state of being insensible to pain while still conscious.

_____ **25.** The group of medications that initiate or alter a cellular activity by attaching to receptor sites, prompting a cellular response.

G. Affinity

H. Agonist medications

I. Analgesia

J. Anaphylaxis

K. Anesthetic

L. Antagonist medications

M. Antibiotics

N. Antifungals

O. Antimicrobials

P. Automaticity

Q. Bioavailability

R. Biotransformation

S. Bronchoconstriction

T. Bronchodilation

U. Chelating agents

V. Cholinergic

W. Class

X. Competitive antagonists

Y. Competitive depolarizing

Part III

Match each of the definitions in the left column to the appropriate term in the right column.

_____ **1.** Use of hydrostatic pressure to force water or dissolved particles through a semipermeable membrane.

_____ **2.** The process in which the rate of elimination is directly influenced by plasma levels of a substance.

_____ **3.** The alteration of a medication via metabolism within the gastrointestinal tract before it reaches the systemic circulation.

_____ **4.** An unusual tolerance to the therapeutic and adverse clinical effects of a medication or chemical.

_____ **5.** The time needed in an average person for metabolism or elimination of 50% of a substance in the plasma.

_____ **6.** The physical, behavioral, or emotional need for a medication or chemical to maintain "normal" physiologic function.

A. Dependence

B. Depolarization

C. Depressant

D. Digitalis preparation

E. Distribution

F. Diuretic

_____ 7. The process of discharging resting cardiac muscle fibers by an electric impulse that causes them to contract.

_____ 8. A chemical or medication that decreases the performance of the central nervous system or sympathetic nervous system.

_____ 9. A drug used in the treatment of heart failure and certain atrial dysrhythmias.

_____ 10. The movement and transportation of a medication throughout the bloodstream to tissues and cells and, ultimately, to its target receptor.

_____ 11. Brief, uncoordinated, visible twitching of small muscle groups; may be caused by the administration of a depolarizing neuromuscular blocking agent (namely, succinylcholine).

_____ 12. The process of medication molecules binding with carrier proteins when no energy is expended.

_____ 13. Seepage of blood and medication into the tissue surrounding the blood vessel.

_____ 14. Originating outside the organism (body).

_____ 15. Originating from within the organism (body).

_____ 16. A chemical that increases urinary output.

_____ 17. A graphic illustration of the response of a drug according to the dose administered.

_____ 18. The specified amount of a medication to be given at specific intervals.

_____ 19. The process in which a mechanism reducing available cell receptors for a particular medication results in tolerance.

_____ 20. A substance that has some therapeutic effect (such as reducing inflammation, fighting bacteria, or producing euphoria) when given in the appropriate circumstances and in the appropriate dose.

_____ 21. In a pharmacologic context, the removal of a medication or its by-products from the body.

_____ 22. In a pharmacologic context, the ability of a medication to produce the desired effect.

_____ 23. Sites of generation of electrical impulses other than normal pacemaker cells.

_____ 24. In a pharmacologic context, the time a medication concentration can be expected to remain above the minimum level needed to provide the intended action.

_____ 25. Pertaining to voluntary muscle movements that are distorted or impaired because of abnormal muscle tone.

G. Dose-response curve

H. Dosing

I. Down-regulation

J. Drug

K. Duration

L. Dystonic

M. Ectopic foci

N. Efficacy

O. Elimination

P. Endogenous

Q. Exogenous

R. Extravasation

S. Facilitated diffusion

T. Fasciculation

U. Filtration

V. First-order elimination

W. First-pass effect

X. Habituation

Y. Half-life

Multiple Choice

Read each item carefully, and then select the best response.

_____ 1. The nonproprietary name is a general name for a drug and is not manufacturer specific. What is another name for nonproprietary drugs?

  A. Chemical

  B. Generic

  C. Trade

  D. Official

_____ 2. What was the first US federal law, legislated in 1906, aimed at protecting the public from mislabeled and harmful drugs?

  A. Food, Drug, and Cosmetic Act

  B. Harrison Narcotic Act

  C. Pure Food and Drug Act

  D. Narcotic Control Act

_____ **3.** Which US government agency has jurisdiction over approving new medications?

   A. Food and Drug Administration

   B. Centers for Disease Control and Prevention

   C. Drug Enforcement Administration

   D. Federal Trade Commission

_____ **4.** What is the medication interaction that is utilized when the emergency department (ED) physician considers administering some ethanol to a patient who has been poisoned due to drinking ethylene glycol (antifreeze)?

   A. Altered absorption

   B. Drug antagonism

   C. Altered metabolism

   D. Neutralization

_____ **5.** The formulation in which a medication is surrounded by a wax-like material that dissolves in a body cavity is called a(n):

   A. capsule.

   B. suppository.

   C. powder.

   D. inhaler.

_____ **6.** Which of the following forms of medication is dissolved or suspended in liquid intended for oral consumption?

   A. Suppository

   B. Inhaler/spray

   C. Drop

   D. Liquid

_____ **7.** What is the name given to the small particles of medication designed to be dissolved or mixed into a solution or liquid?

   A. Tablet

   B. Powder

   C. Pill

   D. Pulvule

_____ **8.** Which receptor sites would have an agonist effect of insulin secretion, uterine relaxation, and bronchiole relaxation?

   A. Alpha-1

   B. Alpha-2

   C. Beta-1

   D. Beta-2

_____ **9.** Certain medications are known to have decreased efficacy or potency when taken repeatedly by a patient. This state is known as:

   A. synergy.

   B. biotransformation.

   C. tolerance.

   D. reabsorption.

_____ **10.** Medications become distributed into each of the following types of body substances, EXCEPT:

   A. oils.

   B. lipids.

   C. water.

   D. proteins.

_____ **11.** The *most basic* concern regarding medication storage is:

   A. ample supply.

   B. need for refrigeration.

   C. integrity of the container.

   D. double-locked cabinetry.

_____ 12. Medications can become unsafe to use if exposed to each of the following, EXCEPT:

   A. direct sunlight.

   B. extreme heat.

   C. IV solutions.

   D. extreme cold.

_____ 13. If there is positive evidence of human fetal risk for a certain medication, but the benefits from use in pregnant women may be acceptable despite the risk, this specific medication is given a pregnancy category of:

   A. A.

   B. B.

   C. C.

   D. D.

_____ 14. Unmatched blood is almost always which of the following?

   A. Type AB, Rh positive

   B. Type O, Rh negative

   C. Type A, Rh negative

   D. Type O, Rh positive

Fill in the Blank

Read each item carefully, and then complete the statement by filling in the missing word(s).

1. A medication's _____ are the reasons or conditions for which the medication is given.

2. Two medications can bind together in the body, creating an inactive substance. This process is referred to as _____.

3. Opiate _____ medication reverses the effects of opioid drugs.

4. When the effect of one medication is greatly enhanced by the presence of another medication, which does not have the ability to produce the same effect, this state is referred to as _____.

5. An agonist that produces vasoconstriction of arteries and veins is called a(n) _____ receptor.

6. An agonist that stimulates bronchus and bronchiole relaxation, as well as insulin secretion and uterine relaxation, is called a(n) _____ receptor.

7. _____ medications cause the kidneys to remove excess amounts of salt and water from the body.

8. Medications that reduce heart rate and blood pressure are called _____ agents.

9. _____ _____ are drugs that decrease the heart rate and improve contractility.

10. Drugs that decrease inflammation and are immunosuppressants are called _____.

Identify

Read the following case study, then list the chief complaint, vital signs, and pertinent negatives.

You are called to a private residence for a 65-year-old woman who has general body weakness. Upon arrival, you find a woman sitting on her couch in the living room. When you ask what the problem is, she tells you that she has heart palpitations. She does not appear to be in distress. Her husband tells you that his wife went to the doctor yesterday for a checkup, and she seemed to be doing okay.

You check the patient's vital signs and find that the pulse is 60 beats/min, regular and weak; respirations are slightly labored at 22 breaths/min; blood pressure (BP) is 90/60 mm Hg; and SpO_2 is 97%. While your partner starts an IV, you listen to the patient's lung sounds, perform a 12-lead electrocardiogram (ECG), and get a SAMPLE history. You observe that the patient seems pale. She tells you that she has no pain or nausea and that she is on medication for hypertension and gastric reflux. She was put on a new medication yesterday for her gastric reflux and an additional medication for her blood pressure. She has had no hospitalizations and has been in relatively good health. The patient was watching TV when her symptoms started.

According to her husband, it is time for the patient's afternoon medications, but you think that she should wait until she gets to the hospital, a 15-minute transport time, and discuss them with the doctor before taking these medications. You transport the patient and reassess her vital signs en route.

1. Chief complaint:

_____

_____

2. Vital signs:

_____

_____

3. Pertinent negatives:

_____

_____

Ambulance Calls

The following case scenarios provide an opportunity to explore the concerns associated with patient management and paramedic care. Read each scenario, and then answer each question.

1. You are on the scene where a 58-year-old man is reporting substernal chest pain rated as 8 out of 10 that came on while he was shoveling snow. You have placed the patient on supplemental oxygen and administered aspirin, and your partner is obtaining vital signs and a 12-lead ECG. You obtain lung sounds and administer nitroglycerin, which has no effect. The patient is now reporting 10 out of 10 for pain. His BP is 160/100 mm Hg, so you decide to administer 5 mg of morphine. The 10 rights for medication administration run through your head as you prepare the drug for administration. What are the 10 rights, and how do they apply?

a. _____

b. _____

c. _____

d. _____

e. _____

f. _____

g. _____

h. _____

i. _____

j. _____

2. Many medications undergo some degree of chemical change by the body, known as biotransformation. What are the four possible effects that this process may have on how a medication is absorbed into the body?

a. _____

b. _____

c. _____

d. _____

3. Very young and very old patients may present with factors that can affect the actions of medications that are administered in the prehospital setting. Which factors should the paramedic consider when providing care to the young and the old, including additional factors that may need to be considered if the patient has underlying medical conditions?

a. _____

b. _____

c. _____

d. _____

e. _____

f. _____

True/False

If you believe the statement to be more true than false, write the letter "T" in the space provided. If you believe the statement to be more false than true, write the letter "F."

_____ 1. The general, nonproprietary name for a drug is its official name.

_____ 2. Schedule V drugs have the highest abuse potential and a propensity for severe dependency.

_____ 3. The changes in pharmacokinetics in geriatric patients are comparable to those observed in young children.

_____ 4. The rate of elimination of a medication is directly influenced by the plasma levels of the substance.

_____ 5. Patients at extremes of age are disproportionately prone to paradoxical medication reactions.

_____ 6. Diuretic medications can help improve the effects of sickle cell disease.

_____ 7. In the cardiac muscle cell, during phases 0, 1, 2, and 3, no additional depolarization may occur because of external stimuli.

_____ 8. Idiosyncrasy is an abnormal reaction by a person to a medication to which most other people do not react.

_____ 9. An unusual tolerance to the therapeutic and adverse clinical effects of a medication or chemical is known as synergism.

_____ 10. Promethazine (Phenergan) is an antidysrhythmic medication taken by cardiac patients.

_____ 11. Disposal of partially used or damaged controlled substances requires verification by an appropriate witness.

_____ 12. Whole blood transfusions are no longer used clinically in the United States.

_____ 13. If studies in animals or humans have demonstrated fetal abnormalities, making the drug contraindicated in women who are pregnant, this is a pregnancy category X drug.

Short Answer

Complete this section with short written answers using the space provided.

1. The medical director of your emergency medical services (EMS) agency announces that a new medication will be introduced into the agency's protocols. As part of an in-service program to learn about this new drug, you are given the pharmaceutical company's drug profile to review. What are the three different names for the medication that will be listed in this literature?

a. _____

b. _____

c. _____

2. What are the components of a drug profile?

a. _____

b. _____

c. _____

d. _____

e. _____

f. _____

g. _____

h. _____

i. _____

j. _____

k. _____

l. _____

3. The Institute for Safe Medication Practices (ISMP) has developed a list of error-prone medication abbreviations. List five potential errors, and explain how they can be avoided.

a. _____

b. _____

c. _____

d. _____

e. _____

4. List eight common adverse effects of medications.

a. _____

b. _____

c. _____

d. _____

e. _____

f. _____

g. _____

h. _____

5. For each of the following medication descriptions, write the medication class next to the common indications or purpose.

a. Treat or prevent nausea and vomiting: _____

b. Decrease gastrointestinal (GI) motility; alter GI secretion activity: _____

c. Treat bacterial infection: _____

d. Neutralize excess acids present in the stomach: _____

e. Block histamine receptors; dry mucous membranes; inhibit immune response in allergic reactions: _____

f. Reduce heart rate and blood pressure: _____

g. Treat anxiety and seizures; provide sedation: _____

h. Decrease inflammation; immunosuppressant: _____

i. Dissolve clots present in blood vessels or vascular access devices: _____

j. Replace hormones; improve bone density that has decreased due to aging and hormone loss: _____

k. Relieve pain and relieve or suppress cough: _____

l. Increase blood pressure, heart rate, and cardiac output; constrict blood vessels: _____

Fill in the Blank

Fill in the missing parts of the tables.

Veins Used During Intraosseous (IO) Infusion	
Intraosseous Site	**Vein**
Proximal tibia	_____
Femur	_____
_____	Great saphenous vein
_____	Axillary vein
Manubrium (sternum)	_____

Gastrointestinal Medication Absorption	
Factor	**Medication Absorption**
_____	Ability of medication to pass through the GI tract into the bloodstream
_____	Perfusion of the GI system (may be decreased during systemic trauma or shock)
_____	Injury or bleeding in the GI system (both can alter GI motility, decreasing the time that oral medications can be absorbed)

Sources of Medications	
Source	**Examples**
_____	Atropine, aspirin, digoxin, morphine
_____	Heparin, antivenom, thyroid preparations, insulin
_____	Streptokinase, numerous antibiotics
_____	Iron, magnesium sulfate, lithium, phosphorus, calcium

Medication Administration

© Jones & Bartlett Learning.

Matching

Part I

In choosing a medication, selecting the route of administration relates to the medication's onset of action. For each of the following, match the onset of action with the route of administration:

_____ **1.** Intramuscular injection

_____ **2.** Nasal mucosal atomization (MAD)

_____ **3.** Endotracheal

_____ **4.** Intraosseous

_____ **5.** Sublingual

_____ **6.** Inhalation

_____ **7.** Intravenous

A. 30–60 seconds

B. 2–3 minutes

C. 3–5 minutes

D. 10–20 minutes

Part II

Match each of the definitions in the left column to the appropriate term in the right column.

_____ **1.** The amount of a drug that the physician orders for the patient.

_____ **2.** Solutions that contain molecules (usually proteins) that are too large to pass out of the capillary membranes and, therefore, remain in the vascular compartment.

_____ **3.** Chemicals used to cleanse an area before performing an invasive procedure, such as starting an IV line; not toxic to living tissues; examples include isopropyl alcohol and iodine.

_____ **4.** Pertaining to the ear.

_____ **5.** The anterior aspect of the elbow.

_____ **6.** Small glass containers that are sealed and the contents sterilized.

_____ **7.** Tubing that connects to the IV bag access port and the catheter to deliver IV fluid.

_____ **8.** A sealed hub on an administration set designed for sterile access to the IV fluid.

_____ **9.** A condition in which a needle is reinserted into the catheter, and it slices through the catheter, creating a free-floating segment.

_____ **10.** The body's natural blood-clotting mechanism.

_____ **11.** The internal diameter of an IV catheter or needle.

_____ **12.** The area of the administration set in which fluid accumulates so that the tubing remains filled with fluid.

A. Access port

B. Administration set

C. Ampules

D. Antecubital

E. Antiseptics

F. Aural

G. Bolus

H. Bone Injection Gun (BIG)

I. Buccal

J. Catheter shear

K. Colloid solutions

L. Desired dose

_____ **13.** A solution (usually water or normal saline) used for diluting a medication.

M. Diluent

_____ **14.** Injecting sterile water or saline from one vial into another vial containing a powdered form of a drug.

N. Drip chamber

_____ **15.** Medication administration that involves the medication passing through a portion of the gastrointestinal tract.

O. Drug reconstitution

_____ **16.** Large neck vein that is lateral to the carotid artery.

P. Enteral medications

_____ **17.** The area of an IV catheter that fills with blood to help indicate when a vein is cannulated.

Q. External jugular (EJ) vein

_____ **18.** Between the cheek and gums.

R. Flash chamber

_____ **19.** A spring-loaded device that is used for inserting an intraosseous needle into the proximal tibia in adult and pediatric patients.

S. Gauge

_____ **20.** A term used to describe "in one mass"; in medication administration, a single dose given by the intravenous or intraosseous route, which may be a small or large quantity of the drug.

T. Hemostasis

Part III

Match each of the definitions in the left column to the appropriate term in the right column.

_____ **1.** A pressurized canister that delivers a specific dose of a medication; commonly used for beta-agonist bronchodilators.

A. Hypotonic solution

_____ **2.** A type of surgical drain often used as a constricting band.

B. Implanted vascular access device

_____ **3.** A device for producing a fine spray or mist that is used to deliver inhaled medications.

C. Infiltration

_____ **4.** A reaction characterized by an abrupt temperature elevation with severe chills, backache, headache, weakness, nausea, and vomiting; a potential complication of intravenous or intraosseous therapy.

D. Infusion pump

_____ **5.** A solution of 0.9% sodium chloride; an isotonic crystalloid.

E. Inhalation

_____ **6.** Blockage, usually of a tubular structure such as a blood vessel or IV catheter.

F. Intradermal

_____ **7.** The ability to influence the movement of water across a semipermeable membrane.

G. Intranasal

_____ **8.** Feature of an IV catheter that allows it to appear on a radiograph.

H. Intraosseous (IO) space

_____ **9.** A Teflon catheter inserted over a hollow needle.

I. Intravenous (IV) therapy

_____ **10.** A solution that has a lower concentration of sodium than does the cell; the increased osmotic pressure lets water flow into the cell, causing it to swell and possibly burst.

J. Isotonic crystalloids

_____ **11.** The escape of fluid into the surrounding tissue; the result of vein perforation during IV cannulation.

K. Isotonic solution

_____ **12.** Devices that are implanted in surgery and sutured under the skin, for the purpose of long-term medication administration, total parenteral nutrition, chemotherapy, blood product administration, or venous blood sampling.

L. Metered-dose inhaler (MDI)

_____ **13.** A mechanical device that infuses a precise intravenous volume programmed by the clinician.

M. Nebulizer

_____ **14.** The layer of the dermis, just beneath the epidermis, a medication delivery route.

N. Normal saline

_____ **15.** Breathing into the lungs; a medication delivery route.

O. Occlusion

_____ **16.** A solution that has the same concentration of sodium as does the cell; in this case, water does not shift, and no change in cell shape occurs.

P. Osmolarity

_____ **17.** Intravenous solutions that do not cause a fluid shift into or out of the cell; examples include normal saline and lactated Ringer solutions.

Q. Over-the-needle catheter

_____ **18.** Cannulation of a vein with an IV catheter to access the patient's vascular system.

R. Penrose drain

_____ **19.** The spongy cancellous bone of the epiphyses and the medullary cavity of the diaphysis, collectively.

S. Pyrogenic reaction

_____ **20.** Within the nose.

T. Radiopaque

Multiple Choice

Read each item carefully, and then select the best response.

_____ **1.** When the patient needs fluid infusion and there are no obvious IV sites available, most emergency medical services (EMS) systems utilize the _____ IO site.

  A. FASTR for the humeral

  B. FAST-1 for the sternal

  C. BIG for the proximal tibial

  D. venous cutdown

_____ **2.** When necessary, medications can be administered via the endotracheal (ET) route. The mnemonic _____ helps the paramedic remember which medications are acceptable.

  A. SOAP

  B. CBERNE

  C. LEAN

  D. MEDS

_____ **3.** Which of the following solutions is the best choice for administration, in the prehospital setting, when the patient needs to have body fluids replaced?

  A. Hypertonic

  B. Hypotonic

  C. Colloid

  D. Crystalloid

_____ **4.** Which administration set will allow for administration of 60 gtt/mL?

  A. Blood tubing

  B. Microdrip set

  C. Macrodrip set

  D. Volutrol administration set

_____ **5.** When inserting an IV catheter, the bevel should be:

  A. facing down.

  B. facing up.

  C. pointed to the side.

  D. rolled as you insert it.

_____ **6.** After starting an IV on a patient, which of the following is NOT necessary to document?

  A. The site of the IV

  B. The gauge of the needle used

  C. The patient's pain scale when you started the IV

  D. The type of fluid you are using

_____ **7.** There are many potential complications with an IV site; _____ means there is an inflammation of the vein.

  A. thrombophlebitis

  B. hematoma

  C. occlusion

  D. vein irritation

_____   **8.** If a sternal IO is used in your EMS system, consideration should be made to review the _____ IO device for this application.
- **A.** BIG
- **B.** FASTR
- **C.** EZ-IO
- **D.** Jamshidi needle

_____   **9.** When taking a blood sample in the field, what is the green-topped tube used for?
- **A.** Determining the patient's blood type
- **B.** Checking glucose and electrolyte levels
- **C.** Determining how long it takes for the patient's blood to clot
- **D.** Checking for alcohol and drugs in the blood system

_____   **10.** Which of the following is an example of an antiseptic?
- **A.** Virex
- **B.** Iodine
- **C.** Cidex
- **D.** Microcide

_____   **11.** Which medication route is usually the fastest and most commonly used in the prehospital setting?
- **A.** Intradermal
- **B.** Subcutaneous
- **C.** Intramuscular
- **D.** Intravenous

_____   **12.** A(n) _____ is a breakable sterile glass container that carries a single dose of medication.
- **A.** vial
- **B.** ampule
- **C.** mix-o-vial
- **D.** prefill

_____   **13.** A(n)_____ injection is given at a 90° angle.
- **A.** subcutaneous
- **B.** intravascular
- **C.** intramuscular
- **D.** bolus

_____   **14.** Which of the following medications is NOT given by the intranasal route?
- **A.** Naloxone
- **B.** Fentanyl
- **C.** Nitroglycerin
- **D.** Glucagon

_____   **15.** How much normal saline should you use as a flush after administering a medication through a gastric tube?
- **A.** 15 to 30 mL
- **B.** 30 to 60 mL
- **C.** 60 to 75 mL
- **D.** You do not use normal saline for a flush.

_____   **16.** Which tool uses the principles of crew resource management by requiring a process for verification for every medication?
- **A.** FMEA
- **B.** CRM
- **C.** MACC
- **D.** MADD

_____ **17.** When using the Medication Administration Cross-Check tool, after the first provider who is going to administer the drug clearly states the dose, drug name, route, rate, and reason, the second provider should state:

    A. contraindications.

    B. quantity.

    C. volume

    D. "Ready."

_____ **18.** Of the following medication routes, which has the slowest onset of action of absorption?

    A. Intraosseous

    B. Inhalation

    C. Oral

    D. Intramuscular injection

_____ **19.** When a patient takes a medication by the _____ route, it is administered between the cheek and the gums.

    A. sublingual

    B. transdermal

    C. aural

    D. buccal

_____ **20.** Which of the following measures will NOT help prevent thrombophlebitis?

    A. Always wear gloves when you are performing a venipuncture.

    B. Anchor the catheter and tubing securely to prevent movement in the vein.

    C. Apply a warm pressure bandage on the extremity into which the catheter is inserted.

    D. Use a povidone-iodine preparation to scrub the skin.

Fill in the Blank

Read each item carefully, and then complete the statement by filling in the missing word(s).

1. An intravenous solution that contains large molecules such as proteins is a(n) _____.

2. An intravenous solution that does not contain large molecules such as proteins is a(n) _____. One example of such a solution is normal _____.

3. When two solutions of different solute concentration are placed on either side of a semipermeable membrane, the more concentrated solution is said to be _____ with respect to the less concentrated solution. Conversely, the less concentrated solution is considered _____ with respect to the more concentrated solution. If the two solutions have the same concentration, they are said to be _____. Thus, for example, 4% saline is _____ with respect to serum; Ringer solution is _____ with respect to serum; and half normal saline (0.45% NaCl) is _____ with respect to serum.

4. When two solutions of different solute concentrations are placed on either side of a semipermeable membrane, water will move from the solution of _____ solute concentration to the solution of _____ solute concentration. The process by which water migrates in that fashion is called _____.

5. The signs and symptoms of circulatory overload include _____, jugular vein distention, and _____.

Labeling

Label the common sites for intramuscular injections.

Ambulance Calls

All of the patients described in the following scenarios are experiencing a problem related to their intravenous therapy. Identify the problem in each case, and explain what you will do to manage it.

1. The patient is a 59-year-old man with severe chest pain on whom you have started a "keep-open" IV. It is a long way to the hospital, and about 10 minutes into the transport, he starts complaining of breathing difficulty. You notice that his respirations have become more rapid, and when you listen to his chest, you can hear crackling (rales) sounds. Meanwhile, you suddenly notice that the liter bag of IV fluid is empty.

   a. What is the patient's problem?

   _____

   _____

   _____

   b. What are you going to do about it?

   _____

   _____

   _____

2. You have started an IV on a frail old woman. After a few minutes, you notice that the IV is infusing more and more slowly. You open the clamp wide, but that does not help. You lower the IV bag below the stretcher; there is no blood return into the tubing. Then you check the IV site. There seems to be a lump in the skin, and the skin feels quite cool.

   a. What is the patient's problem?

   _____

   _____

   _____

b. What are you going to do about it?

_____

_____

_____

c. What other problems might cause an IV to slow down or stop?

_____

_____

_____

3. You are starting an IV near the wrist of a petite 22-year-old woman. When the IV catheter enters the vessel, bright red blood comes spurting back onto your face shield.

a. What is the patient's problem?

_____

_____

_____

b. What are you going to do about it?

_____

_____

_____

4. You are transporting a patient between hospitals. The patient has an IV already running (it was started earlier in the day by the paramedics who brought the patient to the first hospital). The patient complains of pain at the IV site, and you notice that it is red, hot, and swollen.

a. What is the patient's problem?

_____

_____

_____

b. What are you going to do about it?

_____

_____

_____

c. How could this problem have been prevented?

(1)_____

(2)_____

(3)_____

(4)_____

5. A driver is found conscious but very restless. He keeps asking you, "Can't you give me some water? I'm so thirsty—please give me something to drink." His skin is cold and sweaty. You do not see any external signs of serious injury.

a. Do you think this patient has been seriously injured? Explain the reasons for your answer.

_____

_____

_____

b. You decide to start an IV with lactated Ringer solution, which is a _____ (colloid or crystalloid?) solution. Your protocol calls for administering 200 mL/h in these circumstances. You have an administration set that delivers 10 gtt/mL. To set the infusion rate to deliver 200 mL/h, you will need to set the drops per minute at _____ gtt/min. (Show your calculations.)

c. A few minutes after you adjust the IV rate, you notice that the IV has slowed down to the point that it is hardly flowing at all. List the five steps you would take to try to identify and solve the problem with the IV.

(1)_____

(2)_____

(3)_____

(4)_____

(5)_____

True/False

If you believe the statement to be more true than false, write the letter "T" in the space provided. If you believe the statement to be more false than true, write the letter "F."

_____ **1.** MDIs are more reliable than nebulizers for administering beta-agonist medications.

_____ **2.** "Where sodium goes, water follows."

_____ **3.** Calcium is the primary buffer in body fluids.

_____ **4.** A peripheral inserted central catheter (PICC) line is considered a non-tunneling device for long-term use.

_____ **5.** The region between the cheek and gums is highly vascular.

_____ **6.** Nitroglycerin, estrogen, and nicotine are examples of medications that are administered by the intramuscular (IM) route.

_____ **7.** A healthy person will lose up to 1 L of fluid a day as a result of urine output and exhalation.

_____ **8.** Lactated Ringer or normal saline is used for patients who have lost a large amount of blood in the field.

_____ **9.** A crystalloid solution can carry oxygen to the cells.

_____ **10.** A macrodrip administration set delivers 10 or 15 gtt/mL.

_____ **11.** A good thing to do when starting an IV is to work down, in case you miss the first attempt.

_____ **12.** A butterfly catheter has a Teflon catheter over the hollow needle.

_____ **13.** You should always have the bevel to the side when starting an IV.

_____ **14.** When changing an IV bag, you must start all over with the process and restart the IV.

_____ **15.** When an IV infiltrates, you will notice edema at the catheter site.

_____ **16.** When you have cannulated an artery, you must pull the catheter out and apply direct pressure for at least 5 minutes.

_____ **17.** A healthy adult can handle only 1 to 2 extra liters of fluid.

_____ **18.** A red-topped tube is used to determine the blood type of a patient.

_____ **19.** An IO infusion is easier to use, so it should be used as much as possible for the pediatric patient.

_____ **20.** When placing an IO needle, you should feel two "pops."

_____ **21.** The basic unit of weight in the metric system is the gram.

_____ **22.** One pound is equal to 2.2 kg.

_____ **23.** The desired dose is what is ordered to give to the patient.

_____ **24.** Dopamine is delivered to the patient in micrograms.

_____ **25.** The use of Luer-lock IV tubing helps to minimize risks during medication administration.

Short Answer

Complete this section with short written answers using the space provided.

1. Name three ways to make the vein "stand up" so that it is easier to see.

a. _____

b. _____

c. _____

2. List the five things that are a *must* when documenting the IV.

a. _____

b. _____

c. _____

d. _____

e. _____

3. There are seven local reactions that can happen when starting an IV. List three complications and their signs and symptoms.

a. _____

b. _____

c. _____

4. List the six points of information you should document when you administer a medication to a patient.

a. _____

b. _____

c. _____

d. _____

e. _____

f. _____

Fill in the Table

Fill in the missing parts of the table.

Route of Administration	Where in the Body the Medication Goes
Enteral	1.
Oral	2.
Intradermal	3.
Percutaneous	4.
Sublingual	5.
Endotracheal	6.
Buccal	7.
Transdermal	8.
Intramuscular	9.
Rectal	10.
Parenteral	11.
Subcutaneous	12.
Intravenous	13.
Ocular	14.
Aural	15.
Inhalation	16.
Intranasal	17.

Problem Solving

Practice your calculation skills by solving the following math problems.

1. You have started an IV on a bakery worker suffering from heat exhaustion. The physician instructs you to run normal saline by IV at 200 mL/h. Your bag of saline is a 1,000-mL bag. Your administration set delivers 10 gtt/mL. At what rate (how many drops per minute) do you have to run the infusion to give 200 mL/h? (Show your calculations.)

2. You have started a "keep-open" IV with a microdrip infusion set (which delivers 60 gtt/mL). Your instructions are to run the IV at 30 mL/h. At what rate (how many drops per minute) should you set the flow? (Show your calculations.)

3. You are ordered to give a lidocaine drip at a rate of 2 mg/min. You have the following on hand:
   - A vial containing 50 mL of 4% lidocaine
   - A 500-mL bag of D_5W
   - A microdrip administration set that delivers 60 gtt/mL
   a. How many grams of lidocaine are in the vial? _____ g (Show your calculations.)

   b. When you add the contents of the vial to the IV bag, what will be the concentration of lidocaine in the IV bag? _____ mg/mL (Show your calculations.)

   c. How many milliliters per minute (mL/min) will the patient have to receive to get the dosage ordered (2 mg/min)? _____ mL/min (Show your calculations.)

   d. How many drops per minute (gtt/min) is that equivalent to? _____ gtt/min (Show your calculations.)

4. Convert 12 g to milligrams: 12 g × _____ = _____ mg

5. Convert 156 lb to kilograms: 156 lb ÷ _____ = _____ kg (round up)

6. Now use the second method to estimate the patient's weight in kilograms.
   The patient weighs 135 lb.

   Step 1: Divide the patient's weight by 2: _____ ÷ 2 = _____

   Step 2: Take the total from step 1 and multiply it by 10%: _____ × 0.10 = _____ (round up)

   * Remember to round the percentage number for easier subtraction. _____

   Step 3: Take the total of step 1 and subtract the rounded percentage. _____ – _____ = _____ patient's

   weight in kilograms; once again, you may need to round up to _____. What weight would you use for the patient?

   _____ kg

7. You are ordered to give a patient 6 mg of morphine. The morphine comes in 10 mg/mL. How much will you give? _____ mL

8. You are ordered to give 2 mg of diazepam (Valium). Your vial contains 20 mg in 10 mL. What is the concentration on hand? _____ mg/mL
How many mL will you give? _____ mL

9. You are ordered to deliver 10 mcg/kg/min of dopamine for an 80-kg patient. You have mixed 800 mg of dopamine into a 500-mL bag of normal saline. Show your calculations for the following.
   a. What is the desired dose? _____ mcg/min
   b. Determine the dose on hand._____ mg/mL
   c. Convert the mg from answer (b) to mcg. _____ mcg/mL
   d. Determine the amount of volume to infuse per minute. Use the desired dose to calculate this volume. _____ mL/min
   e. Determine how many drops/min will deliver the desired dose, using a microdrip set (60 gtt/mL). _____ gtt/min

10. Fill in the following tables so that each row will contain different ways of representing the same values.

Microgram (mcg)	Milligram (mg)	Gram (g)	Kilogram (kg)
500	0.5	0.0005	0.0000005
_____	_____	1.0	_____
_____	_____	_____	1.0
_____	1.0	_____	_____
1.0	_____	_____	_____
_____	800.0	_____	_____
15.0	_____	_____	_____

Milliliter (mL)	Deciliter (dL)	Liter (L)
5,000.0	50.0	5.0
1.0	_____	_____
10.0	_____	_____
_____	_____	1.0
250.0	_____	0.25

11. Fill in the blanks in the calculations, changing the patient's weight from pounds to kilograms using the "10% trick." Compare your answers using the formula:

$$\text{patient's weight (lb)} \div 2.2 = \text{patient's weight (kg)}$$

Patient's Weight (lb)	Patient's Weight (lb) ÷ 2	Weight (lb) ÷ 2 × 10%	Subtract Your 10% from the Weight ÷ 2	Patient's Weight in Kilograms (kg)	Patient's Weight in lb ÷ 2.2 = Patient's Weight in Kilograms (kg)
60	60 ÷ 2 = 30	30 × 10% = 3	30 − 3 = 27	27	27.27
16	_____	_____	_____	_____	_____
138	_____	_____	_____	_____	_____
8	_____	_____	_____	_____	_____
250	_____	_____	_____	_____	_____
36	_____	_____	_____	_____	_____
82	_____	_____	_____	_____	_____
180	_____	_____	_____	_____	_____
330	_____	_____	_____	_____	_____

12. Volume conversions: Fill in the blanks indicating the amount of medication found in each bag of normal saline (NS), assuming the concentration is the same in each bag. Follow the example in the first row of the table:

1,000 mL NS	500 mL NS	250 mL NS	100 mL NS	50 mL NS
100 g	50 g	25 g	10 g	5 g
_____	800 g	_____	_____	_____
_____	_____	250 g	_____	_____
_____	_____	_____	4 g	_____
_____	50 g	_____	_____	_____

13. Determine the number of milliliters of fluid infused over 1 minute to the patient by filling in the following blanks.
   a. 60-gtt admin set infused 120 gtt/min = _____ mL/min

   b. 15-gtt admin set infused 120 gtt/min = _____ mL/min

   c. 30-gtt admin set infused 120 gtt/min = _____ mL/min

14. Convert the following temperatures from degrees Fahrenheit (°F) to degrees Celsius (°C) by completing the following table. Follow the example in the third row.
   This table is based on the formula $(°F - 32) \times 0.555 = °C$.

Temperature in °F	°F – 32	(°F - 32) × 0.555	Temperature in °C
32			
95.0			
98.6	98.6 - 32 = 66.6	66.6 × 0.555 = 36.96	36.96 (approximately 37)
101.0			
104.0			

15. Determine how much medication is prescribed for the patient by body weight by filling in the following table.

Desired Dose	Patient's Weight in Pounds (lb)	Patient's Weight in Kilograms (kg)	Medication Administered
1 mg/kg lidocaine	90	90 ÷ 2.2 = 40.9 kg (≈ 41 kg)	41 kg × 1 mg lidocaine = 41 mg lidocaine to administer
0.2 mg/kg atropine	30		
0.05 mg/kg lorazepam	180		
30 mg/kg methylprednisolone	220		
15 mg/kg phenobarbital	12		

16. Calculate the volume of normal saline needed to administer to the following trauma patients. Base your calculations on volumes replaced at 20 mL/kg of patient body weight.

Patient's Weight in Pounds (lb)	Patient's Weight in Kilograms: Weight in lb ÷ 2.2 = Weight in kg (or Use the "10% Trick")	Volume to be Infused with First Bolus at 20 mL/kg
60		
80		
100		
125		
150		
175		
190		
220		
300		

17. Find the weight of the following medications in 1 mL of solution.

   a. 100 mg/10 mL lidocaine = _____ mg/1 mL lidocaine

   b. 1 mg/10 mL epinephrine = _____ mg/1 mL epinephrine

   c. 40 mg/14 mL furosemide = _____ mg/1 mL furosemide

   d. 6 mg/2 mL adenosine = _____ mg/1 mL adenosine

   e. 20 mg/5 mL diazepam = _____ mg/1 mL diazepam

   f. 10 mg/5 mL naloxone = _____ mg/1 mL naloxone

   g. 2 mg/5 mL albuterol = _____ mg/1 mL albuterol

   h. 150 mg/3 mL amiodarone = _____ mg/1 mL amiodarone

   i. 25 g/125 mL activated charcoal = _____ g/1 mL activated charcoal = _____ mg/1 mL activated charcoal

18. Find the weight of the following medications in 1 mL of solution.
Follow this example:

50% dextrose = 50 g/100 mL = 0.5 g/1 mL

   a. 1% xylocaine

   b. 10% dextrose

   c. 0.5% albuterol

   d. 10% calcium chloride

   e. 50% magnesium sulfate

   f. 5% Alupent

   g. 0.9% sodium chloride

19. Determine the amount of dopamine in micrograms (mcg) per milliliter when 800 mg of dopamine is added to the following bags of normal saline (NS). (Note: 1 mg = 1,000 mcg)
   a. 800 mg dopamine is added to a 500-mL bag NS = _____ mcg/mL
   b. 800 mg dopamine is added to a 250-mL bag NS = _____ mcg/mL
   c. 800 mg dopamine is added to a 1,000-mL bag NS = _____ mcg/mL
   d. 800 mg dopamine is added to a 100-mL bag NS = _____ mcg/mL

20. Medical control has directed you to administer the correct dosage of medication for your patient (desired dose). The concentration available to you is listed for each calculation. Determine the volume of medication you will administer for each order.

Desired dose in mg ÷ concentration in mg/mL = volume to administer

   a. You are ordered to give 15 mg labetalol. You have a vial with 100 mg/20 mL solution in stock.

b. You are ordered to give 3 mg haloperidol. You have a 1-mL ampule containing 5 mg of medication.

c. You are directed to administer 750 mg calcium chloride. You have a bottle containing 1,000 mg of medication in 10 mL of solution.

Matching

Part I

For each of the following definitions, insert the letter of the appropriate term on the line provided.

_____ **1.** A gradually increasing rate and depth of respirations followed by a gradual decrease with intermittent periods of apnea; associated with brainstem insult.

_____ **2.** The backward, upward, and rightward pressure used during intubation to improve the laryngoscopic view of the glottis opening and vocal cords; also called external laryngoscopic view of the glottis opening and vocal cords; also called external laryngeal manipulation.

_____ **3.** Irregular pattern, rate, and depth of respirations with intermittent periods of apnea; resulting from increased intracranial pressure.

_____ **4.** Prolonged gasping inspirations followed by extremely short, ineffective expirations; associated with brainstem insult.

_____ **5.** The continued alveolar uptake of oxygen, even when the patient is apneic; can be facilitated by administering oxygen via nasal cannula during intubation.

_____ **6.** An inability to remember events after the onset of amnesia.

_____ **7.** A medication that distorts perception of sight and sound and induces a feeling of detachment from environment and self.

_____ **8.** An automatic reaction when something touches an area deep in the oral cavity that helps protect the lower airway from aspiration.

_____ **9.** A leaf-shaped cartilaginous structure that closes over the trachea during swallowing.

_____ **10.** The breath sounds produced as fluid-filled alveoli pop open under increasing inspiratory pressure; can be fine or coarse; formerly called rales.

_____ **11.** A surgical procedure in which the larynx is removed.

_____ **12.** A decrease in arterial oxygen level.

_____ **13.** An approximation of the extent of bronchoconstriction; used to determine whether therapy (such as with inhaled bronchodilators) is effective.

_____ **14.** Drugs that paralyze skeletal muscles; used in emergency situations to facilitate intubation; also called neuromuscular blocking agents.

_____ **15.** A device that measures oxygen saturation level.

_____ **16.** Forcing of air into the lungs.

_____ **17.** In the context of the airway, the resultant orifice of a tracheostomy that connects the trachea to the outside air; located in the midline of the anterior part of the neck.

A. Abdominal thrust maneuver

B. Accessory muscles

C. Agonal gasps

D. Anoxia

E. Apneic oxygenation

F. Apneustic respirations

G. Bimanual laryngoscopy

H. Biot (ataxic) respirations

I. BURP maneuver

J. Cheyne-Stokes respirations

K. Crackles

L. Dissociative anesthetic

M. Epiglottis

N. Gag reflex

O. Hypoxemia

P. Laryngectomy

Q. Orotracheal intubation

_____ **18.** A continuous, low-pitched sound, which indicates the presence of mucus or fluid in the larger lower airways.

_____ **19.** Insertion of an endotracheal tube into the trachea through the mouth.

_____ **20.** Positional dyspnea.

_____ **21.** An absence of oxygen.

_____ **22.** Slow, shallow, irregular respirations or occasional gasping breaths that result from cerebral anoxia.

_____ **23.** Abdominal thrusts performed to relieve a foreign body airway obstruction.

_____ **24.** The muscles not normally used during normal breathing, which include the sternocleidomastoid muscles of the neck and the chest and abdominal muscles.

R. Orthopnea

S. Paralytics

T. Peak expiratory flow

U. Positive pressure ventilation

V. Pulse oximeter

W. Rhonchi

X. Stoma

Part II

Nasotracheal intubation is an excellent technique for establishing control over the airway under select circumstances. In other circumstances, it is preferable to insert the tracheal tube through the mouth; and in yet other limited circumstances, it may be necessary to establish an airway surgically, by cricothyrotomy. For each of the following patients, indicate which of the following intubation methods is preferred.

N   Blind nasotracheal intubation is the preferred technique.

T   Endotracheal intubation is the preferred technique.

C   Cricothyrotomy is the preferred technique.

_____ **1.** A 65-year-old man in cardiac arrest.

_____ **2.** A 28-year-old woman with complete airway obstruction from laryngeal edema.

_____ **3.** A 26-year-old vehicle-collision victim with clear fluid draining from his nose and left ear.

_____ **4.** An 18-year-old woman in a coma from a drug overdose.

_____ **5.** A 48-year-old man extricated from a wrecked car; he is unconscious and has an injury to the back of his head.

_____ **6.** A 58-year-old man with pulmonary edema, who has been taking warfarin (Coumadin; an anticoagulant drug) ever since his heart attack last year.

_____ **7.** A 6-year-old boy who choked on a piece of meat.

_____ **8.** A 52-year-old woman who was given succinylcholine (a paralyzing drug) prior to an intubation attempt; the attempt failed, and afterward, it became impossible to maintain her airway by manual methods.

Part III

For each of the following patients, indicate the most appropriate device for administering supplemental oxygen. (Note: You may use any of the items once, more than once, or not at all.)

_____ **1.** A 63-year-old man in severe respiratory distress from acute pulmonary edema.

_____ **2.** A 56-year-old man complaining of crushing chest pain.

_____ **3.** A car-crash victim in cardiac arrest; you are doing one-rescuer cardiopulmonary resuscitation (CPR) because your partner is busy with another casualty.

_____ **4.** A 78-year-old woman who suddenly stopped speaking this morning and cannot move her left arm or left leg.

_____ **5.** A 26-year-old man who has overdosed on heroin; he is unconscious and breathing shallowly at 6 breaths/min.

_____ **6.** A 26-year-old car-crash victim who was thrown forward against the steering wheel; he is coughing up blood, and his lips look rather blue.

_____ **7.** A 48-year-old man who collapsed in the street; he is in cardiac arrest by the time you arrive.

_____ **8.** An unconscious 10-year-old boy who was rescued from a house fire.

A. Nasal cannula

B. Nonrebreathing mask

C. Pocket mask (mouth-to-mask ventilation) with added supplemental oxygen

D. Bag-mask device with an oxygen reservoir

E. Flow-restricted, oxygen-powered ventilation device (manually triggered ventilation device)

F. Continuous positive airway pressure (CPAP)

Multiple Choice

Read each item carefully, and then select the best response.

_____ 1. What is the leaf-shaped structure that prevents food and liquid from getting into the larynx during swallowing?
   A. Vallecula
   B. Uvula
   C. Epiglottis
   D. Pharynx

_____ 2. Which of the following is the MOST common cause of a partial airway obstruction?
   A. The tongue
   B. Food
   C. Blood
   D. Vomitus

_____ 3. What is the preferred device to deliver supplemental oxygen to the patient who is breathing and has an SpO$_2$ of 93%?
   A. Nasal cannula
   B. Bag-mask device
   C. Simple face mask
   D. Nonrebreathing mask

_____ 4. What is the MOST definitive way to control the airway in an unconscious patient?
   A. Bag-mask device
   B. Endotracheal tube
   C. Oral airway adjunct
   D. Head tilt–chin lift maneuver

_____ 5. In which position should the patient's head be placed when preparing to intubate with a Combitube?
   A. Flexed forward
   B. Neutral position
   C. Hyperextended back
   D. Slightly to the right

_____ 6. Which medication is the only depolarizing neuromuscular blocking agent that is used in the field?
   A. Vecuronium bromide
   B. Pancuronium bromide
   C. Rocuronium bromide
   D. Succinylcholine chloride

_____ 7. How much sterile saline should you have ready when you are performing a needle cricothyrotomy?
   A. 3 mL
   B. 5 mL
   C. 7 mL
   D. 10 mL

_____ 8. The commonly used mnemonic _____ is used to guide assessment of the difficult airway.
   A. SAMPLE
   B. ISTAT
   C. LEMON
   D. CBARR

_____ 9. The clinical finding in which the systolic blood pressure drops more than 10 mm Hg during inhalation is called:
   A. intercostal stimulation.
   B. vagus nerve stimulation.
   C. pulsus paradoxus.
   D. asymmetric movement.

_____ **10.** Which abnormal respiratory pattern do you see in the patient with ketoacidosis?

    A. Cheyne-Stokes

    B. Agonal

    C. Biot

    D. Kussmaul

_____ **11.** What is the major advantage of a multilumen airway device?

    A. It fits all patients, from pediatric to adult.

    B. It prevents all aspiration.

    C. It cannot be placed improperly.

    D. It always provides 100% oxygen to the patient.

_____ **12.** Which of the following is NOT a complication of placing a multilumen airway device?

    A. Vomiting

    B. Unrecognized displacement of the tube

    C. Esophageal trauma

    D. Hyperventilation

_____ **13.** How much air should inflate the proximal balloon on the Combitube?

    A. 15 mL

    B. 25 mL

    C. 100 mL

    D. 150 mL

_____ **14.** When should you use a laryngeal mask airway (LMA) in the field?

    A. When the patient cannot be intubated, as an alternative to the bag-mask device (alone)

    B. When the patient is morbidly obese and has a difficult airway

    C. When the patient has heart failure and is unconscious

    D. When the patient is less than 5 feet tall and needs attention to the airway

_____ **15.** Using the Mallampati classification to predict the relative difficulty of an intubation, if the posterior pharynx cannot be seen, but the base of the uvula is exposed, it is a Class:

    A. I.

    B. II.

    C. III.

    D. IV.

_____ **16.** Complications of the King LT airway may include each of the following, EXCEPT:

    A. possible hypoventilation.

    B. a herniated diaphragm.

    C. vomiting.

    D. laryngospasm.

_____ **17.** Typical rapid sequence intubation (RSI) protocols for a hemodynamically stable patient would include:

    A. immediate sedation.

    B. half the succinylcholine dose.

    C. preoxygenation for 2 to 3 minutes.

    D. administering a polarizing paralytic agent.

_____ **18.** Of the following neuromuscular blocking agents, which has the shortest duration of action?

    A. Vecuronium

    B. Rocuronium

    C. Pancuronium

    D. Succinylcholine

_____ **19.** Which sedative used in airway management is considered a dissociative anesthetic?
  A. Diazepam
  B. Ketamine
  C. Fentanyl
  D. Etomidate

_____ **20.** Tracheobronchial suctioning requires:
  A. a rescue airway in place.
  B. surgical jelly.
  C. a stoma in place.
  D. strict attention to sterile technique.

Fill in the Blank
Read each item carefully, and then complete the statement by filling in the missing word(s).

1. The principal hazard associated with intubation is _____. That hazard can be minimized by _____.

2. For tracheal intubation to proceed smoothly, it is essential to position the patient correctly to bring the trachea into alignment with the mouth and pharynx. To do so, you need to place the patient in the _____ position.

3. An intubation attempt should take no longer than _____ seconds.

4. The _____ features an integral _____ _____, a gastric access _____ that allows for passage of a 12-Fr _____ tube, a supplemental oxygen inlet port to facilitate passive oxygenation, and a(n) _____ strap to secure in position.

5. Foreign body airway obstructions are sometimes the result of decreased airway reflexes, sometimes caused by alcohol consumption or by _____.

6. When you suction the airway, a nonrigid catheter is called a(n) _____ or _____-_____ catheter, but the rigid tip is called a(n) _____-_____ catheter.

7. The _____ on the video laryngoscope is located on the _____ end of the device. You will be unable to obtain a view of the _____ anatomy if the camera becomes _____ by secretions.

8. You should always adequately _____ a patient before you intubate.

9. The King LT airway should not be used in patients with a(n) _____ _____ _____, patients with known esophageal disease, or patients who have ingested a(n) _____ substance.

10. When examining the patient's airway with the mouth wide open, you note that the posterior pharynx is _____ _____. This is considered a Class II in the _____ classification.

Labeling

Label the following diagram with the correct terms.

1. Parts of the larynx

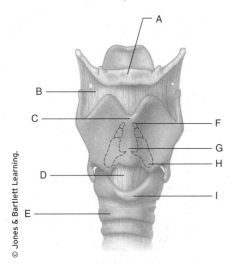

A. _____

B. _____

C. _____

D. _____

E. _____

F. _____

G. _____

H. _____

I. _____

Identify

In the following case study, list the chief complaint, vital signs, and pertinent negatives.

You are called to the high school for a teenager choking. When you arrive, you are directed to a 14-year-old boy who was walking down the hallway when someone scared him from behind. He was chewing on a small cap of a pen when this happened and has sucked the cap into his airway. He is seated in the tripod position and is cyanotic around the lips. You immediately assess that he is breathing because with each breath he makes a whistling noise. A teacher performed the Heimlich maneuver (abdominal thrusts) on him in the hallway initially, and he can at least draw a small breath in. Your partner applies a nonrebreathing mask at 15 L/min. The patient's respirations are 28 breaths/min and shallow. He has decreased lung sounds on the right side and clear sounds on the left. His heart rate is 98 beats/min and regular and his blood pressure (BP) is 128/86 mm Hg. His skin is cyanotic in the face and fingertips and is cool. His oxygen saturation is 90%, and he is a little confused. Because the patient is conscious and you know the cap is in the lungs, and because of the sounds in the lung fields, you position the boy on the cot, sitting up, with oxygen running, and take off for the hospital. You run the unit at Priority 1 (lights and siren) to the emergency department (ED). Later, you learn that the patient had to be taken into surgery to remove the cap.

1. Chief complaint:

_____

_____

2. Vital signs:

_____

_____

3. Pertinent negatives:

_____

_____

Complete the Patient Care Report (PCR)

Reread the incident scenario in the "Identify" section, and then complete the following PCR. Feel free to create the times and numbers, as well as the date of the incident.

EMS Patient Care Report (PCR)				
Date:	Incident No.:	Nature of Call:		Location:
Dispatched:	En Route:	At Scene:	Transport:	At Hospital:	In Service:

Patient Information

Age:	Allergies:
Sex:	Medications:
Weight (in kg [lb]):	Past Medical History:
	Chief Complaint:

Vital Signs

Time:	BP:	Pulse:	Respirations:	SpO$_2$:
Time:	BP:	Pulse:	Respirations:	SpO$_2$:
Time:	BP:	Pulse:	Respirations:	SpO$_2$:

EMS Treatment
(circle all that apply)

Oxygen @ _____ L/min via (circle one): NC NRM Bag-mask device	Assisted Ventilation	Airway Adjunct	CPR
Defibrillation	Bleeding Control	Bandaging	Splinting	Other:

Narrative

Ambulance Calls

The following case scenarios provide an opportunity to explore the concerns associated with patient management and paramedic care. Read each scenario, and then answer each question.

1. You finish a call and return to Joe's Steak 'n' Lobster Shack, where you were having dinner when a previous emergency arose. You hope that they haven't already fed your sirloin to the dog. Happily, Joe has kept your steak waiting for you, and he whips it into the microwave to rewarm it. At last, the steak is back in front of you, along with a generous order of fries. You lift your knife and fork to dig in when, out of the corner of your eye, you see a strange pantomime occurring two tables away. A middle-aged man in a business suit suddenly pushes himself away from the table, clutches his neck, and lurches to his feet. He staggers a few paces and then pitches to the floor—all in complete silence.

   a. The man is showing signs of:

   (1) food poisoning.

   (2) choking.

   (3) strep throat.

   (4) anaphylaxis.

   (5) hysteria.

   b. Which treatment is needed?

   (1) Pump out his stomach.

   (2) Give him manual thrusts.

   (3) Have him gargle with saltwater.

   (4) Give epinephrine 1 mg/mL (1:1,000), 0.5 mL subcutaneously.

   (5) Give diazepam (Valium), 10 mg IM.

2. You are having a barbecue in the backyard one Sunday. The beer has been flowing freely, and everyone is in a jolly mood. You tell a funny story, and everyone present starts laughing uproariously, including one of your friends who had just taken a big bite out of his hot dog. Suddenly, he starts coughing violently. His face gets very red.

   a. At that point, you should take which of the following actions?

   (1) Tilt his head back and attempt to ventilate.

   (2) Perform a quick finger sweep to remove accessible obstructing material.

   (3) Give manual thrusts.

   (4) Reach into his throat with the barbecue tongs and try to snare the hot dog.

   (5) Encourage him to keep coughing.

   b. That course of action does not seem to help. Your friend becomes completely silent, and his face turns a dusky gray as he struggles to breathe. What should you do now?

   (1) Tilt his head back and attempt to ventilate.

   (2) Perform a quick finger sweep to remove accessible obstructing material.

   (3) Do the Heimlich maneuver (abdominal thrusts).

   (4) Reach into his throat with the barbecue tongs and try to snare the hot dog.

   (5) Encourage him to keep coughing.

c. Your friend collapses, unconscious, to the ground. List the next four steps you would take.

(1)_____

(2)_____

(3)_____

(4)_____

d. Meanwhile, an ambulance has arrived (someone had the sense to call 9-1-1), and a couple of paramedics come stampeding through your flower garden carrying what looks like all the equipment from their rig. Now that you have equipment available, which steps will be taken?

(1)_____

(2)_____

(3)_____

(4)_____

3. You are struggling to intubate a 30-year-old male bodybuilder who collapsed while working out at the local health club. You found him in cardiac arrest, and high-quality CPR is in progress. Despite the fact that you have positioned him just as the textbook instructs, you cannot seem to bring his vocal cords into view; they remain hidden just above your laryngoscope blade.

a. To bring the cords into view, you ask your partner to perform the _____ _____, which is _____, _____, _____ pressure on the larynx.

b. That maneuver seems helpful in bringing the vocal cords into view. Another tool that can be useful is the _____ _____ _____, which facilitates entry into the glottis opening and enables you to feel the ridges of the tracheal wall.

c. You finally manage to insert the endotracheal (ET) tube. After confirming proper placement, you secure it with a commercial tube restraint. List some of the specifics you should document on your PCR concerning this intubation.

(1)_____

(2)_____

(3)_____

(4)_____

4. You are attempting a blind nasotracheal intubation on a 60-kg 24-year-old female who took an overdose of sleeping pills. You have succeeded in advancing the tip of the ET tube just beyond the oropharynx.

a. As you continue to advance the tube, how can you tell whether the tip is moving toward the glottis (as opposed to the esophagus)?

(1)_____

(2)_____

(3)_____

b. As you are advancing the tube, you become aware that the bleeps from the cardiac monitor are getting further apart. What has happened?

_____

_____

_____

    c. What should you do about it?

       (1)_____

       (2)_____

       (3)_____

5. You are involved in a search-and-rescue mission to find a 43-year-old male hiker lost in the woods. At last you find him, sitting down, propped against a tree. He tells you that he experienced severe chest pain and could not go on. Because there is a strong possibility that he is experiencing an acute myocardial infarction (AMI), you and your partner will have to carry him the 40-minute walk back to the ambulance. You hook the patient to supplemental oxygen via nasal cannula at a flow rate of 5 L/min. You notice that the pressure gauge on your E cylinder is reading 800 psi.

    a. How long will the oxygen in the E cylinder last?

    _____

    _____

    b. Will that be long enough to get the patient back to the ambulance? (Show your calculations.)

    _____

    _____

6. You are sitting at the movies on your night off when you notice someone a few rows ahead of you suddenly slump over. You leap like a gazelle over several rows of seats to reach the person's side, and you discover that he has stopped breathing. You drag him into an aisle and start mouth-to-mouth ventilation with the barrier device you usually carry in your jacket. How can you tell if you are actually getting air into his lungs?

       (1)_____

       (2)_____

       (3)_____

7. As you continue mouth-to-mouth ventilation on the patient described in question 6, you reflect that you would like to avoid causing gastric distention because you would prefer not to deal with the mess that might follow.

    a. What can you do, that is noninvasive, to minimize gastric distention during artificial ventilation?

       (1)_____

       (2)_____

       (3)_____

    b. Despite your best efforts, you notice that the man's belly is starting to get enlarged. What else should you do (that may be considered invasive)?

    _____

    _____

    _____

8. After your experience in the movie theater, you promise yourself that you will never go anywhere without a pocket mask, or barrier shield, in your pocket, not only to make things more pleasant for yourself, but also because these devices have several advantages over other methods of giving artificial ventilation. List four specific advantages of a pocket mask.

(1)_____

(2)_____

(3)_____

(4)_____

9. A 53-year-old man calls for an ambulance because of shortness of breath. You find him in severe respiratory distress, with foam bubbling out of his mouth. Your examination reveals signs of heart failure (a condition in which fluid backs up into the lungs and interferes with gas exchange).

   a. The patient's pulse oximeter reading when you first arrive shows an oxygen saturation (SpO_2) of 86%. That reading is:

      (1) normal for the patient's age.

      (2) abnormally high.

      (3) abnormally low.

      (4) probably an artifact.

   b. Which measure should you take immediately?

   _____

   c. You treat the patient according to your protocol for heart failure, and his condition improves markedly. Now the SpO_2 reading is 96%. You move the patient to a stretcher and bring him out to the ambulance for transport. When you have him loaded in the ambulance, you notice that the SpO_2 is now reading 85%. The patient, however, still looks comfortable and is not in any respiratory distress, so you conclude that the reading on the pulse oximeter must be an error. List three of the possible causes of the erroneous reading in this patient:

      (1)_____

      (2)_____

      (3)_____

10. You are attempting a blind nasotracheal intubation on an unconscious patient who took an overdose of sleeping pills. When you think you have the tracheal tube in place, you check the end-tidal carbon dioxide monitor that you've snapped onto the tracheal tube. Its color is purple, indicating that the air being exhaled through the tube contains less than 0.5% carbon dioxide.

    a. What can you conclude from that reading?

    _____

    _____

    b. Which actions should you take?

    _____

    _____

11. You are at the scene of a two car collision. A passenger riding in a car #2 is breathing quietly at 12 breaths/min, taking in 500 mL of air with each breath.

   a. What effect do you expect that change in minute volume to have on the patient's arterial P_{CO_2}?

_____

   b. That, in turn, will cause the patient's pH to _____ (rise or fall?).

   c. The resulting derangement in his acid–base balance is called a _____ (respiratory or metabolic?) _____ (acidosis or alkalosis?).

   d. Which treatment is required?

_____

12. Now it's on to a cardiac arrest in a fourth-floor walk-up apartment. You grab the jump kit and the handiest D cylinder from the ambulance while your partner takes the drug box and monitor/defibrillator, and you sprint up the four flights of stairs to the patient's apartment. While your partner starts CPR chest compressions, you "crack" the oxygen cylinder, hook up the oxygen to a bag-mask device, and open the flow control to 10 L/min. As you do so, you notice that the reading on the pressure gauge is 900 psi. How much time do you have before you need to switch to a fresh cylinder? _____ minutes (The cylinder constant for a D cylinder is 0.16. Show your calculations.)

_____

_____

_____

13. A 34-year-old man has been injured in a road collision in which his head apparently struck the windshield with some force. When you first reach the scene, the patient is unconscious. He is breathing 8 breaths/min, inhaling approximately 500 mL of air with each breath.

   a. We can conclude that the patient's arterial P_{CO_2} will tend to _____ (increase or decrease?), so his pH will _____ (increase or decrease?). The net effect will be an acid–base disorder called a _____ (respiratory or metabolic?) _____ (acidosis or alkalosis?). The way you can help correct that abnormality is to _____ _____.

14. The laboratory calls down another blood gas report. "You'd better check on this guy," the lab technician says. "His P_{O_2} is only 48 mm Hg." As you sprint off to alert the doctor about the blood gas results, you review in your mind the conditions that can cause hypoxemia.

   a. List six conditions that can cause respiratory distress and inadequate ventilation.

     (1)_____

     (2)_____

     (3)_____

     (4)_____

     (5)_____

     (6)_____

   b. What is the treatment for hypoxemia?

_____

_____

True/False

If you believe the statement to be more true than false, write the letter "T" in the space provided. If you believe the statement to be more false than true, write the letter "F."

_____   1. Any patient who is to be suctioned should first be preoxygenated.

_____   2. You should not suction while inserting the catheter.

_____   3. Suction a stoma for only 2 minutes at a time.

_____   4. A tonsil-tip catheter is a good choice for suctioning the oropharynx.

_____   5. The Cobra PLA is contraindicated with massive oral cavity trauma.

_____   6. The physical act of moving air into and out of the lungs is oxygenation.

_____   7. The exchange of oxygen and carbon dioxide in the alveoli and the tissues of the body is called ventilation.

_____   8. A barrier to ventilation would include neuromuscular disease.

_____   9. Using the 3-3-2 rule, the mouth should be at least 3 fingerbreadths wide open. The space from the chin to the larynx should be 3 inches, and the distance to the stoma should be 2 fingerbreadths.

_____   10. If your patient weighs over 198 lb (>90 kg), you should use the yellow i-gel.

Short Answer

Complete this section with short written answers using the space provided.

1. Obstruction of the upper airway is an immediate threat to life. The upper airway may become obstructed in several ways. List four causes of upper airway obstruction, and put an asterisk beside the most common cause.

   a. _____

   b. _____

   c. _____

   d. _____

2. Endotracheal intubation has several advantages over other methods of airway control. List three advantages of endotracheal intubation.

   a. _____

   b. _____

   c. _____

3. Despite all its advantages, endotracheal intubation is not for all patients. Like every other medical procedure, it has specific indications. List three indications for endotracheal intubation.

   a. _____

   b. _____

   c. _____

4. Endotracheal intubation is not without potential complications. The most serious acute complications can, however, be avoided by meticulous attention to correct technique.
   a. List a potential complication of endotracheal intubation.

   _____

b. How can it be avoided?

(1)_____

(2)_____

(3)_____

(4)_____

c. How can it be detected and corrected if it does occur?

(1)_____

(2)_____

(3)_____

d. List another potential complication of endotracheal intubation.

_____

e. How can it be avoided?

_____

f. How can it be detected and corrected if it does occur?

_____

_____

5. In some emergency medical services (EMS) systems, paramedics are authorized to use paralyzing drugs to facilitate tracheal intubation. Although such drugs undoubtedly make life easier for the paramedic, they may make life quite precarious for the patient. What is the principal hazard of administering a neuromuscular blocking agent to a patient who needs to be intubated?

_____

_____

6. Oxygen is a drug, and like any other drug, it should be given when there are indications for its use. List five indications for administering supplemental oxygen to a patient.

a. _____

b. _____

c. _____

d. _____

e. _____

7. Sometimes the patient will "tell" you, through his or her symptoms and signs, that either the oxygenation, the ventilation, or both are insufficient—that is, the patient is suffering from acute respiratory insufficiency. List four signs of acute respiratory insufficiency.

a. _____

b. _____

c. _____

d. _____

8. Oxygen is stored in cylinders at pressures up to 2,000 psi, which means that oxygen cylinders have to be treated with respect. List six safety precautions that should be observed when using or storing oxygen cylinders.

a. _____

b. _____

c. _____

d. _____

e. _____

f. _____

9. List three ways of identifying someone in respiratory arrest.

a. _____

b. _____

c. _____

10. A person who has suffered respiratory arrest will need _____ (assisted or artificial?) ventilation.

11. What is the difference between artificial and assisted ventilation?

_____

_____

12. What is the objective of any form of artificial ventilation?

_____

_____

13. List three situations in which information from pulse oximetry could be helpful to you in the field.

a. _____

b. _____

c. _____

14. A car-crash victim who has sustained injury to the cervical spinal cord may develop weakness or paralysis of the respiratory muscles. If so, such a patient may not have the strength to inhale as deeply as he or she otherwise would. Thus, the patient's minute volume will _____ (increase or decrease?), leading to a(n) _____ in the arterial P_{CO_2}.

Fill in the Table

Fill in the missing parts of the table.

1. In mastering the use of any given piece of equipment, it is essential to learn not only how to use the equipment but also when to use it (and when not to use it). Artificial airways can be enormously helpful when applied in the appropriate circumstances; they can be downright dangerous when used in inappropriate circumstances. Fill in the table to summarize the indications and contraindications for the oropharyngeal airway (OPA) and the nasopharyngeal airway (NPA).

	Oropharyngeal Airway	Nasopharyngeal Airway
Use for:		
Do not use for:		

2. Oxygen-delivery devices

Device	Flow Rate (L/min)	Oxygen Delivered (%)
Nasal cannula		
Nonrebreathing mask		
Bag-mask device with reservoir		

3. Airway adjuncts can be very helpful in ensuring a patent air passage, but one needs to use the right adjunct in the right situation. Fill in the following table to remind yourself what to use (and not to use) and when to use it.

Adjunct	Indicated for:	Do Not Use in:
Oropharyngeal airway		
Combitube		
LMA		
Endotracheal intubation		

MEDICAL

Respiratory Emergencies

CHAPTER

16

Matching

Part I

Match each of the items in the left column to the appropriate term in the right column.

_____ **1.** A sitting position with the head elevated to 90 degrees.

_____ **2.** The infiltration of any tissue by air or gas; a chronic obstructive pulmonary disease characterized by distention of the alveoli and destructive changes in the lung parenchyma.

_____ **3.** The production of large amounts of urine by the kidney.

_____ **4.** A common disease of infancy and childhood caused by upper airway obstruction and characterized by stridor, hoarseness, and a barking cough.

_____ **5.** Abnormal breath sounds that have a fine, crackling quality; previously called rales.

_____ **6.** Abnormal breath sounds or noises that occur in addition to the normal breath sounds; examples are crackles and wheezes.

_____ **7.** The saclike units at the end of the bronchioles in which gas exchange takes place.

_____ **8.** The inhalation of anything other than breathable gases.

_____ **9.** Collapse of the alveolar air spaces of the lungs.

_____ **10.** A pharmacologic agent that stimulates the beta-2 receptor sites found in smooth muscle; includes common bronchodilators such as albuterol and levalbuterol.

_____ **11.** An iron-containing protein with red blood cells that has the ability to combine with oxygen.

_____ **12.** A disease of unknown cause characterized by progressive paralysis moving from the feet to the head (ascending paralysis). If paralysis reaches the diaphragm, the patient may require respiratory support.

_____ **13.** A mesh filter placed in the inferior vena cava to catch blood clots in patients who are at high risk of pulmonary embolus.

_____ **14.** A ridgelike projection of tracheal cartilage located where the trachea bifurcates into the right and left mainstem bronchi.

_____ **15.** Deep cyanosis of the face and neck that extends across the chest and back; associated with little or no blood flow; a particularly ominous sign.

_____ **16.** Severe constriction of smooth muscle surrounding the bronchial tree.

A. Adventitious

B. Alveoli

C. Aspiration

D. Atelectasis

E. Beta-2 agonist

F. Botulism

G. Bronchospasm

H. Cape cyanosis

I. Carina

J. Carpopedal spasm

K. Chronic bronchitis

L. Cor pulmonale

M. Crackles

N. Croup

O. Diuresis

P. Emphysema

_____ **17.** Heart disease that develops because of chronic lung disease and affects primarily the right side of the heart.

_____ **18.** A chronic inflammatory condition affecting the bronchi that is characterized by excessive mucus production as a result of overgrowth of the mucous glands in the airways.

_____ **19.** Contorted positioning of the head or foot in which the fingers or toes flex in a clawlike manner; may be caused by hyperventilation.

_____ **20.** Poisoning characterized by severe muscle paralysis and usually caused by eating food containing botulinum toxin.

Q. Fowler position

R. Greenfield filter

S. Guillain-Barré syndrome

T. Hemoglobin

Part II

Match each of the items in the left column to the appropriate term in the right column.

_____ **1.** Excessive accumulation of fluid in the pleural space.

_____ **2.** Severe shortness of breath occurring suddenly at night after several hours of recumbency, as fluid pools in the lungs.

_____ **3.** The functional portions of a gland or solid organ.

_____ **4.** Severe dyspnea experienced when recumbent that is relieved by sitting or standing up.

_____ **5.** The sound of one note during wheezing caused by the vibration of a single bronchus.

_____ **6.** A dangerous condition in which the supply of oxygen to the tissues is reduced.

_____ **7.** To move inadequate volumes of air into the lungs.

_____ **8.** An excess of oxygen.

_____ **9.** Engorgement of the jugular veins when the liver is gently pressed; this finding is specific to right-sided heart failure.

_____ **10.** Coughing up blood in the sputum.

_____ **11.** Full of pus; having the character of pus.

_____ **12.** A false membrane formed by a dead tissue layer; seen in the posterior pharynx of patients with diphtheria.

_____ **13.** The sound of multiple notes during wheezing caused by the vibrations of multiple bronchi.

_____ **14.** The production of too many red blood cells over time, making the blood thick; a characteristic of people with chronic lung disease and chronic hypoxia.

_____ **15.** The transfer of a disease from one organ or part of the body to another that is not directly connected to the original site; often used to describe a cancer that has spread to another part of the body.

_____ **16.** Firming of the lungs as a result of fluid accumulation.

_____ **17.** Inflammation of the larynx, trachea, and bronchi.

_____ **18.** A respiratory pattern characteristic of diabetic ketoacidosis with marked hyperpnea and tachypnea; represents the body's attempt to compensate for the acidosis.

_____ **19.** The visible bulging of the jugular veins when a patient is in a semi-Fowler or full-Fowler position; indicates inadequate blood movement through the heart and/or lungs.

_____ **20.** A state in which the stimulus to breathe comes from a decrease in PaO_2, rather than from the normal stimulus of an increase in $PaCO_2$.

A. Hemoptysis

B. Hepatojugular reflux

C. Hyperoxia

D. Hypoventilate

E. Hypoxia

F. Hypoxic drive

G. Jugular venous distension

H. Kussmaul respirations

I. Laryngotracheo-bronchitis

J. Lung consolidation

K. Metastasis

L. Monophonic

M. Orthopnea

N. Parenchyma

O. Paroxysmal nocturnal dyspnea

P. Pleural effusion

Q. Polycythemia

R. Polyphonic

S. Pseudo-membrane

T. Purulent

Multiple Choice

Read each item carefully, and then select the best response.

_____ 1. The ridgelike point at which the tracheal cartilage bifurcates is called the:

    A. epiglottis.

    B. carina.

    C. larynx.

    D. glottis.

_____ 2. In a pneumothorax, where is air trapped?

    A. Inside the alveoli

    B. In the nasopharynx

    C. Between visceral and parietal pleurae

    D. Between the alveoli

_____ 3. Which of the following substances are thin secretions in the airway that the body can eliminate by coughing?

    A. Antitussives

    B. Corticosteroids

    C. Diuretics

    D. Expectorants

_____ 4. Right-sided heart failure that has been caused by a chronic lung disease is known as:

    A. Guillain-Barré syndrome.

    B. polycythemia.

    C. cor pulmonale.

    D. atelectasis.

_____ 5. Which of the following breathing patterns is characterized by breathing that becomes faster and deeper until there is a period of apnea before the pattern begins again?

    A. Cheyne-Stokes

    B. Kussmaul

    C. Cor pulmonale

    D. Ataxic

_____ 6. What is another name for _rales_?

    A. Rhonchus

    B. Wheezing

    C. Crackles

    D. Death rattle

_____ 7. You respond to a patient who is having difficulty breathing. He is coughing up frothy sputum. What is the classic cause of frothy sputum?

    A. Allergic reaction

    B. Asthma attack

    C. Heart failure

    D. Acute myocardial infarction

_____ 8. Overdose, Lou Gehrig disease, and carbon dioxide narcosis are examples of conditions that affect ventilation through:

    A. upper airway obstruction.

    B. neuromuscular impairment.

    C. chest wall impairment.

    D. lower airway obstruction.

_____ **9.** Which of the following is NOT used to treat asthma as defined in the asthma triad?

    A. Expectorant

    B. Corticosteroid

    C. Bronchodilator

    D. Hyperventilation

_____ **10.** When the body attempts to compensate for acidosis through hyperventilation, this is called:

    A. Kussmaul respirations.

    B. botulism.

    C. Guillain-Barré syndrome.

    D. opioid overdose.

Fill in the Blank

Read each item carefully, and then complete the statement by filling in the missing word(s).

1. Alveolar collapse is known as _____.

2. _____ _____ dyspnea comes on in the middle of the night and may be a sign of _____ heart failure.

3. A surplus of red blood cells that the body makes as a result of a chronic lung disease is called _____.

4. Your patient has two or more ribs, broken in two or more places, that are inhibiting her breathing. In your radio report, you report this as a(n) _____ _____.

5. The medical term for shortness of breath is _____, and the medical term for blue-tinged skin caused by lack of oxygen is _____.

6. Being awakened by difficulty breathing during the night is known as _____ _____ _____.

7. _____ _____ are vibrations felt in the chest when a patient breathes.

8. There are _____ [number] lobes in the right lung and _____ [number] lobes in the left lung.

9. During inhalation, the _____ cartilage is drawn _____, and the area just above the sternal notch is pulled in if there is tracheal tugging.

10. Breathing in a way that allows patients to exhale slowly under controlled pressure is called _____-_____ _____.

Labeling

Label the following diagrams with the correct terms.

1. Respiratory patterns

Normal breathing

ha a   n

nha a   n

Brainstem

hyperpnea

apnea

A

A. _____

B. _____

C. _____

D. _____

E. _____

F. _____

Identify

After reading the following case study, list the chief complaint, vital signs, and pertinent negatives.

You respond to a call for a baby not breathing. As you approach the home, a mother comes running out holding a 1-year-old boy, named Tommy. He is limp in her arms. You immediately jump out and take the child from her, get into the back of the unit, and lay him on the cot. The child is unconscious and blue, and he has no respirations. You begin the steps of cardiopulmonary resuscitation (CPR) by opening the airway and trying to give two breaths. Your partner has crawled into the back along with the mother and is trying to calm her down and help you at the same time. Using a pediatric bag-mask device, you give a breath and notice no chest rise and fall. You reposition the head and try again; once again, there is no rise and fall of the chest. You check the brachial artery and find a faint pulse. Your partner has pulled out the intubation kit and is ready to try to insert an advanced airway. As he looks for the tracheal tube, he reaches for the Magill forceps and suction. After suctioning and using the forceps, he removes a small plastic game piece from the boy. You immediately start to bag the child again with 100% supplemental oxygen. The child's chest rises now. His oxygen saturation is 64%, and the pulse is bradycardic at 46 beats/min. You are unable to get a blood pressure (BP). You manage respirations at one every 3 seconds. After a minute, the child is beginning to "pink up," his "sats" come up to 88%, and his heart rate is steadily climbing and at the moment is 92 beats/min. The child is regaining consciousness and begins to cry and fight you. He is now breathing on his own. His mother wants the child transported to be checked out. Your partner has a pediatric nonrebreathing mask ready with 100% supplemental oxygen. The mother holds the nonrebreathing mask while you strap the child into the special car seat designed for your stretcher and place the mother on the crew bench with the seat belt buckled. By the time you reach the emergency department (ED), little Tommy's heart rate is normal, and his oxygen saturation is 99%; his mother begins to cry with the realization of how close Tommy was to death.

1. Chief complaint:

_____

_____

2. Vital signs:

_____

_____

3. Pertinent negatives:

_____

_____

Ambulance Calls

The following case scenarios provide an opportunity to explore the concerns associated with patient management and paramedic care. Read each scenario, and then answer each question.

1. You are called to an office building for a "possible heart attack." On arriving, you are somewhat surprised to find that the patient is a clerical worker who looks about 22 years old—not at all like the usual heart attack patient. The woman looks pale and anxious, however, and complains of stabbing pains in her chest that came on "out of the blue." She also complains of a "funny tingly feeling in my lips." On examination, her pulse is 110 beats/min and regular, respirations are 30 breaths/min and unlabored, BP is 140/84 mm Hg, and SpO_2 is 93% without significant variation during the respiratory cycle. There are no abnormal physical findings except that the patient's hands look a bit odd, almost like claws.

   a. What is the most probable diagnosis in this case?

   _____

   _____

   _____

   b. Which steps will you take in managing this case?

   (1)_____

   (2)_____

   (3)_____

   c. This woman's arterial P_{CO_2} is probably _____ (higher or lower?) than normal. Explain why.

   _____

   _____

2. You are called late one night to the Smith family residence for a "man who can't breathe." The patient's wife answers the door, quite distraught, and hurries you into the bedroom. She blurts out, "This is the worst it's ever been. I kept telling him to leave those cigarettes alone—the doctor's been saying the same thing—but do you think he listens? Might as well be talking to a brick wall."

   In the bedroom, you find a heavy-set man about 65 years old sitting up at the edge of the bed in obvious respiratory distress. In fact, his "obvious" respiratory distress is obvious only if you know the signs of respiratory distress (increased work of breathing).

   a. List eight signs of respiratory distress or increased work of breathing.

   (1)_____

   (2)_____

   (3)_____

   (4)_____

(5)_____

(6)_____

(7)_____

(8)_____

b. Which steps will you take at this point?

_____

_____

_____

c. In due course, you learn that the patient called for an ambulance because he awoke from sleep unable to breathe. List seven questions you need to ask in taking his history.

(1)_____

(2)_____

(3)_____

(4)_____

(5)_____

(6)_____

(7)_____

d. As you proceed systematically through the secondary assessment of this man, you will be looking for some specific abnormalities at each step. In the following table, indicate what, in particular, you will be looking for as you examine each part of the body indicated.

Part of the Body	What I Am Looking for in Particular
General appearance	
Vital signs	
Head	
Neck	
Chest	
Abdomen	
Extremities	

e. In the course of the focused history, you learn that the patient has been a three-pack-per-day cigarette smoker for about 48 years. He "keeps a cough," but lately it has been worse than usual, and he has been bringing up a lot more sputum. His feet have also begun swelling, to the point that he can hardly get his shoes on. (Most of this you learn from the patient's wife; the patient is too short of breath to provide more than two or three words at a time.)

    (1) This patient most likely has which of the following conditions?

        (a) Pulmonary embolism

        (b) Chronic obstructive pulmonary disease (COPD)

        (c) Pneumonia

        (d) Pickwickian syndrome

        (e) Acute asthmatic attack

    (2) How will you manage this patient?

_____

_____

_____

_____

3. A 56-year-old man calls for an ambulance because of severe dyspnea. His wife greets you at the door. She tells you, "My husband, he's a heart patient. Please get him to the hospital quickly. I think he's having another heart attack."

    You find the patient in the living room, sitting in an armchair and in obvious distress. "Hit me like a ton of bricks," he gasps. "Not like the heart attack"—gasp—"Can't get air"—gasp—"Hurts to breathe."

    On physical examination, his skin is cool and moist. Vital signs are as follows: pulse 120 beats/min and regular, respirations 32 breaths/min and shallow, BP 174/96 mm Hg, and SpO_2 of 94%. The neck veins look a bit distended, but otherwise there are no abnormal findings.

a. This patient is most likely suffering from which of the following conditions?

    (1) Pulmonary embolism

    (2) Decompensated COPD

    (3) Pneumonia

    (4) Pickwickian syndrome

    (5) Acute asthmatic attack

b. Which steps will you take in managing this patient?

    (1)_____

    (2)_____

    (3)_____

    (4)_____

True/False

If you believe the statement to be more true than false, write the letter "T" in the space provided. If you believe the statement to be more false than true, write the letter "F."

_____ **1.** Right-sided heart failure because of chronic lung disease is known as cor pulmonale.

_____ **2.** The right lung has three lobes, whereas the left lung only has two lobes.

_____ **3.** Gas exchange happens only in the alveoli.

_____ **4.** Hiccups, yawns, and sighs are all forms of breathing patterns.

_____ **5.** Laying a patient flat will help the patient breathe better.

_____ **6.** Stridor is a result of a partial obstruction of the upper airway.

_____ **7.** A patient who is sitting in the tripod position (elbows out) and who can speak only in two- or three-word statements is a patient in distress.

_____ **8.** Patients who suffer from severe COPD often have jugular venous distention (JVD).

_____ **9.** The diaphragm of a stethoscope is for listening to high-pitched breath sounds.

_____ **10.** Pulse oximetry is a tool that can give false readings if the patient has a low hemoglobin level.

_____ **11.** An abnormal breathing pattern due to injury to the brainstem is central neurogenic hyperventilation.

_____ **12.** Acute pulmonary edema will sometimes present as a wheeze that sounds like an asthma attack.

_____ **13.** You should withhold high concentrations of oxygen for the patient who breathes with the hypoxic drive.

_____ **14.** An asthmatic who tells you he was previously intubated for his breathing difficulty is at increased risk of death.

_____ **15.** Anticholinergics have emerged as a central component in the management of COPD.

_____ **16.** If you use an aerosol nebulizer to deliver medication, you can expect the patient to benefit from 90% of the medication dose.

_____ **17.** Immediate, fast-acting medications used for bronchodilation are beta-1 agonists.

_____ **18.** When giving a corticosteroid as an IV bolus, you will see immediate results.

_____ **19.** Morphine should be used as the first-line vasodilator in the treatment of pulmonary edema.

_____ **20.** A continuous positive airway pressure (CPAP) machine cannot be used in the field.

Short Answer

Complete this section with short written answers using the space provided.

1. List four things that can cause a pulmonary embolism.

a. _____

b. _____

c. _____

d. _____

2. Discuss the clues to diagnosing a pulmonary embolism.

_____

_____

_____

_____

3. What are the contraindications to supplemental oxygen therapy?

_____

_____

_____

4. Not every patient who presents with dyspnea and wheezing has bronchial asthma. List four other conditions that can produce wheezing.

a. _____

b. _____

c. _____

d. _____

5. Asthma is common in children, so it is important to be able to distinguish a mild asthmatic attack from one that is potentially life threatening. List at least five signs that an asthmatic attack is very severe and warrants urgent transport to the hospital.

a. _____

b. _____

c. _____

d. _____

e. _____

Fill in the Table

Provide the signs and symptoms of the various breathing patterns listed in the following table.

1. Breathing Patterns

Pattern	Comments
Agonal	_____ _____ that are widely spaced; usually represent _____ _____ _____ in a dying patient; occasional agonal gasp not unusual in patients with no pulse; not actually considered a form of breathing
Apneustic	Characterized by a(n) _____ _____ _____ (sometimes called "_____ breathing"); follows damage to the _____ _____ in the brain; an ominous sign of severe _____ _____
Ataxic	Chaotically irregular respirations that indicate _____ brain injury or _____ _____
Biot respirations	Irregular pattern, _____, and depth of respirations, characterized by intermittent patterns of _____; indicates severe brain injury or _____ herniation
Bradypnea	Unusually _____ respirations
Central neurogenic hyperventilation	Tachypneic _____; rapid and deep respirations caused by _____ _____ _____ or direct _____ _____; drives _____ _____ level down and _____ up, resulting in respiratory _____
Cheyne-Stokes respirations	_____-_____ breathing with a period of _____ between cycles; not considered ominous unless grossly _____ or occurs in a patient with brain _____
Cough	Forced exhalation against a closed _____; an airway-clearing maneuver; also seen when _____ _____ irritate the airways; controlled by the cough center in the brain (_____ medications work on the cough center to reduce this sometimes annoying physiologic response)
Eupnea	_____ breathing
Hiccup	Spasmodic contraction of the _____, causing short _____ with a characteristic sound; sometimes seen in cases of diaphragmatic (or _____) nerve irritation from _____ _____ _____, ulcer disease, or _____ _____
Hyperpnea	Abnormally _____ rate and depth of breathing; seen in various _____ or chemical disorders, including overdose with certain drugs
Hypopnea	Abnormally _____ rate and depth of breathing
Kussmaul respirations	The same pattern as in _____ _____ _____, but caused by the body's response to metabolic _____, attempting to rid itself of blood _____ via the lungs; seen in diabetic _____; accompanied by a(n) _____ (acetone) breath odor and, usually, _____ and dry mouth and lips
Sighing	Periodically taking a very deep breath of about _____ the normal volume; forces open _____ that routinely close from time to time
Tachypnea	Unusually _____ breathing; does not reflect _____ of respiration and does not mean a patient is _____ (breathing too rapidly and deeply, resulting in a lowered _____ _____ level); often involves moving only small volumes of air, or _____ (much like a panting dog)
Yawning	Seems beneficial in the same manner as _____

Complete the Patient Care Report (PCR)

Read the incident scenario in the "Identify" exercise, and then complete the following PCR.

EMS Patient Care Report (PCR)					
Date:	Incident No.:	Nature of Call:		Location:	
Dispatched:	En Route:	At Scene:	Transport:	At Hospital:	In Service:

Patient Information	
Age: Sex: Weight (in kg [lb]):	Allergies: Medications: Past Medical History: Chief Complaint:

Vital Signs				
Time:	BP:	Pulse:	Respirations:	SpO$_2$:
Time:	BP:	Pulse:	Respirations:	SpO$_2$:
Time:	BP:	Pulse:	Respirations:	SpO$_2$:

EMS Treatment (circle all that apply)				
Oxygen @ _____ L/min via (circle one): NC NRM Bag-mask device		Assisted Ventilation	Airway Adjunct	CPR
Defibrillation	Bleeding Control	Bandaging	Splinting	Other:

Narrative

Cardiovascular Emergencies

Welcome to the cardiac chapter of the workbook. Because of the length and the amount of material covered in this chapter, it has been divided into three parts to facilitate learning: Part 1 covers cardiac function; Part 2 addresses heart rhythms and the electrocardiogram (ECG), and Part 3 deals with putting it all together and practice ECG strips.

Part 1: Cardiac Function

Matching

Part I

Match each of the definitions in the left column to the appropriate term in the right column.

_____ **1.** An outpouching or bulge in the wall of a portion of the aorta, caused by weakening and dilation of the vessel wall; its rupture is life threatening.

A. Aberration

_____ **2.** A pathologic condition in which the thickening and stiffening of the arterial walls make the arteries less elastic.

B. Absolute refractory period

_____ **3.** The sudden pain that occurs when the oxygen supply to the myocardium is insufficient to meet demand, causing ischemic changes in the tissue.

C. Acute coronary syndromes

_____ **4.** The portion of the conduction system of the heart that consists of the AV node and the nonbranching portion of the bundle of His.

D. Agonal

_____ **5.** An accumulation of fat inside a blood vessel that narrows the diameter of the lumen.

E. Angina pectoris

_____ **6.** A mass of fatty tissue that gradually calcifies, hardening into an atheromatous plaque that infiltrates the arterial wall and diminishes its elasticity.

F. Aortic aneurysm

_____ **7.** A dysrhythmia in which every other complex is a premature complex, causing a normal-early beat-normal-early beat pattern; can be atrial, junctional, or ventricular.

G. Arteriosclerosis

_____ **8.** The classic trio of signs associated with cardiac tamponade: narrowed pulse pressure, muffled heart tones, and jugular vein distention.

H. Artifact

_____ **9.** Movement of the heart's QRS axis to the right or left of its normal position.

I. Asystole

_____ **10.** An intraventricular conduction disturbance involving impedance of electrical impulses from the bundle of His to the right or left bundle branch.

J. Atheroma

_____ **11.** Abnormal whooshing sounds indicating turbulent blood flow within a narrowed vessel; usually heard in the carotid arteries.

K. Atherosclerosis

_____ **12.** On an ECG, leads that contain both a positive pole and a negative pole; leads I, II, and III.

L. Atrioventricular junction

_____ **13.** A term describing the shape of the QRS complex in aberrantly conducted beats.

M. Axis deviation

_____ **14.** The early phase of cardiac repolarization, wherein the heart muscle cannot be stimulated to depolarize; also known as the effective refractory period.

_____ **15.** A series of cardiac conditions caused by an abrupt reduction in coronary artery blood flow.

_____ **16.** Pertaining to the period of dying.

_____ **17.** An artificial product; in cardiology, used to refer to noise or interference in an ECG tracing.

_____ **18.** The absence of ventricular contraction or electrical activity.

_____ **19.** Pathologic process characterized by progressive atherosclerotic narrowing and eventual obstruction of the coronary arteries.

_____ **20.** The blood vessels that supply blood to the tissues of the heart.

_____ **21.** Leads that view geographically similar areas of the myocardium, such as leads II, III, and aVF; useful for localizing areas of ischemia.

_____ **22.** The period from one cardiac contraction to the next; it includes both ventricular contraction (systole) and relaxation (diastole).

_____ **23.** A pathologic condition characterized by restriction of cardiac contraction, falling cardiac output, and shock as a result of pericardial fluid accumulation.

_____ **24.** Pain, cramping, muscle tightness, fatigue, or weakness of the legs during physical activity as a result of increased oxygen demand by the muscle tissue of the legs, hips, and buttocks.

_____ **25.** An ECG pattern in which the QRS complexes are all in the same direction in the precordial leads as a result of improper lead placement, anterior wall myocardial infarction, ventricular tachycardia, or other variables.

N. Beck triad

O. Bigeminy

P. Bipolar leads

Q. Bruits

R. Bundle branch block

S. Cardiac cycle

T. Cardiac tamponade

U. Claudication

V. Concordant precordial pattern

W. Contiguous leads

X. Coronary arteries

Y. Coronary artery disease

Part II

Match each of the definitions in the left column to the appropriate term in the right column.

_____ **1.** Death of a localized area of tissue caused by ischemia.

_____ **2.** Related to only the ventricles; produced by the ventricles.

_____ **3.** A syndrome that occurs when the heart is unable to pump powerfully enough or fast enough to empty its chambers; as a result, blood backs up into the systemic circuit, the pulmonary circuit, or both.

_____ **4.** Inflammation of the endocardium as a result of infection.

_____ **5.** An impulse or rhythm that originates from a site other than the sinoatrial (SA) node.

_____ **6.** Two consecutive (paired) premature ventricular complexes.

_____ **7.** The slurring of the upstroke of the first part of the QRS complex that occurs in Wolff-Parkinson-White syndrome.

_____ **8.** The process of discharging resting cardiac muscle fibers by means of an electrical impulse that stimulates contraction.

_____ **9.** The process by which the intimal and medial layers of a vessel separate after a tear occurs in an aneurysmal portion of the arterial wall; with each ventricular systole, a jet of blood is forced into the torn arterial wall, creating and propagating a false channel.

_____ **10.** Cardiac rhythm disturbances.

_____ **11.** Inflammation of the pericardial sac.

_____ **12.** The first wave of the ECG complex representing depolarization of the ventricles.

_____ **13.** Having a common shape.

_____ **14.** Arising from or pertaining to many foci or locations.

_____ **15.** The death of tissue, usually caused by a cessation of its blood supply.

_____ **16.** The baseline of the ECG, which is neither positive nor negative.

A. Couplet

B. Delta wave

C. Depolarization

D. Dissection

E. Dysrhythmias

F. Ectopic

G. Endocarditis

H. Fascicular block

I. Fibrinolytic therapy

J. First-degree AV block

K. Heart failure

L. Idioventricular

M. Infarction

N. Internodal pathways

O. Ischemia

P. Isoelectric line

_____ **17.** Tissue anoxia caused by diminished blood flow, usually as a result of narrowing or occlusion of an artery.

_____ **18.** The three atrial pathways of electrical conduction that transmit impulses from the SA node to the atrioventricular (AV) node.

_____ **19.** A condition characterized by a QT interval exceeding approximately 0.45 seconds (450 milliseconds).

_____ **20.** A cardiac condition in which the left ventricle becomes enlarged, most often as a result of hypertension.

_____ **21.** One of the two branches of the left main coronary artery; these branches supply the left ventricle, interventricular septum, and part of the right ventricle.

_____ **22.** Failure of the anterior or posterior fascicles of the heart to conduct electrical impulses because of disease or ischemia.

_____ **23.** The use of medications that act to dissolve blood clots.

_____ **24.** A delay in the conduction of the depolarizing impulse from the SA node to the ventricles, prolonging the PR interval.

_____ **25.** Inflammation of the myocardium.

Q. Left anterior descending artery

R. Left ventricular hypertrophy

S. Long QT syndrome

T. Monomorphic

U. Multifocal

V. Myocarditis

W. Necrosis

X. P wave

Y. Pericarditis

Multiple Choice

Read each item carefully, and then select the best response.

_____ **1.** The innermost smooth layer of the heart is called the:
   A. myocardium.
   B. endocardium.
   C. epicardium.
   D. pericardium.

_____ **2.** During the _____ refractory period, cardiac cells are unable to respond to any stimulus.
   A. complete
   B. absolute
   C. relative
   D. nonessential

_____ **3.** The normal dominant pacemaker for the heart is the:
   A. Purkinje fibers.
   B. AV node.
   C. bundle of His.
   D. SA node.

_____ **4.** The _____ component of the ECG represents the depolarization of the ventricles.
   A. P wave
   B. QRS complex
   C. R-R interval
   D. T wave

_____ **5.** The paramedic is palpating the radial pulse while listening to the apical pulse with a stethoscope. Which abnormality is he or she likely to find?
   A. Pulsus paradoxus
   B. Pulse deficit
   C. Pulsus alternans
   D. Pericardial friction rub

_____ **6.** Of the following, which is NOT a cause of a cardiac dysrhythmia?
   A. Myocardial ischemia
   B. Cor pulmonale
   C. Hypoglycemia
   D. Increased vagal tone

_____   **7.** An area of fat in the arteries that has calcified is known as a:

      A. bruit.

      B. phlebitis.

      C. thrombophlebitis.

      D. plaque.

_____   **8.** In a 65-year-old man, a systolic blood pressure of _____ would indicate hypertension.

      A. 120 mm Hg

      B. 130 mm Hg

      C. 140 mm Hg

      D. 150 mm Hg

_____   **9.** Which of the following symptoms is NOT associated with an acute myocardial infarction (AMI) or acute cardiac syndrome (ACS)?

      A. Bulimia

      B. Dizziness

      C. Palpitations

      D. Diaphoresis

_____ **10.** The "M" in the mnemonic MONA stands for:

      A. myocardium.

      B. morphine.

      C. management.

      D. monitor.

Fill in the Blank

Read each item carefully, and then complete the statement by filling in the missing word(s).

1. Alternative routes of blood flow around the heart are known as _____ _____. These are used in case of a blockage.

2. The _____ valve prevents blood from flowing back into the left ventricle.

3. _____ leads refers to leads that view geographically similar areas of myocardium.

4. The _____ _____ consists of the blood vessels between the right ventricle and left atrium, which receive the output of the right side of the heart.

5. Early, _____ advanced airway management is essential for the patient whose cardiac arrest is the result of _____.

6. Because _____-_____ AV block may occur with any _____ in which a(n) _____ wave precedes the _____, the rate associated with it is that of the underlying rhythm.

7. The _____ serves as the gatekeeper to the ventricles.

8. In right _____ hypertrophy the right ventricle becomes _____.

9. During the _____ _____ _____, the heart muscle will not contract because it is drained of all its energy.

10. Repolarization of the ventricles and atria will produce a(n) _____ _____ marking on an ECG.

Labeling

Label the following diagrams with the correct terms.

1. Coronary arteries

Anterior View

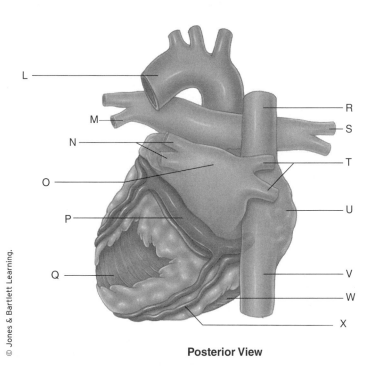

Posterior View

A. _____

B. _____

C. _____

D. _____

E. _____

F. _____

G. _____

H. _____

I. _____

J. _____

K. _____

L. _____

M. _____

N. _____

O. _____

P. _____

Q. _____

R. _____

S. _____

T. _____

U. _____

V. _____

W. _____

X. _____

2. Location of precordial leads

A. _____

B. _____

C. _____

D. _____

E. _____

F. _____

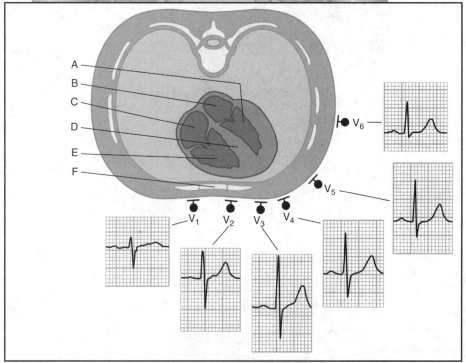

True/False

If you believe the statement to be more true than false, write the letter "T" in the space provided. If you believe the statement to be more false than true, write the letter "F."

_____   **1.** Labetalol and nitroglycerin are drugs that can lower blood pressure.

_____   **2.** The most characteristic physical finding with rupture of an abdominal aortic aneurysm (AAA) is decreased pedal pulse.

_____   **3.** An ECG will be very helpful in diagnosing cardiac tamponade.

_____   **4.** Management of left-sided heart failure should be to decrease preload.

_____   **5.** Furosemide (Lasix) is a diuretic that always helps with left heart failure.

_____   **6.** Percutaneous intervention can be used for a patient who does not qualify for fibrinolytic therapy.

_____   **7.** Fibrinolytic therapy should begin within 2 hours after the AMI has occurred.

_____ **8.** Patients with diabetes experience incredible pain when suffering from ACS.

_____ **9.** The most common symptom of ACS is chest pain.

_____ **10.** Stable angina follows a recurrent pattern and usually occurs after exertion.

Fill in the Table

Fill in the missing parts of the table.

1. Role of electrolytes in cardiac function

Electrolyte	Role in Cardiac Function
_____	Flows into the cell to initiate depolarization
_____	Flows out of the cell to initiate _____ Decreased or increased levels of potassium result in the following: • _____ → increased myocardial irritability • _____ → decreased automaticity/conduction
_____	Has a major role in the depolarization of _____ cells (maintains depolarization) and in myocardial contractility (involved in contraction of heart muscle tissue) Decreased or increased levels of calcium result in the following: • _____ → decreased contractility and increased myocardial irritability • _____ → increased contractility
_____	Stabilizes the cell membrane; acts in concert with _____, and opposes the actions of calcium Decreased or increased levels of magnesium result in the following: • _____ → decreased conduction • _____ → increased myocardial irritability

Part 2: Heart Rhythms and the ECG

Matching

Part I

Match each of the items in the left column to the appropriate term in the right column.

_____ **1.** Where the "RA" (white) or "RL" (green) lead is traditionally placed by paramedics.

_____ **2.** Where the "LL" (red) lead is traditionally placed by paramedics.

_____ **3.** The point where the QRS complex ends and the ST segment begins.

_____ **4.** Represents ventricular repolarization on an ECG.

_____ **5.** A regular rhythm, 60 to 100 beats/min.

_____ **6.** SA node pacemaker with a rate of 100 beats/min or more.

_____ **7.** A rhythm in which the atria are contracting at a rate that is too fast for the ventricles to match.

_____ **8.** When an impulse reaching the AV node is delayed and results in a PR interval longer than 0.20 seconds.

_____ **9.** Rhythm that occurs when the ventricles take over at a rate of 20 to 40 beats/min.

_____ **10.** A delta wave is an indication of this condition.

A. First-degree AV block

B. Heart rate

C. Left lower chest

D. T wave

E. Atrial flutter

F. Tachycardia

G. Right upper shoulder

H. Wolff-Parkinson-White syndrome

I. J point

J. Idioventricular rhythm

Part II

Match each of the definitions in the left column to the appropriate term in the right column.

_____ 1. An inflammatory disease caused by streptococcal bacteria; the disease can cause mitral or aortic valve stenosis.

A. Pulmonary embolism

_____ 2. Dilation of the right atrium that occurs when returning venous pressure is elevated or pulmonary pressure is high.

B. Pulseless electrical activity

_____ 3. Artery that provides oxygenated blood to the walls of the right atrium and ventricle, a portion of the inferior part of the left ventricle, and portions of the conduction system.

C. Purkinje fibers

_____ 4. A condition in which the right side of the heart must work increasingly harder to pump blood into engorged pulmonary vessels; eventually, it is unable to keep up with the increased workload.

D. QRS axis

_____ 5. Treatment intended to facilitate the resumption of blood through a blocked vessel; therapy may be either procedural, such as cardiac catheterization, or pharmacologic, such as administration of a fibrinolytic agent.

E. QRS complex

_____ 6. A short period immediately after depolarization during which the myocytes have not yet repolarized and are unable to fire or conduct an impulse or have partially repolarized and may depolarize in response to an electrical stimulus.

F. Reciprocal changes

_____ 7. Spread of an impulse through tissue already stimulated by that same impulse.

G. Reentry

_____ 8. Mirror-image J-point, ST-segment, and T-wave changes seen on the ECG during ACS.

H. Refractory period

_____ 9. The use of a synchronized direct current electric shock to convert a tachydysrhythmia (such as supraventricular tachycardia) to a normal sinus rhythm.

I. Reperfusion therapy

_____ 10. A type of acute myocardial infarction in which the ischemic process affects only the inner layer of muscle.

J. Rheumatic fever

_____ 11. Angina pectoris characterized by periodic pain with a predictable pattern.

K. Right atrial abnormality

_____ 12. The interval between the end of the QRS complex (the J point) and the beginning of the T wave; when there is significant myocardial ischemia or injury, it is often depressed or elevated with respect to the isoelectric line on the ECG.

L. Right coronary artery

_____ 13. The thick wall that separates the right and left sides of the heart.

M. Right ventricular failure

_____ 14. A disease caused by the bacterium _Streptococcus pyogenes_ and characterized by a sore throat, fever, rash, and "strawberry tongue."

N. Right ventricular hypertrophy

_____ 15. The period between the onset of one QRS complex and the onset of the next QRS complex.

O. R-R interval

_____ 16. A cardiac condition in which the right ventricle becomes enlarged, usually as a result of pulmonary hypertension.

P. Scarlet fever

_____ 17. A single vector that represents the mean (or average) of all vectors created by the ventricles during depolarization.

Q. Septum

_____ 18. A network of cardiac muscle fibers distributed throughout the inner surfaces of the ventricular walls that conducts the excitation impulse from the bundle branches to the ventricular myocardium.

R. Sinoatrial node

_____ 19. An organized cardiac rhythm (other than ventricular tachycardia) on an ECG monitor that is not accompanied by any detectable pulse.

S. Sinus bradycardia

_____ 20. Obstruction in one or more pulmonary arteries by a solid, liquid, or gas that has swept through the right side of the heart into the lungs.

T. Sinus dysrhythmia

_____ 21. A sinus rhythm characterized by a heart rate greater than 100 beats/min.

U. Sinus tachycardia

_____ 22. A variation of cycling of a sinus rhythm that is often associated with respiratory cycle fluctuations; the rate increases during inspiration and decreases during expiration.

V. ST segment

_____ **23.** A sinus rhythm characterized by a heart rate of less than 60 beats/min.

_____ **24.** The dominant pacemaker of the heart, located at the junction of the superior vena cava and the right atrium.

_____ **25.** Deflection of the ECG produced by ventricular depolarization.

W. Stable angina

X. Subendocardial myocardial infarction

Y. Synchronized cardioversion

Multiple Choice

Read each item carefully, and then select the best response.

_____ **1.** _____ is an electrolyte imbalance that causes very tall and pointed T waves.

    A. Hypokalemia

    B. Hyperkalemia

    C. Hyperglycemia

    D. Hypocalcemia

_____ **2.** Lead _____ is NOT a limb lead.

    A. I

    B. aVR

    C. aVF

    D. V_2

_____ **3.** During an AMI, the stage of injury appears as a(n) _____ on the ECG.

    A. T-wave inversion

    B. ST-segment depression

    C. ST-segment elevation

    D. spiked P wave

_____ **4.** Lead V_5 is placed on the patient on the:

    A. anterior axillary line.

    B. midaxillary line.

    C. fourth intercostal space.

    D. left arm.

_____ **5.** _____ is NOT a possible cause of pulseless electrical activity.

    A. Hypovolemia

    B. Hyperthermia

    C. Cardiac tamponade

    D. Pulmonary embolism

_____ **6.** The signs and symptoms of sick sinus syndrome include all of the following, EXCEPT:

    A. dizziness.

    B. palpitation.

    C. bounding pulse.

    D. near-syncope.

_____ **7.** When using an automated external defibrillator (AED) to administer a shock, for safety, do each of the following, EXCEPT:

    A. ensure no one is touching the patient.

    B. do not defibrillate someone who is touching metal.

    C. place the defibrillation pad over the nitroglycerin patch.

    D. if the patient has an implanted pacemaker, place the defibrillation pad below the device.

_____ **8.** The correct term for the use of a defibrillator to end a dysrhythmia other than ventricular fibrillation (VF) or pulseless ventricular tachycardia (VT) is:

    A. cardioversion.

    B. transcutaneous cardiac pacing.

    C. defibrillation.

    D. conversion.

_____　**9.** A genetic condition in which the myocardial wall becomes very thick is called:

    A. Brugada syndrome.

    B. hypertrophic cardiomyopathy.

    C. long Q-T syndrome.

    D. Prinzmetal angina.

_____　**10.** One small box on the ECG strip represents _____ seconds.

    A. 0.04

    B. 0.40

    C. 0.02

    D. 0.20

Fill in the Blank

Read each item carefully, and then complete the statement by filling in the missing word(s).

1. _____ _____ occurs when the SA node fails to fire and initiate an impulse, which in turn eliminates an entire cardiac cycle. After the missed set, the normal function returns.

2. A tachycardic rhythm that begins in the pacemaker above the ventricles is known as a(n) _____ _____.

3. The SA node ceases to fire and the AV node (in the junction) takes over as the pacemaker; however, the rate is greater than 60 beats/min. This is called _____ _____ _____.

4. A(n) _____-_____ heart block occurs when no pulses move between the AV node and the ventricles. In such a case, the junctional or ventricular pacemaker runs the heart.

5. _____ _____ occurs when the entire heart begins to quiver without any organized contractions.

6. The pattern _____ occurs when there is a normal complex followed by a premature ventricular complex (PVC). This pattern repeats itself. If every third beat is a PVC, it is then called _____.

7. _____ occurs when the entire heart is at a standstill and there is no electrical activity.

8. A(n) _____ _____ is an indication of Wolff-Parkinson-White syndrome.

9. When a PVC comes from the same site, it is known as _____, but when the premature ventricular complexes come from different sites in the ventricles, the condition is known as _____.

10. The pacemaker is the SA node, but with a rate of less than 60 beats/min. This is called _____ _____.

True/False

If you believe the statement to be more true than false, write the letter "T" in the space provided. If you believe the statement to be more false than true, write the letter "F."

_____　**1.** When performing an ECG, the electrodes should be attached to the leads prior to placing them on the patient's skin.

_____　**2.** P waves indicate that the pacemaker for the heart is in the AV node.

_____　**3.** The "6-second method" is the simplest, but not the most accurate, method for determining the heart rate when the rhythm is slow.

_____　**4.** A heart rate of more than 100 beats/min is called tachycardia.

_____   **5.** Wandering atrial pacemaker is most commonly seen in patients with diabetes.

_____   **6.** Prehospital treatment of atrial fibrillation is common.

_____   **7.** Mobitz type I occurs when each successive impulse is delayed a little longer, until finally one impulse is not able to continue.

_____   **8.** The ventricles will take over as the pacemaker if the SA node fails.

_____   **9.** Polymorphic VT is more serious than monomorphic VT.

_____   **10.** An agonal rhythm will produce a pulse.

Short Answer

Complete this section with short written answers using the space provided.

1. Discuss the basic principles in placing electrodes on a patient's chest.

_____

_____

_____

2. Explain the causes of the P wave, PR interval, QRS complex, and T wave.

_____

_____

_____

3. Describe how a 12-lead ECG helps to "look" at the heart.

_____

_____

_____

4. What should you do if you find a patient in cardiac arrest?

_____

_____

_____

5. If you are able to terminate cardiopulmonary resuscitation (CPR) in the field, which steps should you and your medical director take before you implement your protocols to do so?

_____

_____

_____

Part 3: Putting It All Together and Practice ECG Strips

Matching

Match the generic name with the trade name for the following drugs.

_____	**1.** Amiodarone	**A.**	Capoten
_____	**2.** Metoprolol	**B.**	Lopressor
_____	**3.** Furosemide	**C.**	Inderal
_____	**4.** Digoxin	**D.**	Coumadin
_____	**5.** Captopril	**E.**	Lasix
_____	**6.** Propranolol	**F.**	Lanoxin
_____	**7.** Atorvastatin	**G.**	Nitrostat
_____	**8.** Warfarin	**H.**	Lipitor
_____	**9.** Verapamil	**I.**	Cordarone
_____	**10.** Nitroglycerin	**J.**	Calan

Labeling

Label the following diagrams with the correct terms.

1. Electrical conduction system

A. _____

B. _____

C. _____

D. _____

E. _____

F. _____

G. _____

© Jones & Bartlett Learning.

Fill in the Table

Fill in the missing parts of the table.

1. Components of the ECG

ECG Representation	Cardiac Event
P wave	Depolarization of the _____
PRI	Depolarization of the atria and delay at the _____ junction
QRS complex	Depolarization of the _____
ST segment	Period between ventricular depolarization and beginning of _____
T wave	Ventricular _____
R-R interval	Time between two _____ ventricular depolarizations

Ambulance Calls

Read each scenario, and then answer all the questions following the scenario.

1. You are called to see a 62-year-old man complaining of severe chest pain. He says that the pain came on an hour earlier and that it feels "like a thousand-pound weight on my chest." The patient is very restless and seems confused, so it is difficult to get much history. On physical examination, he is obviously in marked distress. His skin is pale and cold. His pulse is 82 beats/min and thready, respirations are 32 breaths/min and shallow, and blood pressure (BP) is 90/62 mm Hg. His oxygen saturation is 91% on room air.

   a. Identify the chief complaint and vital signs for this patient.

   Chief complaint:

   _____

   _____

   Vital signs:

   _____

   _____

   b. Which steps would you direct your partner to take at this time of the call?

   (1)_____

   (2)_____

   (3)_____

   (4)_____

   c. After your partner hooks up the monitor, you run a 3-lead ECG strip and see this:

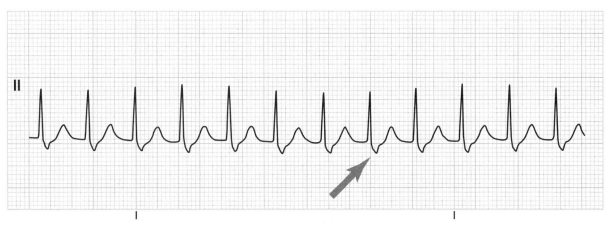

   Reproduced from *Arrhythmia Recognition: The Art of Interpretation*, courtesy of Tomas B.

   (1) Is the rhythm regular? _____

   (2) What is the rate? _____

   (3) Are the P waves present or absent? _____

   (4) If present, is there a P wave before every QRS? _____

   (5) P-R interval: _____ seconds

   (6) QRS complex width: _____

   (7) T waves present or absent? Upright? _____

   (8) What is the name of this rhythm? _____

d. Which field diagnosis will you give this patient and why?

_____

_____

_____

e. Which treatment will you provide for this patient?

_____

_____

_____

2. You are called to see a patient whose chief complaint is dyspnea. He tells you in gasps that for several nights he has been waking up around 0200 hours unable to breathe. He has to get up and sit on the side of the bed to catch his breath. Tonight, sitting up has not helped. "Must be those cigarettes," he wheezes. He tells you that he "keeps a cough," but lately he has been bringing up much more sputum than usual. On physical examination, the patient is in obvious respiratory distress, coughing periodically. His lips look rather blue. His pulse is 102 beats/min and irregular. His respirations are 60 breaths/min and labored, and his BP is 170/94 mm Hg in both arms. His neck veins are distended to the angle of the jaw. His chest is a veritable symphony of crackles and wheezes, and his oxygen saturation is 86% on room air. There is a tender fullness in the right upper quadrant of his abdomen. Both feet are swollen well above the ankles.

a. Identify the chief complaint and vital signs for this patient.
Chief complaint:

_____

Vital signs:

_____

_____

b. Which steps would you take at this point in the call?

(1)_____

(2)_____

(3)_____

(4)_____

c. What do you think the patient is experiencing?

_____

_____

d. What can you do to help this patient?

_____

_____

3. The family of a 76-year-old woman calls for an ambulance after the woman fainted while preparing Sunday dinner. The patient is lying on the sofa when you arrive. She is conscious but somewhat confused. She was unharmed in the fall. Your partner begins to take her vital signs as you try to get a history. The patient's pulse is 44 beats/min and regular, respirations are 22 breaths/min and full, and oxygen saturation is 94%. She says that she is having some pain in her chest but cannot rate the pain because of her confusion. Her BP is 82/40 mm Hg, and her skin is cool. Her lungs are clear, and she seems to be in good health otherwise. She takes a daily vitamin.

a. Identify the chief complaint and vital signs for this patient.

Chief complaint:

_____

_____

Vital signs:

_____

_____

b. List at least four causes of syncopal episodes.

(1)_____

(2)_____

(3)_____

(4)_____

c. You hook up the monitor and see sinus bradycardia. What is your treatment for this patient now?

(1)_____

(2)_____

d. If pharmacologic therapies do not help, what else can you do to raise the heart rate in this patient?

_____

_____

_____

4. A 64-year-old man calls for an ambulance because he has been "feeling poorly." His symptoms are not anything specific; they are nothing he can really pin down. He has just been feeling very weak and washed out for the last few days, so he thought perhaps he ought to go to the hospital and have a doctor take a look at him. There are no striking findings on physical exam except for an irregular heartbeat. The patient's pulse is about 76 beats/min but very irregular so that it is hard to count. His BP is 110/74 mm Hg on both arms. He has no significant history and has not been to a doctor except for a yearly checkup. His lungs are clear, and his oxygen saturation is 97%. His skin is a little cool. You hook up the heart monitor to take a quick peek, and this is what you see.

Reproduced from *Arrhythmia Recognition: The Art of Interpretation*, courtesy of Tomas B. Garcia, MD.

a. Identify the chief complaint and vital signs of this patient.
Chief complaint:

_____

Vital signs:

_____

_____

b. Answer the following questions.

   (1) Is the rhythm regular? _____

   (2) What is the rate? _____

   (3) Are the P waves present or absent? _____

   (4) If present, is there a P before every QRS? _____

   (5) Is there a QRS after every P? _____

   (6) P-R interval: _____

   (7) QRS complexes: _____ normal _____ abnormal

   (8) Name of rhythm: _____

   (9) Treatment: _____

5. You are taking a quick break at the emergency department (ED) after several hectic calls. You have made friends with the nurses, and they let you sit at the desk, where you can see the following heart monitors for different patients. Write the correct name of the rhythm on the line below the strip.

a. _____

b. _____

c. _____

Reproduced from *Arrhythmia Recognition: The Art of Interpretation*, courtesy of Tomas B. Garcia, MD.

d. _____

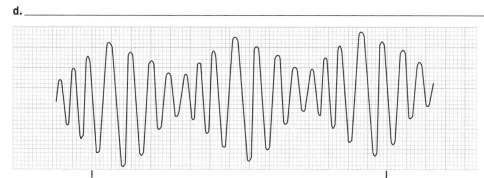

Reproduced from *Arrhythmia Recognition: The Art of Interpretation*, courtesy of Tomas B. Garcia, MD.

e. _____

Reproduced from *Arrhythmia Recognition: The Art of Interpretation*, courtesy of Tomas B. Garcia, MD.

f. _____

Reproduced from *Arrhythmia Recognition: The Art of Interpretation*, courtesy of Tomas B. Garcia, MD.

g. _____

Reproduced from *Arrhythmia Recognition: The Art of Interpretation*, courtesy of Tomas B. Garcia, MD.

h. _____

Modified from *Arrhythmia Recognition: The Art of Interpretation*, courtesy of Tomas B. Garcia, MD.

i. _____

P-P interval

Reproduced from *Arrhythmia Recognition: The Art of Interpretation*, courtesy of Tomas B. Garcia, MD.

j. _____

Reproduced from *Arrhythmia Recognition: The Art of Interpretation*, courtesy of Tomas B. Garcia, MD.

k. _____

l. _____

m. _____

n. _____

o. _____

p. _____

q. _____

r. _____

6. The nurse hands you the following three strips and asks you if you can figure out which type of ectopic beat is present in each strip.

a. _____

b. _____

Reproduced from *Arrhythmia Recognition: The Art of Interpretation*, courtesy of Tomas B. Garcia, MD.

c. _____

Short Answer

1. How many seconds, or portions of a second, does a small box on an ECG graph paper represent? _____

2. How many small boxes does it take to make a large box on the ECG graph paper? _____

3. List the signs and symptoms that are present during a tachycardia that would make the patient "symptomatic" and a candidate for electric cardioversion.

   a. _____

   b. _____

   c. _____

   d. _____

   e. _____

4. What is the initial drug of choice when dealing with patients with a stable tachycardia and a regular rhythm that is not breaking with a trial of vagal maneuvers?

   _____

5. Which drug would be a consideration in a patient with a wide-complex stable tachycardia (ie, possible VT)?

   _____

   _____

6. You are faced with a patient who has a third-degree heart block and a heart rate of 48 beats/min. The patient shows signs of poor perfusion. After starting an IV, what would you do next?

   _____

7. List the initial correct dosage of medication in the following scenarios.
   a. Epinephrine in the care of a patient in cardiac arrest: _____
   b. Epinephrine for a conscious patient with a bradycardia and poor perfusion: _____
   c. Adenosine for a patient with stable, narrow, regular QRS tachycardia with pulses: _____
   d. Amiodarone for a patient with stable, wide-complex tachycardia or PVCs in salvos: _____

8. List the Hs and Ts that you should be thinking about during a cardiac arrest.

H _____   T _____

H _____   T _____

H _____   T _____

H _____   T _____

H _____

H _____

Problem Solving

Practice your calculation skills by solving the following math problems.

1. Suppose a person at rest has a heart rate of 72 beats/min and a stroke volume of 75 mL/beat. What is his cardiac output? _____ mL/min

2. Now that same person is running to catch a bus. His heart speeds up to 100 beats/min, and his stroke volume increases to 90 mL/beat. What is his cardiac output now? _____ mL/min

3. You often need to use your knowledge of anatomy, physiology, and pathophysiology to problem-solve situations you are presented with and arrive at a working field diagnosis. In this case, take the given signs or symptoms and quickly decide if the patient could have left- or right-sided heart failure. Place an L for left-sided and an R for right-sided heart failure before the following signs and symptoms.

a. _____ Dyspnea

b. _____ Jugular vein distention

c. _____ Swelling of the feet

d. _____ Crackles on auscultation

e. _____ Hepatomegaly

f. _____ Sacral edema

g. _____ Pink, frothy sputum

4. Find the MAP for the following blood pressures.

a. 160/94 mm Hg _____

b. 200/126 mm Hg _____

c. 148/86 mm Hg _____

Practice ECG Strips

Examine each of the following ECG strips, and state the rate, the rhythm, and the significant findings for each.

1.

Reproduced from *12-Lead ECG: The Art of Interpretation, courtesy* of Tomas B. Garcia, MD.

Rate: _____

Rhythm: _____

Significant findings: _____

2.

Reproduced from *12-Lead ECG: The Art of Interpretation, courtesy* of Tomas B. Garcia, MD.

Rate: _____

Rhythm: _____

Significant findings: _____

3.

Reproduced from *12-Lead ECG: The Art of Interpretation*, courtesy of Tomas B. Garcia, MD.

Rate: _____

Rhythm: _____

Significant findings: _____

4.

Reproduced from *12-Lead ECG: The Art of Interpretation*, courtesy of Tomas B. Garcia, MD.

Rate: _____

Rhythm: _____

Significant findings: _____

5.

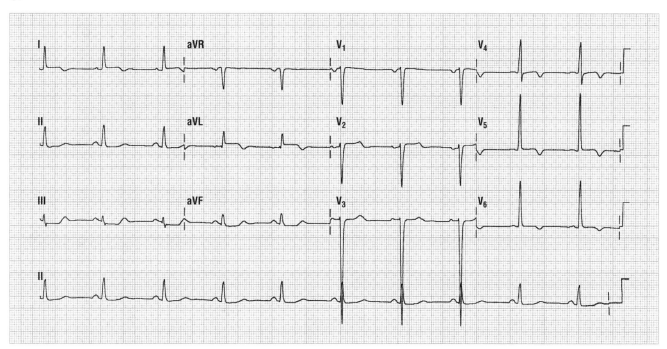

Reproduced from *12-Lead ECG: The Art of Interpretation*, courtesy of Tomas B. Garcia, MD.

Rate: _____

Rhythm: _____

Significant findings: _____

6.

Reproduced from *12-Lead ECG: The Art of Interpretation*, courtesy of Tomas B. Garcia, MD.

Rate: _____

Rhythm: _____

Significant findings: _____

7.

Reproduced from *12-Lead ECG: The Art of Interpretation*, courtesy of Tomas B. Garcia, MD.

Rate: _____

Rhythm: _____

Significant findings: _____

8.

Reproduced from *12-Lead ECG: The Art of Interpretation*, courtesy of Tomas B. Garcia, MD.

Rate: _____

Rhythm: _____

Significant findings: _____

9.

Reproduced from *12-Lead ECG: The Art of Interpretation*, courtesy of Tomas B. Garcia, MD.

Rate: _____

Rhythm: _____

Significant findings: _____

10.

Reproduced from *12-Lead ECG: The Art of Interpretation*, courtesy of Tomas B. Garcia, MD.

Rate: _____

Rhythm: _____

Significant findings: _____

11.

Reproduced from *12-Lead ECG: The Art of Interpretation,* courtesy of Tomas B. Garcia, MD.

Rate: _____

Rhythm: _____

Significant findings: _____

12.

Reproduced from *12-Lead ECG: The Art of Interpretation,* courtesy of Tomas B. Garcia, MD.

Rate: _____

Rhythm: _____

Significant findings: _____

13.

Reproduced from *12-Lead ECG: The Art of Interpretation*, courtesy of Tomas B. Garcia, MD.

Rate: _____

Rhythm: _____

Significant findings: _____

14.

Reproduced from *12-Lead ECG: The Art of Interpretation*, courtesy of Tomas B. Garcia, MD.

Rate: _____

Rhythm: _____

Significant findings: _____

15.

Reproduced from *12-Lead ECG: The Art of Interpretation*, courtesy of Tomas B. Garcia, MD.

Rate: _____

Rhythm: _____

Significant findings: _____

16.

Reproduced from *12-Lead ECG: The Art of Interpretation*, courtesy of Tomas B. Garcia, MD.

Rate: _____

Rhythm: _____

Significant findings: _____

17.

Reproduced from *12-Lead ECG: The Art of Interpretation*, courtesy of Tomas B. Garcia, MD.

Rate: _____

Rhythm: _____

Significant findings: _____

18.

Reproduced from *12-Lead ECG: The Art of Interpretation*, courtesy of Tomas B. Garcia, MD.

Rate: _____

Rhythm: _____

Significant findings: _____

19.

Reproduced from *12-Lead ECG: The Art of Interpretation*, courtesy of Tomas B. Garcia, MD.

Rate: _____

Rhythm: _____

Significant findings: _____

20.

Reproduced from *12-Lead ECG: The Art of Interpretation*, courtesy of Tomas B. Garcia, MD.

Rate: _____

Rhythm: _____

Significant findings: _____

Neurologic Emergencies

Matching

Part I

For each of the following items, indicate the letter that corresponds to each definition.

_____	**1.** A temporary paralysis of the facial nerve (cranial nerve VII), which controls the muscles on each side of the face.	**A.** Abscess
_____	**2.** Sensations commonly experienced before a seizure or migraine headache occurs; may include visual changes in addition to hallucinations.	**B.** Alzheimer disease
_____	**3.** Alteration in the ability to perform coordinated motions such as walking.	**C.** Amyotrophic lateral sclerosis
_____	**4.** Unequal pupils with a difference of greater than 1 mm.	**D.** Anesthesia
_____	**5.** Paralysis of one side of the body.	**E.** Anisocoria
_____	**6.** Weakness of one side of the body.	**F.** Ataxia
_____	**7.** Sensory stimulation that cannot be verified by others.	**G.** Aura
_____	**8.** A rare condition that begins as a sensation of weakness and tingling in the legs, moving to the arms and the thorax; the disorder can lead to paralysis within 2 weeks.	**H.** Bell palsy
_____	**9.** The slow, progressive onset of disorientation, shortened attention span, and loss of cognitive function.	**I.** Bradykinesia
_____	**10.** Thoughts, ideas, or perceived abilities that have no basis in common reality.	**J.** Clonic activity
_____	**11.** Abnormal flexion of the arms toward the chest with the toes pointed; this finding indicates lower cerebral damage.	**K.** Coma
_____	**12.** Abnormal extension of the arms with rotation of the wrists along with the toes pointed; this finding indicates brainstem damage.	**L.** Common reality
_____	**13.** An area in the brain or spinal cord in which cells have been attacked, typically by an infectious agent. To prevent the spread of infection, the immune system "walls off" the area. Pus can collect.	**M.** Corneal reflex
_____	**14.** A progressive, organic condition in which neurons in the brain die, causing dementia.	**N.** Decerebrate posturing
_____	**15.** A condition that strikes the voluntary motor neurons, causing their death. The disease is characterized by fatigue and general weakness of muscle groups; eventually the patient becomes unable to walk, eat, or speak; also known as Lou Gehrig disease.	**O.** Decorticate posturing
_____	**16.** Lack of feeling within a body part.	**P.** Delusions
_____	**17.** A protective movement that results in blinking, moving the head posteriorly, and pupillary constriction.	**Q.** Dementia

_____ **18.** Sensory stimulation that can be verified by others.

_____ **19.** A state in which a person does not respond to either verbal or painful stimuli.

_____ **20.** Type of seizure movement involving the contraction and relaxation of muscle groups.

_____ **21.** Patterns of walking or ambulating.

_____ **22.** The slowing down of voluntary body movements; found in patients with Parkinson disease.

_____ **23.** A toxin released by some bacteria when they die.

_____ **24.** A toxin secreted by living cells to aid in the death and digestion of other cells.

_____ **25.** Contractions of body into bizarre positions.

R. Dystonia

S. Endotoxin

T. Exotoxin

U. Gait

V. Guillain-Barré syndrome

W. Hallucinations

X. Hemiparesis

Y. Hemiplegia

Part II

For each of the following items, indicate the letter that corresponds to each definition.

_____ **1.** A tumor.

_____ **2.** Involuntary jerking motions of the body.

_____ **3.** A condition in which the body generates antibodies against its own acetylcholine receptors, causing muscle weakness, often in the face.

_____ **4.** An autoimmune condition in which the body attacks the myelin that insulates the brain and spinal cord, causing scarring.

_____ **5.** The process by which cells from a malignant neoplasm break away from the site of origin, such as the lung, and move through the bloodstream or lymphatic system to other body sites, such as the brain.

_____ **6.** A tremor that occurs when the body part is not in motion.

_____ **7.** Prolapse of a body part; often refers to drooping of the eyelid.

_____ **8.** Breaking with common reality and existing mainly within an internal world.

_____ **9.** Rotation of the lower arms in a palms-down manner.

_____ **10.** An early sign or symptom that occurs before a disease or condition fully appears (eg, dizziness before fainting).

_____ **11.** A group of conditions in which the nerves that exit the spinal cord are damaged, distorting signals to or from the brain. One type is caused by diabetes; peripheral nerves are damaged as the blood glucose level rises, resulting in lack of sensation, numbness, burning, pain, paresthesia, and muscle weakness.

_____ **12.** A neurologic condition in which the portion of the brain responsible for production of dopamine has been damaged or overused, resulting in tremors.

_____ **13.** Sensation of tingling or numbness in a body part.

14. Involuntary, rhythmic shaking of the eyes.

_____ **15.** Structures within the cerebrum and diencephalon that influence emotions, motivation, mood, and sensations of pain and pleasure.

_____ **16.** The wavelike movement of a seizure from a point of focus to other areas of the brain.

_____ **17.** One of the two main types of stroke, also called an occlusive stroke; occurs when blood flow to a particular part of the brain is cut off by a blockage such as a blood clot, within an artery.

_____ **18.** A tremor that occurs when trying to accomplish a task.

A. Hemorrhagic stroke

B. Idiopathic

C. Intention tremor

D. Ischemic stroke

E. Jacksonian march

F. Limbic system

G. Metastasis

H. Multiple sclerosis

I. Myasthenia gravis

J. Myoclonus

K. Neoplasm

L. Nystagmus

M. Paresthesia

N. Parkinson disease

O. Peripheral neuropathy

P. Poliomyelitis

Q. Postictal

R. Post-polio syndrome

_____ **19.** Of no known cause.

S. Postural tremor

_____ **20.** One of the two main types of stroke; occurs as a result of bleeding inside the brain.

T. Posturing

_____ **21.** Abnormal body positioning that indicates damage to the brain.

U. Prodrome

_____ **22.** A tremor that occurs as the person holds a body part still.

V. Pronation

_____ **23.** The death of nerve fibers as a late consequence of poliomyelitis; characterized by swallowing difficulties, weakness, fatigue, and breathing problems.

W. Psychosis

_____ **24.** A now-rare viral infection that attacks and destroys nerve axons, especially motor axons; the disease can cause weakness, paralysis, and respiratory arrest.

X. Ptosis

_____ **25.** The period after a seizure in which the brain is reorganizing activity.

Y. Rest tremor

Multiple Choice

Read each item carefully, and then select the best response.

_____ **1.** The nervous system is responsible for all of the following functions, EXCEPT:

    A. pulse rate.

    B. blood pressure.

    C. breathing.

    D. heart rhythm.

_____ **2.** What area of the brain acts as a relay center to filter and prioritize the information that you need for conscious thought?

    A. Pons

    B. Medulla oblongata

    C. Diencephalon

    D. Mid stem

_____ **3.** Which of the following acts as "insulation" around the axon?

    A. Myelin

    B. Neuron

    C. Diencephalon

    D. Neurotransmitter

_____ **4.** When the brain receives too much oxygen, it can cause increased intracranial pressure (ICP). What happens to the cerebral arteries during this time?

    A. They vasodilate.

    B. They vasoconstrict.

    C. They leak blood.

    D. They remain normal.

_____ **5.** You respond to a collision in which a woman has been thrown from a vehicle. She is unconscious; her arms are curled to her chest, and her toes are pointed. How would you describe her position?

    A. Trismus posture

    B. Decerebrate posture

    C. Decorticate posture

    D. Pronation posture

_____ **6.** Pupils may be changed by many different things. Which of the following does NOT change the shape of a patient's pupils?

    A. Drugs

    B. Trauma

    C. Seizure

    D. Increased ICP

_____ **7.** You are treating a 22-year-old male who is having a seizure. At this time, he is still except for his left arm, which is rocking back and forth in a rhythmic motion. What is the correct term for this activity?

    A. Clonic activity

    B. Tonic activity

    C. Intension tremors

    D. Paresthesia

_____ **8.** Which subdivision of the brain is responsible for judgment and prediction of the consequences of actions?

    A. Occipital

    B. Temporal

    C. Frontal

    D. Limbic system

_____ **9.** Your patient suffers from an autoimmune disorder in which the body attacks the myelin sheath. What is this called?

    A. Dystonia

    B. Parkinson disease

    C. Trigeminal neuralgia

    D. Multiple sclerosis

_____ **10.** What is the correct term for a temporary paralysis of the seventh cranial nerve?

    A. Guillain-Barré syndrome

    B. Bell palsy

    C. Poliomyelitis

    D. Myasthenia gravis

Labeling

Label the following diagrams with the correct terms.

1. Pupil responses

1. _____

2. _____

3. _____

4. _____

A. Normal
B. Constricted (pinpoint)
C. Dilated
D. Unequal

Fill in the Blank

Read each item carefully, and then complete the statement by filling in the missing word(s).

1. A neurotransmitter is a chemical released into a(n) _____ that helps make the connection between one _____ and another.

2. _____ respirations are gradually _____ and decreases in respirations with periods of _____.

3. When gram-negative bacteria die inside our body, they release a protein that is called a(n) _____.

4. The skull is filled with three substances: the _____, _____, and _____ _____.

5. When a patient has increased ICP, the heart rate and respiratory rate will _____, and the blood pressure (BP) will _____.

6. Kussmaul respirations are _____ tachypnea and _____.

7. _____ activity is a rigid contracted _____ posture.

8. _____ is the fuel for our brain. A normal reading is _____ mg/dL.

9. There are two types of strokes: _____ and _____.

10. There are two types of generalized seizures: _____ and _____.

Identify

After reading the following case study, list the chief complaint, vital signs, and pertinent negatives.

You are called to a middle-class home for a 32-year-old man. He is alert and can answer all your questions. His main complaint is general weakness; he is unable to stand or squeeze your hands. His symptoms started this morning around 0900 hours and have intensified over the last 6 hours. He is having visual disturbances and doesn't want to open his eyes because the double vision he is experiencing is making him nauseous. You begin your assessment with vital signs and a SAMPLE history. His blood pressure (BP) is 128/76 mm Hg, and his pulse is 84 beats/min and regular. He has no allergies and takes no medications. His lungs are clear, and his oxygen saturation is 95% on room air. Because you are still not sure what is going on and his SpO_2 is borderline, you place him on a nasal cannula at 4 L/min. Blood glucose check is 112 mg/dL, and he had a light lunch of a sandwich and soup around noon. He has no history of any illness and appears to be a very healthy individual. You question him about sustaining any trauma, and he denies that he has suffered any in the last year. He does not have a headache or any pain anywhere in his body. He has no signs of any infections. You and your partner have spent a lot of time on scene looking for clues as to what is happening to him. One thing you are both sure of is that he needs to be seen at the emergency department (ED). You provide supportive care and start an IV line as a medication line in case the patient happens to get worse. Later, you check in on the patient and find out they are leaning toward a diagnosis of multiple sclerosis.

1. Chief complaint:

   _____

   _____

2. Vital signs:

   _____

   _____

3. Pertinent negatives:

_____

_____

Complete the Patient Care Report (PCR)

Read the incident scenario in the "Identify" exercise, and then complete the following PCR.

EMS Patient Care Report (PCR)					
Date:	**Incident No.:**	**Nature of Call:**		**Location:**	
Dispatched:	**En Route:**	**At Scene:**	**Transport:**	**At Hospital:**	**In Service:**
Patient Information					
Age: **Sex:** **Weight (in kg [lb]):**		**Allergies:** **Medications:** **Past Medical History:** **Chief Complaint:**			
Vital Signs					
Time:	**BP:**	**Pulse:**	**Respirations:**		**SpO₂:**
Time:	**BP:**	**Pulse:**	**Respirations:**		**SpO₂:**
Time:	**BP:**	**Pulse:**	**Respirations:**		**SpO₂:**
EMS Treatment **(circle all that apply)**					
Oxygen @ _____ L/min via (circle one): **NC NRM Bag-mask device**		**Assisted Ventilation**	**Airway Adjunct**		**CPR**
Defibrillation	**Bleeding Control**	**Bandaging**	**Splinting**		**Other:**
Narrative					

Ambulance Calls

The following case scenarios provide an opportunity to explore the concerns associated with patient management and paramedic care. Read each scenario, and then answer each question.

1. You receive a call for a patient having seizures. This time it is one of the city's homeless whom the police found lying in an alley. He is having a generalized motor seizure when you arrive. It lasts about 3 minutes and then subsides. You quickly open the airway by jaw lift, start supplemental oxygen, and prepare to start an IV line, but before you can do so, the patient has another generalized motor seizure that lasts about 3 minutes.

   a. Urgent treatment measures will take priority over the secondary assessment. When you do get around to examining this patient, what will you look for in particular?

   (1)_____

   (2)_____

   (3)_____

   (4)_____

   (5)_____

   (6)_____

   (7)_____

   (8)_____

   (9)_____

   (10)_____

   b. List the steps in the prehospital management of this patient.

   (1)_____

   (2)_____

   (3)_____

   (4)_____

   c. What medication is given in the field for repeated seizures? (You may need to refer to the Emergency Medications appendix.)

   _____

   _____

   (1) What are the contraindications to this medication?

   _____

   _____

   (2) What is the correct dosage in the present situation, and how is it administered?

   _____

   _____

   (3) What possible adverse side effects might occur when administering this medicine?

   _____

   _____

2. You are called to the home of a 68-year-old woman for a "possible stroke." Arriving at the scene, you are greeted at the door by the woman's daughter. "I phoned and phoned all morning," she says, "and when no one answered, I figured I'd better come and check. I found Mother lying in the bathroom." You proceed to the bathroom, where you find the patient lying on the floor. She is conscious but does not seem to be able to answer your questions—she just makes garbled noises. Her skin is warm and dry. Her vital signs are a pulse of 70 beats/min and slightly irregular, respirations of 20 breaths/min and unlabored, and a BP of 190/120 mm Hg. During the physical exam, you find no evidence of head injury, but the woman's face looks a bit lopsided, and tears are streaming down. The pupils are 4 mm, equal, and reactive. The gag reflex is absent. The right arm and right leg are flaccid. There is no evidence of injury.

a. Do you think the patient is right-handed or left-handed? _____
How did you reach that conclusion?

_____

_____

b. List the steps in treating this patient.

(1)_____

(2)_____

(3)_____

(4)_____

(5)_____

(6)_____

3. You are called to a department store where a woman who appears to be about 60 years old has been found unconscious in the ladies' restroom.

a. List nine possible causes of coma.

(1)_____

(2)_____

(3)_____

(4)_____

(5)_____

(6)_____

(7)_____

(8)_____

(9)_____

b. Now list eight things you would do to manage this comatose woman.

(1)_____

(2)_____

(3)_____

(4)_____

(5)_____

(6)_____

(7)_____

(8)_____

True/False

If you believe the statement to be more true than false, write the letter "T" in the space provided. If you believe the statement to be more false than true, write the letter "F."

_____ 1. The peripheral nervous system is responsible for conducting nerve impulses between the brain and the body.

_____ 2. Normal CPP is 70 to 90 mmHg.

_____ 3. The respiratory pattern that involves extreme tachypnea and hyperpnea is called Cheyne-Stokes.

_____ 4. The medical term for cancer is neoplasm.

_____ 5. The respiratory pattern that involves rapid, regular, deep respirations is called hyperpnea.

_____ 6. The average MAP is 100 to 120 mm Hg.

_____ 7. Trismus may result from head trauma, cerebral hypoxia, and seizures.

_____ 8. When you assess a stroke patient, you can ask the person to smile. This will show if the patient has ptosis.

_____ 9. By stimulating the cough or gag reflex in a patient, you can decrease ICP.

_____ 10. Syncope is caused by a brief interruption in cerebral blood flow.

_____ 11. Hyperglycemic patients do not need any fluid, so you must make sure to give less than 100 mL of fluid.

_____ 12. The Cincinnati Prehospital Stroke Scale uses a six-part criteria scale to assess for a stroke.

_____ 13. A little over one-third of the patients who have a transient ischemic attack (TIA) will have a stroke soon after the initial event.

_____ 14. An aura will usually precede a generalized (grand mal) seizure.

Short Answer

Complete this section with short written answers using the space provided.

1. Define the following vocabulary words:
   a. Hemiparesis

   _____

   _____

   b. Pseudoseizures

   _____

   _____

2. Over the course of a week of ambulance runs, you have found two patients in a coma. You don't have any information about either of them except for the medications found at the scene or on the patient's person. Nonetheless, based on those medications and assessment, you can make an educated guess at least as to each patient's underlying illnesses. For each of the comatose patients whose medications are listed here, indicate the most probable underlying illness(es).

a. Patient 1 is carrying phenobarbital (Luminal) and phenytoin (Dilantin) in her purse.

Probable underlying illness(es): _____

b. Patient 2 is carrying insulin.

Probable underlying illness: _____

Fill in the Table

Fill in the missing parts of the table.

1. Fill in the table with the missing types of dystonias.

Type	Presentation
	Most common form of focal dystonia; intermittent, patterned, repetitive, spasmodic motion of the head in a twisting, flexing, extending, or tilting manner; can involve more than one motion type
	Deviation of the eyes in any direction, usually with eyes strained toward the top of the head
	Forceful contractions of the face, which can involve the tongue darting in and out of the mouth
Blepharospasm	
	Slow, writhing motions commonly involving the face and distal extremities
	Cramping of the hands, elbows, and arms (eg, graphospasm [writer's cramp])
	Quick, jerky, irregular, and unpredictable movements; often found in the face, arms, and hands
Spasmodic dysphonia	

2. Complete the following list of common causes of seizures.

Birth anomaly
Hypertension during pregnancy (eclampsia)
Idiopathic (of no known cause)
Systematic infection

3. Fill in the names of the cranial nerves.

Cranial Nerve	Function
I. _____	Smell
II. _____	Vision
III. _____	Movement of the eye, pupil, and eyelid
IV. _____	Movement of the eye
V. _____	Chewing
	Pain
	Temperature
	Touch of the mouth and face
VI. _____	Movement of the eye
VII. _____	Movement of the face
	Tears
	Salivation and taste
VII. _____	Hearing and balance
IX. _____	Swallowing, taste, and sensation in the mouth and pharynx
X. _____	Sensation and movement of the pharynx, larynx, thorax, and gastrointestinal (GI) system
XI. _____	Movement of the head and shoulders
XII. _____	Movement of the tongue

Problem Solving

Read the following scenario, and then list the portions of the scenario under the correct stroke scale or stroke screen.

You respond to a 69-year-old woman. Her daughter is waiting at the door for you when you arrive. Dispatch information said that the woman might be having a stroke. You enter the room to find "Betty" sitting in her recliner with her feet up. She acknowledges your entrance. "Hi, Mrs. Smith, my name is Jake Johnson, and my partner is Julie Barnes. We are paramedics, and I am here at the request of your daughter. Can you tell me what is wrong today?" Mrs. Smith responds by telling you that her name is Betty, and she doesn't think anything is wrong with her. Her daughter is always fussing over her. You tell Betty that is because her daughter loves her and say that if Betty loves her daughter, she should be smiling about all the attention. Betty does respond with a smile, but the right side of her face doesn't respond as well as the left. Julie asks permission to do a set of vital signs, and Betty says to go right ahead. Julie gets a BP of 136/82 mm Hg, a pulse of 86 beats/min and regular, oxygen saturation of 97% on room air, and respirations of 18 breaths/min. Lung sounds are clear. She checks Betty's blood glucose, which is 110 mg/dL. During this time, you ask Betty to say "You can't teach an old dog new tricks." However, Betty can't seem to get the sentence out very clearly. You proceed by having Betty squeeze both your hands at the same time. Her grip strength is about half strength in the right arm. You then ask her to close her eyes and hold both arms up straight. When she does this, her right arm drifts downward. You then ask Betty and her daughter how long she has been having these symptoms. Betty's daughter says that she had no problems this morning when she was up fixing breakfast at 0800, but she says she began to notice a few minor things around 1100, which is when she decided to call 9-1-1. You take a SAMPLE history and find that Betty has never had any medical problems at all; she takes only a vitamin every morning. Both you and Julie feel she should be seen in the ED, and Betty agrees to go with you. You prepare to take Betty in.

You and Julie did a great job using both the Cincinnati Prehospital Stroke Scale and the Los Angles Prehospital Stroke Screen Assessments. Write the portions of the preceding scenario under the correct assessments. Remember, the same action might be on both assessments.

1. Cincinnati Prehospital Stroke Scale

    a. _____

    b. _____

    c. _____

2. Los Angles Prehospital Stroke Screen

   a. _____

   b. _____

   c. _____

   d. _____

   e. _____

   f. _____

   g. _____

   h. _____

Diseases of the Eyes, Ears, Nose, and Throat

Can you tell me what is wrong?

Maybe we should ask how Mr. Smith likes to communicate?

Can you hear me now?

© Jones & Bartlett Learning.

Matching

Match each of the items in the left column to the appropriate definition in the right column.

_____ 1. Swelling and inflammation of the larynx that is associated with hoarseness or loss of voice.

_____ 2. Irritation and swelling in the inner ear that produces a loss of balance and possibly tinnitus, dizziness, loss of hearing, nausea, and vomiting.

_____ 3. Inflammation of the iris; also called anterior uveitis.

_____ 4. A red, tender lump in the eyelid or at the lid margin; commonly known as a stye.

_____ 5. A group of conditions that lead to increased intraocular pressure, causing damage to the optic nerve; a leading cause of blindness.

_____ 6. A condition that presents as white lesions on the tongue and inner cheeks, caused by the fungus *Candida albicans*; also called thrush.

_____ 7. Either of the second cranial nerves that enter the eyeball posteriorly; through the optic foramen.

_____ 8. A device used to examine the fundus of the eye.

_____ 9. Third cranial nerve; it innervates the muscles that cause motion of the eyeballs and upper eyelids.

_____ 10. An inner ear disorder in which endolymphatic rupture creates increased pressure in the cochlear duct, which then leads to damage to the organ of Corti and the semicircular canal; symptoms include severe vertigo, tinnitus, and sensorineural hearing loss.

_____ 11. A condition in which the pupils are not of equal size.

_____ 12. Bruising over the mastoid bone behind the ear, commonly seen following a basilar skull fracture; also called retroauricular ecchymosis.

_____ 13. A clouding of the lens of the eye that is normally a result of aging.

_____ 14. Cerebrospinal fluid drainage from the nose.

_____ 15. Earwax.

_____ 16. A type of cellulitis that occurs on the floor of the mouth under the tongue; it is caused by bacteria from an infected tooth root (tooth abscess) or mouth injury.

_____ 17. A condition associated with diabetes, in which the small blood vessels of the retina are affected; it can eventually lead to blindness.

_____ 18. Paralysis of gaze or lack of coordination between the movements of the two eyes.

_____ 19. Pain when swallowing.

A. Anisocoria

B. Battle sign

C. Cataract

D. Cerebrospinal rhinorrhea

E. Cerumen

F. Chalazion

G. Conjunctivitis

H. Dental abscess

I. Dentalgia

J. Diabetic retinopathy

K. Dysconjugate gaze

L. Dysphagia

M. Epiglottitis

N. Epistaxis

O. Glaucoma

P. Hordeolum

Q. Iritis

R. Labyrinthitis

S. Laryngitis

_____ **20.** An inflammation of the epiglottis.

_____ **21.** Nosebleed.

_____ **22.** Toothache.

_____ **23.** A collection of pus that forms in the gums, facial tissue, bones, and/or neck.

_____ **24.** An inflammation of the conjunctivae of the eye that usually is caused by bacteria, viruses, allergies, or foreign bodies; it should be considered highly contagious. Also called pinkeye.

_____ **25.** A small, swollen bump or pustule on the external eyelid, which arises when the eyelid's oil glands or ducts become blocked.

T. Ludwig angina

U. Meniere disease

V. Oculomotor nerve

W. Ophthalmoscope

X. Optic nerve

Y. Oral candidiasis

Multiple Choice

Read each item carefully, and then select the best response.

_____ **1.** The nerve that innervates the muscles that cause motion of the eyeballs and upper eyelids, as well as constriction of the pupil, is the _____ nerve.

    A. optic

    B. oculomotor

    C. trigeminal

    D. vagus

_____ **2.** The _____ chamber of the globe is filled with _____ humor, which is a clear, watery fluid.

    A. anterior; vitreous

    B. anterior; aqueous

    C. posterior; vitreous

    D. posterior; aqueous

_____ **3.** Symptoms that may indicate a serious ocular condition include all of the following, EXCEPT:

    A. visual loss.

    B. double vision.

    C. lack of eye pain.

    D. a foreign body sensation.

_____ **4.** Physical exam of the eyes includes assessment of the visible ocular structures, including:

    A. globes.

    B. corneas.

    C. eyelids.

    D. All of the above

_____ **5.** A group of conditions that leads to increased intraocular pressure and that is one of the leading causes of blindness is:

    A. hyphema.

    B. retinal detachment.

    C. glaucoma.

    D. papilledema.

_____ **6.** When examining the eyes, ocular motility involves checking for:

    A. peripheral vision.

    B. dysconjugate gaze.

    C. orbital rim.

    D. visual acuity.

_____ **7.** Of the following components of the ear, which is NOT in the middle ear?

    A. Tympanic membrane

    B. Ossicles

    C. Cochlea

    D. Malleus

_____ **8.** The feeling of vertigo or loss of balance after an ear infection or upper respiratory infection is MOST likely attributable to:

    A. impacted cerumen.

    B. Meniere disease.

    C. otitis.

    D. labyrinthitis.

_____ **9.** An inner ear disorder that usually affects adults and in which there is ultimately damage to the organ of Corti and the semicircular canal is:

    A. Meniere disease.

    B. labyrinthitis.

    C. perforated tympanic membrane.

    D. barotrauma.

_____ **10.** You are treating a 10-year-old boy who has the chills, difficulty opening his mouth, and pain with opening of the mouth. He denies any trauma, although he appears to have facial swelling and is drooling and speaking with a muffled voice. What is MOST likely his condition?

    A. Tonsillitis

    B. Peritonsillar abscess

    C. Pharyngitis

    D. Tracheitis

_____ **11.** All of the following are considered medical conditions of the ear, EXCEPT:

    A. impacted cerumen.

    B. labyrinthitis.

    C. glaucoma.

    D. Meniere disease.

_____ **12.** Which of the following is a specific medical problem related to the nose?

    A. Dentalgia

    B. Thrush

    C. Otitis

    D. Sinusitis

Labeling

Label the following diagrams with the correct terms.

1. Structures of the eye

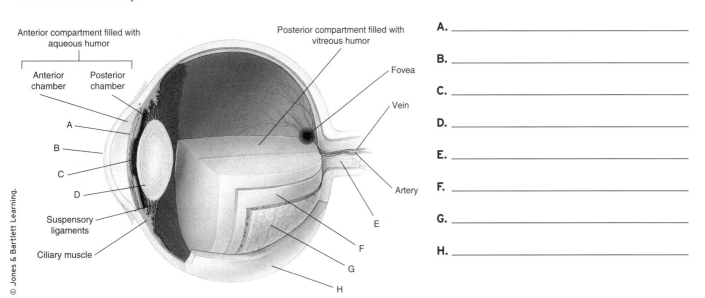

A. _____

B. _____

C. _____

D. _____

E. _____

F. _____

G. _____

H. _____

2. Structures of the ear

A. _____

B. _____

C. _____

D. _____

E. _____

F. _____

G. _____

H. _____

I. _____

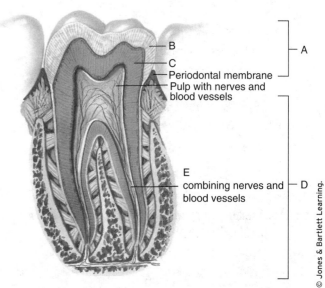

External ear   Middle ear   Inner ear

A

B

C

D

Oval window

Vestibular nerve

Cochlear nerve

E

Vestibule

Round window

F

I   H   G

Ossicles

© Jones & Bartlett Learning.

3. Structure of a tooth

A. _____

B. _____

C. _____

D. _____

E. _____

B

C

Periodontal membrane

Pulp with nerves and blood vessels

A

E

combining nerves and blood vessels

D

© Jones & Bartlett Learning.

Fill in the Blank

Read each item carefully, and then complete the statement by filling in the missing word(s).

1. Assess the _____ for ecchymosis, _____, lacerations, and any abnormalities.

2. You may encounter patients who wear _____ _____. In general, if the eye is injured, you should not attempt to

   _____ contact lenses because you may further aggravate the injury.

3. Practitioners may use a(n) _____ to perform a thorough _____ exam.

4. _____, also known as "pinkeye," is a condition in which the _____ becomes inflamed and red.

5. A(n) _____ is a small, usually _____ lump or _____ on the external eyelid that appears red and swollen.

6. In _____ glaucoma, the aqueous fluid drains too _____.

Identify

After reading the following case studies, list the chief complaint, vital signs, and pertinent negatives.

1. "Medic 620, respond Priority One for a 43-year-old female patient with dizziness. Patient is now conscious and alert." As you enter the apartment, you determine that the scene seems to be safe, and there is only one patient, so you have enough help at this point. The patient is found sitting in a chair in the kitchen. She appears pale and diaphoretic, and you notice that she is drooling. You and your partner lift her off the chair and lay her on the floor, which you have covered with a blanket. Her skin color slightly improves, as does her level of consciousness (LOC). You immediately place the patient on high-flow supplemental oxygen and begin your primary survey. You already have formed your general impression and realize that the patient is suffering from a fever. Her vital signs are a respiratory rate of 20 breaths/min, a pulse oximetry of 89%, a pulse rate (lying flat) of 118 beats/min and regular, and a blood pressure (BP) of 98/P mm Hg. She is complaining of pain when she swallows, which made her nervous, so she asked her husband to call EMS. She denies any loss of consciousness or any pain to her head, chest, or abdomen.

   a. Chief complaint:

   _____

   _____

   b. Vital signs:

   _____

   _____

   c. Pertinent negatives:

   _____

   _____

2. You are dispatched to a reported "nosebleed." On arrival, you find a 78-year-old man standing in the bathroom, spitting blood into the sink. His daughter states that he has been bleeding for hours, and they were not able to stop the nosebleed. She said he is starting to get dizzy and has lost a lot of blood. She also mentions that he is on a "blood thinner" since he had a "mini-stroke" 5 years ago. He has not eaten all day because this nosebleed has been occupying most of his attention. His mental status is alert, and you obtain the following vital signs: respirations of 20 breaths/min and regular, pulse rate of 108 beats/min and irregular, BP of 170/102 mm Hg, and SpO$_2$ of 95%. You check his blood glucose, and it is 110 mg/dL. He states he has a headache and that his doctor told him he has an ECG of A-fib normally. He denies any trauma or shortness of breath. You make an attempt to control the bleeding and prepare to transport him to the hospital.

   a. Chief complaint:

   _____

   _____

b. Vital signs:

_____

_____

c. Pertinent negatives:

_____

_____

Ambulance Calls

The following case scenarios provide an opportunity to explore the concerns associated with patient management and paramedic care. Read each scenario, and then answer each question.

1. You are assessing and treating a conscious, alert 17-year-old boy who was playing baseball in a high school league when he was struck in the right eye with a wild pitch. He is in extreme pain and may have sustained blunt trauma to the globe of the eye. Upon examination of his eye and interviewing the patient, you conclude that he may have sustained a corneal abrasion.

   a. What are five of the signs and symptoms you are likely to find in this patient?

_____

_____

_____

_____

_____

   b. Your patient denies any other previous medical history, he is not on any medications, and he states he has an allergy to sulfa medications. His vital signs are respiratory rate of 20 breaths/min and regular, pulse of 110 beats/min and regular, BP of 120/78 mm Hg, and SpO_2 of 98%. What would be the appropriate treatment for this patient?

_____

_____

_____

2. You are treating a 15-year-old boy whose parent called the ambulance to their home after an accident in their backyard. Your patient states that his eye is burning up. He says he splashed concentrated chlorine into his left eye when he was pouring the chemical into their in-ground pool.

   a. What would your prehospital treatment for this patient include?

_____

_____

_____

True/False

If you believe the statement to be more true than false, write the letter "T" in the space provided. If you believe the statement to be more false than true, write the letter "F."

_____   **1.** Nasal foreign bodies are usually not visible in the anterior nares.

_____   **2.** Certain medications can cause rhinitis.

_____   **3.** Sinusitis occurs when drainage from one or more of the sinuses becomes disrupted.

_____   **4.** Esophageal disorders can also affect the throat.

_____   **5.** The symptoms of vertigo and tinnitus are common with Meniere disease.

_____   **6.** A toothache is also referred to as dentalgia.

_____   **7.** When bacteria growth spreads directly from the cavity into the gums or facial tissue, this can cause a dental abscess.

_____   **8.** Thrush is also called oral candidiasis.

_____   **9.** Oral candidiasis is caused by a virus and is not curable

_____   **10.** Epiglottitis is most commonly found in pediatric patients aged 4 to 9 years.

Gather information about even subtle changes in bowel habits, eating habits, new foods, travel, new medications, or low-grade fevers.

Abdominal and Gastrointestinal Emergencies

Matching

Part I

Match each of the items in the left column to the appropriate definition in the right column.

_____ 1. A weak area in the colon that begins to have small outcroppings that turn into pouches.

_____ 2. Inflammation of pouches in the colon; these pouches form as a result of difficulty moving feces through the colon. Bacteria can become trapped in the pouches, leading to inflammation and infection.

_____ 3. The mechanical and chemical breakdown of the large molecules in food into small molecules that can be absorbed in the gastrointestinal tract and converted to energy for cellular function.

_____ 4. Liquid stool.

_____ 5. A pre-ulcerative state where the stomach is inflamed, but erosions have not yet occurred.

_____ 6. An abnormal connection between two cavities.

_____ 7. Smelling of feces.

_____ 8. Dilated blood vessels of the esophagus, commonly caused by difficulty in blood flow through the liver; the presence of these can lead to vessel rupture.

_____ 9. A bowel sound characterized by increased activity within the bowel; also called hyperperistalsis.

_____ 10. Forceful vomiting that results in a tear in the esophagus that extends entirely through the esophageal wall, creating a hole.

_____ 10. A group of disorders that involve inflammation of the gallbladder; these include cholangitis, cholelithiasis, cholecystitis, and acalculous cholecystitis.

_____ 12. Abdominal edema typically signaling liver failure.

_____ 13. A condition of sudden onset of pain within the abdomen, usually indicating peritonitis; demands immediate medical or surgical treatment.

_____ 14. Light, clay-colored stools indicative of liver failure.

_____ 15. Inflammation of the ileum and possibly other portions of the gastrointestinal tract, in which the immune system attacks portions of the intestinal walls, causing them to become scarred, narrowed, stiff, and weakened.

_____ 16. Early failure of the liver; characterized by portal hypertension, coagulation deficiencies, and diminished detoxification.

A. Acholic stools

B. Acute abdomen

C. Acute gastroenteritis

D. Anal fissures

E. Appendicitis

F. Ascites

G. Biliary tract disorders

H. Boerhaave syndrome

I. Borborygmi

J. Cholangitis

K. Cholelithiasis

L. Cholecystitis

M. Cirrhosis

N. Crohn disease

O. Diarrhea

P. Digestion

_____ **17.** An inflammation of the esophagus.

Q. Diverticulitis

_____ **18.** The region of the abdomen directly inferior to the xiphoid process and superior to the umbilicus.

R. Diverticulum

_____ **19.** Insertion of a flexible fiber-optic tube into the esophagus to visualize, remove, or repair damaged or diseased tissue.

S. Endoscopy

_____ **20.** A family of conditions that revolve around a central theme of infection with fever, abdominal pain, diarrhea, nausea, and vomiting.

T. Epigastric

_____ **21.** Linear tears to the mucosal lining in and near the anus, possibly caused by the passage of large, hard stools; a cause of lower gastrointestinal (GI) bleeding.

U. Esophagitis

_____ **22.** Inflammation of the appendix.

V. Esophagogastric varices

_____ **23.** Inflammation of the gallbladder.

W. Feculent

_____ **24.** The presence of stones within the gallbladder.

X. Fistula

_____ **25.** Inflammation of the bile duct.

Y. Gastritis

Part II

Match each of the items in the left column to the appropriate definition in the right column.

_____ **1.** Dark, tarry, malodorous stools caused by upper gastrointestinal bleeding.

A. Gastroesophageal reflux disease

_____ **2.** A condition in which the junction between the esophagus and the stomach tears, causing severe bleeding and, potentially, death.

B. Hematemesis

_____ **3.** The sphincter between the esophagus and the stomach; controls the amount of food that moves up the esophagus; also called the cardiac sphincter.

C. Hematochezia

_____ **4.** A condition in which patients have abdominal pain and changes in their bowel habits; generally, the pain and accompanying changes in bowel habits must be present for at least 3 days a month for at least 3 months to be considered this disease.

D. Hepatic encephalopathy

_____ **5.** Increased pressure in the portal veins; caused by the inability of blood to flow normally through the liver; can lead to rupture of these vessels.

E. Hepatitis

_____ **6.** Inflammation of the peritoneum, the protective membrane that lines the abdominal and pelvic cavities.

F. Hernia

_____ **7.** A disease in which the mucous lining of the stomach and duodenum have been eroded, allowing the acid to eat into these organs.

G. Hiatal hernia

_____ **8.** Pain caused by inflammation of the parietal peritoneum that is generally described as steady, aching, and aggravated by movement.

H. Hyperperistalsis

_____ **9.** A condition in which the sphincter between the esophagus and the stomach opens, allowing stomach acid to move superiorly; can cause a burning sensation within the chest (heartburn); also called acid reflux disease.

I. Hypoperistalsis

_____ **10.** Vomit with blood; can either look like coffee grounds, or contain bright red blood, indicating active bleeding.

J. Icteric

_____ **11.** The passage of stool in which bright red blood can be distinguished; caused by lower GI bleeding.

K. Incarcerated

_____ **12.** Impairment of brain function resulting from failure of the liver.

L. Incisional

_____ **13.** Inflammation of the liver, usually caused by a virus, that causes fever, loss of appetite, jaundice, fatigue, and altered liver function.

M. Inflammatory bowel disease

_____ **14.** Telescoping of the intestines into themselves.

N. Intussusception

_____ **15.** Chronic inflammation of all or part of the gastrointestinal tract.

O. Irritable bowel syndrome

_____ **16.** Inflammation of the pancreas.

P. Lower esophageal sphincter

_____ **17.** A mass of tissue produced by abnormal cell growth and division that may be malignant (cancerous) or benign.

_____ **18.** An interruption of the blood supply to the mesentery.

_____ **19.** A type of hernia in which intestinal contents herniate through an incision, for example, after abdominal surgery.

_____ **20.** A type of hernia in which an organ is trapped in the new location; most commonly obstructs the bowel.

_____ **21.** Yellowish coloration of the conjunctiva (the whites of the eyes) caused by the buildup of bilirubin in the blood during liver failure.

_____ **22.** The protrusion of a loop of an organ or tissue through an abnormal body opening.

_____ **23.** A protrusion of a portion of the stomach through the diaphragm.

_____ **24.** Increased activity within the bowel; also called borborygmi.

_____ **25.** Decreased activity in the bowel.

Q. Mallory-Weiss syndrome

R. Melena

S. Mesenteric ischemia

T. Neoplasm

U. Pancreatitis

V. Parietal pain

W. Peptic ulcer disease

X. Peritonitis

Y. Portal hypertension

Multiple Choice

Read each item carefully, and then select the best response.

_____ **1.** A 45-year-old woman calls for an ambulance because of "burning" epigastric pain of several hours' duration. She says that yesterday she noticed her bowel movement was "black as pitch," and about an hour ago she vomited some "stuff that looked like coffee grounds." She also feels quite dizzy. She takes no medications except Mylanta (alumina/magnesia/simethicone) "for my heartburn." On physical examination, she looks pale and anxious, and she sits leaning forward. Her skin is cold and sweaty. Her pulse is 140 beats/min and regular; her respirations are 20 breaths/min and slightly labored; her blood pressure (BP) is 90/60 mm Hg. Her abdomen is diffusely tender, especially over the epigastrium. There is guarding but no real rigidity. Peripheral pulses are intact. This patient's findings are most consistent with which of the following conditions?

    A. Peptic ulcer disease

    B. Diverticulitis

    C. Mesenteric ischemia

    D. A leaking abdominal aortic aneurysm

_____ **2.** A 70-year-old woman calls for an ambulance because of abdominal pain of 4 hours' duration. "I just knew I shouldn't have eaten all that rich, fatty food," she says. "It never agrees with me. Oh, I hate to cause everyone so much bother." And she starts to cry. On questioning, she says she had some diarrhea, but it didn't relieve the pain. Her past medical history is notable for two previous acute myocardial infarctions. On physical examination, the woman appears to be in considerable distress. Pulse is 108 beats/min and slightly irregular; respirations are 20 breaths/min and shallow; BP is 160/100 mm Hg in both arms. The chest is clear. The patient has a positive Murphy sign. This patient most likely has which of the following conditions?

    A. Peptic ulcer disease

    B. Diverticulitis

    C. Cholecystitis

    D. A leaking abdominal aortic aneurysm

_____ **3.** A 52-year-old woman called for an ambulance because of severe abdominal pain. She says the pain started a couple of days ago as a kind of steady ache (she points to the left lower quadrant), and it just kept getting worse and worse. Now her whole abdomen hurts. It's been 2 days since she had a bowel movement, and that one may have had some blood in it. On physical examination, the patient is in obvious distress. She lies very still on the stretcher and cries out with pain when your partner accidentally bumps the stretcher. Her pulse is 128 beats/min and regular; respirations are 28 breaths/min and shallow; BP is 150/80 mm Hg. The abdomen is slightly distended, and it does not move with respiration. On palpation, it feels like a slab of concrete. The pedal pulses are equal. You are told that the patient has a history of underlying thrombotic disease. This patient's findings are most consistent with which of the following conditions?

    A. Peptic ulcer disease

    B. Diverticulitis

    C. Mesenteric ischemia

    D. A leaking abdominal aortic aneurysm

_____ **4.** A 30-year-old man contacts calls 9-1-1 and states he has severe abdominal pain in the lower right quadrant. He states a history of rectal bleeding, diarrhea, arthritis, and fever. He further states episodic periods of similar symptoms. This patient's findings are most consistent with which of the following conditions?

    A. Peptic ulcer disease

    B. Diverticulitis

    C. Crohn disease

    D. A leaking abdominal aortic aneurysm

_____ **5.** Pain that originates in the abdomen and causes pain in a distant location as a result of similar paths for the peripheral nerves of the abdomen and the distant location is considered _____ pain.

    A. referred

    B. parietal

    C. somatic

    D. rebound

_____ **6.** On arrival, you discover that your patient is a 28-year-old woman complaining of severe vomiting. She explains that she is in the first trimester of pregnancy and has been suffering from morning sickness. Her vomiting is so severe that she is now vomiting blood. She most likely has which of the following conditions?

    A. Peptic ulcer disease

    B. Hemorrhoids

    C. Pancreatitis

    D. Mallory-Weiss syndrome

_____ **7.** The proper treatment for esophageal varices includes:

    A. narcotic pain relief.

    B. treatment with 5% dextrose and water.

    C. fluid resuscitation.

    D. placement of a laryngeal mask airway (LMA) to prevent aspiration.

_____ **8.** Pain that is difficult to localize and is described as a burning, cramping, gnawing, or aching is called _____ pain.

    A. referred

    B. visceral

    C. somatic

    D. parietal

_____ **9.** You receive an emergency call for a conscious, alert 26-year-old man with a sudden onset of severe abdominal pain. He is complaining of an associated fever, nausea, and vomiting. The pain appears isolated to the right lower quadrant (RLQ). Your patient most likely has which of the following conditions?

    A. Hypovolemia

    B. Inflammation of the interstitial lining

    C. Esophageal varices

    D. Appendicitis

_____ **10.** Which of the following would NOT cause a bowel obstruction?

    A. Paralysis of the intestines

    B. An immune attack against the GI tract

    C. Infection

    D. Kidney disease

Fill in the Blank
Read each item carefully, and then complete the statement by filling in the missing word(s).

1. When patients have _____, any drug that is given may remain active within the body for _____ than anticipated.

2. Chronic consumption of _____ or _____ may increase the acidity in the stomach beyond the limits of the protective _____ layer.

3. The _____ vein transports _____ blood from the GI tract directly to the liver for processing of the nutrients that have been _____.

4. The medication ketorolac (Toradol) is a(n) _____ and, therefore, does not tend to cause _____ and respiratory depression.

5. People who are _____ are more likely to have a poor outcome from _____-_____ illness.

6. Most peptic ulcers are the result of infection of the stomach with _____ _____. Another major cause is chronic use of _____ anti-inflammatory drugs.

7. _____ _____ _____ involve inflammation of the gallbladder.

8. Ulcerative _____ is caused by inflammation of the colon.

9. _____ _____ is a disease of the young; most patients are between 15 and 30 years of age. It occurs with equal incidence in men and women. There is a strong _____ component to this disease.

10. The presentation of appendicitis can be divided into the following three stages: _____, _____, and _____.

Labeling
Label the following diagrams with the correct terms.

1. Normal versus hiatal hernia

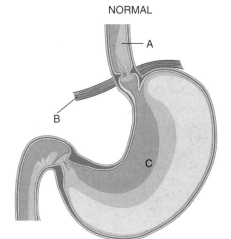

NORMAL

Normal:

A. _____

B. _____

C. _____

HIATAL HERNIA

Hiatal hernia:

A. _____

B. _____

C. _____

2. Common locations of abdominal hernias

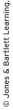

A. _____

B. _____

C. _____

D. _____

E. _____

Identify

In the following case studies, list the chief complaint, vital signs, and pertinent negatives.

1. "Medic 640, respond Priority One for a 63-year-old male patient, near syncope. Patient is now conscious and alert." As you enter the apartment, you recognize the odor. It smells as though the patient has melena stools. Your paramedic instructor was right; it's an unforgettable smell even for a brand-new, inexperienced paramedic. The patient is found to be sitting on the commode in the bathroom. He appears ashen, diaphoretic, and barely able to sit up. You and your partner lift him off the commode and lay him on the floor, which you have covered with towels. His skin color slightly improves, and his level of consciousness (LOC) improves as well. You immediately place the patient on high-flow supplemental oxygen and begin your primary survey. You already have formed your general impression and realize that the patient is suffering from a GI bleed. His vital signs are a pulse oximetry of 89%, a pulse rate (lying flat) of 118 beats/min, and BP of 88/P mm Hg. His abdomen is slightly distended. The patient tells you that he has an extensive history of rectal bleeding.

a. Chief complaint:

_____

_____

b. Vital signs:

_____

_____

c. Pertinent negatives:

_____

_____

2. You are dispatched to a reported "man down." On arrival, you find law enforcement standing next to a man who presents as very unkempt. He has an empty bottle of Wild Irish something in his hands. You assume that this is a street person. Regardless of your feelings, you understand the importance of remaining professional. Law enforcement explains that the patient is highly intoxicated, is a danger to himself, and needs to be transported to a detox unit. You begin to assess the patient and decide that he looks much older than his real age of 42. Assessment reveals a male patient with an odor of ETOH and urine. He is conscious and alert but slurring his words. He is mostly cooperative. The patient has icteric sclera and right upper quadrant (RUQ) pain on palpation. His blood glucose is 110 mg/dL. His oxygen saturation level is 94%, pulse rate is 104 beats/min and regular, and BP is 142/86 mm Hg. His skin is jaundiced but cool and dry. He has equal bilateral motor neurologic function to all extremities. His lungs are essentially clear and equal bilaterally. The patient has slightly delayed capillary refill. He has sinus tachycardia on the monitor and appears to have had several bowel movements that appear to have been alcoholic in nature. The patient denies any recent injury or falls. He's not a very good historian.

a. Chief complaint:

_____

_____

b. Vital signs:

_____

_____

c. Pertinent negatives:

_____

_____

3. It's New Year's Eve, and your patient is a 45-year-old slightly overweight woman. She is complaining of severe RUQ pain. She states that she knows better than to eat fatty foods, but after all, it's New Year's Eve. She is in pain that she describes as "worse than childbirth." She is slightly nauseated and complains of gas pains. She denies any recent injury or trauma. She states a history of gallbladder disease that is usually controlled by diet. But tonight the pain is "unbearable." She further states that tonight's episode is consistent with other bouts of gallbladder attack. She says that after tonight she is going to "finally have it taken out." Her vital signs are as follows: Her pulse is 92 beats/min, strong and regular. She has equal bilateral radial pulses. The abdomen is tender in the RUQ. Her oxygen saturation is 99%. Electrocardiogram (ECG) reveals sinus rhythm. Capillary refill is normal. Skin color is normal, and skin is warm and slightly diaphoretic. Your patient is crying for pain relief.

a. Chief complaint:

_____

_____

b. Vital signs:

_____

_____

c. Pertinent negatives:

_____

_____

Ambulance Calls

The following case scenarios provide an opportunity to explore the concerns associated with patient management and paramedic care. Read each scenario, and then answer each question.

1. You are assessing and treating a conscious, alert 23-year-old man with a sudden severe onset of periumbilical pain that migrates to the right lower quadrant. He states that he can't find a position of comfort and feels slightly nauseated and febrile.

a. What is your initial impression of this patient's presentation?

_____

_____

b. Your patient denies any other previous medical history, he is not on any medications, and he denies allergies to medications. His vital signs would be considered within normal limits. How would you treat this patient?

(1)_____

(2)_____

(3)_____

(4)_____

(5)_____

(6)_____

c. Your patient is very nauseated and is vomiting frequently. You have a choice of the following standing-order medications in your drug box: ondansetron (Zofran), diphenhydramine (Benadryl), hydroxyzine (Vistaril), and promethazine (Phenergan). List the cautions of each.

(1)   Ondansetron (Zofran):

_____

_____

(2)   Diphenhydramine (Benadryl):

_____

_____

(3)   Hydroxyzine (Vistaril):

_____

_____

(4)   Promethazine (Phenergan):

_____

2. Your patient presents with a history of esophageal varices. He is vomiting copious amounts of undigested blood. What would your prehospital treatment for this patient include?

a. _____

b. _____

c. _____

d. _____

3. You respond to a call for a 76-year-old woman with a possible bowel obstruction. In the prehospital setting, there might not be much you can do to treat this particular patient. List the general treatment guidelines for patients with GI disease.

a. _____

b. _____

c. _____

d. _____

e. _____

f. _____

g. _____

True/False
If you believe the statement to be more true than false, write the letter "T" in the space provided. If you believe the statement to be more false than true, write the letter "F."

_____ **1.** Promethazine is a drug for managing patients with nausea and vomiting.

_____ **2.** Ulcerative colitis presents with a chronic complaint of abdominal pain, often in the lower right area. This pain corresponds to the location of the ileum. Rectal bleeding, weight loss, and diarrhea are some symptoms of this condition.

_____ **3.** All types of severe liver damage will lead to liver failure.

_____ **4.** Patients with peptic ulcers experience a classic sequence of burning or gnawing pain in the stomach that subsides or diminishes immediately after eating and then reemerges 2 to 3 hours later.

_____ **5.** Deep palpation can help you discern some of the organs and structures in the cavity and requires a level of technique usually employed in the prehospital setting.

_____ **6.** Pain is often an unimportant finding with GI patients. The patient's complaint of pain is something that a paramedic must learn to expect.

_____ **7.** The major presenting problems from GI diseases typically result in pain, hypovolemia, and infection.

_____ **8.** True absent bowel sounds, which are characterized by no sounds heard for 2 minutes, are typically not practical to discover in the prehospital setting.

_____ **9.** The foul-smelling stools that accompany GI emergencies are to be expected.

_____ **10.** Orthostatic vital signs are only relevant when dealing with abdominal trauma.

Short Answer
Complete this section with short written answers using the space provided.

1. Define the following vocabulary words:

a. Borborygmi:

_____

_____

b. Cholecystitis:

_____

_____

c. Scaphoid:

_____

_____

d. Mallory-Weiss syndrome:

_____

_____

2. A 15-year-old girl complains of sharp pain in the right lower quadrant. The pain is made worse by coughing or moving around. The spot she points to is the spot that is most tender to palpation. She lies very still, with her right leg flexed at the hip and knee.

a. What type of abdominal pain is this?

_____

b. What mechanism is most likely to produce this type of pain?

_____

c. Describe the causes of this type of pain.

_____

3. Your patient is complaining of pain localized to the right upper abdomen. The patient describes the pain as sharp and as the worst pain he's ever felt. He also states that he is nauseous and has vomited several times. Physical exam reveals fever, tachycardia, hypotension, and muscle spasms in the extremities.

a. What type of abdominal pain is this?

_____

b. When does this type of pain usually occur?

_____

Fill in the Table
Fill in the missing parts of the table.

1. In the course of a busy week (is there any other kind?), you have several calls for patients with abdominal pain. Each time you have to evaluate a different story and a different set of physical findings. Among the findings in the patients you cared for were those listed here. For each finding, explain its clinical significance.

Finding	What the Finding Tells Me
Coffee-ground vomitus	
Melena	
Tenting of the skin	
Patient very still	

Genitourinary and Renal Emergencies

The kidneys work best if you keep putting fluid in and out!

TM3

According to the National Institutes of Health, there are more than 600,000 emergency department visits for renal calculi.

Matching

Part I

Match each of the items in the left column to the appropriate term in the right column.

_____ **1.** A double-layered cup with the inner layer infiltrating and surrounding the capillaries of the glomerulus.

_____ **2.** A condition that results from bacteria entering the skin of the scrotum or perineum, causing infection and subsequent necrosis of the subcutaneal tissue and muscle in the scrotum.

_____ **3.** A surgically created connection between an artery and a vein, usually in the arm, for dialysis access.

_____ **4.** An infection that causes inflammation of the epididymis along the posterior border of the testis; a possible complication of male urinary tract infection.

_____ **5.** A condition in which the kidneys are unable to function, and toxic waste materials build up in the patient's blood; occurs after acute or chronic kidney injury.

_____ **6.** The U-shaped portion of the renal tubule that extends from the proximal to the distal convoluted tubule; concentrates the filtrate and converts it to urine.

_____ **7.** Solid crystalline masses formed in the kidney, resulting from an excess of insoluble salts or uric acid crystallizing in the urine; may become trapped anywhere along the urinary tract.

_____ **8.** Solid, bean-shaped organs housed in the retroperitoneal space that filter blood and excrete body wastes in the form of urine.

_____ **9.** A type of acute kidney injury characterized by damage in the kidney itself. Often caused by immune-mediated diseases, prerenal acute kidney injury, toxins, heavy metals, some medications, or some organic compounds.

_____ **10.** A chronic inflammation of the interstitial cells surrounding the nephrons.

_____ **11.** The presence of blood in the urine.

_____ **12.** Connects with the kidney's collecting tubules.

_____ **13.** A condition characterized by nausea, vomiting, headache, and confusion, which results when, as a consequence of dialysis, water initially shifts from the bloodstream into the cerebrospinal fluid, mildly increasing intracranial pressure (ICP).

A. Acute kidney injury

B. Air embolism

C. Anuria

D. Arteriovenous graft

E. Azotemia

F. Benign prostate hypertrophy

G. Chronic kidney disease

H. Disequilibrium syndrome

I. Distal convoluted tubule

J. End-stage renal disease

K. Epididymitis

L. Fistula

M. Fournier gangrene

_____ **14.** Progressive and irreversible inadequate kidney function caused by the prostate gland.

N. Glomerular (Bowman) capsule

_____ **15.** Age-related nonmalignant enlargement of the prostate gland.

O. Hematuria

_____ **16.** A sudden decrease in filtration through the glomeruli.

P. Interstitial nephritis

_____ **17.** The presence of air in the venous circulation, which forms a gas bubble that can block the outflow of blood from the right ventricle to the lung; can lead to cardiac arrest, shock, or other life-threatening complications.

Q. Intrarenal acute kidney injury

_____ **18.** A complete cessation of urine production.

R. Kidneys

_____ **19.** A surgical connection between an artery and a vein.

S. Kidney stones

_____ **20.** Increased nitrogenous wastes in the blood.

T. Loop of Henle

Part II

Match each of the items in the left column to the appropriate term in the right column.

_____ **1.** A pair of thick-walled, hollow tubes that transport urine from the kidneys to the bladder.

A. Nephrons

_____ **2.** A hollow tubular structure that drains urine from the bladder, expelling it from the body.

B. Oliguria

_____ **3.** A hollow muscular sac in the midline of the lower abdominal area that stores urine until it is released from the body.

C. Orchitis

_____ **4.** The inability to control the release of urine from the bladder.

D. Paraphimosis

_____ **5.** A connection between the arterial and venous system in which no gas exchange occurs.

E. Phimosis

_____ **6.** Twisting of the testicle on the spermatic cord, from which it is suspended; associated with scrotal pain and swelling, and is a medical emergency.

F. Postrenal acute kidney injury

_____ **7.** The presence of excessive amounts of urea and other waste products in the blood.

G. Prerenal acute kidney injury

_____ **8.** A powdery buildup of uric acid, especially on the skin of the face.

H. Priapism

_____ **9.** A technique for filtering the blood of its toxic wastes, removing excess fluids, and restoring the normal balance of electrolytes.

I. Prostatitis

_____ **10.** An upper urinary tract infection in which the kidneys are involved.

J. Proximal convoluted tubule

_____ **11.** One of the two complex sections of the nephron: includes an enlargement at the end called the glomerular capsule.

K. Pyelonephritis

_____ **12.** Inflammation of the prostate gland.

L. Renal dialysis

_____ **13.** A condition that results when the foreskin is retracted over the glans penis and becomes entrapped; constriction of the glans causes it to swell even further.

M. Shunt

_____ **14.** A complication of a male urinary tract infection in which one or both testes become infected, enlarged, and tender, causing pain and swelling in the scrotum.

N. Testicular torsion

_____ **15.** Urine output of less than 500 mL/day.

O. Uremia

_____ **16.** The structural and functional units of the kidney that form urine, composed of the glomerulus, the glomerular (Bowman) capsule, the proximal convoluted tubule, the loop of Henle, and the distal convoluted tubule.

P. Uremic frost

_____ **17.** Inability to retract the distal foreskin over the glans penis.

Q. Ureters

_____ **18.** A type of acute kidney injury caused by obstruction of urine flow from the kidneys, commonly caused by a blockage of the urethra by an enlarged prostate gland, blood clots, or strictures.

R. Urethra

_____ 19. A type of acute kidney injury that is caused by hypoperfusion of the kidneys, resulting from hypovolemia (hemorrhage, dehydration), trauma, shock, sepsis, and heart failure (secondary to myocardial infarction); often reversible if the underlying condition can be found and perfusion restored to the kidney.

S. Urinary bladder

_____ 20. A painful, tender, persistent erection of the penis; can result from spinal cord injury; erectile dysfunction drugs, or sickle cell disease.

T. Urinary incontinence

Multiple Choice

Read each item carefully, and then select the best response.

_____ 1. Which of the following is NOT considered part of the urinary system?
   A. Ureters
   B. Kidney
   C. Liver
   D. Bladder

_____ 2. Excessive amounts of urea and other waste products cause a condition called:
   A. hypoxia.
   B. sepsis.
   C. uremia.
   D. hypovolemia.

_____ 3. Inflammation of the kidney linings is caused by:
   A. sepsis.
   B. urinary tract infection.
   C. uremia.
   D. hypoxia.

_____ 4. Treatment options for kidney stones include each of the following, EXCEPT:
   A. extracorporeal lithotripsy.
   B. cystoscopy with stent placement.
   C. smooth muscle constriction.
   D. percutaneous nephrostomy tube.

_____ 5. What is the most common composition of kidney stones?
   A. Calcium
   B. Salt
   C. Glucose
   D. Fat

_____ 6. When a patient is suffering pain from a kidney stone, it is important to remember that the greater the pain, the:
   A. lower the BP and pulse will be.
   B. higher the BP and pulse will be.
   C. higher the BP will be and the lower the pulse will be.
   D. lower the BP will be and the higher the pulse will be.

_____ 7. What is the name of the condition when urine output stops completely?
   A. Oliguria
   B. Uremia
   C. Anuria
   D. Hematuria

_____ 8. When reading an electrocardiogram (ECG), what is a classic finding of hyperkalemia?
   A. Peaked T waves
   B. Inverted T waves
   C. Atrial flutter
   D. No T waves at all

_____ **9.** Which of the following is NOT a sign of air embolism caused by a loose dialysis system?

    A. Cyanosis

    B. Hypertension

    C. Hypotension

    D. Dyspnea

_____ **10.** How should pain be managed in the 25-year-old man whom you suspect has a kidney stone?

    A. Conservatively administer low doses of Valium.

    B. Aggressively administer a narcotic analgesic with medical control's permission.

    C. Administer oxygen and acetylsalicylic acid (ASA).

    D. Withhold pain medications until arrival at the emergency department (ED).

Labeling

Label the following diagrams with the correct terms.

1. The urinary system

A. _____

B. _____

C. _____

D. _____

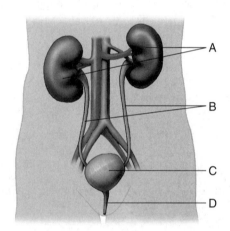

2. The four-quadrant system

A. _____

B. _____

C. _____

D. _____

E. _____

F. _____

G. _____

H. _____

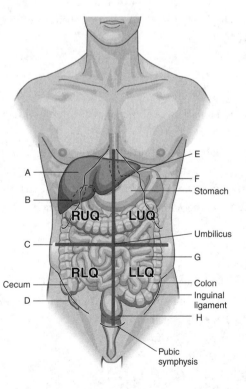

3. The nine-section system

A. _____

B. _____

C. _____

D. _____

E. _____

F. _____

© Jones & Bartlett Learning.

Fill in the Blank

Read each item carefully, and then complete the statement by filling in the missing word(s).

1. When managing a patient whose chief complaint is renal calculi, your focus should be on _____ and _____.

2. The kidneys' internal anatomy is divided into three regions: the _____, the _____, and the _____.

3. _____ _____ _____ is a sudden decrease in the rate of filtration through the glomeruli.

4. During _____, the patient's blood circulates through a dialysis machine that works the same way the patient's kidneys function.

5. _____ _____ occurs during dialysis and happens because of the water shifting from the bloodstream into the cerebrospinal fluid.

6. Leukemia and tumors, blunt penetrating trauma, cocaine abuse, and spinal cord injury can cause _____ in the male patient.

7. _____ pain is usually associated with hollow organs and presents with a crampy, aching pain deep within the body.

8. You should always monitor the patient's fluid imbalances, electrolyte abnormalities, and _____ function when dealing with an end-stage renal patient.

9. Treatment of kidney stones in the prehospital setting should revolve around _____ _____ for the patient.

10. Urinary tract infections usually occur in the _____ urinary tract.

Identify

After reading the following case study, list the chief complaint, vital signs, and pertinent negatives.

You're just about to hit the hay after a long day at the fire station. Unfortunately, Bill, the paramedic on duty, is not feeling very well, and so you have to fill in for him. He has had a crampy pain in his lower back all day, and he is worried he is coming down with the flu. At about 0100 hours, Bill wakes you and tells you something is really wrong. He is having pain in his lower quadrants, and he can't take it anymore. You give him a little ribbing about all the potato chips he has been eating and the gallons of sports drink he drinks each day. You tell him to go back to sleep. It is just an upset stomach. He tells you he is about to jump through his skin because it hurts so badly and asks you to get up and haul him to the ED. You decide that maybe Bill is having some problems, so you wake up the other emergency medical technician (EMT) and start an assessment on Bill. He is 47 years old, he is alert, and his oxygen saturation is 98%. You put him on a nasal cannula at 4 L/min just for good measure. Your partner takes his pulse, which is 104 beats/min, and the heart monitor shows a sinus tachycardia with no ectopy. BP is 148/94 mm Hg, respirations are 18 breaths/min, and all lung fields are clear. His skin is warm and dry, and he has a normal temperature. Not wanting to miss anything on Bill, you measure his blood glucose, which is 96 mg/dL. His pain is a 10 on a scale of 1 to 10, and he is really hurting. Bill doesn't smoke and, other than a fast-food diet, he keeps in good shape.

Both you and Bill are now suspecting a kidney stone. You start an IV line and give him a 500-mL bolus of normal saline on the way to the hospital. Medical direction agrees with you about the possibility of a stone and orders 5 mg morphine for the pain. Bill is feeling a lot better when you reach the ED. His pain is down to a 4 out of 10. You check back with him in the morning when you get off shift. He says that he passed a stone about 4 hours after you brought him in. They will run a few more tests, but he thinks he will be out of the hospital around noon. He is now swearing off sports drinks and promises water is his new buddy.

1. Chief complaint:

_____

_____

_____

2. Vital signs:

_____

_____

_____

3. Pertinent negatives:

_____

_____

_____

Ambulance Calls

The following case scenarios provide an opportunity to explore the concerns associated with patient management and paramedic care. Read each scenario, and then answer each question.

1. A 52-year-old man complains of crampy abdominal pain that builds up to a peak, subsides, and then builds again. When you ask where the pain is, he points to the general area of the umbilicus, but when you palpate his abdomen, the part that is tender is in the left lower quadrant. He tells you that he has been vomiting nearly constantly since the pain started, about 6 hours ago.

a. What type of abdominal pain is this?

_____

_____

_____

b. What mechanism is most likely to produce this type of pain?

_____

_____

_____

c. Describe the causes of this type of pain.

_____

_____

_____

2. On the first hot day of the summer, a 35-year-old construction worker calls for an ambulance because of "excruciating" abdominal pain. He was hit in the back lower right quadrant by a steel beam that was being moved into place by a crane. It knocked him down, but he didn't want to appear hurt to his coworkers. So, after catching his breath, he went back to work. He has come home for lunch and now is hurting badly. His wife admits you to the house, where you find the patient in the bedroom, writhing about on the bed, tears rolling down his face. "I can't take it. I can't take it," he says. "Please give me something for the pain." His wife says that he came home from work complaining of back pain and then pain in his groin, and it just got worse and worse. He has been vomiting for the past hour or so. On physical examination, he is clearly in severe distress. His pulse is 124 beats/min and regular, respirations are 30 breaths/min, and BP is 160/80 mm Hg. There is some guarding in the abdomen and tenderness on the left side, but no rigidity. This patient's findings are most consistent with which of the following conditions? Please explain.

   A. Peptic ulcer disease

   B. Diverticulitis

   C. Mesenteric ischemia

   D. Leaking abdominal aortic aneurysm

   E. Trauma to the kidneys

   F. None of the above

_____

_____

_____

3. The following ambulance calls involve dialysis patients. For each situation described, indicate what you think is the problem and what you would do about it.

   a. A patient is due for dialysis today but says he feels "too weak and dizzy even to get out of bed." His ECG shows a rate of 40 beats/min; flattened P waves; wide QRS complexes; and tall, pointy T waves. You are 30 minutes from the hospital ED.

   (1) What do you think is the problem?

_____

   (2) What steps will you take to manage the problem?

   (a) _____

   (b) _____

   (c) _____

   (d) _____

   (e) _____

b. The patient just got home from a dialysis session at the local kidney center. He complains of a severe headache and nausea. He has vomited twice since getting home. On physical examination, he seems a little confused. His pulse is 56 beats/min and regular, respirations are 16 breaths/min, and BP is 180/102 mm Hg.
(1) What do you think is the problem?

_____

True/False

If you believe the statement to be more true than false, write the letter "T" in the space provided. If you believe the statement to be more false than true, write the letter "F."

_____   **1.** Prerenal acute kidney injury is caused by hyperperfusion of the kidneys.

_____   **2.** Hyperkalemia presents with an inverted T wave on the ECG.

_____   **3.** Chronic inflammation of the interstitial cells surrounding the nephrons can produce intrarenal acute kidney injury (IAKI).

_____   **4.** Nephrons are the functioning units inside the kidney that form urine.

_____   **5.** Patients with chronic kidney disease exhibit edema in the extremities and face.

_____   **6.** In hemodialysis, the patient's blood circulates through a dialysis machine that functions as a normal liver.

_____   **7.** Dialysis patients are more vulnerable to heart failure.

_____   **8.** The female urethra is much shorter than the male urethra.

_____   **9.** Men are more prone to urinary tract infections than women are because of the length of their urethra.

_____   **10.** Prerenal acute kidney injury is caused by a lack of blood flow to the kidneys.

Short Answer

Complete this section with short written answers using the space provided.

1. Many patients with chronic kidney disease are kept alive by periodic hemodialysis. Although dialysis does remove toxic wastes from the blood and helps restore fluid and electrolyte balance, it does not by any means solve all the patient's problems. Patients maintained on long-term dialysis for chronic kidney disease are much more vulnerable than patients with normal kidneys. List five medical problems to which patients with chronic kidney disease, who are taking dialysis treatments, are more vulnerable:

a. _____

b. _____

c. _____

d. _____

e. _____

Fill in the Table

Fill in the missing parts of the table.

| Signs and Symptoms of Acute Kidney Injury ||
Type of Acute Kidney Injury	Signs and Symptoms
Prerenal	_____
Intrarenal	_____
Postrenal	_____

Gynecologic Emergencies

© Jones & Bartlett Learning.

Matching

Part I

Match each of the items in the left column to the appropriate term in the right column.

_____	**1.** A pregnancy in which the fertilized oocyte implants somewhere other than the uterus.	**A.** Amenorrhea
_____	**2.** Uterine bleeding that is abnormal in amount or frequency (more than every 21 days).	**B.** Bartholin glands
_____	**3.** Infection caused by bacteria that travel from the perineum, through the genital tract, into the urethral opening; also called bladder infection.	**C.** Cervix
_____	**4.** A small, cylindrical mass of erectile tissue and nerves located at the anterior junction of the labia minora, similar to the glans penis of the male.	**D.** Clitoris
_____	**5.** A fluid-filled sac that forms on or within an ovary.	**E.** Cystitis
_____	**6.** A rounded pad of fatty tissue that overlies the symphysis pubis and is anterior to the urethral and vaginal openings.	**F.** Dysfunctional uterine bleeding
_____	**7.** Cyclical shedding of the endometrial lining from the uterine cavity.	**G.** Ectopic pregnancy
_____	**8.** The period when a woman's reproductive cycle ceases; also called the female climacteric.	**H.** Embryo
_____	**9.** The inner layer of the uterine wall.	**I.** Endometriosis
_____	**10.** An inflammation of the endometrium that is often associated with a bacterial infection.	**J.** Endometritis
_____	**11.** The presence of tissue outside the uterus that resembles the endometrium in both structure and function.	**K.** Endometrium
_____	**12.** Fertilized egg.	**L.** Fallopian tube
_____	**13.** The narrowest portion (lower third of the neck) of the uterus that opens into the vagina.	**M.** Hymen
_____	**14.** The glands that secrete mucus for sexual lubrication.	**N.** Labia majora
_____	**15.** Absence of menstruation.	**O.** Labia minora
_____	**16.** The first menstrual cycle; the onset of menses.	**P.** Menarche
_____	**17.** A pair of skin folds devoid of pubic hair that protects the vagina.	**Q.** Menopause
_____	**18.** A pair of prominent, rounded folds of skin covered with pubic hair that protects the vagina.	**R.** Menstruation
_____	**19.** A membrane that protects the vaginal orifice before first intercourse.	**S.** Mons pubis
_____	**20.** The anatomic structure that connects each ovary with the uterus and provides a passageway for the ova.	**T.** Ovarian cyst

Part II

Match each of the items in the left column to the appropriate term in the right column.

_____ 1. The muscular, inverted, pear-shaped organ where the fetus grows.

_____ 2. A condition in which the uterus moves or drops into the vagina.

_____ 3. An inflammation of the external vulva.

_____ 4. An inflammation of the vagina.

_____ 5. An infection cause by the fungus *Candida albicans*, in which fungi overpopulate the vagina.

_____ 6. Any type of sexual contact or behavior that occurs without the explicit consent of the recipient.

_____ 7. A fluid-filled sac within the ovary that bursts from internal pressure.

_____ 8. Nonconsensual oral, anal, or vaginal penetration of the victim by body parts or objects using force, threats of bodily harm, or taking advantage of a victim who is incapacitated or otherwise incapable of giving consent.

_____ 9. Kidney infection.

_____ 10. The genital canal in the female that serves as a passageway for the elimination of menstrual fluids, receives the penis during sexual intercourse, holds the spermatozoa before their passage into the uterus, and serves as the passageway for childbirth.

_____ 11. The area between the vaginal opening and the anus.

_____ 12. An infection of the female reproductive organs.

_____ 13. Midcycle release of an egg (ovum) during the menstrual cycle.

_____ 14. A pair of female reproductive organs that release eggs (ova) that, if fertilized, will develop into a fetus.

_____ 15. A painful condition in which the ovary becomes twisted.

A. Ovarian torsion

B. Ovaries

C. Ovulation

D. Pelvic inflammatory disease (PID)

E. Perineum

F. Pyelonephritis

G. Rape

H. Ruptured ovarian cyst

I. Sexual assault

J. Uterine prolapse

K. Uterus

L. Vagina

M. Vaginal yeast infection

N. Vaginitis

O. Vulvovaginitis

Multiple Choice

Read each item carefully, and then select the best response.

_____ 1. How many days is the average "cycle" of a woman?

  A. 5 days

  B. 10 days

  C. 28 days

  D. 30 days

_____ 2. What is the onset of the first menses called?

  A. Menopause

  B. Premenstrual syndrome

  C. Menstruation

  D. Menarche

_____ 3. During an ectopic pregnancy, where do most eggs implant?

  A. In the uterus

  B. In the fallopian tube

  C. In the ovary

  D. In the cervical opening

_____ 4. Which of the following is the most common cause of amenorrhea?

  A. Exercise

  B. Pregnancy

  C. A low body fat percentage

  D. Anorexia nervosa

_____ **5.** Which of the following is NOT one of the classic diagnostic triad for ectopic pregnancy?

    A. Vaginal bleeding

    B. Anxiety and decreased pulse pressure

    C. Amenorrhea

    D. Abdominal pain

_____ **6.** Which of the following is NOT considered a life-threatening gynecologic condition?

    A. Childbirth

    B. Ectopic pregnancy

    C. Tubo-ovarian abscess

    D. Ruptured ovarian cyst

_____ **7.** Each of the following drugs is considered a "club drug" and has been used to facilitate a sexual rape, EXCEPT:

    A. Rohypnol.

    B. GHB.

    C. naloxone.

    D. ketamine.

_____ **8.** Which of the following is a cause of an ectopic pregnancy?

    A. Pelvic inflammatory disease

    B. IUD use

    C. Pelvic surgery

    D. All of the above

_____ **9.** When dealing with a victim of sexual assault, which of the following statements is true?

    A. You should try to obtain as much information as possible about the assault.

    B. You should place the patient's articles in a paper bag.

    C. You should place the patient's articles in a plastic bag to preserve DNA.

    D. You should allow the patient time to wash himself or herself.

_____ **10.** Which condition involves the presence of tissue outside the uterus that resembles the endometrium in both structure and function?

    A. Ovarian cyst

    B. Ovarian torsion

    C. Endometriosis

    D. Endometritis

Labeling

Label the following diagrams with the correct terms.

1. Anatomy of the female genital tract and pelvis

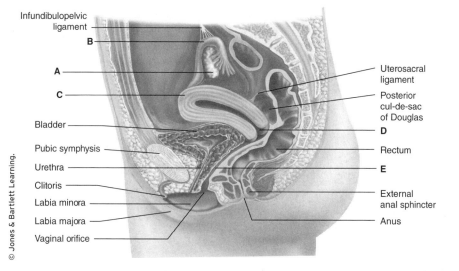

A. _____

B. _____

C. _____

D. _____

E. _____

2. Reproductive system with an ectopic pregnancy

A. _____

B. _____

C. _____

D. _____

Fill in the Blank

Read each item carefully, and then complete the statement by filling in the missing word(s).

1. The lower portion of the birth canal is also called the _____.

2. In some cases, a(n) _____ _____ will completely cover the vaginal orifice.

3. The cessation of menses is known as _____.

4. _____ is cessation of ovarian function and of the menstrual cycle such that a woman is no longer able to bear children.

5. Endometrial tissue grows outside the uterus and causes _____.

6. In _____ pregnancy, bleeding usually occurs _____ the onset of pain.

7. _____ _____ is the first thing to ensure when called to a gynecologic emergency.

8. At all times, you should try to protect a patient's _____ when treating a gynecologic emergency.

9. _____ sign or _____ _____ sign may indicate internal bleeding.

10. _____ is usually caused by _____ that ascend from the _____ through the genital tract into the urethral opening.

Identify

Read the following case study, and then list the chief complaint, vital signs, and pertinent negatives.

Your unit has been called to the local high school for a young woman with severe abdominal pain. When you arrive, the 16-year-old patient, Lucy, is doubled up in pain. She is crying. You begin your primary survey (ABCDE) and apply supplemental oxygen via a nonrebreathing mask. Lucy rates her pain as 10 on a scale of 1 to 10. Your partner Abe begins with her baseline vital signs as you gather a personal history. Lucy's heart rate is 120 beats/min, her electrocardiogram (ECG) rhythm is sinus tachycardia, and her blood pressure (BP) is 140/92 mm Hg. Her oxygen saturation is 94%, and respirations are 20 breaths/min. Her skin is very warm, and her temperature is 102°F. Pupils are equal, round, and reactive to light and accommodation (PERRLA). Lung sounds are clear. The patient has no history of illness or trauma. She denies being sexually active yet. A physical examination reveals guarding of the abdomen. She has rebound tenderness, and her abdomen is distended. She says she is going to be sick and then begins to vomit. You believe that she is a load-and-go priority patient, so your partner gets an IV line started, and you load the patient quickly and get to the emergency department (ED) as quickly as possible.

1. Chief complaint:

_____

_____

2. Vital signs:

_____

_____

3. Pertinent negatives:

_____

_____

Ambulance Calls

The following case scenarios provide an opportunity to explore the concerns associated with patient management and paramedic care. Read each scenario, and then answer each question.

1. A 25-year-old woman calls for an ambulance because of abdominal pain. She says the pain started yesterday and has just gotten worse and worse. It is a "heavy," aching pain in the lower abdomen. This afternoon, she started having chills as well, and she threw up once. Her last menstrual period was 5 days ago and was normal. She uses an intrauterine device (IUD) for contraception. On physical examination, the patient looks ill. Her skin feels hot and dry. Her pulse is 110 beats/min and regular while sitting, 116 beats/min while standing; her respirations are 24 breaths/min and unlabored; and her BP is 122/74 mm Hg. The abdomen is very tender to palpation in all quadrants.
   a. This patient is most likely experiencing which of the following conditions?
      A. A threatened abortion
      B. An inevitable abortion
      C. A septic abortion
      D. An ectopic pregnancy
      E. Pelvic inflammatory disease (PID)

   b. List the steps you would take in managing this patient.

      (1)_____

      (2)_____

2. A 24-year-old woman calls for an ambulance because she says, "I think I have appendicitis." She has been having some crampy pain in the right lower quadrant for a couple of days, but today it got much worse. She cannot remember exactly when her last menstrual period was and says, "But I think I'm getting my period now because I had some spotting this morning." She is certain, in any case, that she could not possibly be pregnant. On physical examination, she appears anxious and in moderate distress. Her skin is cool and moist. Her pulse is 100 beats/min and regular while sitting, and 124 beats/min while standing; her respirations are 24 breaths/min and regular; and her BP is 110/70 mm Hg. Her abdomen is very tender to palpation.
   a. What is your field diagnosis of this patient?
      A. A threatened abortion
      B. An inevitable abortion
      C. A septic abortion
      D. An ectopic pregnancy
      E. Pelvic inflammatory disease (PID)

b. List the steps you would take in managing this patient.

(1)_____

(2)_____

(3)_____

(4)_____

(5)_____

(6)_____

(7)_____

(8)_____

True/False

If you believe the statement to be more true than false, write the letter "T" in the space provided. If you believe the statement to be more false than true, write the letter "F."

_____　　**1.** The paramedic should take a detailed history of a rape incident to enable the victim to vent her feelings about what happened.

_____　　**2.** An inflammation of the bladder that is caused by a yeast infection is called a Bartholin abscess.

_____　　**3.** The patient who has experienced a rape should be discouraged from cleaning up before being examined in the ED.

_____　　**4.** The rape victim's external genitalia should be routinely inspected for injury.

_____　　**5.** The insertion of an IUD can increase a woman's risk of developing PID.

_____　　**6.** Infection can cause the Bartholin glands to become cystic and abscessed.

_____　　**7.** Menarche is when a woman reaches menopause.

_____　　**8.** Endometritis is hereditary and runs in families.

_____　　**9.** The region of sexual stimulation is called the hymen.

_____　　**10.** The menstrual cycle is divided into the ovarian and the uterine cycles.

Short Answer

Complete this section with short written answers using the space provided.

1. You are summoned to a downtown apartment for a "sick woman." On arrival, you find a 24-year-old woman complaining of severe abdominal pain.

a. List 10 questions you would ask in taking this woman's history.

(1) _____

(2) _____

(3) _____

(4) _____

(5) _____

(6) _____

(7) _____

(8) _____

(9) _____

(10) _____

b. List two things you would look for in particular in performing the physical examination.

(1) _____

(2) _____

2. Ectopic pregnancy is more likely in some women than in others. List two factors that predispose a woman to ectopic pregnancy.

a. _____

b. _____

3. Three findings in the history make up the classic diagnostic triad for ectopic pregnancy, and a woman who has those three findings must be considered to be experiencing an ectopic pregnancy until proven otherwise. Which three findings make up the classic triad for ectopic pregnancy?

a. _____

b. _____

c. _____

Fill in the Table
Fill in the missing parts of the table.

Elements of the Gynecologic History
Current symptoms: Vaginal bleeding? Amount? Any tissue passed?
Current symptoms: Vaginal discharge? Color, amount, odor, itching?
Current sexual activity? Birth control?
Prior pregnancies (gravidity)
Prior pregnancy complications or losses?
Other past medical history, medications, allergies

Endocrine Emergencies

Prescription bottles can help pinpoint the patient's underlying medical problems and identify his or her physician.

Matching

Part I

Match each of the definitions in the left column to the appropriate terms in the right column.

_____ **1.** A hormone produced by the pancreas that is vital to the control of the body's metabolism and blood glucose level. Glucagon stimulates the breakdown of glycogen to glucose.

_____ **2.** Diabetes that develops during pregnancy in women who did not have diabetes before pregnancy.

_____ **3.** Protrusion of the eyes from the normal position within the socket.

_____ **4.** One of the three major female hormones at puberty; it brings about the secondary sex characteristics.

_____ **5.** A hormone produced by the adrenal medulla that plays a vital role in the function of the sympathetic nervous system.

_____ **6.** A hormone secreted by the thyroid gland that helps maintain normal calcium levels in the blood.

_____ **7.** A hormone secreted by the posterior pituitary lobe of the pituitary gland, which constricts blood vessels and raises the blood pressure; also called vasopressin.

_____ **8.** Male sex hormones that regulate body changes associated with sexual development (puberty), including growth spurts, deepening of the voice, growth of facial and pubic hair, and muscle growth and strength.

_____ **9.** A hormone that stimulates the kidneys to reabsorb sodium from the uterine and excrete potassium by altering the osmotic gradient in the blood.

_____ **10.** A hormone that targets the adrenal cortex to secrete cortisol (a glucocorticoid).

_____ **11.** Abnormally high blood glucose level.

_____ **12.** A type of hyperthyroidism in which the thyroid gland becomes enlarged as it is infiltrated by T lymphocytes and plasma cells.

_____ **13.** An autoimmune disorder that causes thyroid gland hypertrophy and severe hyperthyroidism.

_____ **14.** A visible mass in the anterior part of the neck caused by enlargement of the thyroid gland.

_____ **15.** The passage of large quantities of urine containing glucose.

_____ **16.** Acute adrenal insufficiency.

A. Addisonian crisis

B. Adrenocorticotrophic hormone (ACTH)

C. Aldosterone

D. Androgens

E. Antidiuretic hormone (ADH)

F. Calcitonin

G. Corticosteroids

H. Cortisol

I. Cushing syndrome

J. Diabetes

K. Diabetes insipidus (DI)

L. Diabetes mellitus

M. Diabetic ketoacidosis (DKA)

N. Diuresis

O. Dyslipidemia

P. Epinephrine

_____ **17.** An excessive level of lipids (fats) circulating in the blood, which increases the risk of atherosclerosis and coronary artery disease.

_____ **18.** The production of large amounts of urine by the kidney.

_____ **19.** A form of acidosis in uncontrolled diabetes in which certain acids accumulate when insulin is not available.

_____ **20.** Disease characterized by the body's inability to sufficiently metabolize glucose; it occurs either because the pancreas does not produce enough insulin or because the cells do not respond to the effects of the insulin that is produced.

_____ **21.** A group of complex metabolic disorders with many causes, which include diabetes mellitus, gestational diabetes, hypoglycemia/hyperglycemia, diabetic ketoacidosis, and hyperosmolar hyperglycemic syndrome.

_____ **22.** A condition caused by an excess of cortisol production by the adrenal glands or by excessive use of cortisol or other similar corticosteroid (glucocorticoid) hormones.

_____ **23.** Hormones that stimulates most body cells to increase their energy production.

_____ **24.** Hormones that regulate the body's metabolism, the balance of salt and water in the body, the immune system, and sexual function.

_____ **25.** A relatively uncommon disorder that has some of the same characteristics as diabetes, such as polyuria and polydipsia, in which the body is unable to regulate fluid owing to a lack of antidiuretic hormone or the kidneys are unable to respond appropriately.

Q. Estrogen

R. Exophthalmos

S. Gestational diabetes

T. Glucagon

U. Glycosuria

V. Goiter

W. Graves disease

X. Hashimoto disease

Y. Hyperglycemia

Part II

Match each of the definitions in the left column to the appropriate terms in the right column.

_____ **1.** An "orange peel" appearance and nonpitting edema of the skin on the anterior part of the leg below the knee.

_____ **2.** A condition identified in people who have certain risk factors associated with type 2 diabetes that exists when blood glucose levels or hemoglobin A1c levels are above normal levels, yet not high enough to be diagnosed as diabetes.

_____ **3.** Frequent and plentiful urination.

_____ **4.** Increased appetite.

_____ **5.** Significant thirst.

_____ **6.** An endocrine disorder in which an excess of antidiuretic hormone results in a decrease in urinary output and, therefore, systemic fluid overload.

_____ **7.** A hormone that inhibits insulin and glucagon secretion by the pancreas.

_____ **8.** A common condition characterized by a lack of adrenocorticotropic hormone (also called corticotrophin).

_____ **9.** Also known as Addison disease; a rare condition in which the adrenal glands produce an insufficient amount of adrenal hormones.

_____ **10.** A hormone secreted by the parathyroid glands that acts as an antagonist to calcitonin; secreted when calcium blood levels are low.

_____ **11.** The inadequate production or absence of the pituitary hormones, including adrenocorticotropic hormone (ACTH), cortisol, thyroxine, luteinizing hormone (LH), follicle-stimulating hormone (FSH), estrogen, testosterone, growth hormone, and antidiuretic hormone (ADH).

_____ **12.** A hormone produced by the adrenal glands that is vital in the function of the sympathetic nervous system.

A. Hyperosmolar hyperglycemic syndrome (HHS)

B. Hyperosmolar nonketotic coma (HONK)

C. Hypoglycemia

D. Insulin

E. Insulin resistance

F. Islets of Langerhans

G. Ketonemia

H. Lipolysis

I. Luteinizing hormone

J. Microangiopathy

K. Myxedema coma

L. Testosterone

_____ **13.** The most important androgen in men.

_____ **14.** A rare condition that can occur in patients who have severe, untreated hypothyroidism.

_____ **15.** Microscopic deterioration of vessel walls caused primarily by adherence of blood lipids to vessel walls.

_____ **16.** A metabolic derangement that occurs principally in patients with type 2 diabetes; it is characterized by hyperglycemia and hyperosmolarity, in absence of significant ketosis; also known as hyperosmolar nonketotic coma.

_____ **17.** Another name for hyperosmolar hyperglycemic syndrome.

_____ **18.** Abnormally low blood glucose level.

_____ **19.** A hormone produced by the pancreas that is vital to the control of the body's metabolism and blood glucose level; it causes sugar, fatty acids, and amino acids to be absorbed and metabolized by cells.

_____ **20.** Condition in which the pancreas produces enough insulin but the body cannot effectively use it.

_____ **21.** A hormone that regulates the production of both eggs and sperm, as well as the production of reproductive hormones.

_____ **22.** The metabolism (breakdown or destruction) of stored fat that has been released into the circulation.

_____ **23.** Excess amounts of ketone bodies in the blood.

_____ **24.** A specialized group of cells in the pancreas in which insulin and glucagon are produced.

_____ **25.** A tumor of the adrenal gland, usually in the medulla, that causes excessive release of the hormones epinephrine and norepinephrine.

M. Norepinephrine

N. Panhypopituitarism

O. Parathyroid hormone

P. Pheochromocytoma

Q. Polydipsia

R. Polyphagia

S. Polyuria

T. Prediabetes

U. Pretibial myxedema

V. Primary adrenal insufficiency

W. Progesterone

X. Somatostatin

Y. Syndrome of inappropriate antidiuretic hormone secretion (SIADH)

Multiple Choice

Read each item carefully, and then select the best response.

_____ **1.** The endocrine system is made up of a network of glands that produce:

    A. homeostasis.

    B. glucose.

    C. calcium.

    D. hormones.

_____ **2.** The parathyroid glands assist in the regulation of:

    A. sodium.

    B. potassium.

    C. calcium.

    D. iron.

_____ **3.** Which part of the endocrine system has a role in hormone production as well as in digestion?

    A. Hypothalamus

    B. Pancreas

    C. Thyroid

    D. Parathyroid

_____ **4.** The pituitary gland stimulates other endocrine glands, including each of the following, EXCEPT:

    A. calcitonin.

    B. ACTH.

    C. luteinizing hormone.

    D. thyroid-stimulating hormone.

_____ **5.** The thyroid secretes:

    A. iodine.

    B. calcitonin.

    C. cardiac enzymes.

    D. norepinephrine.

_____ **6.** The adrenal glands consist of two parts: an outer part, called the adrenal cortex, and an inner part, called the:

    A. adrenal cortex.

    B. adrenal medulla.

    C. posterior adrenal cortex.

    D. inferior medulla.

_____ **7.** Epinephrine stimulates _____ nervous system receptors throughout the body.

    A. parasympathetic

    B. sympathetic

    C. dopamine

    D. neuron

_____ **8.** In the past, type 2 diabetes mellitus was called:

    A. juvenile diabetes.

    B. adult-onset diabetes.

    C. diabetic hypoglycemia.

    D. sweet diabetes.

_____ **9.** The most common form of diabetes is type 2 diabetes, also known as:

    A. insulin intolerance.

    B. insulin tolerance.

    C. insulin resistance.

    D. insulin opposition.

_____ **10.** Patients in diabetic ketoacidosis (DKA) are seldom:

    A. comatose.

    B. asymptomatic.

    C. hyperglycemic.

    D. hypoglycemic.

_____ **11.** Which of the following conditions is characterized by hyperglycemia, hyperosmolarity, and the absence of ketosis?

    A. Hyperosmolar nonketotic coma (HONK)

    B. Hyperosmolar hyperglycemic syndrome (HHS)

    C. Cardiometabolic syndrome

    D. Both A and B

_____ **12.** Signs and symptoms of acute adrenal insufficiency may appear suddenly and are commonly referred to as:

    A. addisonian crisis.

    B. adrenal insufficiency.

    C. severe infection.

    D. None of the above

_____ **13.** Cushing syndrome is caused by:

    A. an excess of cortisol production.

    B. an excess of glucocorticoid hormones.

    C. tumors of the pituitary gland or adrenal cortex.

    D. All of the above

_____ **14.** An extreme manifestation of untreated hypothyroidism that is accompanied by physiologic decompensation is called:

    A. myxedema coma.

    B. thyroid storm.

    C. Cushing syndrome.

    D. diabetic ketoacidosis.

_____ **15.** Thyrotoxicosis may be caused by all of the following, EXCEPT:

    A. goiters.

    B. Graves disease.

    C. thyroid cancer.

    D. ketoacidosis.

Labeling

Label the following diagrams with the correct terms.

1. Diabetic emergencies

Blood Glucose Level (mg/dL)   **Diabetic Emergency**

A. _____

B. _____

C. _____

D. _____

E. _____

A

400

B

120

C

80

D

40

E

© Jones & Bartlett Learning.

Fill in the Blank

Read each item carefully, and then complete the statement by filling in the missing word(s).

1. _____ coma is a metabolic and cardiovascular emergency. If not diagnosed and treated immediately, the mortality rate is approximately 40%.

2. The anterior pituitary gland secretes _____-_____ _____ in response to secretion of thyrotropin-releasing hormone by the hypothalamus.

3. Aldosterone regulates and maintains the _____ and _____ balance in the blood.

4. The goals of prehospital treatment for diabetic ketoacidosis are to begin _____ and to correct the patient's _____ and acid–base abnormalities.

5. Hyperglycemia usually progresses slowly, over a period of _____ to _____ hours, with the patient's level of consciousness _____ only gradually.

6. Symptoms of type 2 diabetes may include _____, _____, nausea, frequent urination, unexplained weight loss, blurred vision, unresponsiveness, and thirst

7. Two forms of diabetes exist: _____ _____ and _____ _____. Both types are serious conditions that affect many tissues and functions other than the glucose-regulating mechanism, and both require lifelong medical management.

8. The endocrine component of the pancreas is made up of the _____ _____ _____. These cell groups in the pancreas act like "an organ within an organ." The main hormones they secrete are _____, _____, and somatostatin, which are responsible for the regulation of blood glucose levels.

9. The pituitary gland secretions control, or regulate, the secretions of other _____ glands.

10. HHS, which stands for _____ hyperglycemic syndrome and is also called _____ nonketotic _____ (HONK), is a metabolic derangement that occurs principally in patients with type 2 diabetes.

Identify

Read the following case studies, and then list the chief complaint, vital signs, and pertinent negatives. Also identify the possible nature of the endocrine disorder.

1. It is a sunny but very cold and windy mid-February day. You and your partner would be content to remain inside the station practicing your advanced life support (ALS) skills. The silence is broken with a dispatch to a priority 1 call for an unconscious, unresponsive patient waiting for a prescription at the neighborhood pharmacy. On arrival, you find the 29-year-old woman being attended by the pharmacist, who states the patient was waiting for an insulin prescription. The patient is unresponsive. You note that respirations are shallow, and the patient is diaphoretic. Her radial pulse is 118 beats/min. Her blood pressure (BP) is 104/88 mm Hg. Her blood glucose is 48 mg/dL. As you prepare the electrocardiogram (ECG) monitor and intravenous (IV) equipment, the pharmacist pulls her history.

   a. Chief complaint:

   _____

   _____

   b. Vital signs:

   _____

   _____

   c. Pertinent negatives:

   _____

   _____

d. Nature of the endocrine disorder:

_____

_____

2. It is cold and flu season, and today is no exception. It seems these ailments are what everyone is calling in for. On arrival at the scene, you locate an elderly man sitting in his rocker, apparently short of breath. He states that he has had the flu for a number of days and cannot stop vomiting. He speaks in full, complete sentences, but he has an unusual breathing pattern and fruity breath odor. You quickly place the pulse oximeter probe on his finger. Surprisingly, his oxygen saturation is 95% on room air. You immediately follow up with high-flow supplemental oxygen as you begin your assessment. The patient states that he has a long history of diabetes. He further states that he has not been able to keep food down for several days but has been taking all of his medications. His blood glucose is 405 mg/dL. He is tachycardic, with a BP of 108/82 mm Hg. He has poor skin turgor, and skin tenting is present. The monitor is showing a sinus tachycardia. The patient complains of thirst.

a. Chief complaint:

_____

_____

b. Vital signs:

_____

_____

c. Pertinent negatives:

_____

_____

d. Nature of the endocrine disorder:

_____

_____

3. Once again today, you are requested to respond to a call to the local nursing home for a "routine" transport to the emergency department (ED). You are met by family members, who are concerned that Grandma's mental status has been rapidly deteriorating; she also appears to be cold. The family states that the patient has suddenly become confused and psychotic. The nursing home chart indicates a history of hypothyroidism. Her pulse rate is slightly bradycardic. She is also hypotensive. You cannot get an accurate pulse oximeter reading because of poor peripheral perfusion.

a. Chief complaint:

_____

_____

b. Vital signs:

_____

_____

c. Pertinent negatives:

_____

_____

d. Nature of the endocrine disorder:

_____

_____

Ambulance Calls

The following case scenarios provide an opportunity to explore the concerns associated with patient management and paramedic care. Read each scenario, and then answer each question.

1. A 22-year-old woman is found unconscious in her apartment. Her roommate, who is nearly hysterical, tells you between sobs, "I went away for the weekend, and when I got back tonight, I found her like this. She won't die, will she?" A neighbor arrives and helps calm the roommate while you and your partner carry out the primary assessment. That accomplished, you proceed to the secondary assessment. You find that the patient wakens to a painful stimulus but rapidly returns to sleep. Her skin is warm and flushed and tents when you pinch it. Her vital signs are as follows: Pulse is 110 beats/min and regular, respirations are 30 breaths/min and deep, and BP is 90/60 mm Hg. The patient's eyes look sunken, and her pupils are 5 mm and equal, round, and reactive to light and accommodation (PERRLA). The patient's breath smells like fruit-flavored gum (or nail polish remover). Her neck is not rigid, her chest is clear, and her abdomen is soft. There are multiple needle marks and skin changes over the anterior thighs. Completing your examination, you ask the patient's roommate, "Miss, does your friend by chance have diabetes?"

"Oh, didn't I mention that?" the roommate sniffles.

List the steps in treating this patient.

a. _____

b. _____

c. _____

d. _____

2. Over the course of a week of ambulance runs, four patients are found in a coma. You do not have any information about any of them except for the medications found at the scene or on the patient's person. Nonetheless, based on those medications, you can make an educated guess at least as to each patient's underlying illness(es). For each of the comatose patients whose medications are listed as follows, indicate the most probable underlying illness(es).

a. Patient 1 has glyburide (Micronase) on his bedside table.

Probable underlying illness(es):

_____

b. A vial of insulin is found in patient 2's refrigerator.

Probable underlying illness(es):

_____

c. Patient 3 has what appears to be an insulin pump. The patient's medical identification bracelet confirms your suspicion.

Probable underlying illness(es):

_____

d. Patient 4, a 35-year-old insulin-dependent woman, had a sudden onset of a severe headache and blurred vision before she became unconscious and fell to the floor, striking her head on a concrete surface.

Probable underlying illness(es):

_____

Chapter 23

Complete the Patient Care Report (PCR)

Read the first incident scenario in the preceding Ambulance Calls section, and then complete the following patient care report (PCR).

EMS Patient Care Report (PCR)					
Date:	**Incident No.:**	**Nature of Call:**		**Location:**	
Dispatched:	**En Route:**	**At Scene:**	**Transport:**	**At Hospital:**	**In Service:**
Patient Information					
Age: **Sex:** **Weight (in kg [lb]):**		**Allergies:** **Medications:** **Past Medical History:** **Chief Complaint:**			
Vital Signs					
Time:	**BP:**	**Pulse:**	**Respirations:**		**SpO$_2$:**
Time:	**BP:**	**Pulse:**	**Respirations:**		**SpO$_2$:**
Time:	**BP:**	**Pulse:**	**Respirations:**		**SpO$_2$:**
EMS Treatment **(circle all that apply)**					
Oxygen @ _____ L/min via (circle one): NC NRM Bag-mask device		**Assisted Ventilation**	**Airway Adjunct**		**CPR**
Defibrillation	**Bleeding Control**	**Bandaging**	**Splinting**		**Other:**
Narrative					

True/False

If you believe the statement to be more true than false, write the letter "T" in the space provided. If you believe the statement to be more false than true, write the letter "F."

_____   **1.** Cold, clammy skin is classically a sign of shock but may also signal severe hypoglycemia, as from an insulin reaction.

_____   **2.** Aldosterone stimulates the bladder to eliminate large quantities of potassium.

_____   **3.** Adult hypothyroidism is sometimes called myxedema.

_____   **4.** The anterior pituitary gland secretes thyroid-stimulating hormone (TSH) in response to the hypothalamus's secretion of thyrotropin-releasing hormone (TRH).

_____   **5.** The primary clinical manifestation of adrenal crisis is atrial fibrillation.

_____   **6.** The signs and symptoms of hypoglycemia and hyperglycemia can be quite similar.

_____   **7.** Normal blood glucose is approximately 70 to 120 mg/dL; hypoglycemia occurs when blood glucose drops to 35 mg/dL.

_____   **8.** Type 2 diabetes may be related to metabolic syndrome.

_____   **9.** Symptoms of type 2 diabetes may include fatigue; nausea; frequent urination; thirst; unexplained weight loss; blurred vision; frequent infections and slow healing of wounds; crankiness, confusion, or shakiness; unresponsiveness; and seizure.

_____   **10.** Most patients with diabetes do not live a normal life span, even if they adjust their lives to the demands of the disease, especially their eating habits and activities.

_____   **11.** Endocrine disorders can be caused by either hypersecretion or insufficient secretion of a gland.

_____   **12.** In addition to secreting somatostatin, the islets of Langerhans secrete glucagon and insulin, which are responsible for the regulation of blood glucose levels.

_____   **13.** When sodium is reabsorbed into the blood, water is secreted; this action decreases both blood volume and blood pressure.

_____   **14.** Iodine is an important component of thyroxine. Without the proper level of dietary iodine intake, thyroxine cannot be produced.

_____   **15.** Cushing syndrome is caused by an excess of testosterone.

Short Answer

Complete this section with short written answers using the space provided.

1. Define the following vocabulary words:
   a. Hypoglycemia:

_____

_____

_____

   b. Diabetic ketoacidosis (DKA):

_____

_____

_____

c. Thyrotoxicosis:

_____

_____

_____

d. Insulin:

_____

_____

_____

e. Cushing syndrome:

_____

_____

_____

2. Explain the treatment for the following conditions:

a. Myxedema coma:

_____

_____

_____

_____

_____

b. Adrenal insufficiency:

_____

_____

_____

_____

_____

c. Hyperosmolar nonketotic coma:

_____

_____

_____

_____

Fill in the Table

Fill in the missing parts of the table.

Oral Agents Used to Treat Type 2 Diabetes Mellitus		
Medication Class	**Function**	**Examples**
Sulfonylureas		Chlorpropamide (Diabinese)
		Glipizide (Glucotrol)
		Glyburide (Micronase, Glynase, DiaBeta)
		Glimepiride (Amaryl)
	Stimulate beta cells to produce more insulin	Repaglinide (Prandin)
		Nateglinide (Starlix)
Biguanides		Metformin (Glucophage)
	Increase insulin effectiveness in the muscle and decrease liver glucose production	Rosiglitazone (Avandia)
		Pioglitazone (ACTOS)
Alpha-glucosidase inhibitors		Acarbose (Precose)
		Miglitol (Glyset)
DPP-4 inhibitors	Inhibit the breakdown of GLP-1, a naturally occurring compound in the body that reduces blood glucose levels	Sitagliptin (Januvia)
		Saxagliptin (Onglyza)

Hematologic Emergencies

Your patient did not choose to have a disorder.
Treat all of your patients with compassion.

Matching

Part I

Match each of the items in the left column to the appropriate definition in the right column.

_____ 1. The most common type of anemia.

_____ 2. A bleeding and clotting abnormality.

_____ 3. The body's natural blood-clotting mechanism.

_____ 4. A bleeding disorder relating to the breakdown of red blood cells.

_____ 5. A disorder that is primarily hereditary, in which clotting does not occur or occurs insufficiently.

_____ 6. Any disorder of the blood.

_____ 7. The proportion of red blood cells in the total blood volume.

_____ 8. Red blood cells.

_____ 9. A condition that begins with widespread activation of the clotting cascade, which depletes the clotting factors and platelets and eventually results in uncontrolled hemorrhage.

_____ 10. Any type of bleeding disorder that interferes with the activation or continuation of the clotting cascade or hemostasis.

_____ 11. A condition in which red blood cells break down quickly; it may occur as a result of sickle cell disease.

_____ 12. The iron-rich protein in the blood that carries oxygen.

_____ 13. The system that includes all blood components and the organs involved in their development and production.

_____ 14. The study of the physiology of blood.

_____ 15. Substances in the blood that are necessary for clotting; also called coagulation factors.

_____ 16. A vasoocclusive crisis that can be associated with pneumonia; common signs and symptoms include chest pain, fever, and cough; associated with sickle cell disease.

_____ 17. A condition in which red blood cells become trapped in the spleen, causing a dramatic fall in hemoglobin available in the circulation; it usually occurs in infants or toddlers.

_____ 18. A lower-than-normal hemoglobin or erythrocyte level.

A. Acute chest syndrome

B. Acute splenic sequestration syndrome

C. Anemia

D. Aplastic crisis

E. Clotting cascade

F. Clotting factors

G. Coagulopathy

H. Disseminated intravascular coagulation (DIC)

I. Erythrocytes

J. Hematocrit

K. Hematologic disorder

L. Hematology

M. Hematopoietic system

N. Hemoglobin

O. Hemolytic crisis

P. Hemolytic disorder

Q. Hemophilia

R. Hemostasis

_____ **19.** A temporary halt in the production of red blood cells; it may occur as a result of sickle cell disease.

_____ **20.** Lymphocytes that have been transformed because of stimulation by an antigen.

_____ **21.** A reduction in the number of white blood cells.

_____ **22.** An increase in the total number of white blood cells.

_____ **23.** White blood cells.

_____ **24.** The process by which clotting factors work together to ultimately form fibrin.

_____ **25.** A cancer or malignancy of the blood-forming organs that particularly affects the white blood cells, which develop abnormally and/or excessively at the expense of normal blood cells.

S. Hemostatic disorder

T. Iron-deficiency anemia

U. Leukemia

V. Leukocytes

W. Leukocytosis

X. Leukopenia

Y. Lymphoblasts

Part II

Match each of the items in the left column to the appropriate definition in the right column.

_____ **1.** Coagulation or clotting of blood in a blood vessel.

_____ **2.** A condition in which the body produces too many platelets.

_____ **3.** The system in the body that is primarily used to defend against infection.

_____ **4.** Platelets.

_____ **5.** A type of anemia in which either not enough hemoglobin is produced or the hemoglobin is defective.

_____ **6.** Ischemia and pain caused by sickle-shaped red blood cells that obstruct blood flow to a portion of the body.

_____ **7.** A transfusion reaction characterized by increased pulmonary capillary permeability resulting in noncardiogenic pulmonary edema.

_____ **8.** A physiologic response that is similar to an anaphylactic reaction, in which the body reacts to the infusion of blood; it occurs rapidly and can cause severe circulatory collapse and death.

_____ **9.** An overabundance or overproduction of red blood cells, white blood cells, and platelets.

_____ **10.** The system primarily made up of bone marrow, lymph nodes, and spleen, which participates in the formation of lymphocytes and immune responses.

_____ **11.** Malignant diseases that arise within the lymphoid system; they include non-Hodgkin and Hodgkin lymphomas.

_____ **12.** A disease in which the number of plasma cells in the bone marrow increases abnormally, causing tumors to form in the bones.

_____ **13.** Cells that can develop into other types of cells in the body.

_____ **14.** An acute, painful enlargement of the spleen caused by sickle cell disease.

_____ **15.** A disease that causes the red blood cells to be misshapen, resulting in poor oxygen-carrying capability and potentially resulting in lodging of the red blood cells in blood vessels or the spleen.

_____ **16.** A component of blood, made of 92% water and 6% to 7% proteins, as well as electrolytes, clotting factors, and glucose; this component accounts for 55% of the total blood volume.

_____ **17.** An abnormally low number of neutrophils.

_____ **18.** A condition in which a patient with sickle cell disease experiences significant pain due to insufficient passage of oxygen and nutrients into tissues and joints because of vessel congestion.

A. Lymphoid system

B. Lymphomas

C. Multiple myeloma

D. Neutropenia

E. Plasma

F. Polycythemia

G. Reticuloendothelial system

H. Sickle cell crisis

I. Sickle cell disease

J. Splenic sequestration crisis

K. Stem cells

L. Thalassemia

M. Thrombocytes

N. Thrombocytosis

O. Thrombosis

P. Transfusion reaction

Q. Transfusion-related lung injury

R. Vasoocclusive crisis

Multiple Choice

Read each item carefully, and then select the best response.

_____ 1. During the history taking and secondary assessment of a patient with a hematologic emergency, it is important to do all of the following, EXCEPT:

   A. look for changes in level of consciousness.

   B. obtain a SAMPLE history.

   C. check for skin color changes and itching.

   D. interview the family; confidentiality rules dictate that the family not be present.

_____ 2. Common findings with patients with blood disorders include which of the following?

   A. Bone fractures

   B. Mental health disorders

   C. "Clubbed" nails

   D. Epistaxis

_____ 3. Assessment and management of patients with hemophilia include which of the following procedures?

   A. Controlling bleeding

   B. Administering high-flow supplemental oxygen

   C. Administering an analgesic

   D. All of the above

_____ 4. All of the following organs assist in the production of red blood cells (RBCs), EXCEPT the:

   A. medulla.

   B. liver.

   C. spleen.

   D. bone marrow.

_____ 5. Sickle cell disease is associated with low readings of:

   A. RBCs.

   B. hematocrit.

   C. thrombocytes.

   D. hemoglobin.

_____ 6. Which blood type is considered the universal donor?

   A. AB

   B. A

   C. O

   D. B

_____ 7. Patients with leukemia may have which of the following signs and symptoms?

   A. Frequent urinary tract infections

   B. No symptoms

   C. Unexplained bleeding

   D. Spontaneous pneumothorax

_____ 8. Disseminated intravascular coagulopathy (DIC):

   A. has a mortality rate of 60% to 65%.

   B. has a mortality rate of 10% to 15%.

   C. is rarely fatal.

   D. can be prevented with a large fluid bolus.

_____ 9. Assessment and management of patients with multiple myeloma include which of the following procedures?

   A. IV therapy using a Bone Injection Gun (BIG) device

   B. Pain management

   C. Supplemental oxygen via continuous positive airway pressure (CPAP)

   D. Transport with multiple IV lines in place

_____ **10.** Blood performs which of the following functions?
   A. Transports oxygen from the lungs to the tissues
   B. Ferries waste products of metabolism
   C. Carries hormones from the endocrine glands to target tissues
   D. All of the above

Labeling

Label the following diagrams with the correct terms.

1. Major organs for producing and regulating the blood

A. _____

B. _____

C. _____

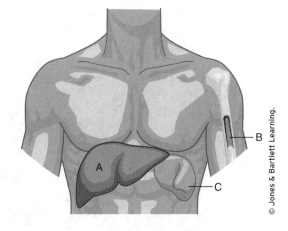

© Jones & Bartlett Learning.

Fill in the Blank

Read each item carefully, and then complete the statement by filling in the missing word(s).

1. Blood is a(n) _____ tissue.

2. The _____ system includes blood components and the organs involved in their development and production.

3. The formed elements of blood include red _____ _____, white _____ _____, and _____.

4. Red blood cell production occurs within _____ _____.

5. _____ _____, _____ _____, and _____ are three common laboratory tests done on blood samples.

6. _____ are the smallest of the formed elements and are responsible for the clotting of blood.

7. _____ _____ is a painless, progressive enlargement of the lymphoid glands, most commonly affecting the spleen and the lymph nodes.

8. The most common inherited blood disorder is called _____ _____ _____.

9. Patients with leukemia frequently present with _____, _____, or _____.

10. Patients with lymphoma may require _____ management.

11. In _____, the body's ability to clot is decreased due to the absence of a key protein that is necessary for platelet adhesion.

12. The phenomenon in which oxygen-rich RBCs release oxygen as a result of being in an environment that contains higher concentrations of carbon dioxide is called the _____.

Identify

Read the following case studies, and then list the chief complaint, vital signs, and pertinent negatives.

1. You are called to the home of a 42-year-old woman with a history of metastatic cancer and bone marrow transplant. Her chief complaint is extreme weakness, fatigue, and exertional dyspnea. You find the patient lying in bed conscious and alert, although she appears very "withdrawn" and weighs about 90 lb. She denies chest pain or shortness of breath. She tells you that she does not have any energy, and the doctor's office wants her back in the hospital. Her vital signs are as follows: Pulse is 86 beats/min, slightly irregular, and difficult to palpate; blood pressure (BP) is also difficult to auscultate but appears to be 92/P mm Hg. The patient's skin is pale, warm, and dry. She has an oxygen saturation of 91% on ambient air. Her pupils are equal, round, and reactive to light and accommodation (PERRLA). She has a central IV port in place.

   a. Chief complaint:

   _____

   _____

   b. Vital signs:

   _____

   _____

   c. Pertinent negatives:

   _____

   _____

2. Your unit is dispatched to a high-priority "Charlie" response to Middle Road Elementary School. The dispatch information indicates the patient is a 10-year-old boy with near syncope. Once inside the nurse's office, you recognize your patient—you have transported him several times in the past. For years, he has been treated for leukemia. His mother is on the scene, and she appears comforted to see a familiar face. She explains that her son just returned to school full time after his latest round of treatments. As you speak to the patient, it is apparent that his mental status is slightly altered. However, when you ask him about his favorite topic, baseball, he becomes quite talkative. En route to the hospital, his vital signs indicate that he is now conscious and alert. He does not remember the near syncope. His radial pulses are equal bilaterally and regular at 86 beats/min. He currently denies any complaints as the baseball conversation continues. BP is 98/64 mm Hg. His skin is jaundiced but cool and dry. Pupils are PERRLA. The oxygen saturation is 98% on a nonrebreathing mask. The patient has central IV access. You contact medical control for direction and are told to continue transport while monitoring his ABCs. His IV will be activated in the emergency department (ED).

   a. Chief complaint:

   _____

   _____

   b. Vital signs:

   _____

   _____

   c. Pertinent negatives:

   _____

   _____

3. It has been a rather busy day, with mostly routine emergency calls. However, this call is a little different. A man with a history of sickle cell disease is having an acute crisis and is in extreme pain. He states that the pain is breaking through his oral morphine tablets and fentanyl transdermal patch. He reports his pain as a 9 on a scale of 1 to 10. According to the patient, this is the worst sickle cell pain that he has ever had. His vital signs are as follows: Pulse is 112 beats/min and regular; skin is pale, warm, and moist; and BP is 148/96 mm Hg. Pupils are PERRLA. His pulse oximetry reading is 91%. The patient is anxious and keeps telling you to "get the rubber on the road."

a. Chief complaint:

_____

_____

b. Vital signs:

_____

_____

c. Pertinent negatives:

_____

_____

Ambulance Calls

The following case scenarios provide an opportunity to explore the concerns associated with patient management and paramedic care. Read each scenario, and then answer each question.

1. You are transporting a patient from the local community hospital to a regional trauma center. The patient's vital signs are stable when you start the transport. He has a unit of blood running. Shortly after you set out, the patient begins complaining of severe back pain. Soon thereafter he breaks out in a cold sweat, his lips take on a bluish tinge, and his neck veins seem to bulge out. You check his pulse, and it is 60 beats/min. A few minutes later, when you check it again, it is 110 beats/min.

a. The patient is showing signs of a(n):
   (1) allergic reaction to the transfusion.
   (2) hemolytic reaction to the transfusion.
   (3) air embolism.
   (4) pyrogenic reaction to the transfusion.
   (5) thrombophlebitis.

b. List the steps you will take to deal with the situation.

   (1)_____

   (2)_____

   (3)_____

   (4)_____

2. You and your partner receive a call for a 76-year-old man with a severe hemorrhage. On arrival, you find the patient's 49-year-old daughter hysterical on the front porch. She states that her father is "bleeding to death." She is too excited and emotional to provide any additional information. You enter the house and are directed to the bathroom. You are met by a rather pleasant but obviously frustrated 76-year-old man. There is a minimal amount of blood in the sink. He is holding a tissue to his carotid region and states that he cut himself shaving. He is very apologetic for and embarrassed about his daughter's behavior. He states that he has a history of a blood disorder called polycythemia, and he wears a medical identification bracelet.

a. What is polycythemia, and what are some of the symptoms?

_____

_____

_____

b. How would you treat a patient who exhibits signs and symptoms of polycythemia?

_____

_____

_____

True/False

If you believe the statement to be more true than false, write the letter "T" in the space provided. If you believe the statement to be more false than true, write the letter "F."

_____   **1.** White blood cells are responsible for transporting oxygenated blood.

_____   **2.** Red blood cell production occurs in the pancreas.

_____   **3.** "Clot busters" activate the fibrinolytic system, resulting in clot decomposition.

_____   **4.** The "universal donor" is a person with AB blood type.

_____   **5.** Malignant diseases that occur within the lymphoid system are called lymphomas.

_____   **6.** Phlebotomy is the treatment of choice for patients with disseminated intravascular coagulopathy.

_____   **7.** In multiple myeloma, abnormal plasma cells infiltrate the bone marrow.

_____   **8.** Patients with hematologic diseases might have symptoms that include vertigo, fatigue, or syncopal episodes.

_____   **9.** Oxygen is generally contraindicated for patients with red blood cell abnormalities.

_____   **10.** Paramedics should be supportive and communicate therapeutically with the patient with a suspected blood disorder.

Short Answer

Complete this section with short written answers using the space provided.

1. Blood disorders present differently from other typical injuries and diseases encountered by paramedics. Provide some of the common findings as they relate to the following:

a. Level of consciousness

_____

_____

_____

b. Skin

_____

_____

_____

c. Visual disturbances

_____

_____

_____

d. Gastrointestinal system

_____

_____

_____

e. Skeletal system

_____

_____

_____

f. Cardiovascular system

_____

_____

_____

g. Genitourinary system

_____

_____

_____

2. Assessment and treatment of patients with blood disorders may differ slightly from assessment and treatment of patients with more typical diseases encountered by paramedics. Describe how the treatment and assessment of the following diseases differ.

    a. Leukemia

        (1) _____

        (2) _____

        (3) _____

        (4) _____

        (5) _____

    b. Hemophilia

        (1) _____

        (2) _____

        (3) _____

        (4) _____

   c. Polycythemia

     (1) _____

     (2) _____

     (3) _____

     (4) _____

     (5) _____

     (6) _____

3. Define the following vocabulary words:

   a. Leukopenia:

_____

   b. Polycythemia:

_____

   c. Reticuloendothelial system:

_____

   d. Pruritus:

_____

   e. Hematocrit:

_____

   f. Melena:

_____

Fill in the Table

Fill in the missing parts of the table.

ABO Rh Type and Preferred and Alternative Donor Types		
Recipient Blood Type	**Preferred Donor Type**	**Additional Permissible Types**
A+	A+	A–, O+, O–
AB+	AB+	AB–, A+, A–, B+, B–, O+, O–
B+	B+	B–, O+, O–
O+	O+	O–

Data from: Applegate EJ. *The Anatomy and Physiology Learning System*. 4th ed. Philadelphia, PA: Saunders; 2011.

© Jones & Bartlett Learning.

My neck hurts. It feels really stiff and hard to move.

Translation—point tenderness at C4 and C5 and limited range of motion with left-side rotation.

Immunologic Emergencies

Matching

Part I

Match each of the items in the left column to the appropriate definition in the right column.

_____ **1.** A group of autoimmune disorders that affect the collagen in tendons, bones, and connective tissues.

_____ **2.** A chemical found in mast cells that, when released, causes vasodilation, capillary leaking, and bronchiole constriction.

_____ **3.** Occurs when a patient reacts with exaggerated or inappropriate allergic symptoms after coming into contact with a substance the body perceives as harmful.

_____ **4.** White blood cells that work to produce chemical mediators during an immune response.

_____ **5.** A two-phase allergic reaction in which the patient's symptoms improve and then reappear without being exposed to the trigger (allergen) a second time; the symptoms can resurface up to 8 or more hours after the initial incident.

_____ **6.** Chemicals that work to cause the immune or allergic response; for example, histamine.

_____ **7.** Eating or drinking materials for absorption through the gastrointestinal tract.

_____ **8.** In allergic reactions, foreign substances are breathed in through the respiratory system.

_____ **9.** In allergic reactions, when foreign material is deposited on and moves into the skin.

_____ **10.** A substance that produces allergic symptoms in a patient.

_____ **11.** An abnormal immune response the body develops when reexposed to a substance or allergen.

_____ **12.** An agent that, when taken into the body, stimulates the formation of specific protective proteins called antibodies.

_____ **13.** A protein the body produces ion response to an antigen; an immunoglobulin.

_____ **14.** An extreme systemic form of an allergic reaction involving one, two, or more body systems.

_____ **15.** An extreme allergic response that does not involve IgE antibody mediation. The exact mechanism is unknown, but an event of this type may occur without the patient being previously exposed to the offending agent.

A. Absorption

B. Allergen

C. Allergic reaction

D. Anaphylactoid reaction

E. Anaphylaxis

F. Antibody

G. Antigen

H. Basophils

I. Biphasic reaction

J. Chemical mediators

K. Collagen vascular diseases

L. Histamine

M. Hypersensitivity

N. Ingestion

O. Inhalation

Part II

Match each of the items in the left column to the appropriate definition in the right column.

_____ **1.** The ability to recognize a foreign substance the next time it is encountered.

_____ **2.** The body's reaction when it is exposed to an antigen for which it already has antibodies, in which it responds by killing the invading substance.

_____ **3.** An autoimmune connective tissue disease that causes fibrotic (scar tissue-like) changes to the skin, blood vessels, muscles, and internal organs.

_____ **4.** Hives or reddened elevated patches on the skin.

_____ **5.** A reaction that occurs throughout the body, possibly affecting multiple body systems.

_____ **6.** A multisystem autoimmune disease.

_____ **7.** Itching.

_____ **8.** Anaphylaxis symptoms that continue over time, with time frames anywhere from 5 to 32 hours.

_____ **9.** The first encounter with the foreign substance to begin the immune response.

_____ **10.** In allergic reactions, when the skin is pierced, and foreign material is deposited into the skin.

_____ **11.** When the body limits a response to a specific area after being exposed to a foreign substance.

_____ **12.** Basophils that are located in the tissues.

A. Injection

B. Local reaction

C. Mast cells

D. Primary response

E. Prolonged (persistent) reaction

F. Pruritus

G. Scleroderma

H. Secondary response

I. Sensitivity

J. Systemic lupus erythematosus

K. Systemic reaction

L. Urticaria

Multiple Choice

For the following questions, select the best response based on the scenario provided.

It's been a slow shift, so you decide to grab a quick dinner at Bill's Steak 'n Lobster. You park your ambulance outside and find a table near the door, in case you have to leave in a hurry on a call. You've just had your medium-rare sirloin placed in front of you when you notice a woman at the next table who does not look well. You ask her if there is anything the matter. "I don't know," she says in a very squeaky voice. "I have this lump in my throat, and I feel like I'm going to die," whereupon she collapses to the floor.

_____ **1.** This woman is MOST likely experiencing:

    A. food poisoning.

    B. choking.

    C. strep throat.

    D. anaphylaxis.

_____ **2.** The treatment you need to give MOST urgently is:

    A. pumping out her stomach.

    B. administering 6 to 10 manual abdominal thrusts.

    C. having her gargle with saltwater.

    D. administering epinephrine.

_____ **3.** Assuming the patient is having an acute anaphylactic reaction, what other medications might be helpful?

    A. Nitroglycerin sublingual

    B. Corticosteroids

    C. Morphine sulfate

    D. Narcan

_____ **4.** You decide to administer diphenhydramine (Benadryl) to your patient as well. You determine that Benadryl may also be helpful at this time because it blocks:

    A. beta receptor sites.

    B. alpha receptor sites.

    C. neurotransmitters that cause respiratory distress.

    D. histamine receptors.

_____ 5. While assessing and treating your patient, you discover a used EpiPen next to her collapsed body. The EpiPen auto-injector (if used properly) would have administered:

  A. 1 mg of solution IM.

  B. 1 mg of solution IV.

  C. 0.5 mg of solution subcutaneously.

  D. 0.3 mg of solution IM.

_____ 6. The patient is responding slowly to the epinephrine. Which of the following medications may also be helpful if medical control concurs?

  A. Glucagon

  B. Albuterol

  C. A corticosteroid

  D. All of the above

The patient's mother explains that the baby had been up all night tugging at her ear and crying inconsolably. She has been running a low-grade fever that appears to respond well to pediatric Tylenol (acetaminophen). Today the baby went to the pediatrician, who prescribed liquid amoxicillin for an ear infection. After the first dose of the strawberry-flavored antibiotic, the baby began to vomit and appeared to stop breathing. Emergency Medical Services (EMS) was called. On your arrival, the child appeared conscious and alert and was acting appropriately for her age.

_____ 7. The baby was MOST likely suffering from:

  A. an anaphylactic reaction.

  B. a localized reaction.

  C. no reaction; sometimes sick children vomit and appear to hold their breath.

  D. a systemic reaction.

_____ 8. If the small child were having a reaction to the antibiotic, what would be the correct course of treatment?

  A. Secure the ABCs, consider pharmacologic intervention in concert with medical control, and assess the need for rapid but safe transport to an appropriate facility.

  B. Initiate rapid transport, and perform all assessment and treatment modalities en route.

  C. After securing the patient's ABCs, administer IM Benadryl (diphenhydramine) immediately.

  D. Contact medical control for further instructions.

_____ 9. What was the "route" of exposure?

  A. Exposure

  B. Inhalation

  C. Ingestion

  D. Injection

_____ 10. Of the following substances, which is NOT considered one of the body's chemical weapons designed to fight off the antigen?

  A. Kinins

  B. Serotonin

  C. Norepinephrine

  D. Prostaglandin

_____ 11. What would be the prehospital implication for the paramedic caring for a lupus patient exhibiting symptoms of pneumonia?

  A. You should assess for history of renal failure and electrolyte imbalance.

  B. You should assess for a fever, tachypnea, cough, and/or worsening of chest pain.

  C. You should monitor the patient for stroke and seizure precautions.

  D. Be sure to collect a history that includes bloody stools and gastrointestinal (GI) distress.

_____ 12. What is the MOST common type of transplant patient in the United States?

  A. Liver

  B. Heart

  C. Skin

  D. Kidney

Labeling

Use the following figure to answer the questions regarding anaphylaxis.

1. What is the first form of attack on the human body?

_____

2. What types of cells are released?

_____

3. What signs and symptoms may be present in the respiratory system?

_____

4. What are the negative cardiovascular signs/symptoms that may be present?

_____

5. Are there any effects to the circulatory system? If so, list them.

_____

6. The skin is often the first place to show signs/symptoms; what are they?

_____

Fill in the Blank

Read each item carefully, and then complete the statement by filling in the missing word(s).

1. Through the _____ response, the body develops _____, that is, the ability to recognize the antigen the next time it

   is encountered.

2. The _____ response occurs with _____ to a foreign substance.

3. A protein the body produces in response to an antigen is a(n) _____.

4. _____ cells meet and greet invaders.

5. _____ is a chemical found in mast cells.

6. A(n) _____ _____ airway is an early sign of impending airway occlusion due to swelling.

7. A(n) _____ reaction occurs throughout the body, possibly affecting _____ body systems.

8. _____ occurs when a person's _____ system reacts with _____ or inappropriate symptoms after coming into contact with a substance perceived by the body to be harmful.

9. _____ vascular diseases are considered _____ diseases, which means that the body perceives its own tissues or cells as a dangerous invader.

10. High-flow _____ should be given to each anaphylactic patient.

Identify

In the following case studies, list the chief complaint, vital signs, and pertinent negatives.

1. You are treating a 16-year-old girl who was stung by a bee at her pool. She complains of hives and itching at the sting site. She denies respiratory distress or trouble swallowing. She states that she has never been stung before and doesn't carry an EpiPen. She is conscious and alert. Her skin color is normal, warm, and dry. Capillary refill is normal. Her oxygen saturation is 99%, blood pressure (BP) is 112/68 mm Hg, and pupils are equal, round, and reactive to light and accommodation (PERRLA).

a. Chief complaint:

_____

_____

b. Vital signs:

_____

_____

c. Pertinent negatives:

_____

_____

2. You are called to a rural location for a 23-year-old man who states that he was bitten by a tick. He appears scared, but other than being "grossed-out," he has no complaint. The tick is still attached to his leg. After removing the tick, you assess his vital signs. He is conscious and alert. His pulse is 110 beats/min and regular, BP is 142/84 mm Hg, PERRLA, and skin is warm and moist. The patient has no previous medical history, no allergies, and no known drug allergies.

a. Chief complaint:

_____

_____

b. Vital signs:

_____

_____

c. Pertinent negatives:

_____

_____

3. A Priority One response directs you to Uptown Elementary School for an eighth grader complaining of trouble breathing and swallowing after ingesting brownies brought by a classmate. The student is in a class that has signs posted designating it as a "peanut-free" environment. The student has a medical identification bracelet indicating a severe allergy to peanuts and any by-products. The school nurse believes that the student accidentally ingested peanuts that were ingredients in the brownies. The student is conscious and alert, anxious, and speaking in a raspy voice. He has redness around his face and neck. Vital signs are pulse of 124 beats/min, oxygen saturation of 90%, and BP of 90/62 mm Hg.

a. Chief complaint:

_____

_____

b. Vital signs:

_____

_____

c. Pertinent negatives:

_____

_____

4. It's about 2200 hours. You respond to a call for an allergic reaction to seafood. On arrival, you are met by a 32-year-old woman who states that she's allergic to shellfish and iodine. She speaks in complete full sentences and complains of nausea and vomiting. While giving her medical history, she indicates that she has never had a reaction previously to eating fish. While assessing your patient, you note the following vital signs: Her pulse is 124 beats/min and regular, oxygen saturation is 90% on ambient air, and BP is easily auscultated at 112/62 mm Hg.

a. Chief complaint:

_____

_____

b. Vital signs:

_____

_____

c. Pertinent negatives:

_____

_____

5. It's late in the morning, and you are responding to a reported allergic reaction in a 10-month-old boy. Dispatch advises that the child was at the pediatrician today for a well-baby check. While there, the child received several immunizations. The child is now lethargic and gasping for breath. The child presents with urticaria all over. The baby has no other reported medical history or reported allergies. The apical pulse is 190 beats/min. The infant has delayed capillary refill and mottled skin.

a. Chief complaint:

_____

_____

b. Vital signs:

_____

_____

c. Pertinent negatives:

_____

_____

Ambulance Calls

The following case scenarios provide an opportunity to explore the concerns associated with patient management and paramedic care. Read each scenario, and then answer each question.

1. You are called to the suburban home of a 58-year-old man with "shortness of breath." You learn that while gardening, the patient was stung by numerous bees; within minutes, he noticed a tight feeling in his chest and started to wheeze. Now, 10 minutes after the sting, he looks flushed and very apprehensive and has a rash on the front of his chest. His vital signs are a pulse of 124 beats/min and slightly irregular, respirations of 36 breaths/min and shallow, and BP of 86/50 mm Hg. His SpO_2 is 93%.

   a. List the steps in managing this patient.

   (1)_____

   (2)_____

   (3)_____

   (4)_____

   (5)_____

   (6)_____

   (7)_____

   (8)_____

   b. One of the drugs that you will be giving is epinephrine. List the possible adverse effects or side effects of epinephrine.

   (1)_____

   (2)_____

   (3)_____

   (4)_____

   (5)_____

2. You are dining out on your night off at Fish Fare, a local restaurant. As you are just about to dig into your red snapper, you notice a woman at a nearby table looking distressed. "Aunt Gertrude, what's the matter?" asks another woman at the table.

   "I don't know," squeaks the distressed woman. "I feel so peculiar. Like there's a lump in my throat. And my chest feels so tight."

   Without waiting to hear another word, you bolt over to the telephone, dial 9-1-1, and ask for an ambulance posthaste. Then you go over to the woman in distress and introduce yourself as a paramedic. You notice that the woman's face is very flushed, and her eyes look puffy. Her pulse is weak and rapid.

"Oh, dear, I think I'm going to be sick," she says.

Just then, the ambulance pulls up. List the steps in treating this patient.

a. _____

b. _____

c. _____

d. _____

e. _____

3. Which of the following patients is most likely to be experiencing an anaphylactic reaction? (For those who are not, indicate what you think they are suffering from.)

    a. A 45-year-old man is dining at a fast-food joint. Suddenly he grows very pale and lurches back from the table, clutching his throat, with his eyes popping. He staggers to his feet and then collapses to the floor—all in complete silence. His problem is most likely:

    _____

    b. You are summoned for a 60-year-old man having a "bad reaction" to a medicine. Earlier in the day, the patient was prescribed erythromycin for a respiratory infection. Now he complains of severe abdominal distress and nausea. On physical examination, his skin is slightly pale and cool. His pulse is 72 beats/min and regular, his respirations are 22 breaths/min and unlabored, and his BP is 160/94 mm Hg. His problem is most likely:

    _____

    c. A 22-year-old man is found sitting on the sidewalk in marked distress. He tells you hoarsely that he just got "a shot" at the venereal disease (VD) clinic down the street, and right after he was given the shot and sent home, he started to feel "real strange." He says he got hot and itchy all over, and now he feels like he's going to die. On physical examination, his face looks quite flushed and puffy. His pulse is 140 beats/min and thready, his respirations are 32 breaths/min and shallow, and his BP is 110/60 mm Hg. His problem is most likely:

    _____

4. List the steps you would take to manage the patient described in Question 3.

    a. _____

    b. _____

    c. _____

    d. _____

    e. _____

5. After you report to medical control regarding the patient in Question 3, the physician instructs you to give diphenhydramine (Benadryl) as well. Per the Volume 1 Appendix, *Emergency Medications*, what are the contraindications to giving diphenhydramine?

    a. _____

    b. _____

    c. _____

    d. _____

    e. _____

6. What are the correct dosage and route of administration in this case?

_____

Complete the Patient Care Report (PCR)

Read the first incident scenario in the Ambulance Calls section, and then complete the following PCR.

EMS Patient Care Report (PCR)					
Date:	**Incident No.:**	**Nature of Call:**		**Location:**	
Dispatched:	**En Route:**	**At Scene:**	**Transport:**	**At Hospital:**	**In Service:**
Patient Information					
Age:		**Allergies:**			
Sex:		**Medications:**			
Weight (in kg [lb]):		**Past Medical History:**			
		Chief Complaint:			

Vital Signs				
Time:	**BP:**	**Pulse:**	**Respirations:**	**SpO$_2$:**
Time:	**BP:**	**Pulse:**	**Respirations:**	**SpO$_2$:**
Time:	**BP:**	**Pulse:**	**Respirations:**	**SpO$_2$:**

EMS Treatment (circle all that apply)				
Oxygen @ _____ L/min via (circle one): NC NRM Bag-mask device		**Assisted Ventilation**	**Airway Adjunct**	**CPR**
Defibrillation	**Bleeding Control**	**Bandaging**	**Splinting**	**Other:**

Narrative

True/False

If you believe the statement to be more true than false, write the letter "T" in the space provided. If you believe the statement to be more false than true, write the letter "F."

_____ **1.** All patients who exhibit signs and symptoms of allergic reaction should receive epinephrine.

_____ **2.** Patients should be educated to wear medical identification tags and carry their prescribed anaphylaxis kit.

_____ **3.** Corticosteroids can be used for anaphylaxis.

_____ **4.** Epinephrine has beta-1 properties that cause the blood vessels to constrict, reducing vasodilation.

_____ **5.** Bee stingers are best removed with sharp, pointy tweezers.

_____ **6.** Millions of Americans are at risk for anaphylaxis.

_____ **7.** Allergens can invade the body through the skin, respiratory tract, or GI tract.

_____ **8.** The respiratory system usually protects the human body from substances and organisms that are considered foreign to the body.

_____ **9.** An inhaled beta-adrenergic agent can be used for a patient with an allergic reaction with bronchospasm.

_____ **10.** The time of onset after administration of corticosteroids is 4 to 6 hours.

Short Answer

Complete this section with short written answers using the space provided.

1. When an antigen combines with a specific antibody on the surface of a mast cell, the mast cell loses its chemical bombs ("degranulates," to use the technical term), releasing a variety of powerful mediators, such as histamine and serotonin. List seven effects produced by the mediator "histamine."

a. _____

b. _____

c. _____

d. _____

e. _____

f. _____

g. _____

2. Besides bees, what other agents are commonly responsible for anaphylactic reactions? List at least four.

a. _____

b. _____

c. _____

d. _____

Fill in the Table

Fill in the missing parts of the table with examples of the common substances associated with anaphylaxis.

Causes of Anaphylactic Reactions	
Antigen, General Category	**Comments**
Foods	
Medications	
Insect stings	
Anti-cancer drugs	
Latex	
Animals	

Data from Mustafa S. Anaphylaxis. Medscape website. http://emedicine.medscape.com/article/135065-overview#a4. Updated February 22, 2017. Accessed March 31, 2017; and Peroni DG, Sansotta N, Bernardini R, et al. Muscle relaxants allergy. Int J Immunopathol Pharmacol. 2011;24(3 Suppl):S35-46. Pub Med Abstract. https://www.ncbi.nlm.nih.gov/pubmed/22014924. Accessed January 17, 2017.

The cycle of infection can often be easily broken by handwashing.

Infectious Diseases

Matching

Part I

Match each of the items in the left column to the appropriate term in the right column.

_____ **1.** A sexually transmitted disease caused by the bacterium *Chlamydia trachomatis*; has the highest incidence in sexually transmitted diseases; signs and symptoms include inflammation of the urethra, epididymis, cervix, and fallopian tubes and discharge from the urethra.

_____ **2.** A pathogen is present but has produced no illness in the host; often progresses to active infection; a colonized host is often called a carrier because he or she can transmit the pathogen to others.

_____ **3.** An infectious disease that can be transmitted from one person to another by direct contact or by indirect contact through a vector or fomite; also called contagious disease.

_____ **4.** A virus that originated in Africa and is transmitted by the *Aedes aegypti* mosquito; signs and symptoms include fever that typically lasts from 5 to 7 days, and possibly incapacitating joint pain.

_____ **5.** A highly contagious sexually transmitted disease caused by the bacteria *Haemophilus ducreyi,* which causes painful sores (ulcers), usually of the genitals.

_____ **6.** Consistently present or prevalent in a population or geographic area.

_____ **7.** A virus formerly limited to West Africa, spread through direct contact through nonintact skin or mucous membranes, and whose initial symptoms include fever, intense weakness, muscle pain, headaches, and sore throat; both contact and droplet precautions are needed with this disease; approximately 10% of infected people experience internal or external bleeding.

_____ **8.** The transmission of an infectious agent by inhalation of relatively large particles generated when an infected person coughs or sneezes; these particles travel a short distance through the air before falling to the ground.

_____ **9.** Use of a surgical mask on the patient and airflow measures to prevent droplet transmission; used for patients with possible influenza, meningitis, pertussis (whooping cough), mumps, rubella (German measles), and Ebola.

_____ **10.** A person trained to ensure that proper postexposure medical treatment and counseling are provided to an exposure employee or volunteer.

_____ **11.** An overgrowth of bacteria in the vagina, characterized by itching, burning, or pain and possibly a fishy-smelling discharge.

A. Acquired immunodeficiency syndrome (AIDS)

B. Airborne precautions

C. Airborne transmission

D. Avian (bird) flu

E. Bacteria

F. Bacterial vaginosis

G. Bloodborne pathogens

H. Candidiasis

I. Carriers

J. Chancre

K. Chancroid

_____ **12.** Small organisms that can grow and reproduce outside the human cell in the presence of the needed temperature and nutrients and cause disease by invading and multiplying in the tissues of the host.

_____ **13.** A disease caused by a virus that occurs naturally in the bird population; signs and symptoms include fever, sore throat, cough, and muscle aches.

_____ **14.** The transmission of an infectious agent by inhalation of small particles that become aerosolized when the infected person coughs, sneezes, talks, or exhales; particles remain suspended in this vapor and can be carried a short distance, usually 3 feet (1 m) to 6 feet (2 m).

_____ **15.** The use of a surgical mask on the patient and the use of airflow measures to prevent airborne transmission; apply to diseases that are large particle and can travel a distance of 6 feet (2 m), then drop to the floor.

_____ **16.** A virus transmitted by the mosquitos *Aedes aegypti* and *Aedes albopictus*, found throughout the world, in which the majority of people are asymptomatic; if the severe form develops, it is characterized by hypovolemic shock, hemorrhage, and potentially death.

_____ **17.** The presence of blood or other potentially infectious materials on an item or surface.

_____ **18.** The transmission of an infectious agent by means of direct or indirect contact with the infected persons, such as skin-to-skin contact or contact with the patient's environment and/or equipment.

_____ **19.** The use of precautions (gloves, gown, good handwashing, and cleaning of high-touch items) to prevent contact transmission; used for patients presenting with draining wounds, multidrug-resistant infection, lice, norovirus, and Ebola.

_____ **20.** The period during which an infected person can transmit a communicable disease to someone else.

_____ **21.** The end-stage disease process caused by the human immunodeficiency virus; results in extreme vulnerability to numerous opportunistic bacterial, viral, and fungal infections that would not affect a person with an intact immune system.

_____ **22.** The primary hard lesion or ulcer of syphilis that occurs at the entry site of the infection.

_____ **23.** People who harbor an infectious agent and, although not personally ill, can transmit the infection to other people.

_____ **24.** A vaginal infection that is not technically a sexually transmitted infection, and that can occur in a pregnant or nonpregnant female, but is more common in pregnancy; also called thrush or a yeast infection.

_____ **25.** Pathogenic microorganisms that are present in human blood and can cause disease in humans. These pathogens include, but are not limited to, hepatitis B virus, human immunodeficiency virus, hepatitis C virus, and syphilis.

L. Chikungunya

M. Chlamydia

N. Colonized

O. Communicable disease

P. Communicable period

Q. Contact precautions

R. Contact transmission

S. Contaminated

T. Dengue

U. Designated infection control officer (DICO)

V. Droplet precautions

W. Droplet transmission

X. Ebola

Y. Endemic

Part II

Match each of the items in the left column to the appropriate term in the right column.

_____ **1.** An infectious viral disease that occurs most often in late winter and spring; begins with a fever followed by a cough, running nose; and pinkeye; a rash spreads from the face and neck down the back and trunk.

_____ **2.** A tick-borne disease that primarily affects the skin, heart, joints, and nervous system and is characterized by a round, red lesion or bull's-eye rash.

_____ **3.** Tiny, wingless, parasitic insects that feed on blood; an infestation is easily spread through close personal contact; types include head, body, and pubic lice.

A. Epidemic

B. Enterococcus

C. Fomites

_____ **4.** The presence of excessive bile pigments in the bloodstream that give the skin, mucous membranes, and eyes a distinct yellow color; often associated with liver disease.

D. Fungi

_____ **5.** A disease originating from the Arabian peninsula, transmitted by close contact with camel urine or nasal secretions. Symptoms include fever, cough, and shortness of breath, and gastrointestinal disturbances; there is very low risk to health care providers and the general public in the United States.

E. Gastroenteritis

_____ **6.** A type of meningitis caused by the meningococcal bacterium, *Neisseria meningitidis.*

F. Genital warts

_____ **7.** An inflammation of the meningeal coverings of the brain and spinal cord; usually caused by a virus or bacterium; the viral type is not communicable and is less severe than the bacterial type, which can result in brain damage, hearing loss, learning disability, or death.

G. Gonorrhea

_____ **8.** The period between exposure to an organism and the first symptoms of illness, during which the organism multiplies within the body and starts to produce symptoms. This period is when the disease can be transmitted to another person.

H. Hantavirus

_____ **9.** The process of producing widespread immunity to a specific infectious disease among a targeted group by inoculating individual members of the population; can also refer to a set of vaccinations given together or on a recommended schedule.

I. Health care–associated infection

_____ **10.** The yellow appearance of the skin and other tissues caused by an accumulation of bile pigments.

J. Host resistance

_____ **11.** The most common sexually transmitted disease that can cause genital warts and some types of cancer.

K. Human immunodeficiency virus (HIV)

_____ **12.** The virus that may lead to acquired immunodeficiency syndrome; cells in the immune system are killed or damaged so that the body is unable to fight infections and certain cancers.

L. Human papilloma virus (HPV)

_____ **13.** A term that comprises many types of infections and irritations of the gastrointestinal tract; symptoms include nausea and vomiting, fever, abdominal cramps, and diarrhea; also called stomach flu.

M. Icterus jaundice

_____ **14.** Small organisms that can grow rapidly in the presence of the needed nutrients and organic material and can cause infection related to contact with decaying organic matter or from airborne spores in the environment such as molds.

N. Immunization

_____ **15.** Inanimate objects contaminated with microorganisms that serve as a means of transmitting an illness.

O. Incubation period

_____ **16.** A common, normal organism of the gastrointestinal tract, urinary tract, and genitourinary tract that can be pathogenic and become resistant to vancomycin.

P. Infectious disease

_____ **17.** An outbreak of disease that substantially exceeds what is expected based on recent experience.

Q. Infectious hepatitis

_____ **18.** A sexually transmitted disease that results in infection caused by the gonococcal bacteria *Neisseria gonorrhea*; signs and symptoms include pus-containing discharge from the urethra and painful urination in males and signs and symptoms of an acute abdomen in females.

R. Influenza

_____ **19.** Warts caused by the human papillomavirus, a sexually transmitted disease; also called condylomata acuminata or venereal warts.

S. Jaundice

_____ **20.** A type of virus found in wild rodents, which can also cause disease in humans, characterized by fever, headache, abdominal pain, loss of appetite, and vomiting; diseases caused are hemorrhagic fever with renal syndrome and hantavirus pulmonary syndrome.

T. Lice

_____ **21.** An infection acquired 2 days after admission to a health care setting or 30 days after discharge from one.

_____ **22.** One's ability to fight off infection.

_____ **23.** The flu, a respiratory infection caused by a variety of viruses; differs from the common cold in that the flu involves a fever, headache, and extreme exhaustion.

_____ **24.** Another name for hepatitis A; an inflammation from a virus that causes mild fatigue, loss of appetite, fever, nausea, abdominal pain, and, eventually, jaundice, dark-colored urine, and pale, clay-colored stools.

_____ **25.** A disease caused by pathogenic organisms.

U. Lyme disease

V. Measles

W. Meningitis

X. Meningococcal meningitis

Y. Middle East respiratory syndrome (MERS)

Multiple Choice

Read each item carefully, and then select the best response.

_____ **1.** Agencies responsible for protecting public health include the following, EXCEPT:

    A. Occupational Safety and Health Administration (OSHA).

    B. Centers for Disease Control and Prevention (CDC).

    C. state health departments.

    D. National Sanitary Foundation.

_____ **2.** Communicable diseases may be transmitted by:

    A. droplets.

    B. airborne particles.

    C. vectors.

    D. All of the above

_____ **3.** Host resistance refers to:

    A. drug-resistant antibiotics.

    B. the body's ability to fight off infection.

    C. virulence of the invading microorganism.

    D. the period of contagiousness.

_____ **4.** Which of the following best defines the key element of the Ryan White Comprehensive AIDS Resources Emergency Act?

    A. A designated infection control officer (DICO) is required by federal law in each county.

    B. The medical facility must release source patient tests to the DICO.

    C. Emergency response personnel must be notified within 48 hours after a workplace exposure to tuberculosis.

    D. Patients' health records are protected by federal law.

_____ **5.** Personal protective equipment (PPE) needs to be worn by a paramedic:

    A. at all collision scenes.

    B. at any multiple-casualty incident.

    C. only while working in a contaminated environment.

    D. according to your department's exposure control plan.

_____ **6.** No matter how high-tech PPE may be, it is only effective if:

    A. proper removal techniques are employed.

    B. it is used prior to the 36-month expiration.

    C. the patient is in the incubation period.

    D. the patient gives permission for you to use it.

_____ **7.** An inflammation of the membranes that cover the brain and spinal cord is called:
- **A.** influenza.
- **B.** pertussis.
- **C.** meningitis.
- **D.** tuberculosis.

_____ **8.** Most droplets and airborne disease exposures can be prevented by:
- **A.** placing a mask on patients with fevers and rashes.
- **B.** doing nothing; confining the patient's face may exacerbate secretions.
- **C.** the crew wearing level III biohazard suits.
- **D.** notifying the hospital in advance and having the patient decontaminated prior to admission.

_____ **9.** All of the following are highly communicable viral diseases, EXCEPT:
- **A.** measles.
- **B.** mumps.
- **C.** pertussis.
- **D.** meningitis.

_____ **10.** Lice and scabies infections may affect:
- **A.** patients.
- **B.** families.
- **C.** crews.
- **D.** All of the above

Fill in the Blank

Read each item carefully, and then complete the statement by filling in the missing word(s).

1. _____ _____ is the term used to describe infection control practices that reduce the opportunity of an exposure to occur in the daily care of patients.

2. A paramedic's major protective measure is _____.

3. Unfortunately, paramedics get exposed to communicable diseases. The third line of defense is considered _____ _____ _____-_____.

4. _____ _____ include bacteria, viruses, fungi, and parasites.

5. Mononucleosis is caused by the _____-_____ virus. Transmission occurs via direct contact with _____ secretions.

6. _____ _____ is caused when a deer tick's bite injects a bacterium into the bloodstream of the human host.

7. Gonorrhea, syphilis, and herpes are all considered _____ _____ _____.

8. An inflammation of the liver that may be produced by five distinct forms of virus is called _____ _____.

9. Methicillin-resistant *Staphylococcus aureus* (MRSA) is believed to be transmitted from _____ to _____ via _____ hands.

10. Severe acute respiratory syndrome (SARS) arose from the merger of viruses from _____ and _____.

Identify

Read the following case studies, and then list the chief complaint, vital signs, and pertinent negatives.

1. Your unit is called to the airport to meet an inbound flight. There is a patient reported to have flu-like symptoms that include fever, chills, and dry cough. The patient is conscious and alert but very weak. He is assisted from the aircraft when it arrives at the terminal gate. You note that the flight appears to be domestic in origin. While you are taking the patient's history, he denies any type of international travel but has been traveling extensively with very little sleep this past week. He denies other previous medical history. He denies medications and allergies to medications or prescription drugs. His skin is warm and dry. He feels febrile. After further discussion, you discover that his school-aged children were recently sick with a viral infection. His vital signs are as follows: Respiratory rate is 20 breaths/min, oxygen saturation on ambient air is 95%, pulse is 106 beats/min and regular, and blood pressure (BP) is 128/68 mm Hg.

   a. Chief complaint:

   _____

   _____

   b. Vital signs:

   _____

   _____

   c. Pertinent negatives:

   _____

   _____

2. It's a hot, humid day in the mid-90s and your advanced life support (ALS) unit is dispatched to assist the police department. You arrive on scene to discover several patrol vehicles located outside an unkempt house. You are met by one of the officers, who explains that the police department received a call from an out-of-town relative to check on the welfare of the elderly resident. Once inside the house, the police officers noticed a severe lice infestation. Many of the officers are exposed to the nasty critters. Although the exposure is not life threatening, the officers appear very annoyed. They describe the conditions as squalid. You request that the exposed officers assist the elderly patient out to his front yard so that you can properly decontaminate him and minimize the lice exposure to any additional providers and equipment. Once outside, the patient appears emaciated and is wearing soiled clothing, yet states he just put on the clean clothes the other morning. He has a bag of prescription medications that seem to indicate a mental health and cardiac history but says he rarely needs to take any pills. His vital signs are as follows: Pulse is 88 beats/min and irregular, BP is 98/72 mm Hg, and oxygen saturation is 88%. He is tachypneic, and there is obvious skin tenting and delayed capillary refill.

   a. Chief complaint:

   _____

   _____

   b. Vital signs:

   _____

   _____

   c. Pertinent negatives:

   _____

   _____

3. While preparing for an ALS interfacility transport, you are told by the nurse's station that the patient has MRSA. The patient has a number of drip medications, along with strict respiratory precautions. You are told that the patient is "stable" for transport. He is also on a nonrebreathing face mask and is conscious and alert. The patient is on a cardiac monitor and is in a sinus rhythm. His BP as noted on the noninvasive monitor is 98/54 mm Hg, and his heart rate is 62 beats/min. He has a lengthy medical history, including kidney transplant. He is on several immunosuppressants.

   a. Chief complaint:

_____

_____

   b. Vital signs:

_____

_____

   c. Pertinent negatives:

_____

_____

Ambulance Calls

The following case scenarios provide an opportunity to explore the concerns associated with patient management and paramedic care. Read each scenario, and then answer each question.

1. You are called to transport a 22-year-old college student from the college infirmary to the hospital. The nurse tells you that the student has a high fever. He complains of a severe headache and stiff neck, and he seems rather confused. He vomits twice en route to the hospital.

   a. What is the patient experiencing?

_____

_____

   b. How can the paramedic minimize the risk of catching the illness?

_____

_____

2. A 54-year-old man calls for an ambulance after he coughed up some blood. He says that over the past several weeks he has been waking up in the middle of the night with his pajamas and bedclothes soaked through with sweat. He has lost about 25 pounds in the last 2 or 3 months, and today he started noticing some blood in his sputum.

   a. What is the patient experiencing?

_____

_____

   b. How can the paramedic minimize the risk of catching the illness?

_____

_____

3. A 28-year-old man calls for an ambulance because he "feels lousy." He says that for a week or so, he hasn't had any energy at all. He doesn't feel like eating or doing anything; he just feels "done in." Even cigarettes "taste like cow dung." This morning, he noticed that his urine was very dark, and he got panicky. On examination, you observe that his eyes have a yellow tinge; he has a low-grade fever and aching joints. There are also needle tracks on both of his arms.

a. What is the patient experiencing?

_____

_____

b. How can the paramedic minimize the risk of catching the illness?

_____

_____

4. You are called to transport an 8-year-old boy who fell and sustained a laceration to his forehead. "I told him to stay in bed," his mother says, "but no, he has to go horsing around with his brother." According to the mother, both children have been sick for a week, with a fever, no appetite, and soreness under their ears. On examining the 8-year-old, you find a 2-inch laceration on the left side of the forehead, and you control the bleeding with pressure. He does seem a little warm to the touch and has a headache.

a. Aside from the soft-tissue injury, what is the patient likely experiencing?

_____

_____

b. How can the paramedic minimize the risk of catching the illness?

_____

_____

5. It's back to the college infirmary for another patient with a fever—this time a 19-year-old woman. She complains of headache and says the light bothers her a lot. Her eyes are reddened, and she is coughing. She has a blotchy, red rash over her face and neck, and when you examine her throat, you notice some little white spots on the mucous membranes in her mouth.

a. What is the patient experiencing?

_____

_____

b. How can the paramedic minimize the risk of catching the illness?

_____

_____

Complete the Patient Care Report (PCR)

Read the second scenario in the Ambulance Calls section, and then complete the following PCR.

EMS Patient Care Report (PCR)			
Date:	**Incident No.:**	**Nature of Call:**	**Location:**
Dispatched:	**En Route:**	**At Scene:**	**Transport:** **At Hospital:** **In Service:**

Patient Information			
Age:		**Allergies:**	
Sex:		**Medications:**	
Weight (in kg [lb]):		**Past Medical History:**	
		Chief Complaint:	

Vital Signs				
Time:	**BP:**	**Pulse:**	**Respirations:**	**SpO$_2$:**
Time:	**BP:**	**Pulse:**	**Respirations:**	**SpO$_2$:**
Time:	**BP:**	**Pulse:**	**Respirations:**	**SpO$_2$:**

EMS Treatment (circle all that apply)				
Oxygen @ _____ L/min via (circle one): NC NRM Bag-mask device		**Assisted Ventilation**	**Airway Adjunct**	**CPR**
Defibrillation	**Bleeding Control**	**Bandaging**	**Splinting**	**Other:**

Narrative

True/False

If you believe the statement to be more true than false, write the letter "T" in the space provided. If you believe the statement to be more false than true, write the letter "F."

_____ **1.** Ebola is a virus spread through direct contact with nonintact skin or mucous membranes.

_____ **2.** Patients with AIDS are abnormally susceptible to many opportunistic infections.

_____ **3.** AIDS can be acquired through casual contact, such as shaking hands with an HIV-positive patient.

_____ **4.** HIV is transmitted by airborne means.

_____ **5.** HIV type 1 was first identified in the late 1970s.

_____ **6.** Many health care workers have acquired HIV through contact with the blood or body fluids of patients.

_____ **7.** The majority of AIDS cases that have occurred in health care workers as a result of occupational exposure have been among emergency medical services (EMS) personnel.

_____ **8.** Complications of syphilis can include cardiac, ophthalmic, auditory, and central nervous system complications.

_____ **9.** Sexually transmitted diseases (STDs) require special standard precautions.

_____ **10.** The incubation period of genital herpes is 3 to 4 weeks.

Short Answer

Complete this section with short written answers using the space provided.

1. Carry out the following research project before you begin employment as a paramedic.

a. Check off the illnesses you had as a child or up to this point:

_____ Measles

_____ Mumps

_____ Chickenpox

_____ German measles (rubella)

_____ Polio

_____ Hepatitis B

b. Check off the immunizations you have had up to this point, and fill in the dates (obtain the records from your family doctor or the clinic where you received your immunizations):

_____ Measles   Date immunized: _____

_____ Mumps   Date immunized: _____

_____ Rubella   Date immunized: _____

_____ DPT (diphtheria/pertussis/tetanus)

        #1   Date immunized: _____

        #2   Date immunized: _____

        #3   Date immunized: _____

_____ Most recent tetanus booster   Date immunized: _____

_____ Oral polio #1   Date immunized: _____

_____ Oral polio #2   Date immunized: _____

_____ Oral polio #3   Date immunized: _____

_____ Hepatitis B   Date immunized: _____

c. Based on the preceding data you have compiled, what immunizations do you need to get before you start work?

_____

_____

a. List three ways that HIV can be transmitted from one person to another.

(1)_____

(2)_____

(3)_____

b. List three things you can do to minimize the risk of acquiring HIV from a patient.

(1)_____

(2)_____

(3)_____

Fill in the Table

Fill in the missing parts of the table.

1. Complete the following table, which outlines the PPE necessary in preventing transmission of HIV and HBV. Indicate "yes" or "no" for each task or activity.

Recommended Personal Protective Equipment for Preventing Transmission of Human Immunodeficiency Virus and Hepatitis B Virus in the Prehospital Setting				
Task or Activity	Disposable Gloves	Gown	Mask	Protective Eyewear
Bleeding control with spurting blood	Yes		Yes	
Bleeding control with minimal bleeding	Yes		No	
Emergency childbirth	Yes		Yes, if spatter	
Drawing blood samples	Yes		No	
Inserting an IV line	Yes		No	
Advanced airway insertion (eg, endotracheal intubation, laryngeal mask airway, Combitube)	Yes		No, unless spatter is likely[a]	
Oral/nasal suctioning, manually cleaning airway	Yes		No, unless spatter is likely[a]	
Handling and cleaning instruments with microbial contamination	Yes		No	
Measuring blood pressure	No		No	

Task or Activity	Disposable Gloves	Gown	Mask	Protective Eyewear
Measuring temperature	No		No	
Giving an injection	No		No	
ªSpatter is often likely, so use personal protective equipment accordingly.				

Data from Centers for Disease Control and Prevention (CDC): Guidelines for prevention of transmission of human immunodeficiency virus and hepatitis B virus to health-care and public-safety workers: A response to P.L. 100-607 The Health Omnibus Programs Extention Act of 1988. MMWR. 1989;38(S-6):Table 4, (d)(3)(ix)(A)-(C). Available at: http://wonder.cdc.gov/wonder/prevguid/p0000114/p0000114.asp. Accessed November 10, 2011; and Ask the expert: gloves for injections. HCPro OSHA Heathcare Advisor website. http://blogs.hcpro.com/osha/2012/01/ask-the-expert-gloves-for-injections/; and Standard interpretations. United States Department of Labor, OSHA website. https://www.osha.gov/pls/oshaweb/owadisp.show_document?p_table=INTERPRETATIONS&p_id=20819

2. Indicate the mode(s) of transmission and recommended protective measures for each of the diseases in the following table.

Disease	Mode(s) of Transmission	Protective Measures
AIDS		
HAV		
HBV		
Meningitis		
Mumps		
Syphilis		
Tuberculosis		
MERS		
SARS		

Toxicology

Matching

Part I

Match the definitions in the left column to the appropriate terms in the right column.

_____ **1.** Any use of drugs that causes physical psychological, economic, legal, or social harm to the user or others affected by the user's behavior.

_____ **2.** Substance that has some therapeutic effect (such as reducing inflammation, fighting bacteria, or producing euphoria) when given in the appropriate circumstances and in the appropriate dose.

_____ **3.** A common houseplant that is also called dumb cane; ingestion leads to burns of the mouth and tongue and, possibly, paralysis of the vocal cords and nausea and vomiting; in severe cases, causes edema of the tongue and larynx, leading to airway compromise.

_____ **4.** A severe withdrawal syndrome seen in people with alcoholism who are deprived of ethyl alcohol; characterized by restlessness, fever, sweating, disorientation, agitation, and seizures; can be fatal if untreated.

_____ **5.** The dried leaves and flower buds of the *Cannabis sativa* plant that are smoked to achieve a high.

_____ **6.** A common mood stabilizer used in the treatment of bipolar disorder.

_____ **7.** In relation to drugs, legalized drugs such as coffee, alcohol, and tobacco.

_____ **8.** A perennial flowering shrub with clusters of red berries that can lead to serious and even fatal poisoning. Also known as red sage or wild sage; ingestion causes stomach upset, muscle weakness, shock, and, sometimes, death.

_____ **9.** A method of suicide that involves mixing certain household chemicals in an enclosed space to create toxic gases, such as hydrogen sulfide and hydrogen cyanide, as the chemicals combine; also called detergent suicide.

_____ **10.** Chemicals that are acids or alkalis; cause direct chemical injury to the tissues they contact.

_____ **11.** A seed that contains the poison ricin; causes a variety of toxic effects; burning of the mouth and throat; nausea, vomiting, diarrhea, and severe stomach pains; prostration; failing vision; and kidney failure, which is the usual cause of death.

_____ **12.** A common houseplant that contains calcium oxalate crystals; ingestion leads to nausea, vomiting, and diarrhea.

A. Alcoholism

B. Amphetamines

C. Antagonist

D. Antidote

E. Barbiturate

F. Benzodiazepines

G. Caladium

H. Castor bean

I. Caustics

J. Chemical suicide

K. Cocaine

L. Delirium tremens (DTs)

_____ **13.** In relation to drugs, illegal drugs such as marijuana, cocaine, and lysergic acid diethylamide.

_____ **14.** Compounds made up principally of hydrogen and carbon atoms mostly obtained from the distillation of petroleum.

_____ **15.** An agent that produces false perceptions in any one of the five senses.

_____ **16.** A physical tolerance and psychological dependence on a drug or drugs.

_____ **17.** The family of sedative-hypnotics that provide muscle relaxation and mild sedation; most commonly used to treat anxiety, seizures, and alcohol withdrawal; include drugs such as diazepam (Valium) and midazolam (Versed).

_____ **18.** Potent sedative-hypnotics historically used as sleep aids, antianxiety drugs, and as part of the regimen for seizure control; include drugs such as thiopental (Pentothal, Trapanal) and methohexital (Brevital).

_____ **19.** Something to counteract the effect of a poison.

_____ **20.** A molecule that blocks the ability of a given chemical to bind to its receptor, preventing a biologic response.

_____ **21.** A plant that contains cardiac glycosides used in making digitalis; ingestion of leaves causes nausea, vomiting, diarrhea, abdominal cramps, hyperkalemia, and a variety of dysrhythmias.

_____ **22.** A chronic disorder characterized by the compulsive use of a substance that results in physical, psychological, or social harm to the user, who continues to use the substance despite the harm.

_____ **23.** A stimulant; a naturally occurring alkaloid that is extracted from the _Erythroxylon coca_ plant leaves found in South America.

_____ **24.** A disorder characterized by a physical and psychological addiction to ethanol.

_____ **25.** A class of drugs that increase alertness and excitation (stimulants); including methamphetamine (crank or ice), methylenedioxyamphetamine (MDA, Adam), and methylenedioxymethamphetamine (MDMA, Eve, Ecstasy).

M. Dieffenbachia

N. Drug

O. Drug abuse

P. Drug addiction

Q. Foxglove

R. Habituation

S. Hallucinogen

T. Hydrocarbons

U. Illicit

V. Lantana

W. Licit

X. Lithium

Y. Marijuana

Part II

Match the definitions in the left column to the appropriate terms in the right column.

_____ **1.** A physiologic state of adaption to a drug, usually characterized by tolerance to the effects of the drug and a withdrawal syndrome if use of the drug is stopped, especially abruptly.

_____ **2.** A substance whose chemical action could damage structures or impair function when introduced into the body.

_____ **3.** Enhancement of the effect of one drug by another drug.

_____ **4.** The emotional state of craving a drug to maintain a feeling of well-being.

_____ **5.** A predictable set of signs and symptoms, usually involving altered central nervous system activity that occurs after the abrupt cessation of a drug or after rapidly decreasing the usual dosage of a drug.

_____ **6.** A group of drugs used to treat severe depression and manage pain; minimal dosing errors can cause toxic results.

_____ **7.** A poison or harmful substance produced by bacteria, animals, or plants.

_____ **8.** The syndrome-like symptoms of any given class or group of poisonous agents.

_____ **9.** A highly addictive drug in the amphetamine family.

_____ **10.** Psychiatric medication used primarily to treat atypical depression by increasing norepinephrine and serotonin levels in the central nervous system.

A. Methamphetamine

B. Monoamine oxidase inhibitors (MAOIs)

C. Narcotic

D. Opiate

E. Opioid

F. Organophosphates

G. Overdose

H. Physical dependence

I. Poison

J. Potentiation

_____ **11.** The generic term for opiates and opioids, drugs that act as a central nervous system depressant and produce insensibility or stupor.

_____ **12.** Various alkaloids derived from the opium or poppy plant.

_____ **13.** The study of toxic or poisonous substances.

_____ **14.** Medical emergencies caused by toxic agents such as poison; may be intentional or unintentional.

_____ **15.** Physiologic adaptation to the effects of a drug such that increasingly larger doses of the drug are required to achieve the same effect.

_____ **16.** The action of two substances, such as drugs, in which the total effects are greater than the sum of the independent effects of the two substances.

_____ **17.** A synthetic narcotic not derived from opium, with sedative properties; examples are fentanyl (Sublimaze) and alfentanil (Alfenta); also called narcotics.

_____ **18.** A class of chemical found in many insecticides used in agriculture and in the home.

_____ **19.** A condition that occurs when a drug (either licit or illicit) is taken in excess; can have toxic or lethal consequences.

_____ **20.** The destruction of muscle tissue leading to a release of potassium and myoglobin.

_____ **21.** A primary ingredient in aspirin.

_____ **22.** A drug used to reduce anxiety, calm agitated patients, and help produce drowsiness and sleep (central nervous system depressants).

_____ **23.** A class of antidepressants that inhibit the reuptake of serotonin.

_____ **24.** An idiosyncratic complication that occurs with antidepressant therapy in which patients have lower extremity muscle rigidity, confusion or disorientation, and/or agitation.

_____ **25.** An illicit drug consisting of a blend of synthetic cannabinoids; it can produce delirium and short- and long-term psychotic effects.

K. Psychological dependence

L. Rhabdomyolysis

M. Salicylates

N. Sedative-hypnotic

O. Selective serotonin reuptake inhibitors (SSRIs)

P. Serotonin syndrome

Q. Spice

R. Synergism

S. Tolerance

T. Toxicologic emergencies

U. Toxicology

V. Toxidrome

W. Toxin

X. Tricyclic antidepressants (TCAs)

Y. Withdrawal syndrome

Multiple Choice

Read each item carefully, and then select the best response.

_____ **1.** Poisoning by ingestion, in adults, is usually a result of:
- **A.** improperly labeled over-the-counter medications.
- **B.** improperly dispensed prescribed medications.
- **C.** suicide attempts or unintentional overdose.
- **D.** workplace mishaps involving chemicals and toxic exposures.

_____ **2.** All of the following are common routes of poisoning, EXCEPT:
- **A.** inhalation.
- **B.** ingestion.
- **C.** injection.
- **D.** excretion.

_____ **3.** Alcoholism is usually diagnosed when the patient has a demonstrated:
- **A.** problem handling his or her drinks in public.
- **B.** physical and psychological addiction to ethanol.
- **C.** medicinal need to relieve pain with alcohol.
- **D.** binge drinking at least two times in the last month.

_____ **4.** Alcohol abuse may cause a number of medical consequences, including:
- **A.** subdural hematoma.
- **B.** GI bleeding.
- **C.** a higher risk of burns.
- **D.** All of the above

5. Alcohol withdrawal may have life-threatening consequences, including delirium tremens. Delirium tremens, or the "DTs," are best characterized by:
   A. tremors and diaphoresis.
   B. confusion and fever.
   C. restlessness and tachycardia.
   D. All of the above

6. The general assessment approach for toxicologic emergencies includes all of the following tasks, EXCEPT:
   A. primary survey.
   B. scene size-up.
   C. physical exam.
   D. There is no "general assessment"; these patients should receive a secondary assessment.

7. You are called to the scene of a 4-year-old who ingested a common houseplant. The best source of information regarding the accidental ingestion is:
   A. referring to the *Emergency Response Guidebook (ERG)*.
   B. contacting the Poison Center.
   C. contacting CHEMTREC.
   D. contacting medical control.

8. A chronic disorder characterized by the compulsive use of a substance resulting in physical, psychological, economic, legal, or social harm to the user who continues to use the substance despite the harm is considered:
   A. tolerance.
   B. drug addiction.
   C. substance abuse.
   D. antagonist.

9. The treatment for patients abusing cocaine, amphetamine, or methamphetamine is fundamentally the same. This treatment includes the following tasks, EXCEPT:
   A. establishing and maintaining the airway; consider an advanced airway as needed.
   B. establishing vascular access.
   C. administering morphine for pain relief.
   D. contacting medical control for sedation when behavior is violent.

10. Signs and symptoms of overdose with cardiac drugs may include:
    A. hypotension.
    B. weakness or confusion.
    C. nausea and vomiting.
    D. All of the above

11. Diarrhea, urination, miosis, muscle weakness, bradycardia, bronchospasm, bronchorrhea, emesis, lacrimation, seizures, salivation, and sweating are symptoms associated with a toxic exposure to:
    A. psychedelics.
    B. narcotics.
    C. ketamine.
    D. organophosphates.

12. Physical examination of a patient who has been poisoned with cyanide may reveal each of the following, EXCEPT:
    A. an altered mental state.
    B. respirations that are rapid and labored and that become slow and gasping.
    C. a slow and thready pulse.
    D. a bitter almond scent.

_____   **13.** The common symptoms of a tricyclic antidepressant overdose are:
   A. tachycardia, tachypnea, and hypotension.
   B. abdominal pain and nausea.
   C. internal bleeding and mottled skin.
   D. burning of the eyes, nose, and throat.

_____   **14.** An adult presenting with a potential salicylate overdose is likely to have:
   A. mistakenly taken too much Pepto-Bismol for a stomach ache.
   B. ingested a couple of extra Tylenol.
   C. a history of drug abuse or a psychiatric condition.
   D. a history of seizures or diabetes.

_____   **15.** Death from ingestion of large amounts of the plant foxglove usually occurs as a result of:
   A. acute respiratory distress.
   B. psychogenic shock.
   C. cardiac dysrhythmias.
   D. anaphylactic shock.

Fill in the Blank

Read each item carefully, and then complete the statement by filling in the missing word(s).

1. A(n) _____ is a substance that is toxic by nature, no matter how it gets into the body or in what quantities it is

   taken. By contrast, a(n) _____ is a substance that has some therapeutic effect when given in the appropriate dose.

2. _____ _____ usually fall under one of two general headings: _____ and _____.

3. Toxins cannot exert their effects until they enter the body. The four primary methods of entry are _____,

   _____, _____, and _____.

4. _____ are useful for remembering the assessment and management of different substances that fall under the same

   _____ _____.

5. The _____ effects of alcohol on the _____ produce a variety of _____, such as coagulopathies, hypoglycemia,

   and ____ bleeding.

6. _____, in both licit and illicit forms, can have devastating effects on those who _____ them. From smokable cocaine

   or _____ and methamphetamine to _____ diet aids and medications for attention deficit disorder (ADD), you will

   at some point care for a patient who is under the influence of _____.

7. Shortly after injecting _____, a user will appear to pass out. However, the user is typically quiet _____ and

   remains aware of what is being done or said.

8. Overdoses of cardiac medications are usually _____.

9. Treatment of carbon monoxide (CO) _____ in the field is aimed at providing the highest concentration of

   _____ possible to attempt to displace CO molecules from the _____.

10. Acids tend to be more _____-_____ than _____, and so they are often diluted relatively quickly. With _____,

   it is more important to keep water continually flowing because it usually takes much longer to rinse away the substance.

11. _____ is an analog of methamphetamine, and it may have similar toxic effects on the smaller scale.

12. Huffing _____ _____ can produce euphoria, anesthesia, weakness, _____, abdominal cramps, loss of coordination, neuropathy, blindness, and cardiac dysrhythmias.

13. Hydrocarbon products cause _____ _____, which results in severe abdominal _____, diarrhea, and belching. At the other end of the spectrum, just a single hydrocarbon substance exposure may cause life-threatening _____.

14. With a serious tricyclic antidepressant (TCA) overdose, be alert for electrocardiogram (ECG) changes, including a(n)_____ PR interval, _____, widening QRS, a terminal R wave greater than 3 mm in aVR, and a prolonged _____ interval.

15. Organic _____ is lipid soluble and quickly _____ in the _____.

Identify

In the following case studies, identify the appropriate toxidrome, and list two drugs associated with it.

1. You arrive on scene to find a 22-year-old woman who appears confused, has a blood pressure (BP) of 88/60 mm Hg, is slurring her speech, and is somewhat sleepy.
   a. Identify the appropriate toxidrome:

   _____

   b. Name two drugs that may fit this toxidrome.

   (1)_____

   (2)_____

2. Your advanced life support (ALS) ambulance arrives on scene at the request of law enforcement for a very agitated 42-year-old man. He won't stop talking and is paranoid.
   a. Identify the appropriate toxidrome:

   _____

   b. Name two drugs that may fit this toxidrome.

   (1)_____

   (2)_____

In the following case studies, identify the possible causative agent based on the presenting symptoms.

3. On arrival, you discover a 16-year-old boy with severe nausea and vomiting. You begin assessing the patient and immediately notice an odor that appears to be alcohol.

   _____

4. You are dispatched to a "delta" response (high priority) for a patient seizing. On arrival, you discover a 56-year-old man who is actively seizing and has snoring respirations. Family members state the patient has been recently depressed and withdrawn.

   _____

Ambulance Calls

The following case scenarios provide an opportunity to explore the concerns associated with patient management and paramedic care. Read each scenario, and then answer each question.

1. You are called to a somewhat rundown apartment building where the police have forcibly entered an apartment after neighbors reported that the occupant of the apartment has not been seen for a few days and has not answered his telephone. Inside, you find a man who looks to be about 30 years old lying unresponsive on a sofa in the living room. Some neighbors are milling around, giving information to the police officers.

   a. List six questions you would ask the neighbors about the patient.

      (1)_____

      (2)_____

      (3)_____

      (4)_____

      (5)_____

      (6)_____

   b. Besides the neighbors, what other sources of information might be present? What places in the apartment would you check? What would you be looking for?

      (1)_____

      (2)_____

      (3)_____

   c. When you examine the patient, you detect the following findings. For each finding listed, indicate its possible diagnostic significance.

Finding	Possible Diagnostic Significance
Cold, dry skin	
Pulse = 110 beats/min, thready	
BP = 90/60 mm Hg	
Respirations = 12 breaths/min and shallow	
Pupils dilated and not reactive to light	
Breath smells of alcohol (ETOH)	

   d. In assessing this patient's mental status, you find the following:
   • He does not open his eyes.
   • His arms flex when you pinch his leg.
   • He does not make any sound in response to your calling his name or pinching him.
   In view of those findings, he is best described as which of the following?
      (1)   Drowsy
      (2)   Lethargic
      (3)   Comatose
      (4)   Stuporous
      (5)   Obtunded

e. List steps in managing this patient.

(1)_____

(2)_____

(3)_____

(4)_____

(5)_____

(6)_____

(7)_____

(8)_____

(9)_____

(10)_____

2. You are called to the home of a frantic young couple who discovered their 3-year-old happily consuming the contents of a bottle from the cleaning cupboard. List five questions you would ask in taking the history of the incident.

a. _____

b. _____

c. _____

d. _____

e. _____

3. A middle-aged man is found unconscious in his garage. He has left a suicide note on the car windshield, but the hood of the car is cold, so you are reasonably sure the engine has not been run recently. List five things to which you would give particular attention in the physical examination of this patient.

a. _____

b. _____

c. _____

d. _____

e. _____

4. A 15-year-old boy swallowed about 20 of his father's tricyclic antidepressant pills in a suicide gesture after a family argument. You arrive at the scene, some 30 minutes distant from the nearest hospital, about 15 minutes after the ingestion. In a telephone consultation, Poison Control advises you to administer activated charcoal (if available) and monitor the airway and electrocardiogram (ECG) for dysrhythmias. The boy is alert, and vital signs are all within normal limits at this point.

a. What is the purpose of giving activated charcoal? That is, what is the therapeutic effect?

_____

b. List poisonings in which activated charcoal is contraindicated.

(1)_____

c. List the steps in treating this patient.

(1)_____

(2)_____

(3)_____

(4)_____

(5)_____

(6)_____

(7)_____

(8)_____

(9)_____

(10)_____

(11)_____

(12)_____

5. A 35-year-old man ingested "about a tablespoon" of drain buildup remover (Drano) crystals 10 to 15 minutes before your arrival. He is fully alert and complaining of severe pain in his throat and chest. His lips and mouth are very red, and there are still crystals sticking to the mucous membranes in his mouth.

a. From a management perspective, advanced life support care for a toxicologic emergency builds on the following basics:

(1)_____

(2)_____

(3)_____

(4)_____

(5)_____

(6)_____

(7)_____

(8)_____

(9)_____

6. You are summoned to a location near the railway tracks where the local "down-and-outs" gather. A police officer at the scene gestures you toward two of the group members congregated there. "They looked in pretty bad shape," he says, "so I thought I'd better call EMS."

"Been drinking real bad stuff," one of the group chimes in. "Told 'em to stay away from that rotgut—you can go blind from drinkin' stuff like that."

The first patient is in severe respiratory distress. He says he hasn't had a drink since the previous day, when he drank "some stuff they left lying around the gas station—I don't know what it was—tasted pretty good." He says he threw up a few times about 6 hours after that. On physical examination, the patient is alert. There is no alcohol odor on his breath. His vital signs are a pulse of 120 beats/min and regular, respirations of 36 breaths/min and noisy, and BP of 180/105 mm Hg. The pupils are midposition, equal, and reactive to light. The gag reflex is present. The chest is full of crackles.

a. What do you think is this patient's problem?

_____

b. List the steps you would take in managing this patient.

(1)_____

(2)_____

(3)_____

(4)_____

(5)_____

The second patient appears intoxicated. His speech is slurred, and he can scarcely walk. "Why ish it shnowing in Sheptember?" he mumbles. His breath smells of alcohol. His pulse is 108 beats/min and regular, his respirations are 30 breaths/min and deep, and his BP is 140/86 mm Hg. There is no evidence of head injury. The pupils are about 6 mm and equal and react sluggishly to light. The gag reflex is present. The chest is clear. The abdomen is very tender and nearly rigid to palpation.

c. What do you think is this patient's problem?

_____

d. List the steps you would take in managing this patient.

(1)_____

(2)_____

(3)_____

(4)_____

(5)_____

7. You are staying with friends at their cabin in the mountains for a nice ski weekend. Your host takes considerable pride in the cabin, which he built himself. "Snug as a bug in a rug," he says. "Not a draft in the place." You have to admit that he did a good insulation job and that the place is nice and cozy with the Franklin stove in the corner.

When you get up the next morning, your friend's wife, asks, "Will you have a look at the baby? She's sick with something. She's been throwing up all morning." You don't know much about babies, and you don't feel so hot yourself, but you take a look at the baby. You find her pale and dehydrated, with a bounding pulse but no fever. As you are examining her, she has a grand mal seizure. "It must be the flu," says the baby's mother, "because I'm coming down with something, too. I feel really sick to my stomach." Meanwhile, your friend, just getting up, says, "Boy, do I have a headache; it's like Niagara Falls roaring through my skull."

a. What do you think is the baby's problem?

_____

b. What steps should you take in this situation?

(1)_____

(2)_____

(3)_____

(4)_____

(5)_____

(6)_____

(7)_____

8. One fine Sunday afternoon, you are called to a suburban home for a "possible heart attack." On arrival, you find a middle-aged man, clad in shorts and a T-shirt, sprawled out on the sofa in the living room. "I don't know what happened," he says. "I was just sitting outside on the lawn, and I started to feel real dizzy and sick to my stomach, and real weak. And there's this tight feeling in my chest—"

"It's that stuff Mr. Greenthumb was spraying," his wife chimes in. "I'm sure of it. Why he has to spray his precious roses precisely when we're sitting in the garden is beyond me."

While you begin your assessment of the patient, your partner goes next door to talk with Mr. Greenthumb. You find the patient in considerable distress. His skin is pale and diaphoretic. His vital signs are a pulse of 42 beats/min and regular, respirations are 28 breaths/min and labored, and BP is 140/80 mm Hg. The pupils are very constricted. The patient is salivating profusely, and his breath smells like garlic. The neck veins are flat. The chest is full of wheezes. As you are completing the examination, your partner returns carrying a bottle labeled "parathion."

a. What do you think is this patient's problem?

_____

b. What drug is used to treat this problem?

_____

c. What is the correct dosage in this situation?

_____

d. List the steps in treating this patient.

(1)_____

(2)_____

(3)_____

(4)_____

(5)_____

(6)_____

(7)_____

(8)_____

(9)_____

9. You are called to a local junior high school where a 12-year-old boy had a grand mal seizure. The school nurse, who is kneeling on the floor of the boys' restroom beside the boy, tells you that the boy has no known seizure history. The boy is unconscious but can be roused by painful stimuli. You cannot find any abnormalities on physical examination save for signs that he indeed just had a seizure (slight bleeding of the tongue, incontinence). A search of his pockets, however, reveals a few small bottles of typewriter correction fluid. What steps will you take in managing this patient?

a. _____

b. _____

c. _____

d. _____

e. _____

f. _____

g. _____

Complete the Patient Care Report (PCR)

Read the ninth incident scenario in the Ambulance Calls section, and then complete the following PCR.

EMS Patient Care Report (PCR)				
Date:	**Incident No.:**	**Nature of Call:**		**Location:**
Dispatched:	**En Route:**	**At Scene:**	**Transport:**	**At Hospital:**	**In Service:**

Patient Information

Age:	**Allergies:**
Sex:	**Medications:**
Weight (in kg [lb]):	**Past Medical History:**
	Chief Complaint:

Vital Signs

Time:	BP:	Pulse:	Respirations:	SpO$_2$:
Time:	BP:	Pulse:	Respirations:	SpO$_2$:
Time:	BP:	Pulse:	Respirations:	SpO$_2$:

EMS Treatment
(circle all that apply)

Oxygen @ _____ L/min via (circle one): NC NRM Bag-mask device		Assisted Ventilation	Airway Adjunct	CPR
Defibrillation	Bleeding Control	Bandaging	Splinting	Other:

Narrative

True/False

If you believe the statement to be more true than false, write the letter "T" in the space provided. If you believe the statement to be more false than true, write the letter "F."

_____ **1.** Your call to the Poison Control Center helps the center collect data on poisonings in your region. These data may be analyzed to help detect trends, spot developing public health problems, and evaluate current treatment protocols for different poisonings.

_____ **2.** Oxygen has a greater affinity than carbon monoxide (CO) to bind to hemoglobin on the red blood cells.

_____ **3.** There is an increasing trend of patients attempting suicide by mixing certain household chemicals while in a parked vehicle, which can be very dangerous to emergency response personnel.

_____ **4.** The major toxidromes are produced by stimulants, narcotics, cholinergics, anticholinergics, sympathomimetics, sedatives, and hypnotics.

_____ **5.** The more frequently consumption of alcohol takes place, the greater the irritation of the digestive system.

_____ **6.** The severity of alcohol withdrawal can vary according to the length and intensity of the patient's alcoholism. Minor withdrawal is characterized by restlessness, anxiousness, sleeping problems, agitation, and tremors.

_____ **7.** Prolonged heavy use of alcohol may cause ulcers, gastric esophageal reflux, and cancers of the mouth and throat.

_____ **8.** In a poisoning, the container and the remaining contents should never be taken with the patient to the hospital for fear of contaminating the emergency department.

_____ **9.** The trends in prevalence of cocaine use between 2013 and 2015 show that use is increasing.

_____ **10.** Patients who take lithium and nonsteroidal anti-inflammatory drugs (NSAIDs) have slowed renal clearance of the lithium, increasing the likelihood that they will inadvertently reach a toxic lithium level.

_____ **11.** Most patients who have swallowed caustic substances present with severe respiratory distress and pain in the mouth, throat, or chest.

_____ **12.** The primary goals when dealing with a patient who has inhaled hydrocarbons are to remove the patient from the noxious environment, give high-concentration supplemental oxygen, and promptly transport to the appropriate facility.

_____ **13.** Synthetic cathinones, also known as bath salts, refer to an emerging group of drugs similar to MDMA.

_____ **14.** Field treatment of a salicylate overdose should include the "universal antidote."

Short Answer

Complete this section with short written answers using the space provided.

1. List 10 medical problems to which alcoholics are particularly susceptible.

a. _____

b. _____

c. _____

d. _____

e. _____

f. _____

g. _____

h. _____

i. _____

j. _____

Fill in the Table

Fill in the missing parts of the table.

1. Although it is advisable to consult Poison Control for definitive identification of any ingested substance, it is nonetheless worthwhile to have a general knowledge of the categories of poisons and some of the more commonly encountered examples of each category. Fill in the following table with examples of each type of poison mentioned.

Common Poisons	
Type of Poison	Examples
Strong acid	
Strong alkali	
Hydrocarbons	
Toxic plants	

2. Fill in the amount of time it takes for the four stages of acetaminophen toxicity.

Signs and Symptoms of Acetaminophen Toxicity		
Stage	Time Frame	Signs and Symptoms
I		Nausea, vomiting, loss of appetite, pallor, malaise
II		Right upper quadrant abdominal pain; abdomen tender to palpation
III		Metabolic acidosis, renal failure, coagulopathies, recurring gastrointestinal (GI) symptoms
IV		Recovery slowly begins, or liver failure progresses, and the patient dies

© Jones & Bartlett Learning.

Psychiatric Emergencies

Matching

Part I

Match each of the descriptions in the left column to the appropriate item in the right column.

_____ **1.** A fixed belief that is not shared by others of a person's culture or background and that cannot be changed by reasonable argument; a false belief.

_____ **2.** The slow onset of progressive disorientation, shortened attention span, and loss of cognitive function.

_____ **3.** A mental health disorder characterized by a persistent mood of sadness, despair, and discouragement; it may be a symptom of many different mental and physical disorders, or it may be a disorder on its own.

_____ **4.** A condition in which a person is characterized by uncontrolled and disconnected thought, is usually incoherent or rambling in speech, and may or may not be oriented to person and place.

_____ **5.** A condition in which a person may be confused about his or her identity, the location, and the time of day; one of the ways in which various conditions, such as schizophrenia or organic brain syndrome may present.

_____ **6.** The basic activities a person usually accomplishes during a normal day, such as eating, dressing, and washing.

_____ **7.** A syndrome that may occur in patients taking typical antipsychotic agents. The patient develops muscle spasms of the neck, face, and back within a few days of starting treatment with the medication.

_____ **8.** The outward expression of a person's inner feelings (eg, happy, sad, angry, fearful, withdrawn).

_____ **9.** An acute confrontational state characterized by global impairment of thinking, perception, judgment, and memory.

_____ **10.** Literally, "fear of the marketplace"; fear of entering a public place from which escape may be impeded.

_____ **11.** The use of medication to subdue a patient.

_____ **12.** Lacking expression or movement, or appearing rigid.

_____ **13.** An eating disorder characterized by consumption of large amounts of food, for which the patient often compensates by using purging techniques.

_____ **14.** A disorder characterized by disordered images of self, impulsive and unpredictable behavior, marked shifts in mood, and instability in relationships with others.

A. Activities of daily living (ADLs)

B. Acute dystonic reaction

C. Affect

D. Agitated delirium

E. Agoraphobia

F. Anorexia nervosa

G. Anxiety disorder

H. Atropine-like effects

I. Behavior

J. Behavioral emergency

K. Bipolar mood disorder

L. Borderline personality disorder

M. Bulimia nervosa

N. Catatonic

_____ 15. A disorder in which a person alternates between mania and depression.

_____ 16. Behavior that has a hidden meaning or intention that only the person understands.

_____ 17. Act of pointing out something of interest in the patient's conversation or behavior, thereby directing the patient's attention to something of which he or she may have been unaware.

_____ 18. The invention of experiences to cover gaps in memory; seen in patients with certain organic brain syndromes.

_____ 19. Repetitive actions carried out to relieve the anxiety of obsessive thoughts.

_____ 20. Situation in which the patient includes many irrelevant details in his or her account of things.

_____ 21. An eating disorder in which a person diets by exerting extraordinary control over his or her eating and loses weight to the point of jeopardizing his or her health and life.

_____ 22. A mental disorder in which the dominant mood is fear and apprehension.

_____ 23. Results of some antipsychotic medications that include adverse effects similar to atropine, resulting in dry mouth, blurred vision, urinary retention, and cardiac dysrhythmias.

_____ 24. How a person functions or acts in response to his or her environment.

_____ 25. The point at which a person's reactions to events interfere with activities of daily living; becomes a psychiatric emergency when it causes a major life interruption, such as attempted suicide.

O. Chemical restraint

P. Circumstantial thinking

Q. Compulsions

R. Confabulation

S. Confrontation

T. Covert behavior

U. Delusion

V. Dementia

W. Depression

X. Disorganization

Y. Disorientation

Part II

Match each of the descriptions in the left column to the appropriate item in the right column.

_____ 1. Temporary or permanent dysfunction of the brain, caused by a disturbance in the physical or physiologic functioning of brain tissue.

_____ 2. A collection of psychiatric disorders without psychotic symptoms and lacking the intense psychopathology or other mood disorders; includes anxiety disorders, phobias, and panic disorder.

_____ 3. A sense perception not founded on objective reality; a false perception.

_____ 4. The absence of speech.

_____ 5. A group of disorders in which the disturbance of mood is accompanied by full or partial manic or depressive syndrome.

_____ 6. A severe form of anxiety that stems from a traumatic experience; characterized by the reliving of the stress and nightmares of the original situation.

_____ 7. Disorders involving an unreasonable fear, apprehension, or dread of a specific situation or thing.

_____ 8. An abnormal and persistent dread of a specific object or situation.

_____ 9. The condition in which a person behaves or thinks in a way that is dysfunctional or causes distress to other people.

_____ 10. Repeating the same idea over and over again.

_____ 11. Meaningless echoing of the interviewer's words by the patient.

_____ 12. A disorder in which a person wishes to be sick and intentionally produces or feigns physical or psychological signs or symptoms. Symptoms are under voluntary control, with no obvious physiologic reason.

_____ 13. The absence of emotion; appearing to feel no emotion at all.

_____ 14. Accelerated thinking in which the mind skips very rapidly from one thought to the next.

A. Echolalia

B. Factitious disorder

C. Flat affect

D. Flight of ideas

E. Generalized anxiety disorder (GAD)

F. Hallucination

G. Impulse control disorder

H. Inappropriate affect

I. Labile

J. Loosening of associations

K. Mania

L. Manic-depressive illness

M. Medication noncompliance

N. Mental status exam (MSE)

_____ **15.** A disorder in which a person worries about everything for no particular reason, or in which the worrying is unproductive and the person cannot decide what to do about an upcoming situation.

_____ **16.** Behavior that is open and generally understood by those around the person.

_____ **17.** A disorder characterized by sudden, usually unexpected, and overwhelming feelings of fear and dread, accompanied by a variety of other symptoms produced by a massive activation of the autonomic nervous system.

_____ **18.** A bipolar disorder in which mood fluctuates between depression and mania. The alterations in mood are usually episodic and recurrent.

_____ **19.** A situation in which a patient chooses to not take his or her medications as prescribed, for reasons that may include undesirable adverse effects or prohibitive cost.

_____ **20.** A tool for measuring the "mental vital signs" in a patient who is disturbed. The mnemonic COASTMAP can be used to conduct this exam, assessing consciousness, orientation, activity, speech, thought, memory, affect and mood, and perception.

_____ **21.** A mental disorder characterized by abnormally exaggerated happiness, joy, or euphoria with hyperactivity, insomnia, and grandiose ideas.

_____ **22.** A situation in which the logical connection between one idea and the next becomes obscure, at least to the listener.

_____ **23.** Rapidly shifting among different emotional states.

_____ **24.** Emotion that is out of sync with the situation (eg, wearing a smile while discussing a parent's death).

_____ **25.** A condition in which a person lacks the ability to resist a temptation or cannot stop acting on a drive.

O. Mood disorder

P. Mutism

Q. Neurotic disorders

R. Organic brain syndrome

S. Overt behavior

T. Panic disorder

U. Perseveration

V. Personality disorder

W. Phobia

X. Phobic disorders

Y. Posttraumatic stress disorder (PTSD)

Part III

For each of the following signs and symptoms, indicate whether it is:

O: More typical of organic brain syndrome

P: More typical of psychiatric illness

B: Apt to be seen in both organic and psychiatric illnesses

_____ **1.** Obsessional thinking

_____ **2.** Flat affect

_____ **3.** Delirium

_____ **4.** Distractibility

_____ **5.** Compulsions

_____ **6.** Visual hallucinations

_____ **7.** Confabulation

_____ **8.** Anxiety

_____ **9.** Coma

_____ **10.** Circumstantial thinking

Part IV

For each of the psychiatric signs and symptoms listed, indicate whether it is a disturbance of:

A. Consciousness

B. Motor activity

C. Speech

D. Thinking

E. Affect or mood

F. Memory

G. Orientation

H. Perception

_____ **1.** The patient cannot name three objects that you listed out loud 5 minutes earlier.

_____ **2.** The patient is pacing back and forth.

_____ **3.** The patient smiles pleasantly as he tells you that his daughter was run over by a truck.

_____ **4.** The patient keeps shifting his attention from you to the television or to the window.

_____ **5.** The patient seems to be having a conversation with an invisible friend.

_____ **6.** The patient thinks the current year is 1931.

_____ **7.** The patient thinks he is Albert Einstein.

_____ **8.** The patient tells you, "All the world is my kingdumbell, and I'm the pellmellery scullop."

_____ **9.** The patient is terrified of spiders.

_____ **10.** The patient puts two fingers to his forehead in a salute every time he finishes speaking.

_____ **11.** The patient complains of palpitations, nausea, tightness in his chest, and numbness around his lips.

_____ **12.** The patient thinks that the sound of the wind is someone calling his name.

Multiple Choice

Read each item carefully, and then select the best response.

_____ **1.** In an acute behavioral emergency, which of the following disease states may produce psychotic symptoms resulting from alcohol abuse, kidney failure, liver failure, and amphetamines?

 A. Toxic or deficiency states

 B. Infections

 C. Neurologic disease

 D. Endocrine disorders

_____ **2.** Pressured speech, neologisms, echolalia, and mutism are examples of:

 A. disorders of thinking.

 B. disorders of mood and affect.

 C. disorders of motor activity.

 D. disorders of speech.

_____ **3.** During the primary survey of patients with behavioral disorders, it is important for a paramedic to:

 A. hurry the call; you can't really assist the patient.

 B. assess the patient only en route to the hospital.

 C. convey that you have the time and concern.

 D. not gain consent because consent is never required.

_____ **4.** The mental status exam includes:

 A. perception.

 B. affect and mood.

 C. memory.

 D. All of the above

_____ **5.** Guilt, depressed appetite, sleep disturbances, lack of interest, low energy, and suicidal thoughts are diagnostic features of:

 A. depression.

 B. anxiety.

 C. mood disorders.

 D. manic-depressive illness.

_____ **6.** Paramedics always need to take scene safety seriously. All of the following are risk factors for violence, EXCEPT:

 A. posture.

 B. speech.

 C. motor activity.

 D. prescription medication.

_____   **7.** Restraining a violent patient should include:
      A. a law enforcement presence.
      B. a Reeves stretcher.
      C. lots of duct tape.
      D. no more than two paramedics.

_____   **8.** A psychiatric emergency exists when a patient:
      A. threatens to harm himself or herself.
      B. threatens to harm other people.
      C. is delusional.
      D. All of the above

_____   **9.** All of the following drugs may sometimes cause a psychotic state, EXCEPT:
      A. steroids.
      B. Wellbutrin (bupropion).
      C. digitalis.
      D. LSD and PCP.

_____   **10.** Which of the following is considered a disturbance of behavior?
      A. Generalized anxiety disorder
      B. Organic brain syndrome
      C. Head injury
      D. Stroke

_____   **11.** The following are appropriate guidelines for the care of any patient with a psychiatric emergency, EXCEPT:
      A. being as calm and direct as possible.
      B. asking all the other disruptive family members to participate in the interview.
      C. maintaining a nonjudgmental attitude.
      D. developing a plan of action.

_____   **12.** A patient who has been diagnosed as having bipolar disorder, manic behavior, and depression is categorized as having what type of psychiatric disorder?
      A. Cognitive disorder
      B. Neurotic disorder
      C. Mood disorder
      D. Somatoform disorder

Fill in the Blank

Read each item carefully, and then complete the statement by filling in the missing word(s).

1. The causes of abnormal behavior can be classified into four broad categories: (1) causes that are _____ or _____ in nature, (2) causes resulting from a person's _____, (3) causes resulting from acute _____ or _____, and (4) causes that are _____-_____.

2. Identify yourself _____. Tell the patient who you are and what you are trying to do. If the patient is _____ or _____, you may have to explain yourself at _____ intervals.

3. Overwhelming feelings of _____ and _____, accompanied by a variety of other symptoms produced by a massive activation of the _____ nervous system, characterize panic disorder.

4. There are two major types of eating disorders: _____ _____ and _____ _____.

5. _____, _____, and _____ are common trade names for heterocyclic (tricyclic and tetracyclic) antidepressants.

6. One potential adverse effect of monoamine oxidase (MAO) inhibitors when taken by patients with a history of depression would be _____ _____, which although occasionally severe, usually responds to _____ therapy.

7. _____ is the second-leading cause of death among people aged 10 to 34 years and the fourth-leading cause of death among 35- to 54-year-olds.

8. One in _____ people will be affected by _____ in their lifetimes.

Identify

List the behavioral medications in the following scenarios.

1. You respond to a domestic dispute. When you arrive on scene, you are told by law enforcement that the scene is secure and safe. You and your partner proceed inside. The patient's wife is holding a bag of the patient's medications. The patient denies any complaint and simply states that he has a cardiac history and takes furosemide (Lasix) and digoxin. While you calm the patient, your partner reviews the bag of medications. He finds the furosemide and digoxin along with glyburide, fluoxetine (Prozac), and diazepam (Valium).

   _____

   _____

2. You are called to an outpatient mental health clinic for a patient requiring voluntary in-patient hospitalization. The patient has a history of hypercholesterolemia and depression. The patient is taking over-the-counter omega-3 and garlic. The patient is on the following prescription medications: phenelzine (Nardil), bupropion (Wellbutrin), simvastatin (Zocor), and atorvastatin (Lipitor).

   _____

   _____

3. You receive an emergency call for a "psychotic" patient. As you evaluate your patient, you review her medication list and discover the following prescriptions: tamoxifen, niacin (Niaspan), fluticasone/salmeterol inhaled (Advair), aripiprazole (Abilify), and famotidine (Pepcid).

   _____

   _____

Ambulance Calls

The following case scenarios provide an opportunity to explore the concerns associated with patient management and paramedic care. Read each scenario, and then answer each question.

1. The following is the transcript of an interview between an inexperienced paramedic and a disturbed patient. The interview illustrates several errors in approach. Read through the interview. Then, list the points in the interview that you think could have been handled or phrased in a better way.

   Paramedic (entering an apartment in which there is a lot of noise and confusion): Okay, which one of you is the patient?

   (Someone points to a young woman crouching in a corner, crying.)

   Paramedic (approaching the woman and standing in front of her): Now, dearie, what's the trouble?

   (Patient continues crying.)

   Paramedic: Now come on, get hold of yourself. Big girls don't cry.

   Patient (sobbing): Everything's just so hopeless.

   Paramedic: Things are never hopeless. You're probably just making a mountain out of a molehill, and by tomorrow, you'll wonder what you were making such a big fuss about.

   (Patient sits crying to herself.)

Paramedic: Well, if you don't want to tell me what's wrong, maybe one of your friends here can tell me. Is there anyone here who can tell me what's going on?

(Immediately the noise and confusion resume, as everyone starts talking at once. The patient huddles farther into the corner.)

List the things you think were done incorrectly in this interview, including errors of omission and errors of commission.

a. _____

b. _____

c. _____

d. _____

e. _____

f. _____

g. _____

h. _____

2. You are called to a downtown apartment building for a "sick man." Reaching the corridor outside the man's apartment, you are intercepted by a neighbor who had called for the ambulance. "I feel a little silly troubling you folks," she says, "but Mr. Crosby next door—he's just not himself lately—doesn't even poke his head out of that apartment. Doesn't want to see no one. He just says, 'Go away,' when I knock. So I got to worrying. I mean, I don't even think he's got himself anything to eat in there."

"Who's there?" someone finally says.

"We're paramedics, from the city ambulance service."

"Well, what do you want with me?"

"We just want to talk with you a bit," you say. "There are folks worried about you."

It takes some persuading, but finally, Mr. Crosby opens the door and admits you into his apartment. The place is in complete disarray, and it appears as if no one has washed a dish or tidied up in months. Here and there you note an empty liquor bottle lying on the floor.

So what do you want?" Mr. Crosby asks listlessly.

    a. Where would you go from here? List some of the questions you would ask Mr. Crosby at this point.

_____

_____

_____

_____

    b. In the course of your interview with Mr. Crosby, which seems to go very slowly, you learn that he is a 62-year-old widower. He has one son and says, "I never hear from him." He used to be a watchmaker, he says, "but I haven't been worth anything since I got this arthritis 10 years ago." In response to your query about why he has stopped going out of the apartment, he says, "What's there to go out for? Anyway, I don't have the energy to go rambling around the city."

    "Don't you have to shop for food?" you ask.

    "What for? I don't feel much like eating these days anyway."

    This patient is showing clear symptoms of depression. List the symptoms of depression present in this case.

    (1)_____

    (2)_____

    (3)_____

    (4)_____

c. List four other symptoms or signs of depression.

(1)_____

(2)_____

(3)_____

(4)_____

d. List the risk factors for suicide present in this patient's history.

(1)_____

(2)_____

(3)_____

(4)_____

(5)_____

e. List six other risk factors for suicide.

(1)_____

(2)_____

(3)_____

(4)_____

(5)_____

(6)_____

f. List three questions you would ask to try to evaluate the patient's risk of suicide.

(1)_____

(2)_____

(3)_____

3. You are called to a downtown office building for a "possible heart attack." When you reach the building, you are escorted into an office by a harried-looking businessman. "It's my secretary," he says. "She's having some kind of cardiac attack." In the midst of a buzzing group of people, you see a woman who looks to be about 24 years old sitting wide-eyed and pale. People are fanning her with file folders and trying to get her to drink some water. You make your way through the crowd and ask the woman what her problem is.

"Can't breathe," she gasps. "Chest all tight (gasp). Feel like I'm going to pass out (gasp). Everything is unreal (gasp), like I'm dying (gasp)."

"Quick! Quick!" squeaks one of the bystanders. "Get her to the hospital!"

Ignoring the chorus demanding that you leave immediately for the hospital, you begin taking the woman's vital signs. Her pulse is 112 beats/min and regular, her respirations are 30 breaths/min and deep, and her blood pressure (BP) is 160/88 mm Hg. You notice that her skin is cold and sweaty and her hands are shaking.

a. What do you think is this patient's problem?

_____

b. What signs and symptoms led you to that conclusion?

(1)_____

(2)_____

(3)_____

(4)_____

(5)_____

(6)_____

(7)_____

c. Are there any other diagnoses you need to take into consideration? If so, what are they?

(1)_____

(2)_____

(3)_____

(4)_____

(5)_____

d. How will you attempt to control the situation quickly?

(1)_____

(2)_____

(3)_____

(4)_____

(5)_____

(6)_____

4. You and your partner are called to a downtown bar to see a man who has apparently become disruptive there. A police officer meets you at the entrance to the bar. "Listen," he says, "the barkeeper called us to deal with an unruly customer, but personally, I think the guy's a psycho case—so I thought maybe you folks ought to take a look at him."

You enter the bar and find a well-dressed but disheveled man pacing rapidly up and down. "One week from today," he is announcing, "one week from today, I'll be one of the richest men in America. I'm putting together a business empire now that will rule Wall Street." He is talking a mile a minute, cracking jokes, and gesturing extravagantly. He catches sight of you and your partner and says, "Well, hello, fellas. Bartender, give these fine young people a drink, on me. They do a great public service. This country was built on public service—yes indeed, it was. So give them a public service drink."

"You haven't paid for the drinks you already ordered," says the bartender.

"Listen, fathead, I said give these nice people a drink."

"Uh, sir," you break in, "we're not allowed to drink while on duty. And we thought maybe you'd like to take a little ride with us to the hospital."

"Hospital? What do I need to go to the hospital for? Never felt better in my life. By next week, I'll be able to buy the hospital, buy this bar too, buy the whole damned town."

The police officer says, "Maybe you ought to go with them, sir, just to get a checkup."

"Any of you puts a hand on me," replies the man, "I'll sue the whole lot of you. Assault. Battery. False imprisonment. I'll sue you for the whole lot, and let me tell you, you don't want to tangle with my team of lawyers. Best legal talent in the country. You wouldn't stand a chance."

a. What do you think is this man's problem?

_____

b. What symptoms and signs led you to that conclusion?

(1)_____

(2)_____

(3)_____

(4)_____

c. How will you manage this patient?

_____

_____

5. You are called to a downtown street corner where several police officers are standing around, apparently trying to talk to a somewhat wild-eyed man who could be anywhere from 55 to 75 years old. He is dressed in about six layers of tattered clothes and wearing a naval officer's cap. He clearly hasn't had a bath, shave, or haircut in weeks. "He was just walking down the middle of Main Street," says one of the police officers, "as if he didn't even notice the traffic—and all those horns blowing, people screeching on their brakes."

You introduce yourself to the man and ask whether you can be of help. He mumbles something that sounds like, "Dogs and cats."

"Sorry," you say, "I didn't quite catch what you said."

"Salt and pepper," he says. "Black and blue, I didn't, don't 'ya know, I didn't."

The police officer gives you a meaningful look.

How will you manage this case?

_____

_____

_____

_____

6. A middle-aged woman calls for an ambulance because "my son is acting real strange." When you arrive at the designated address, the woman greets you at the door. She tells you that her 20-year-old son won't come out of his room. He's been in there for 2 days now. Sometimes she hears him talking to someone, but there isn't anyone else there. "I'm sure it's all that karate stuff," she says. "It just went to his head, made him crazy, all that black-belt business."
You go up to the son's room and knock on the door.

"You're not going to get me," says a voice from the other side of the door. "You won't take me alive."

"Sir, we're paramedics. We've just come to talk with you."

"You can't fool me. I know you're from the FBI. Well, you'll have to shoot me to take me."

You try the door and find it's unlocked. Inside, a young man clothed in karate garb is sitting in an armchair, gripping the armrests.

You introduce yourselves again. The patient looks away.

"You won't take me alive," he says again in a monotone. He looks suddenly toward the wall. "I know, I know," he says to the wall.

"Who are you talking to?" you ask.

He looks startled. "The voices said you would come. They killed John Lennon, and the FBI is after me. The voices said not to let you take me alive."

a. This patient is showing signs of:

(1) a panic attack.

(2) psychosis.

(3) depression.

(4) mania.

(5) disorganization.

b. Are there any indications that he might become violent?

_____

c. If so, what are four indications?

(1)_____

(2)_____

(3)_____

(4)_____

d. How will you attempt to manage this case?

_____

_____

_____

_____

_____

_____

True/False

If you believe the statement to be more true than false, write the letter "T" in the space provided. If you believe the statement to be more false than true, write the letter "F."

_____　**1.** The most important thing a paramedic can do to help a disturbed patient is to remain calm and steady.

_____　**2.** There should be a maximum sense of urgency in evacuating a disturbed patient to the hospital because there is nothing that can be done to help the patient in the field.

_____　**3.** It is essential to correct a patient's misinterpretations of reality.

_____　**4.** The disturbed patient should be reassured that everything will turn out all right.

_____　**5.** The paramedic should remain with the disturbed patient at all times until the emergency department (ED) staff takes over the patient's care.

_____　**6.** Police intervention is usually required to transport a disturbed patient against his or her will.

Short Answer

Complete this section with short written answers using the space provided.

1. Certain situations have a higher potential for violence than others do. List three scenarios that should activate the paramedic's "nose for danger."

   a. _____

   b. _____

   c. _____

2. List four diagnostic groups that would activate the paramedic's "nose for danger."

   a. _____

   b. _____

   c. _____

   d. _____

Fill in the Table

Fill in the missing parts of the table with the conditions and substances that can produce psychotic symptoms.

Selected Disease States That May Produce Psychotic Symptoms	
Disease State	**Psychotic Symptoms**
	Drug-induced psychoses, especially from: • Digitalis • Steroids • Disulfiram • Amphetamines • LSD, PCP, and other psychedelics Nutrition disorders: • Alcohol abuse • Vitamin deficiencies Poisoning with bromide or other heavy metals • Kidney failure • Liver failure
	Syphilis Parasites Viral encephalitis (eg, after measles) Brain abscess
	Seizure disorders (especially temporal lobe seizures) Primary and metastatic tumors of the brain Dementia Stroke Closed head injury
	Low cardiac output (eg, in heart failure)
	Thyroid hyperfunction (thyrotoxicosis) Adrenal hyperfunction (Cushing syndrome)
	Electrolyte imbalances (eg, after severe diarrhea) Hypoglycemia Diabetic ketoacidosis

CHAPTER

Trauma Systems and Mechanism of Injury

29

Matching

Part I

For each of the injuries listed in the left column, indicate which incident from the right column it is likely to be associated with. (Note: Some injuries may be associated with more than one type of mechanism.)

_____ **1.** "Whiplash" injury

_____ **2.** Multiple rib fractures

_____ **3.** Fracture of the tibia/fibula

_____ **4.** Fracture of the patella

_____ **5.** Fracture of the humerus

_____ **6.** Skull fracture

_____ **7.** Laryngeal fracture

_____ **8.** Flail chest

_____ **9.** Pelvic fracture

_____ **10.** Cervical spine injury

A. Head-on collision (unrestrained driver)

B. Lateral impact (unrestrained front-seat passenger)

C. Rear-impact collision (unrestrained driver)

D. Pedestrian struck by an oncoming car

Part II

Match each of the terms in the right column to the appropriate definition in the left column.

_____ **1.** The shattering effect of a shock wave and its ability to cause disruption of tissues and structures.

_____ **2.** An impact on the body by objects that cause injury without penetrating soft tissues or internal organs and cavities.

_____ **3.** The leading edge of the shock wave.

_____ **4.** The study of the physiology and mechanics of a living organism using the tools of mechanical engineering.

_____ **5.** The energy that results from sudden changes in pressure as may occur in a diving accident or sudden decompression in an airplane.

_____ **6.** A primary mechanism of tissue disruption from certain rifles in which pieces of the projectile break apart, allowing the pieces to create their own separate paths through tissues.

_____ **7.** The way in which traumatic injuries occur; the forces that act on the body to cause damage.

A. Acceleration

B. Angle of impact

C. Arterial air embolism

D. Avulsing

E. Ballistics

F. Barometric energy

G. Biomechanics

_____ **8.** The energy that results from motion (kinetic energy) or that is stored in an object (potential energy).

_____ **9.** The law of physics stating that energy can be neither created nor destroyed; it can only change form.

_____ **10.** The study of the relationships among speed, mass, vector direction, and physical injury.

_____ **11.** The rate of change in velocity; speeding up.

_____ **12.** The angle at which an object hits another; it characterizes the force vectors involved and has a bearing on patterns of energy dissipation.

_____ **13.** Air bubbles in the arterial blood vessels.

_____ **14.** A tearing away or forcible separation.

_____ **15.** The study of nonpowered objects in flight; most often associated with rifle or handgun bullet travel.

_____ **16.** The energy delivered in the form of high voltage.

_____ **17.** The point at which a penetrating object enters the body.

_____ **18.** The point at which a penetrating object leaves the body, which may or may not be in a straight line from the entry wound.

_____ **19.** The acceleration of a body by the attraction of the earth's gravitational force, normally 32.2 ft/sec^2.

_____ **20.** A bursting inward.

_____ **21.** Cavity formation; shock waves that push tissues in front of and lateral to the projectile and may not necessarily increase the wound size or cause permanent injury but can result in cavitation.

_____ **22.** The energy released as a result of a chemical reaction.

_____ **23.** A negative acceleration; slowing down.

_____ **24.** Anticipating the possibility of specific types of injury.

_____ **25.** The energy associated with bodies in motion, expressed mathematically as half the mass times the square of the velocity.

H. Blast front

I. Blunt trauma

J. Brisance

K. Cavitation

L. Chemical energy

M. Deceleration

N. Electrical energy

O. Entrance wound

P. Exit wound

Q. Gravity

R. Implosion

S. Index of suspicion

T. Kinetic energy (KE)

U. Kinetics

V. Law of conservation of energy

W. Mechanical energy

X. Mechanism of injury (MOI)

Y. Missile fragmentation

Part III

Match each of the terms in the right column to the appropriate definition in the left column.

_____ **1.** A score that relates to the likelihood of patient survival with the exception of a severe head injury. It is calculated on a scale from 1 to 16, with 16 being the best possible score. It takes into account the Glasgow Coma Scale (GCS) score, respiratory rate, respiratory expansion, systolic blood pressure, and capillary refill.

A. Multisystem trauma

_____ **2.** A combination of hypothermia, coagulopathy (poor blood clotting), and acidosis that is a major contributor to death in patients with severe traumatic bleeding.

B. Negative wave pulse

_____ **3.** Acute physiologic and structural change (injury) that occurs in a person's body as a result of the rapid dissipation of energy delivered by an external source.

C. Newton's first law of motion

_____ **4.** Energy transferred from sources that are hotter than the body, such as a flame, hot water, and steam.

D. Newton's second law of motion

_____ **5.** An applied force or pressure exerted against the surface and layers of the skin as tissues slide in opposite but parallel planes.

_____ **6.** The path of crushed tissue produced by a missile traversing part of the body.

_____ **7.** Injury caused by objects that pierce the surface of the body, such as knives and bullets, and damage internal tissues and organs.

_____ **8.** The tissue displacement that occurs as a result of low-displacement shock waves that travel at the speed of sound in tissue.

_____ **9.** The law of motion stating that the force that an object can exert is the product of its mass times its acceleration.

_____ **10.** The law of motion stating that a body at rest will remain at rest unless acted on by an outside force.

_____ **11.** An injury to the cervical vertebrae or its supporting ligaments and muscles, usually resulting from sudden acceleration or deceleration.

_____ **12.** A pattern of vehicle-versus-pedestrian injuries in children and people of short stature in which (1) the bumper hits pelvis and femur, (2) the chest and abdomen hit the grille or low hood, and (3) the head strikes the ground.

_____ **13.** The distance an object travels per unit time.

_____ **14.** The eardrum; a thin, semitransparent membrane in the middle ear that transmits sound vibrations to the internal ear by means of the auditory ossicles.

_____ **15.** The phase of an explosion in which pressure from the blast is less than atmospheric pressure.

_____ **16.** Trauma caused by generalized mechanisms that affect numerous body systems.

_____ **17.** A scoring system used for patients with head trauma.

_____ **18.** Pulmonary trauma resulting from short-range exposure to the detonation of high explosives.

_____ **19.** The amount of energy stored in an object, which is the product of mass, gravity, and height, and which is converted into kinetic energy and results in injury, such as from a fall.

_____ **20.** The phase of the explosion in which there is a pressure front with a pressure higher than atmospheric pressure.

E. Pathway expansion

F. Penetrating trauma

G. Permanent cavity

H. Positive wave pulse

I. Potential energy

J. Pulmonary blast injuries

K. Revised Trauma Score (RTS)

L. Shearing

M. Thermal energy

N. Trauma

O. Trauma lethal triad

P. Trauma score

Q. Tympanic membrane

R. Velocity (V)

S. Waddell triad

T. Whiplash

Multiple Choice

Read each item carefully, and then select the best response.

_____ **1.** Which of the following is NOT a criterion for referral to a regional trauma center?

    A. 45-year-old patient restrained in a low-speed auto crash

    B. Pelvic fracture

    C. Motorcycle crash at a speed greater than 20 mph

    D. A pregnant patient

_____ **2.** The "platinum 10 minutes" refers to the:

    A. amount of time taken to extricate a patient from a motor vehicle crash.

    B. total response time to a traumatic incident.

    C. goal of the maximum time spent at a scene for a critical trauma patient.

    D. time deciding on your "transport decision."

_____ 3. Which level of trauma center would be able to provide Advanced Trauma Life Support (ATLS) before transfer of patients to a higher-level trauma center?

    A. Level I

    B. Level II

    C. Level III

    D. Level IV

_____ 4. Pediatric pedestrian injuries differ from adult pedestrian injuries because:

    A. the skulls of children are not fused, which allows for energy absorption.

    B. children are shorter, so they are more likely to be run over by the vehicle.

    C. children are more likely to "fly over" the vehicle.

    D. the bumper is more likely to strike children's femurs rather than their lower extremities.

_____ 5. All of the following are important information to provide to the trauma team, EXCEPT the:

    A. name of the street gang.

    B. range at which the firearm was fired.

    C. kind of bullet or projectile.

    D. type of weapon used.

_____ 6. Blast injuries may be seen in which of the following scenarios?

    A. Mining mishaps

    B. Chemical plants

    C. Terrorist activities

    D. All of the above

_____ 7. All of the following are factors in the seriousness of firearms injuries, EXCEPT:

    A. the type of tissue penetrated.

    B. missile velocity.

    C. fragmentation.

    D. the firearm manufacturer.

_____ 8. Which of the following is one type of mechanical energy?

    A. Kinetic energy

    B. Barometric energy

    C. Electrical energy

    D. Chemical energy

_____ 9. Criteria for transport of an adult patient to a trauma center as defined by the American College of Surgeons Committee on Trauma (ACS-COT) and the Centers for Disease Control and Prevention (CDC) include all of the following, EXCEPT:

    A. Glasgow Coma Scale score of 13 or less.

    B. amputation proximal to the wrist or ankle.

    C. ejection from an automobile.

    D. falls from a height greater than 10 feet.

_____ 10. A combination of facial injuries, pulmonary contusions, flail chest, ruptured aorta, and fractured sternum is an example of which of the following?

    A. "Ring" of chest injuries

    B. Typical injuries from lateral impacts

    C. Typical injuries from head-on crashes

    D. "Down and under pathway"

Labeling

Label the following diagram with the correct mechanisms of blast injuries.

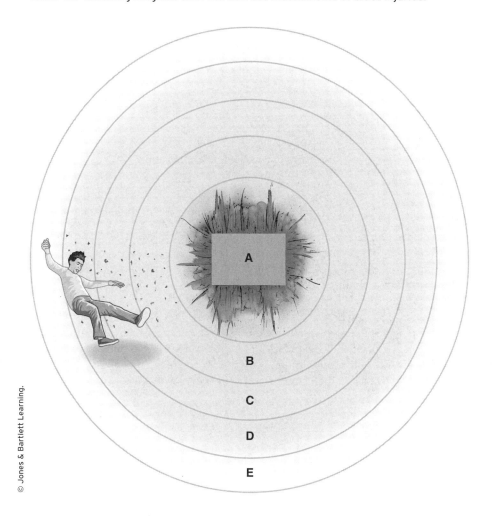

A. _____

B. _____

C. _____

D. _____

E. _____

Fill in the Blank

Read each item carefully, and then complete the statement by filling in the missing word(s).

1. The speed, duration, and pressure of the shock wave from an explosion are affected by the following factors:

   a. _____

   b. _____

   c. _____

   d. _____

2. The severity of a stab wound depends on the _____ area involved, depth of _____, blade length, and angle of

   penetration.

3. _____ _____ _____ is one of the most concerning of pulmonary blast injuries.

4. Severity of injuries in falls from heights depend on the following factors:

a. _____

b. _____

c. _____

d. _____

e. _____

5. Specific injuries associated with seat belt use include _____ fractures due to flexion stresses and _____ sprains.

Identify

Read the following case studies, and then list the mechanism of injury, chief complaint, vital signs, and pertinent negatives.

1. While working in a paramedic first-response vehicle, you receive a call for a motor vehicle crash. On arrival, you find two patients who are out of the vehicle and standing along the roadside. You notice that the vehicle appears to have rolled over onto its side. No other patients are involved, and the scene is deemed safe for patient contact and treatment. One occupant denies any complaint and does not want anything to do with emergency medical services (EMS). The other patient is holding his right forearm and complains of neck pain. The injured occupant states that he had his seat belt on. You notice that the airbag deployed. The injured man denies loss of consciousness (LOC), shortness of breath, or other complaints. Your physical examination indicates that the patient is slightly ashen and has an obvious bruising and deformity to his right midshaft radius/ulna. He has positive distal pulses and motor and sensory function (PMS), along with the following findings: pulse is 110 beats/min and regular, respirations are 16 breaths/min and unlabored, blood pressure (BP) is 106/96 mm Hg, and SpO$_2$ is 98%. The patient denies significant previous medical history.

   a. Mechanism of injury:

   _____

   _____

   b. Chief complaint:

   _____

   _____

   c. Vital signs:

   _____

   _____

   d. Pertinent negatives:

   _____

   _____

2. Today you are assigned to work on an advanced life support (ALS) ambulance. Your response area includes many high-speed interstate highways. It is toward the end of your shift and, until now, the day has been uneventful. Medcom dispatches you, Priority 1 (a Charlie response), to a reported motorcycle crash with one critical injury. On arrival, you notice a long line of stopped traffic and concerned bystanders. They are frantically waving you toward the injured patient. You notice a one-vehicle, motorcycle-versus-guardrail collision. The patient appears to be talking, but you notice a pool of blood alongside him as well as a cracked helmet. He has a badly deformed lower leg that you quickly conclude is fractured or dislocated. The patient is in obvious pain and is able to communicate that he "hurts all over."

You quickly begin to assess the patient, and he appears agitated, ashen, diaphoretic, and slightly short of breath. He has delayed (more than 2 seconds) capillary refill, and he has diminished left-side breath sounds and no tracheal deviation. His pulse is 120 beats/min, respiratory rate is 28 breaths/min, BP is unobtainable, and SpO$_2$ is 92%. You note that the patient has a palpable femoral pulse but no radial or brachial pulse.

a. Mechanism of injury:

_____

_____

b. Chief complaint:

_____

_____

c. Vital signs:

_____

_____

d. Pertinent negatives:

_____

_____

3. You respond to a "routine" call at an adult care facility for a "fall." Your patient is an 82-year-old woman who is lying on a carpeted floor with a walker positioned beside her. She appears conscious but slightly confused. She does not really know why she fell or how she ended up on the ground. She asks you to help her up. You begin your primary survey of the patient, and she denies any knowledge of the incident. During the secondary assessment, she denies any chest discomfort, shortness of breath, or neck or back pain. You note some deformity and rotation of her right lower extremity. On palpation, it is tender to the touch. The patient is confused regarding her previous medical history. The staff tells you that she has a history of transient ischemic attacks (TIAs) and heart problems. She is on multiple medications and is allergic to morphine sulfate. Her abdomen is soft and nontender. Her vital signs are as follows: pulse 58 beats/min and irregular; BP 158/110 mm Hg; SpO$_2$ 95%. Her skin is pale, cool, and dry.

a. Mechanism of injury:

_____

_____

b. Chief complaint:

_____

_____

c. Vital signs:

_____

_____

d. Pertinent negatives:

_____

_____

Complete the Patient Care Report

Reread the second case study in the preceding Identify exercise and then complete the following patient care report (PCR). Feel free to create the times and numbers as well as the date of the incident.

EMS Patient Care Report (PCR)					
Date:	**Incident No.:**	**Nature of Call:**		**Location:**	
Dispatched:	**En Route:**	**At Scene:**	**Transport:**	**At Hospital:**	**In Service:**
Patient Information					
Age: **Sex:** **Weight (in kg [lb]):**		**Allergies:** **Medications:** **Past Medical History:** **Chief Complaint:**			
Vital Signs					
Time:	**BP:**	**Pulse:**	**Respirations:**		**SpO₂:**
Time:	**BP:**	**Pulse:**	**Respirations:**		**SpO₂:**
Time:	**BP:**	**Pulse:**	**Respirations:**		**SpO₂:**
EMS Treatment (circle all that apply)					
Oxygen @ _____ L/min via (circle one): NC NRM Bag-mask device		**Assisted Ventilation**	**Airway Adjunct**		**CPR**
Defibrillation	**Bleeding Control**	**Bandaging**	**Splinting**		**Other:**
Narrative					

Ambulance Calls

The following case scenarios provide an opportunity to explore the concerns associated with the mechanism of injury and trauma systems. Read each scenario, and then answer each question.

1. You are called to the scene of a backroad single-vehicle collision in which a car plowed into a utility pole. The driver of the car is sitting on the grass beside his wrecked vehicle, looking dazed and confused. Which parameters would you use to assess the mechanism of injury and suspected injuries and/or injury patterns?

   a. _____

   b. _____

   c. _____

   d. _____

   e. _____

   f. _____

2. You are summoned to the scene of a smoky apartment-house fire. When you arrive, one of the firefighters directs you to a casualty who has been carried to a spot just beyond the fire lines. The firefighter tells you that the man jumped from a window.

   a. Which further information do you need to obtain about this patient to evaluate the potential seriousness of the injuries he might have sustained in making that jump?

   _____

   _____

   _____

   _____

   _____

   b. Assuming the patient landed on his feet, which injuries might you expect him to have suffered?

   _____

   _____

3. On your next call, you are summoned to a housing project where a 2-year-old child managed to crawl over the edge of a second-story balcony and fall into the playground below. Which sort of injuries would this child most likely have sustained, and why?

   _____

   _____

4. You are called to a somewhat disreputable downtown area for a "man shot." You arrive on the scene to see the patient lying on the ground in the center of a small group of men, some of whom are apparently intoxicated and all of whom are talking at once.

a. What is the *first* action you will take before entering the scene?

_____

b. Which information do you need to obtain regarding the shooting incident?

(1)_____

(2)_____

(3)_____

(4)_____

(5)_____

5. A fire at a warehouse of a large construction company ignites the stock of dynamite and produces an explosion that shatters windows for blocks around. As you respond to the scene, you review in your mind the different kinds of injuries you might soon have to deal with. List the four *mechanisms* of injury that can be produced by an explosion, and describe each one.

a. _____

b. _____

c. _____

d. _____

6. Among the patients whom you treat at the scene of the explosion is a young man who had been taking a walk about half a block from the construction company when the explosion occurred. The man states that the blast "knocked me clear off my feet." He complains of a "tight feeling in my chest" and blurry vision. On physical examination, he appears somewhat confused; he cannot tell you the date or what day of the week it is. His vital signs are as follows: pulse 100 beats/min, full and regular; respirations 30 breaths/min and somewhat shallow; BP 120/80 mm Hg. His skin is warm and dry. Aside from a little dried blood in the left ear canal, there are no other physical findings. Which tissues are at risk? What is the evidence for you thinking so?

Tissues at Risk	Evidence
1.	
2.	
3.	

True/False

If you believe the statement to be more true than false, write the letter "T" in the space provided. If you believe the statement to be more false than true, write the letter "F."

_____ **1.** Solid organs are relatively protected from shock-wave injury but may be injured by secondary missiles or a hurled body.

_____ **2.** A Level IV trauma center provides the most comprehensive trauma care possible.

_____ **3.** Transport considerations are not necessary if the patient is seriously hurt.

_____ **4.** Blunt trauma typically occurs in motor vehicle crashes.

_____ **5.** The "paper-bag syndrome" can result in a pneumothorax.

_____   **6.** Small children should be seated in the front seats of motor vehicles so that they will benefit from the protection offered by airbags.

_____   **7.** Evaluation of the patient's GCS score is a component of step 1 in the 2011 CDC decision scheme for field trauma of injured patients.

_____   **8.** If a patient was riding a motorcycle and was involved in a crash at about 15 mph, he should automatically be taken to a trauma center based on the 2011 CDC decision scheme for field trauma of injured patients.

Short Answer

Complete this section with short written answers using the space provided.

1. A 2,000-lb automobile is traveling at 20 mph when it strikes a pedestrian.

a. What happens to the kinetic energy of the vehicle at the moment of impact?

_____

_____

_____

b. If the vehicle weighed 6,000 lb instead of 2,000 lb, what difference would that make in terms of its kinetic energy?

_____

_____

_____

c. If the vehicle were traveling at 60 mph rather than 20 mph, what difference would that make in terms of its kinetic energy?

_____

_____

_____

2. A car traveling at 50 mph goes out of control and slams into a concrete wall. That sequence of events involves five phases of deceleration, each of which proceeds like a separate collision and each of which involves a transfer of kinetic energy (KE). Which objects are involved in each of the first three collisions, and what happens to the KE in each case?

a. Collision 1:

_____

_____

b. Collision 2:

_____

_____

c. Collision 3:

_____

_____

_____

3. Careful inspection of a wrecked vehicle can enable the rescuer to detect injuries among the patients that might not otherwise be obvious. For each of the vehicular findings mentioned in the following list, list the injuries that are likely to be associated.

   a. Deformed dashboard

     (1)_____

     (2)_____

     (3)_____

     (4)_____

     (5)_____

   b. Deformed steering column

     (1)_____

     (2)_____

     (3)_____

     (4)_____

     (5)_____

     (6)_____

   c. Cracked windshield

     (1)_____

     (2)_____

     (3)_____

     (4)_____

   d. Door smashed in

     (1)_____

     (2)_____

     (3)_____

4. One of the most lethal objects in a motor vehicle is the steering wheel. Whenever you find structural damage to a steering wheel—indeed, whenever there is significant deformity to the front end of a car involved in a collision—you must be alert for the presence of the "ring of injuries" impact that the steering wheel may have produced in the driver of the car. List six injuries that may be associated with steering wheel trauma.

   a._____

b. _____

c. _____

d. _____

e. _____

f. _____

Fill in the Table

Fill in the missing parts of the table.

1. Fill in the key elements for the corresponding definition.

Key Elements for Trauma Centers		
Level	**Definition**	**Key Elements**
Level I	A comprehensive regional resource that is a tertiary care facility. Capable of providing total care for every aspect of injury—from prevention through rehabilitation.	1. 2. 3. 4. 5.
Level II	Able to initiate definitive care for all injured patients.	1. 2. 3. 4. 5.
Level III	Able to provide prompt assessment, resuscitation, and stabilization of injured patients and emergency operations.	1. 2. 3. 4. 5.

Level IV	Able to provide ATLS before transfer of patients to a higher-level trauma center.	1.
		2.
		3.
		4.

2. List the "ring" of chest injuries from impacting the steering wheel or dashboard.

"Ring" of Chest Injuries From Impact With the Steering Wheel or Dashboard

- _____
- Soft-tissue neck trauma
- Larynx and tracheal trauma
- _____
- _____
- _____
- Pulmonary contusion
- Hemothorax, rib fractures
- _____
- _____
- Intra-abdominal injuries

Problem Solving

Use the formula for kinetic energy to answer the following questions.

$$KE = M/2 \times V^2$$

You have responded to a motor vehicle crash. This was a collision involving a car and a stationary bridge abutment. There are two patients. Your patient appears to be a 6-feet man who weighs approximately 200 lb. The patient is conscious and alert. While talking to him, you discover that he was not wearing a seat belt, and his vehicle was traveling at 50 mph.

1. Use the formula for calculating kinetic energy (KE) to determine the KE units involved in this crash. The second passenger in the vehicle was also unbelted, and she weighs 120 lb.

2. How many KE units are involved for the second passenger?

Bleeding

Left shoulder pain after a sports injury can signify a spleen injury.

Matching

Match each of the definitions in the left column to the appropriate term in the right column.

_____ **1.** A mass of blood in the soft tissues beneath the skin; it indicates bleeding into soft tissues and may be the result of a minor or a severe injury.

_____ **2.** Blood in the urine.

_____ **3.** The proportion of red blood cells in the total blood volume.

_____ **4.** Passage of stools containing bright red blood.

_____ **5.** Vomited blood.

_____ **6.** The body's natural blood-clotting mechanism.

_____ **7.** A condition in which volume is lost in the form of blood.

_____ **8.** Bleeding.

_____ **9.** Coughed-up blood.

_____ **10.** A bleeding disorder that is primarily hereditary, in which clotting does not occur or occurs insufficiently.

_____ **11.** An abnormal state associated with inadequate oxygen and nutrient delivery to the metabolic apparatus of the cell.

_____ **12.** The precontraction pressure in the heart, which increases as the volume of blood builds up.

_____ **13.** Small cells in the blood that are essential for clot formation.

_____ **14.** A component of blood; made of 92% water, 6% to 7% proteins, and electrolytes, clotting factors, and glucose.

_____ **15.** The delivery of oxygen and nutrients to the cells, organs, and tissues of the body.

_____ **16.** The pressure in the aorta against which the left ventricle must pump blood; increasing this pressure can decrease cardiac output.

_____ **17.** The fluid tissue that is pumped by the heart through the arteries, veins, and capillaries; it consists of plasma and formed elements or cells, such as red blood cells, white blood cells, and platelets.

_____ **18.** The amount of blood pumped by the heart per minute; calculated by multiplying the stroke volume by the pulse rate per minute.

A. Afterload

B. Blood

C. Cardiac output

D. Compensated shock

E. Decompensated (hypotensive) shock

F. Ejection fraction

G. Exsanguination

H. Hematemesis

I. Hematochezia

J. Hematocrit

K. Hematoma

L. Hematuria

M. Hemophilia

N. Hemoptysis

O. Hemorrhage

P. Hemorrhagic shock

Q. Hemostasis

R. Hypoperfusion

_____ **19.** The early stage of shock, in which the body can still compensate for blood loss. The systolic blood pressure and brain perfusion are maintained.

_____ **20.** The late stage of shock, when blood pressure is falling.

_____ **21.** The loss of the total blood volume, resulting in death.

_____ **22.** The percentage of blood that leaves the heart each time it contracts.

_____ **23.** Passage of dark, tarry stools.

_____ **24.** A condition that occurs when the circulating blood volume is inadequate to deliver adequate oxygen and nutrients to the body.

_____ **25.** A condition that occurs when the level of tissue perfusion decreases below that needed to maintain normal cellular functions.

S. Hypovolemic shock

T. Melena

U. Perfusion

V. Plasma

W. Platelets

X. Preload

Y. Shock

Multiple Choice

Read each item carefully, and then select the best response.

_____ **1.** _____ is a blood test that measures the portion of red blood cells (RBCs) in the whole blood.
   A. Plasma count
   B. Hematocrit
   C. Cardiac output
   D. Ejection fraction

_____ **2.** Which of the following substances accounts for more than half of the body's blood volume?
   A. Erythrocytes
   B. Leukocytes
   C. Plasma
   D. Hemoglobin

_____ **3.** A laceration or tear of a large artery can cause a patient to exsanguinate in as little as _____ minutes.
   A. 2
   B. 3
   C. 5
   D. 10

_____ **4.** The body cannot tolerate an acute blood loss of _____. This loss will produce a significant change in vital signs of the adult patient, referred to as a Class III hemorrhage.
   A. less than 5%
   B. less than 15%
   C. 15% to 30%
   D. 30% to 40%

_____ **5.** When you encounter a patient who is bleeding, the first thing you should do is:
   A. estimate the blood loss.
   B. apply direct pressure.
   C. check for breathing.
   D. don personal protective equipment.

_____ **6.** A stool that contains bright red blood is called:
   A. hematochezia.
   B. melena.
   C. hematuria.
   D. epistaxis.

_____ **7.** The coughing up of blood is referred to as:
   A. hematemesis.
   B. hematuria.
   C. hemoptysis.
   D. melena.

8. The initial stage of hemorrhagic shock is characterized by low circulating blood volume with:

    A. a respiratory rate of 30 to 40 breaths/min.

    B. minimal signs of hypoperfusion.

    C. absent capillary refill.

    D. a heart rate of more than 120 beats/min.

9. Which of the following statements about the use of an arterial tourniquet is correct?

    A. It is rarely used in the field today.

    B. It can be used only for arterial bleeding.

    C. It should be placed proximal to the injury on the extremity.

    D. It should be applied on and off every 20 minutes to save the limb.

10. A patient has the signs and symptoms of shock from a fracture or a burn. This is MOST likely due to which cause of shock?

    A. Poor vessel function

    B. Low fluid volume

    C. Respiratory failure

    D. Pump failure

Labeling

Label the following diagram with the correct terms.

1. The circulatory system

A. _____

B. _____

C. _____

D. _____

E. _____

F. _____

G. _____

H. _____

I. _____

J. _____

Fill in the Blank

Read each item carefully, and then complete the statement by filling in the missing word(s).

1. Red blood cells contain _____, a protein that gives blood its reddish color.

2. Blood circulation through an organ or tissue that meets the cells' current needs for oxygen, nutrients, and waste removal is known as _____.

3. _____ is the process in which platelets aggregate at the site, plugging the hole and sealing injured portions of the vessel.

4. A lower gastrointestinal (GI) bleed is indicated with the passing of _____, which is a dark, tarry-looking stool.

5. _____ is bleeding from the nose.

6. _____ happens when the level of tissue perfusion drops below normal limits.

7. When a patient is passing a bloody stool, this is referred to as _____ and can indicate hemorrhage near the external opening of the anus.

8. A small portion of the population lacks one or more of the blood's _____ factors. This condition is called _____.

9. As _____ increases and _____ drops, patients in shock develop cold, mottled, and pulseless extremities with _____ mental status.

10. The organs and organ systems with a high incidence of exsanguination from penetrating injuries include the _____, thoracic vascular system, abdominal vascular system, venous system, and _____.

11. The three phases of shock are _____, _____, and _____ shock.

12. The IV fluid of choice when replacing lost blood volume is either _____ _____ or _____ _____.

13. Do not give the patient with suspected hypovolemia anything by _____ because he or she is likely to _____.

14. Solutions that do not contain proteins or any other large molecules, and that are typically used in shock fluid resuscitation, are known as _____.

Identify

Read the following case study, and then list the chief complaint, vital signs, and pertinent negatives.

You are called to the scene of a local gas station where the 44-year-old man behind the counter was shot during a robbery. He is experiencing abdominal pain with a small bullet wound in the umbilical area. Upon arrival, the police determine that the perpetrator has fled the scene, so the scene is safe for you to proceed with your trauma assessment. John, the patient, is clutching his belly with a towel for bleeding control. You note there is no radial pulse, yet John is still alert and oriented. Your partner quickly places John on high-flow supplemental oxygen by a nonrebreathing mask and applies an occlusive dressing to the wound. You determine that John has no obvious injury to his chest, and his lung sounds are equal in both lungs. As he is being packaged to go to the trauma center, an electrocardiogram (ECG) monitor is applied, and you determine that John's heart is in a sinus tachycardia with a rate of 120 beats/min and no ectopy. He is breathing at 24 breaths/min, and his room air saturation is 92%. He is very anxious but comes around with the oxygen and is able to answer all your questions. His pupils are equal, round, and reactive to light and accommodation (PERRLA). His blood pressure (BP) is 80/56 mm Hg, and his skin is pale, cool, and diaphoretic. You determine that there are no other injuries, although you know that an abdominal gunshot wound (GSW) is significant, and it is difficult to tell how much internal bleeding he may have so far. En route to the trauma center, you start two large-bore IV lines of normal saline. You call ahead to prepare the emergency department (ED) for your arrival and then begin reassessment.

1. Chief complaint:

   _____

   _____

2. Vital signs:

   _____

   _____

3. Pertinent negatives:

_____

_____

Complete the Patient Care Report

Reread the case study in the preceding Identify exercise, and then complete the following patient care report (PCR) for the patient.

EMS Patient Care Report (PCR)					
Date:	Incident No.:	Nature of Call:		Location:	
Dispatched:	En Route:	At Scene:	Transport:	At Hospital:	In Service:
Patient Information					
Age: Sex: Weight (in kg [lb]):		Allergies: Medications: Past Medical History: Chief Complaint:			
Vital Signs					
Time:	BP:	Pulse:	Respirations:		SpO_2:
Time:	BP:	Pulse:	Respirations:		SpO_2:
Time:	BP:	Pulse:	Respirations:		SpO_2:
EMS Treatment (circle all that apply)					
Oxygen @ _____ L/min via (circle one): NC NRM Bag-mask device		Assisted Ventilation	Airway Adjunct		CPR
Defibrillation	Bleeding Control	Bandaging	Splinting		Other:
Narrative					

Ambulance Calls

The following case scenarios provide an opportunity to explore the concerns associated with patient management and paramedic care. Read each scenario, and then answer each question.

1. A middle-aged man was struck by a car as he was crossing the street. You find him lying by the side of the road, complaining of severe pain in his abdomen, where the car hit him. You would like to make an assessment of his state of perfusion. How will you assess the following?

   a. His *peripheral* perfusion:

   _____

   _____

   b. The perfusion to his *brain*:

   _____

   _____

2. You are called to a downtown bar where firearms were used to settle a difference of opinion. You find a man lying on the floor of the bar, unconscious, his trouser leg soaked in blood. In the correct sequence, list the steps you would take in treating this patient.

   a. _____

   b. _____

   c. _____

   d. _____

   e. _____

   f. _____

3. One rainy day, a car bomb was detonated in front of a foreign consulate. Some bystanders were injured by flying debris, including jagged pieces of metal torn from the car's body. The first patient you come upon is bleeding from multiple sites, including a deep gash on the right side of the neck and a laceration that has partially severed the right leg at the groin. The leg laceration is gushing blood; it is too proximal to benefit from a tourniquet. It is difficult to evaluate the patient's skin condition in the rain. Pulse is around 100 beats/min and somewhat weak; respirations are 30 breaths/min.

   a. Which steps would you take at the scene?

   (1)_____

   (2)_____

   (3)_____

   (4)_____

   b. Which steps would you take during transport?

   (1)_____

   (2)_____

   (3)_____

4. A second patient from the car bombing, a young man, was sideswiped by a piece of flying debris, which made a clean 14-inch incision straight across his abdomen. He is conscious and in moderate distress. Pulse is 104 beats/min and regular, respirations are 28 breaths/min and slightly labored, and BP is 104/70 mm Hg. What looks to be a major portion of the patient's intestines is outside the abdomen.

a. Which steps would you take at the scene?

(1)_____

(2)_____

(3)_____

b. Which steps would you take during transport?

(1)_____

(2)_____

(3)_____

True/False

If you believe the statement to be more true than false, write the letter "T" in the space provided. If you believe the statement to be more false than true, write the letter "F."

_____ **1.** One of the earliest signs of hypovolemic shock is a fall in the blood pressure.

_____ **2.** Patients in hemorrhagic shock tend to have a normal pulse rate.

_____ **3.** The IV fluid of choice to provide volume to a patient in hypovolemic shock is 5% dextrose in water (D_5W).

_____ **4.** A patient may go into shock without losing any blood or fluid from the body.

_____ **5.** The amount of blood pumped through the circulatory system in 1 minute is known as the cardiac output.

_____ **6.** The function of plasma is to produce red blood cells (RBCs) and white blood cells (WBCs).

_____ **7.** Nontraumatic internal bleeding usually happens in the gastrointestinal tract.

_____ **8.** A 1-year-old child has a blood volume of approximately 800 mL.

_____ **9.** You can use a wire, rope, or any narrow material as a tourniquet.

_____ **10.** Definitive management for internal hemorrhage is in the hospital.

Short Answer

Complete this section with short written answers using the space provided.

1. Three components are required for a functioning circulatory system. If any one of those components is impaired, shock may result. List the three necessary components.

a. _____

b. _____

c. _____

2. The type of shock you will see most frequently in the prehospital setting is hemorrhagic shock. It is very important to detect hypovolemic shock early and to start treatment early. To do so, you must have a high index of suspicion in assessing patients at risk of hypovolemic shock, which means you must be aware of the situations in which hypovolemia is likely to occur. List four causes of hypovolemic shock.

a. _____

b. _____

c. _____

d. _____

3. Knowing the findings in hemorrhagic shock is important for you as a paramedic. For each of the following findings, note whether the value is increased, decreased, flat, or changed during suspected Class II fluid and blood loss.

Estimated Fluid and Blood Loss (for Class II)	
Heart rate (beats/min)	
Systolic blood pressure (mm Hg)	
Pulse pressure (mm Hg)	
Respiratory rate (breaths/min)	
Central nervous system/mental status	
Skin condition	
Urine output (mL/h)	

4. It is not necessary in the field to make a specific diagnosis of a patient's abdominal pain, but it is necessary to be able to recognize when a potentially life-threatening situation exists. Any patient with abdominal pain showing symptoms or signs of shock must be considered to be in danger. To recognize that danger, you must be able to spot the symptoms and signs of shock. List six symptoms and signs of shock.

a. _____

b. _____

c. _____

d. _____

e. _____

f. _____

5. List the four steps in managing external hemorrhage.

a. _____

b. _____

c. _____

d. _____

Fill in the Table

Fill in the missing parts of the table.

Compensated Versus Decompensated Shock	
Compensated	**Decompensated**
• _____	• Altered mental status (verbal to unresponsive)
• Sense of impending doom	• _____
• _____	• Labored or irregular breathing
• Clammy (cool, moist) skin	• _____
• _____	• Ashen, mottled, or cyanotic skin
• Shortness of breath	• _____
• _____	• Diminished urine output (oliguria)
• Delayed capillary refill in infants and children	• _____
• _____	
• Normal systolic blood pressure	

Soft-Tissue Trauma

The paramedic is asked to be an island of calm and authority.

© Jones & Bartlett Learning.

Matching

Part I

Match each of the terms in the right column to the appropriate definition in the left column.

_____ **1.** Protein that gives tensile strength to the connective tissues of the body.

_____ **2.** A bruise; an injury that causes bleeding beneath the skin but does not break the skin.

_____ **3.** A traumatic injury that results in the soft tissue of a part of the body being drawn downward like a glove being removed.

_____ **4.** The tendency toward constancy or stability in the body's internal environment.

_____ **5.** A type of injury that occurs when a foreign material is forcefully injected into soft tissue.

_____ **6.** A localized collection of blood in the soft tissues as a result of injury or a broken blood vessel.

_____ **7.** The continual shedding of the dead cells on the surface of the skin.

_____ **8.** Material used to directly cover a wound.

_____ **9.** Extravasation of blood under the skin, producing a "black-and-blue" mark.

_____ **10.** The outermost layer of the skin.

_____ **11.** Cells that contain granules.

_____ **12.** An infection commonly caused by *Clostridium perfringens*, which results in tissue destruction and gas production that may lead to death.

_____ **13.** An injury in which a portion of the body is denuded of the epidermis by scraping or rubbing.

_____ **14.** An injury in which part of the body is completely or partially severed.

_____ **15.** An injury that leaves a piece of skin or other tissue partially or completely torn away from the body.

_____ **16.** The inner layer of skin, containing hair follicle roots, sweat glands, blood vessels, nerve endings, and sebaceous glands.

_____ **17.** The formation of fresh epithelial tissue to heal a wound.

_____ **18.** Material used to secure a dressing in place.

_____ **19.** The factors that cause cells to migrate into an area.

A. Abrasion

B. Amputation

C. Avulsion

D. Bandage

E. Chemotactic factors

F. Closed wound

G. Collagen

H. Contusion

I. Degloving

J. Dermis

K. Desquamation

L. Dressing

M. Ecchymosis

N. High-pressure injection injury

O. Epidermis

P. Epithelialization

Q. Erythema

R. Fasciitis

S. Flexor tenosynovitis of the hand

_____ **20.** An injury in which damage occurs beneath the skin or mucous membrane but the surface remains intact.

T. Gangrene

_____ **21.** A closed-space infection of the hand.

U. Granulocytes

_____ **22.** Inflammation of the fascia.

V. Homeostasis

_____ **23.** Reddening of the skin.

W. Hematoma

Part II

Match each of the terms in the right column to the appropriate definition in the left column.

_____ **1.** Death of tissue from bacterial infection caused by more than one infecting organism—most commonly, *Staphylococcus aureus* and hemolytic streptococci; this condition has a high mortality rate.

A. Hypertrophic scar

_____ **2.** Inflammation of the muscle, usually caused by infection.

B. Incision

_____ **3.** A wound made by tearing or cutting tissues.

C. Integument

_____ **4.** Inflammation of a lymph channel.

D. Keloid scar

_____ **5.** The process by which the body maintains temperature through a combination of heat gain by metabolic processes and muscular movement and heat loss through breathing, evaporation, conduction, convection, and perspiration.

E. Laceration

_____ **6.** A disease caused by spores that enter the body through a puncture wound contaminated with animal feces, street dust, or soil or that enter through contaminated street drugs.

F. Lymphangitis

_____ **7.** The pattern of tautness of the skin, which is arranged over body structures and affects how well wounds heal.

G. Tetanus

_____ **8.** A surgical procedure to improve the appearance of a scar, reestablish function, or correct disfigurement from soft-tissue damage, surgical incision, or lesion.

H. Myositis

_____ **9.** Development of new blood vessels to aid in healing injured soft tissue.

I. Necrotizing fasciitis

_____ **10.** An injury in which there is a break in the surface of the skin or the mucous membrane, exposing deeper tissue to potential contamination.

J. Neovascularization

_____ **11.** Infection of the area around the fingernail bed.

K. Open wound

_____ **12.** A narrow strip of tissue by which an avulsed piece of tissue remains connected to the body.

L. Paronychia

_____ **13.** An abnormal scar with excess collagen that does not extend over the wound margins.

M. Pedicle

_____ **14.** A wound usually made deliberately, as in surgery; a clean cut, as opposed to a laceration.

N. Phagocytosis

_____ **15.** The skin.

O. Puncture wound

_____ **16.** An abnormal scar commonly found in people with darkly pigmented skin, which extends over a wound's margins.

P. Rabid

_____ **17.** Describes an animal that is infected with rabies.

Q. Scar revision

_____ **18.** An injury resulting from a piercing object, such as a nail or a knife; also referred to as a penetrating wound.

R. Thermoregulation

_____ **19.** The process in which one cell "eats" or engulfs a foreign substance to destroy it.

S. Tension lines

Multiple Choice

Read each item carefully, and then select the best response.

_____ 1. The injury that occurs when high-pressure injected material enters the soft tissues can result in:

    A. no pain, initially.

    B. acute inflammation.

    C. chronic inflammation.

    D. All of the above

_____ 2. Blood vessels, nerves, tendons, muscles, and internal organs can all be damaged by:

    A. compartment syndrome.

    B. improperly applied dressings.

    C. use of a wet dressing instead of a dry dressing.

    D. application of a tourniquet.

_____ 3. When should the paramedic remove an impaled object in a patient's abdomen?

    A. When the object affects packaging and transport

    B. When the object does not stand up straight on its own

    C. When bleeding cannot be successfully controlled

    D. The paramedic should never remove an impaled object from that location.

_____ 4. When a foreign material is forcefully injected into soft tissue, the resulting injury is called a(n):

    A. high-pressure injection injury.

    B. amputation.

    C. tympanic membrane rupture.

    D. blast injury.

_____ 5. Patients with soft-tissue injuries:

    A. rarely have life-threatening injuries.

    B. should be "signed off" to save emergency medical services (EMS) system resources.

    C. should be treated with aggressive advanced life support (ALS) treatment in the event of unforeseen injury.

    D. have a high incidence of morbidity and mortality.

_____ 6. The guidelines for the management of an amputation include each of the following, EXCEPT:

    A. do not place the amputated part in water.

    B. do not use dry ice to cool the part.

    C. keep the amputated part warm.

    D. wrap the part loosely in saline-moistened sterile gauze.

_____ 7. There are numerous types of soft-tissue injuries. Many of them are relatively minor, but some have potentially serious outcomes. Which of the following injuries requires transportation?

    A. Abrasion

    B. Laceration

    C. Necrotizing fasciitis

    D. Incision

_____ 8. Soft-tissue injuries often involve external hemorrhaging. All of the following measures would be considered appropriate bleeding management, EXCEPT:

    A. direct pressure with thick, bulky dressings.

    B. pressure with elastic bandages.

    C. "wet" dressings applied to the wound.

    D. tourniquet on a severely bleeding extremity.

_____ 9. Soft-tissue injuries to the neck may lead to which of the following complications?

    A. Air embolism

    B. Spinal injury

    C. Airway disruption

    D. All of the above

_____ **10.** Which of the following can interfere with normal wound healing?
  A. An underlying cardiac history
  B. A seizure disorder
  C. Carpal tunnel syndrome
  D. A history of diabetes

Labeling

1. Label the components of the skin in the following diagram.

A. _____   G. _____

B. _____   H. _____

C. _____   I. _____

D. _____   J. _____

E. _____   K. _____

F. _____   L. _____

2. Determine which types of open wounds are shown in each of the following photos.

A. _____

B. _____

C. _____

D. _____

E. _____

Fill in the Blank

Read each item carefully, and then complete the statement by filling in the missing word(s).

1. _____ injuries require substantial irrigation and _____ before closing by an emergency practitioner.

2. Visible clues of infection include _____, _____, _____, _____, and _____ _____.

3. *Clostridium tetani* causes the body to produce a potent _____, which results in painful muscle _____ that are strong enough to fracture bones.

4. _____ is dead tissue. It is caused when _____ supply delivery to tissue is interrupted or stopped.

5. _____ is the most common infection of the hand in the United States.

6. Excessive _____ formation can occur if the healing process is not balanced between the building-up and breaking-down phases of healing.

7. Wet dressings have limited use in the field but are used in the care of _____ burns.

Identify

Read the following case studies, and then identify the type of soft-tissue injury and the care that you would provide.

1. You are called to the scene of a local campsite where a 10-year-old boy was playing with his pocket knife, whittling some wood, when he cut himself. The injury is a jagged incision to his right forearm. There is moderate darkish-red blood oozing from the site.

_____

_____

_____

2. A patient was working in his home shop when he became distracted while using a circular saw. He inadvertently cut the fingers on his left hand. When you arrive, the patient is sitting in a chair, conscious and alert. He appears pale and sweaty. He has several blood-soaked towels covering his hand. You notice that his left middle and ring fingers are sitting on his wood-crafting bench.

_____

_____

_____

3. It is a busy shift. On this call you are dispatched to a bar fight. On arrival, there is a crowd hovering around a woman who complains of pain in her right side and moderate shortness of breath. Her companion states that she was involved in a dispute and felt a sharp object impact her right side. The patient is somewhat angry and combative and wants to continue the dispute. As you examine the injury, you notice a minimal amount of bleeding that appears to have stopped. The patient has a quarter-inch circular opening to her chest. There appears to be a small amount of swelling and a rush of air when she breathes.

_____

_____

_____

Ambulance Calls

The following case scenarios provide an opportunity to explore the concerns associated with patient management and paramedic care. Read each scenario, and then answer each question.

1. You are summoned to Bugsy's Butcher Shop to tend to the proprietor, Bugsy Butterfingers, who dropped a meat cleaver on his left leg. There is a large gash in the left calf, and it is bleeding profusely.

a. List three methods you might use to try to control the bleeding, and put an asterisk next to the method likely to be the most effective. Please note that standard precautions are being done appropriately.

(1)_____

(2)_____

(3)_____

b. Suppose Bugsy's wound had been on the forearm rather than on the leg. Which artery is most likely the cause of severe bleeding in the arm?

_____

_____

2. One of Bugsy's employees, Frank Fillet, becomes so distracted watching you care for his boss that he accidentally chops off two of his fingers while preparing an order of steaks.

a. How will you treat Frank's injury?

_____

_____

b. What will you do with the two fingers lying on the chopping board?

_____

_____

3. Yet another worker in the butcher shop, Hercules Hamburger, had been watching, slack-jawed and transfixed, as this drama was unfolding. So intent was he on the spectacle that he did not realize his right hand had entered the meat grinder—at least not until his hand became engaged in the grinding blades. Hearing his screams, a customer rushes over to where Hercules is standing and manages to shut off the meat grinder, but not before Hercules's hand and forearm have been badly mangled. You already have your hands full with Bugsy and Frank, so you instruct the Good Samaritan who shut off the meat grinder, "Have him lie down, and try to control the bleeding—I'll be with him in just a minute." Obligingly, the customer grabs a piece of rope that he finds behind the counter, winds it around Hercules's upper arm, and slips a ballpoint pen into the knot to serve as a tourniquet. He twists the rope as tightly as he possibly can, secures the pen, and uses the butcher's apron to wrap the entire hand and arm.

Although the customer was trying to be helpful, in fact, he made several very serious mistakes. List the mistakes.

a. _____

b. _____

c. _____

d. _____

4. During deer-hunting season, two young backpackers were strolling through the woods when hunters, mistaking the pair for deer, discharged their crossbows at them. One arrow entered the eye of the first backpacker, while another arrow went straight through the cheek of the second backpacker.

a. Describe the steps you would take in treating the backpacker with the arrow in his eye. Please note that standard precautions are being done appropriately.

_____

_____

_____

_____

_____

_____

b. Describe the steps you would take in treating the backpacker who has an arrow impaled in his cheek.

_____

_____

_____

_____

_____

5. You are folding up your deck chair when you happen to see a jogger running erratically down the beach toward you. His shorts are torn, and there is blood trickling down one leg. "What happened to you?" you ask.

"Some big Doberman tackled me as I was running. I figured the best thing to do was keep running to where I left my car." You note the tooth marks and a laceration on the runner's left leg.

How would you manage this patient? Please note that standard precautions are being done appropriately.

a. _____

b. _____

c. _____

d. _____

True/False

If you believe the statement to be more true than false, write the letter "T" in the space provided. If you believe the statement to be more false than true, write the letter "F."

_____ 1. Amputation is a form of avulsion.

_____ 2. Soft-tissue trauma is the leading form of injury.

_____ 3. Sweating is regulated through the parasympathetic nervous system.

_____ 4. Subcutaneous blood vessels have a crucial role in regulating body temperature.

_____ 5. An incision is a clean (linear), intentional cut.

_____ 6. Human bites carry a higher risk of infection than animal bites do.

_____ 7. Keloid scars typically develop in areas of high tissue stress.

_____ 8. Tetanus infection causes the body to produce a potent toxin that results in lockjaw.

_____ 9. It is important to remove all other dressings before applying a hemostatic dressing.

_____ 10. Bleeding control is a key principle in treating open wounds.

Short Answer

Complete this section with short written answers using the space provided.

1. You can appreciate the possible consequences of injury to the skin if you understand which functions healthy, intact skin performs. List four functions performed by the skin in a healthy person.

   a. _____

   b. _____

   c. _____

   d. _____

2. Healing of wounds is a natural process that involves several overlapping stages. List the five stages of wound healing.

   a. _____

   b. _____

   c. _____

   d. _____

   e. _____

3. Wounds are characterized as either closed or open. List the characteristics of closed wounds.

   a. _____

   b. _____

   c. _____

Burns

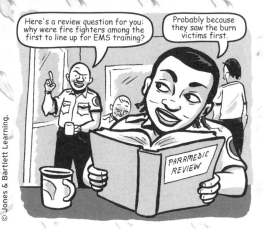

Here's a review question for you: why were fire fighters among the first to line up for EMS training?

Probably because they saw the burn victims first.

PARAMEDIC REVIEW

© Jones & Bartlett Learning.

Matching

Part I

Match each of the patients with the appropriate treatment in question 1 and with the appropriate sequence in question 2.

1. In the course of a busy week, you are called on to treat eight burn victims in a variety of circumstances. In each case, you have to determine whether the patient has suffered a critical burn because, if so, he or she must be evacuated directly to the regional burn center, which is 24 miles away; noncritical burns, in contrast, can be managed by the community hospital right in town. A description of the patients you saw follows. Beside each description, indicate whether:

   A. The patient has a critical burn and should be brought to a regional burn center.

   B. The patient does not have a critical burn and can be managed in the community hospital.

   _____ (1) A 2-year-old boy who overturned a pot of soup from the stovetop onto himself; both legs and the anterior trunk are burned.

   _____ (2) A 57-year-old woman with diabetes and a scald burn of her left lower leg.

   _____ (3) A 28-year-old woman with a scald burn of her entire right arm.

   _____ (4) A lineman who suffered an electric shock. There is a small bull's-eye entrance wound on the left hand; you cannot find the exit wound. The lineman did not fall. His left leg feels rock hard.

   _____ (5) A 22-year-old male short-order cook with partial-thickness (second-degree) burns over both anterior thighs, sustained when he spilled a pot of soup.

   _____ (6) A 34-year-old woman rescued from a burning building, where she had been trapped in her smoke-filled bedroom. She has partial-thickness burns of the right forearm. She is coughing up sooty sputum.

   _____ (7) A 25-year-old man who tripped and fell onto the hibachi on the back porch as he was preparing to grill some steaks. His hand went straight into the bed of red-hot charcoal, and his shirt caught fire. He has full-thickness (third-degree) burns of the left hand and forearm and partial-thickness burns of the anterior chest.

   _____ (8) A plumber who spilled a bottle of industrial-strength liquid drain cleaner down the front of his pants.

2. You are called to treat a patient who was in a tenement fire. He is a middle-aged man who apparently fell asleep in an armchair while holding a lit cigarette. You arrive at the scene just as he is being carried, unresponsive, from the building and note that his clothes are still smoldering. Following, in random order, are the steps you will have to take in managing this patient. Arrange the steps in the correct sequence.

   A. Administer supplemental oxygen.

   B. Start an IV.

   C. Open the airway manually.

   D. Put out the fire.

   E. Remove the patient's clothing.

   F. Pass a nasogastric tube into his stomach.

   G. Determine the extent and depth of the burn.

   H. Intubate the trachea (if a basic life support [BLS] airway is not adequate).

   I. Cover the burns with sterile dressings.

J. Obtain a set of baseline vital signs.

(1) _____   (6) _____

(2) _____   (7) _____

(3) _____   (8) _____

(4) _____   (9) _____

(5) _____   (10) _____

Part II

Match each of the terms in the right column to the appropriate definition in the left column.

_____ 1. The skin.

_____ 2. Also referred to as burn shock; the shock or hypoperfusion caused by a burn injury and the tremendous loss of fluids; capillaries leak, resulting in intravascular fluid volume oozing out of the circulation and into the interstitial spaces, and cells take in increased amounts of salt and water.

_____ 3. A tendency toward constancy or stability in the body's internal environment.

_____ 4. A burn that extends through the epidermis and dermis into the subcutaneous tissues beneath; previously called a third-degree burn.

_____ 5. An electrothermal injury caused by arcing of electric current.

_____ 6. One of the complex materials found, along with collagen fibers and elastin fibers, in the dermis of the skin.

_____ 7. A detailed version of the rule of nines chart that takes into consideration the changes in total body surface area that occur with growth.

_____ 8. A form of necrosis that results from the transformation of tissue into a liquid viscous mass (pus).

_____ 9. A description of the relationship between heat production, current, and resistance.

_____ 10. The clinical course that usually begins within hours of exposure to a radiation source. Symptoms include nausea, vomiting, diarrhea, fatigue, fever, and headache. The long-term symptoms are dose related and are hematopoietic and gastrointestinal in nature.

_____ 11. A burn produced by touching a hot object.

_____ 12. A formula that recommends giving 2 to 4 mL of normal saline for each kilogram of body weight, multiplied by the percentage of total body surface area burned; sometimes used to calculate fluid needs during lengthy transport times; formerly called the Parkland formula.

_____ 13. A protein that gives tensile strength to the connective tissues of the body.

_____ 14. Cell death typically caused by ischemia or infarction.

_____ 15. A burn on the neck or chest, which may compress the airway, or on an extremity, which might act like a tourniquet.

_____ 16. A thermal burn caused by flames touching the skin.

_____ 17. A surgical cut through the eschar or leathery covering of a burn injury to allow for swelling and minimize the potential for development of compartment syndrome in a circumferentially burned limb or the thorax.

_____ 18. The outermost layer of the skin.

_____ 19. The inner layer of skin containing hair follicle roots, glands, blood vessels, and nerves.

_____ 20. A protein that gives the skin its elasticity.

A. Acute radiation syndrome

B. Circumferential burn

C. Coagulation necrosis

D. Collagen

E. Consensus formula

F. Contact burn

G. Dermis

H. Elastin

I. Epidermis

J. Escharotomy

K. Flame burn

L. Flash burn

M. Full-thickness burn

N. Homeostasis

O. Hypovolemic shock

P. Integument

Q. Joule's law

R. Liquefaction necrosis

S. Lund-Browder chart

T. Mucopolysaccharide gel

Part III

Match each of the terms in the right column to the appropriate definition in the left column.

_____ **1.** An injury caused by radiation or direct contact with a heat source on the skin.

_____ **2.** Located above the glottis opening, as in the upper airway structures.

_____ **3.** A burn involving only the epidermis, which produces very red, painful skin; previously called a first-degree burn.

_____ **4.** Located below the glottis opening, as in the lower airway structures.

_____ **5.** A burn that has been caused by direct exposure to hot steam exhaust, as from a broken pipe.

_____ **6.** The peripheral area surrounding the zone of coagulation that has decreased blood flow and inflammation; it can undergo necrosis within 24 to 48 hours after the injury, particularly if perfusion is compromised due to burn shock.

_____ **7.** In a thermal burn, the area that is least affected by the burn injury; an area of increased blood flow where the body is attempting to repair injured but otherwise viable tissue.

_____ **8.** The reddened area surrounding the leathery and sometimes charred tissue that has sustained a full-thickness burn.

_____ **9.** The formula that describes the relationship between voltage and resistance: Current (I) = Voltage (V) divided by Resistance (R).

_____ **10.** A burn that involves the epidermis and part of the dermis, characterized by pain and blistering; previously called a second-degree burn.

_____ **11.** A system that assigns percentages to sections of the body, allowing for calculation of the amount of total body surface area burned.

_____ **12.** A system that estimates the total body surface area burned by comparing the affected area with the size of the patient's palm, which is roughly equal to 1% of the patient's total body surface area.

_____ **13.** A burn produced by hot liquids.

A. Ohm's law

B. Partial-thickness burn

C. Rule of nines

D. Rule of palms

E. Scald burn

F. Steam burn

G. Subglottic

H. Superficial burn

I. Supraglottic

J. Thermal burn

K. Zone of coagulation

L. Zone of hyperemia

M. Zone of stasis

Multiple Choice

Read each item carefully, and then select the best response.

_____ **1.** What is the second "rule" when in a lightning storm?
  A. Take shelter in a structure.
  B. Avoid touching a conductor.
  C. Don't be the smallest conductor.
  D. Don't stand near the tallest conductor.

_____ **2.** When dealing with acute radiation syndrome, which of the following is NOT likely to happen to the patient?
  A. Central nervous system changes
  B. Urinary changes
  C. Gastrointestinal changes
  D. Hematologic changes

_____ **3.** There are three methods of calculating an area of burned skin. Which method is the fastest and most universally used?
  A. Rule of nines
  B. The Lund-Browder chart
  C. Rule of palms
  D. A Broselow tape

_____ 4. You have arrived on scene to find a 12-year-old girl who has been burned by chicken noodle soup from the stove. She has blisters and redness on her chest. How would you classify this burn?

  A. Full-thickness burn

  B. First-degree burn

  C. Partial-thickness burn

  D. Superficial burn

_____ 5. An adult man's entire back is worth what percentage when using the rule of nines?

  A. 9%

  B. 18%

  C. 27%

  D. 36%

_____ 6. What is the *immediate management* when dealing with a 45-year-old woman who fell asleep with a cigarette in her hand?

  A. Managing the airway

  B. Starting fluid resuscitation

  C. Extinguishing the fire

  D. Keeping the patient warm

_____ 7. The Consensus (Parkland) formula determines how much fluid a burn patient should receive:

  A. during the first hour.

  B. during transport to the hospital.

  C. during the first 12 hours.

  D. during the first 24 hours.

_____ 8. What is the BEST way to give pain medication to the burn patient?

  A. IV route

  B. Subcutaneous injection

  C. By mouth

  D. Intramuscular injection

_____ 9. What should you do first when treating a patient with a chemical burn?

  A. Remove all the patient's clothing.

  B. Begin flushing with copious amounts of water.

  C. Brush the chemicals off the skin.

  D. Wait for a hazardous materials team to arrive.

_____ 10. You arrive on the scene to find a child engaged in an electrical outlet. The child is "held" by the electricity. What should you do?

  A. Use a wooden pole to push the child away from the source.

  B. Throw a rope to the child and pull him away from the source.

  C. Wait until someone shuts off the power to the source.

  D. Cut the wires inside the electrical box.

Labeling

1. Label the layers of the skin in the following diagram.

Hair
Pore
Germinal layer of epidermis
Sebaceous gland
Nerve (sensory)
Sweat gland
Hair follicle
Blood vessel
Subcutaneous fat
Fascia
Muscle

A. _____

B. _____

C. _____

2. Classify the following images as superficial, partial-thickness, or full-thickness burns.

A. _____

B. _____

C. _____

Fill in the Blank

Read each item carefully, and then complete the statement by filling in the missing word(s).

1. The _____, or outermost layer, is the body's first line of defense, constituting the major barrier against water, dust, microorganisms, and mechanical stress.
2. Sweat glands are found in the _____.
3. A(n) _____ burn is most commonly seen in children and physically or developmentally challenged adults.
4. Chemical burns can occur when the skin comes in contact with _____, _____, or _____, or other corrosive materials.
5. _____ _____ cause exothermic reaction in addition to tissue destruction. They can also cause systemic poisoning.
6. You should always make sure the _____ _____ _____ before beginning any management of a patient struck by lightning.
7. There are three types of ionizing radiation: _____, _____, and _____.
8. The central area of a burn that has suffered the most damage is known as the _____ _____ _____.
9. When treating a full-thickness burn, you should apply a(n) _____ _____ to the area that has been burned.
10. A patient with a radiation burn must be _____ before being transported to the emergency department (ED).

Identify

Read the following case study, and then list the chief complaint, vital signs, and pertinent negatives.

Around noon, you are called to the local burger joint for a 56-year-old woman who has been burned by oil from a hot fryer. Upon arrival, you find her with holes in her jeans on the top of both thighs. She is crying and immediately rates her pain as unbearable. You cut the jeans away to find that there is an area covering most of the front of both thighs that is blistering and very red. The patient is breathing at 22 breaths/min, her oxygen saturation is 97%, and lung sounds are clear bilaterally. You apply supplemental oxygen via a nonrebreathing mask at 15 L/min. You have your partner take the rest of the vital signs as you apply a Water-Jel dressing to the burned areas. The patient's blood pressure is 150/100 mm Hg, her pulse is 114 beats/min, and her rhythm on the monitor is sinus tachycardia. You do catch a premature ventricular contraction on the monitor but do not see another after watching for a full minute. The patient's skin is cool to the touch, and you believe she might be going into shock. You cover her with a blanket and start an IV line of normal saline. The patient is able to answer all your questions, and she has no medical history or allergies. You find no other areas of burns as you do a secondary trauma assessment. The patient states she slipped on the floor when carrying the hot oil to the disposal. She splashed the oil on the front of her legs. She does rate her pain 10/10, so you give her 5 mg of morphine for the pain en route to the hospital. When you arrive at the hospital, which is only 10 minutes from the burger joint, her pain has dropped to a 3/10.

1. Chief complaint:

_____

_____

2. Vital signs:

_____

_____

3. Pertinent negatives:

_____

_____

Complete the Patient Care Report

Reread the case study in the preceding Identify exercise and then complete the following patient care report (PCR) for the patient.

EMS Patient Care Report (PCR)					
Date:	Incident No.:	Nature of Call:		Location:	
Dispatched:	En Route:	At Scene:	Transport:	At Hospital:	In Service:
Patient Information					
Age: Sex: Weight (in kg [lb]):			Allergies: Medications: Past Medical History: Chief Complaint:		
Vital Signs					
Time:	BP:	Pulse:		Respirations:	SpO$_2$:
Time:	BP:	Pulse:		Respirations:	SpO$_2$:
Time:	BP:	Pulse:		Respirations:	SpO$_2$:
EMS Treatment (circle all that apply)					
Oxygen @ _____ L/min via (circle one): NC NRM Bag-mask device		Assisted Ventilation	Airway Adjunct		CPR
Defibrillation	Bleeding Control	Bandaging	Splinting		Other:
Narrative					

Ambulance Calls

The following case scenarios provide an opportunity to explore the concerns associated with patient management and paramedic care. Read each scenario, and then answer each question.

1. You are called to the scene of a smoky apartment-house fire to treat a man who jumped from his bedroom window approximately 15 feet above the ground. What you observe at first glance is the following: The patient is now lying unresponsive on the ground. His trousers are smoldering. His beard is partly burned off, and his lips are swollen. His left leg is splayed out at a peculiar angle. List, in the correct sequence, the steps you would take in managing this patient.

   a. _____

   b. _____

   c. _____

   d. _____

   e. _____

   f. _____

   g. _____

   h. _____

2. While you are securing the IV line on the patient described in question 1, firefighters lead the patient's wife over to you (they just rescued her from another room). A quick check does not reveal any injuries, but you give her supplemental oxygen by nasal cannula anyway because of her exposure to smoke. Meanwhile, you take advantage of the opportunity to get some information about her husband. List five questions you would ask this woman regarding her husband and what happened to him.

   a. _____

   b. _____

   c. _____

   d. _____

   e. _____

3. Meanwhile, the firefighters bring you yet another victim of the fire, a college student who climbed down a fire escape in the back of the building. He has burns to the right side of his body and complains of severe pain in the right arm. On examination you find the following:
   - The *right arm* is mottled red and exquisitely sensitive to the lightest touch (even the breeze blowing past it causes pain).
   - The *right flank* is fiery red and very painful.
   - The *right lower leg* has a leathery appearance. In places, you can see thrombosed veins beneath the surface. When you touch the skin with a sterile needle, the patient does not feel the pinprick.
   a. The burn on the right arm is probably a(n) _____ burn.
   The appropriate treatment for that burn is:

   _____

   _____

   b. The burn on the flank is probably a(n) _____ burn.
   The appropriate treatment for that burn is:

   _____

   _____

c. The burn on the right leg is probably a(n) _____ burn.
The appropriate treatment for that burn is:

_____

_____

4. You are called to a construction site 20 miles out of town for a "man electrocuted." According to the person who telephoned your dispatcher, one of the construction workers apparently bulldozed through a buried electric cable. He dismounted his bulldozer and picked up the cable to toss it aside, not realizing that it was live, and his hand "froze" to the cable.

a. En route to the call, you review in your mind the types of injuries that may occur in connection with electrocution. You remember that there may be four different types of burns:

(1)_____

(2)_____

(3)_____

(4)_____

b. You also recall that high-voltage electricity may cause a variety of nonburn injuries. List six possible injuries or abnormal conditions that you need to be alert for in this patient.

(1)_____

(2)_____

(3)_____

(4)_____

(5)_____

(6)_____

c. When you reach the construction site, you see a knot of agitated people at one end of the site. One of them is holding a long two-by-four, with which he apparently jarred the victim loose from the cable. The victim is lying very still and appears to be unresponsive. The free end of the cable is now arcing along the ground like an angry snake. List the steps you will take in dealing with this situation in the sequence in which you will perform them.

(1)_____

(2)_____

(3)_____

(4)_____

(5)_____

(6)_____

(7)_____

(8)_____

(9)_____

(10)_____

5. You are summoned to a house fire where the firefighters have just rescued a young man from a particularly smoky part of the building. He is unresponsive, and you notice that his clothes are smoldering.

  a. Whenever a person has been unresponsive in a smoky environment, you have to worry about the possibility of respiratory injury. List seven signs that should lead you to suspect the presence of respiratory injury in a burned patient.

  (1)_____

  (2)_____

  (3)_____

  (4)_____

  (5)_____

  (6)_____

  (7)_____

  b. What is the *first* step you should take in dealing with this patient?

  _____

  _____

  c. In due course, you remove the patient's clothing and examine him from head to toe to evaluate the depth and extent of the burn. You find the following:
  • Full-thickness burns of the posterior surfaces of both legs, extending well into the buttocks and groin
  • Partial-thickness burns of the entire left arm and a hand-sized patch of the left flank
  (1) What percentage of the patient's body has been burned? _____%
  (2) Does the patient have a critical burn? _____ If yes, according to which criteria?

  (a) _____

  (b) _____

  (c) _____

  d. Use the Consensus formula to calculate the rate at which you should run the patient's IV infusion. Assume that he weighs 70 kg and that your infusion set delivers 10 gtt/mL. (Show your calculations.)

  The IV infusion should be run at _____ gtt/min.

  e. After a few minutes of oxygen therapy, the patient regains consciousness and begins complaining of excruciating pain, especially in his groin and left arm. Medical control instructs you to administer morphine.

  1. What is the correct dosage of morphine for this patient?

  _____

  2. By which route should it be given?

  _____

3. List three possible adverse side effects that you should be ready to deal with.

(a) _____

(b) _____

(c) _____

6. In examining a patient, you find that he has mixed partial- and full-thickness burns of his entire left leg and posterior right leg, extending into his groin. There are also partial-thickness burns over most of the left forearm.
 a. What percentage of his body is burned? (Show your calculations.) _____%

 b. Does he have a critical burn? _____ Explain the reason for your answer.

 (1)_____

 (2)_____

 c. In doing the rapid trauma assessment, you are unable to detect either a dorsalis pedis pulse or an anterior tibial pulse in the left foot. What do you think is the most likely reason?

 _____

 _____

 d. What are you going to do about it?

 _____

 _____

True/False

If you believe the statement to be more true than false, write the letter "T" in the space provided. If you believe the statement to be more false than true, write the letter "F."

_____ **1.** If you know the identity of the chemical that caused a burn, it is preferable to start treatment with a chemical antidote (eg, applying a weak acid to an alkali burn, and vice versa).

_____ **2.** When a person has been burned by a chemical agent, the skin should be flushed with copious amounts of water.

_____ **3.** It is important to use only sterile water to flush a chemical burn, lest you contaminate the burn wound.

_____ **4.** In burns caused by hot tar, it is crucial to remove the tar from contact with the skin as quickly as possible to prevent systemic tar poisoning.

_____ **5.** If chemicals have splashed into a patient's eyes, the eyes should be continuously irrigated with a steady stream of water.

_____ **6.** Burn shock occurs because of the fluid loss across the damaged skin and the volume shifts within the rest of the body.

_____ **7.** Although fire deaths continue to decrease, children younger than 5 years continue to be at a high risk of dying in a fire.

_____ **8.** Carbon monoxide binds to the hemoglobin 500 times faster than oxygen does.

_____ **9.** Currents as small as 0.1 A may cause ventricular fibrillation if the current passes through the heart.

_____ **10.** You should peel away clothing that has "melted" into the flesh of a burn patient.

Short Answer

Complete this section with short written answers using the space provided.

1. Discuss the four rules that can help you avoid being struck by lightning.

a. _____

_____

b. _____

_____

c. _____

_____

d. _____

_____

2. You would suspect that a patient with flame burns has a respiratory injury if any of the following signs are present:

a. _____

b. _____

c. _____

d. _____

e. _____

f. _____

g. _____

3. Injury from a high-voltage electric source or from lightning may produce any of the following conditions:

a. _____

b. _____

c. _____

d. _____

e. _____

f. _____

Fill in the Table

Fill in the missing columns of the table.

Approximate the amount of fluid the burned patient will need by using the Consensus formula. During the first 24 hours, the burned patient will need:

$$2\text{–}4 \text{ mL} \times \text{body weight (in kg)} \times \text{percentage of body surface burned}$$

				Consensus Formula Chart							
% Burn	10 kg	20 kg	30 kg	40 kg	50 kg	60 kg	70 kg	80 kg	90 kg	100 kg
10	25			100	125	150	175		225	250
20	50			200	250	300	350		450	500
30	75			300	375	450	525		675	750
40	100			400	500	600	700		900	1,000
50	125			500	625	750	875		1,125	1,250
60	150			600	750	900	1,050		1,350	1,500
70	175			700	875	1,050	1,225		1,575	1,750
80	200			800	1,000	1,200	1,400		1,800	2,000
90	225			900	1,125	1,350	1,575		2,025	2,250
20 mL/kg	200			800	1,000	1,200	1,400		1,800	2,000

This table represents the fluid recommended in the *first hour* (one-eighth of the initial 8-hour dose) by the Consensus formula. The final row represents the amount of a 20-mL/kg bolus.

Note: Values in this table are based on the high end of the 2- to 4-mL range in the formula.

Problem Solving

Practice your calculation skills by solving the following math problems.

1. On examining the patient, you find burns covering the following areas:
   - The whole right leg (front and back)
   - The anterior left leg
   - The anterior trunk
   - The whole right arm

   a. Use the rule of nines to calculate what percentage of the patient's body surface area is burned: _____ %. (Show your calculations.)

   b. If the patient weighs 154 lb, at what rate should you run his IV infusion? Use the Consensus formula to calculate the rate (do not forget to convert the patient's weight to kilograms first!). (Show your calculations.)
   IV infusion rate = _____ mL/h

   c. If you have a standard infusion set that delivers 10 gtt/mL, at how many drops per minute do you have to run the IV infusion to deliver the volume you calculated?
   IV infusion rate = _____ gtt/min

   d. Which IV fluid will you use?

Face and Neck Trauma

Matching

Part I

Match each of the terms in the right column to the appropriate definition in the left column.

_____ **1.** An inflammation of the conjunctivae that usually is caused by bacteria, viruses, allergies, or foreign bodies; should be considered highly contagious if infectious in origin; also called pinkeye.

A. Adnexa

_____ **2.** A thin, transparent membrane that covers the sclera and internal surfaces of the eyelids.

B. Alveoli

_____ **3.** A fracture to the floor of the orbit, usually caused by a blow to the eye.

C. Le Fort fractures

_____ **4.** Nosebleed.

D. Anterior chamber

_____ **5.** Difficulty swallowing.

E. Blowout fracture

_____ **6.** Paralysis of gaze or lack of coordination between the movements of the two eyes.

F. Conjunctiva

_____ **7.** One of the three anatomic parts of the ear; the external portion of the tympanic membrane.

G. Conjunctivitis

_____ **8.** Small pits or cavities, such as the sockets for the teeth.

H. Cornea

_____ **9.** The surrounding structures and accessories of an organ; for the eye, these parts include the eyelids, lashes, and lacrimal structures.

I. Craniofacial disjunction

_____ **10.** The anterior area of the globe between the lens and the cornea, which is filled with aqueous humor.

J. Crown

_____ **11.** Maxillary fractures that are classified into three categories based on their anatomic location.

K. Cusps

_____ **12.** The colored portion of the eye.

L. Dentin

_____ **13.** One of the three anatomic parts of the ear; it consists of the cochlea and semicircular canals.

M. Diplopia

_____ **14.** The eyeball.

N. Dysconjugate gaze

_____ **15.** The bony anterior part of the palate that forms the roof of the mouth.

O. Dysphagia

_____ **16.** Coughing up blood.

P. Epistaxis

_____ **17.** Double vision.

Q. External ear

_____ **18.** The principal mass of the tooth.

R. Globe

_____ **19.** Points at the top of a tooth.

S. Hard palate

_____ **20.** A Le Fort III fracture that involves a fracture of all of the midface bones, which separates the entire midface from the cranium.

T. Hemoptysis

_____	**21.** The transparent anterior portion of the eye that overlies the iris and pupil.	**U.** Hyoid bone
_____	**22.** Bleeding into the anterior chamber of the eye, resulting from direct ocular trauma.	**V.** Hyphema
_____	**23.** A bone at the base of the tongue that supports the tongue and its muscles.	**W.** Inner ear
_____	**24.** The part of the tooth that is external to the gum.	**X.** Iris

Part II

Match each of the terms in the right column to the appropriate definition in the left column.

_____	**1.** Traumatic separation of the trachea from the layers.	**A.** Malocclusion
_____	**2.** A thin membrane that separates the middle ear from the outer ear and sets up vibrations in the ossicles; also called the eardrum.	**B.** Mandible
_____	**3.** A jellylike substance found in the posterior compartment of the eye between the lens and the retina.	**C.** Mediastinitis
_____	**4.** An injury to the neck in which hyperextension occurs as a result of the head moving abruptly forward or backward; it can be difficult to differentiate from injuries that involve cervical bony structures and the spine.	**D.** Middle ear
_____	**5.** The joint between the temporal bone and the posterior condyle that allows for movements of the mandible.	**E.** Oculomotor nerve
_____	**6.** The movement of both eyes in unison.	**F.** Optic nerve
_____	**7.** Stretching or tearing of a muscle or tendon.	**G.** Orbits
_____	**8.** Stretching or tearing of ligaments.	**H.** Pinna
_____	**9.** The act of declaring that a spinal injury is not present.	**I.** Pulp
_____	**10.** The white part of the eye.	**J.** Pupil
_____	**11.** Misalignment of the teeth.	**K.** Retina
_____	**12.** The movable lower jaw bone.	**L.** Retinal detachment
_____	**13.** Inflammation of the mediastinum, often a result of the gastric contents leaking into the thoracic cavity after esophageal perforation.	**M.** Sclera
_____	**14.** A delicate, 10-layered structure of nervous tissue located in the rear of the interior of the globe; it receives light and generates nerve signals that are transmitted to the brain through the optic nerve.	**N.** Spinal clearance
_____	**15.** The circular opening in the center of the eye through which light passes to the lens.	**O.** Sprain
_____	**16.** Specialized connective tissue within the cavity of a tooth.	**P.** Strain
_____	**17.** The third cranial nerve; it innervates the muscles that cause motion of the eyeballs and upper eyelid.	**Q.** Sympathetic eye movement
_____	**18.** One of the three anatomic parts of the ear; it consists of the inner portion of the tympanic membrane and the ossicles.	**R.** Temporomandibular joint (TMJ)
_____	**19.** The large outside portion of the ear through which sound waves enter the ear; also called the auricle.	**S.** Tracheal transection
_____	**20.** Bony cavities in the frontal part of the skull that enclose and protect the eyes.	**T.** Tympanic membrane
_____	**21.** Either of the secondary cranial nerves that enter the eyeball posteriorly, through the optic foramen.	**U.** Vitreous humor
_____	**22.** Separation of the inner layers of the retina from the underlying choroid, the vascular membrane that nourishes the retina.	**V.** Whiplash

Multiple Choice

Read each item carefully, and then select the best response.

_____   1. In addition to causing massive bleeding and shock, injury to the major arteries in the neck can cause:

      A. air embolism.

      B. cerebral infarct.

      C. cerebral hypoxia.

      D. All of the above

_____   2. There are _____ facial bones that form the structure of the face.

      A. 6

      B. 14

      C. 9

      D. 21

_____   3. How many adult teeth does the average adult have?

      A. 32

      B. 34

      C. 30

      D. 36

_____   4. The large cartilaginous external portion of the ear is called the:

      A. organ of Corti.

      B. pinna.

      C. tympanic membrane.

      D. cochlea.

_____   5. What is the name of the substance that forms the principal mass of the tooth?

      A. Alveolar ridge

      B. Cusp

      C. Pulp

      D. Dentin

_____   6. What is the function of the oculomotor nerve?

      A. Causes motor function of the tongue

      B. Causes motion of eyeballs and upper eyelids

      C. Slows down the heart rate

      D. Causes the motor function of mastication

_____   7. You are treating a patient who appears to have a fracture that has affected the upper jaw and the hard palate. What is the name for this fracture?

      A. Le Fort I

      B. Le Fort II

      C. Nasal fracture

      D. Mandibular fracture

_____   8. Which of the following materials is NOT advisable for use when covering an injured eye?

      A. Aluminum eye shield

      B. Gauze

      C. Sterile dressing

      D. Cup

_____ **9.** A patient who has a maxillofacial fracture may have all of the following signs and symptoms, EXCEPT:

    A. dental malocclusion.

    B. swelling.

    C. Battle sign.

    D. blood or fluid running from the nose.

_____ **10.** What is the name of the fracture resulting from blunt trauma to the face that causes the face to appear flattened?

    A. Hyoid bone fracture

    B. Zygomatic bone fracture

    C. Le Fort I fracture

    D. Orbital bone injury

_____ **11.** You are treating a patient who sustained a blunt injury to his right eye from a fight. The patient reports that he is seeing flashing lights and specks. He MOST likely has the condition called:

    A. diplopia.

    B. hyphema.

    C. retinal detachment.

    D. conjunctivitis.

_____ **12.** The physical examination of the eyes involves evaluating the patient for all of the following, EXCEPT:

    A. ecchymosis of the eyelids.

    B. sympathetic eye movements.

    C. redness of the globes.

    D. foreign bodies in the cornea.

_____ **13.** When assessing a patient's eyes, you find visual field defects, which are also referred to as:

    A. dysconjugate gaze.

    B. hemianopsia.

    C. conjunctivitis.

    D. globe disruption.

_____ **14.** Which of the following is NOT a type of contact lens?

    A. Rigid gas-permeable

    B. Soft hydrophilic

    C. Hard

    D. Chemical

_____ **15.** You are treating a patient who has an injury to the anterior neck. She reports difficulty swallowing, hematemesis, and hemoptysis. What is her MOST likely injury?

    A. Esophageal perforation

    B. Neurologic impairment

    C. Vascular injury

    D. Laryngeal fracture

Labeling

Label the following diagrams with the correct terms.

1. Structures of the eye

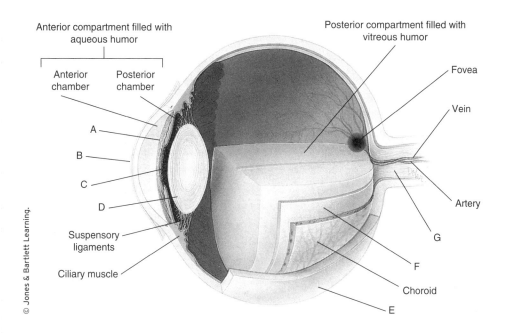

Anterior compartment filled with aqueous humor

Posterior compartment filled with vitreous humor

Anterior chamber

Posterior chamber

Fovea

Vein

A

B

C

D

Artery

Suspensory ligaments

Ciliary muscle

G

F

Choroid

E

A. _____

B. _____

C. _____

D. _____

E. _____

F. _____

G. _____

© Jones & Bartlett Learning.

2. Structures of the anterior neck

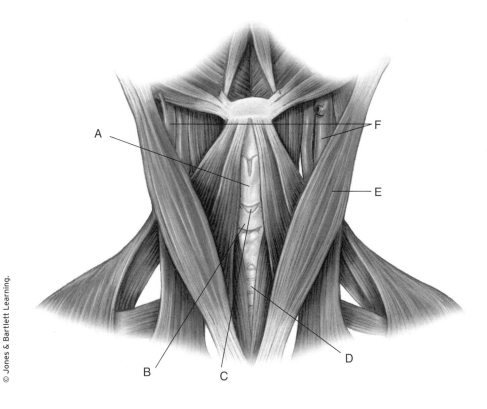

A

F

E

B

C

D

A. _____

B. _____

C. _____

D. _____

E. _____

F. _____

© Jones & Bartlett Learning.

3. Arteries of the neck

A. _____

B. _____

C. _____

D. _____

E. _____

F. _____

G. _____

H. _____

I. _____

© Jones & Bartlett Learning.

Fill in the Blank
Read each item carefully, and then complete the statement by filling in the missing word(s).

1. The most common cervical strain is often called a(n) _____ injury.

2. A(n) _____ is a stretching or tearing of muscle or tendon.

3. The bones around the eye are thin, and with significant trauma to the face, the eye can be dislodged. This is called a(n) _____ fracture.

4. When assessing the ears, look for _____ from the ears and note if it is clear or _____.

5. Note the presence of enlarged _____ nodes on the neck on your assessment.

6. A(n) _____ fracture of the maxilla that involves the _____ _____ and the inferior maxilla, separating them from the rest of the skull, is called a Le Fort I fracture.

7. Massive _____ discharge of blood and possibly _____ may occur with an orbital fracture, and vision is often impaired.

8. The _____ _____ consists of the cochlea and semicircular canals.

9. When dealing with an impaled object in the face, the only time you should remove the object is when the patient has

   _____ complications.

10. Bleeding into the anterior chamber of the eye is called _____.

11. _____, _____, and _____ rays can burn the delicate tissues of the eyes.

12. If a patient has a burn to the eyes caused by a strong alkali or acid, you should irrigate the eye for _____ minutes.

13. The only indication for removing a contact lens in the field is a(n) _____ _____.

14. Reimplantation of a tooth may be successful for up to _____ hour(s) after it has been avulsed from the mouth.

15. Any open neck wounds should be covered with a(n) _____ dressing.

16. Chemicals, heat, and _____ rays can all burn the delicate tissues of the eye and _____ (the surrounding structures and

   accessories), often causing permanent damage.

17. When a patient has a facial injury, because _____ irritates the gastric lining, the risks of vomiting and aspiration

   are significant.

18. When a patient has a protruding eye, you should cover it with a moist, sterile dressing and stabilize it along with the

   uninjured eye to prevent further injury due to _____ _____ _____, the movement of both eyes in

   unison.

19. The paramedic should never exert _____ on or manipulate a patient's injured globe in any way.

20. A patient who has sustained a fracture of all midface bones, separating the entire midface from the cranium, has

   sustained a Le Fort III fracture, also called a(n) _____ _____.

Identify

Read the following case study, and then list the chief complaint, vital signs, and pertinent negatives; then answer the additional questions.

Tom and Dan arrive at the scene of a collision as additional help. It is 0030 hours, and a carload of teenagers has rolled into a cornfield. The corn is about shoulder high, and nobody can say for sure how many kids were in the car. Tom begins a search around the crash site as Dan helps with a patient. Tom hears something to his left and finds a 17-year-old girl on the ground.

The girl is lying face down, and when Tom carefully rolls her over, maintaining in-line manual stabilization with the assistance of two firefighters, he notices that she has severe facial injuries. The primary survey shows no life-threatening bleeding once her airway has been opened by positioning and the blood has been suctioned from her throat. The girl is a U on the AVPU scale, and Tom suspects that she may have gone through the windshield. Her respirations are 34 breaths/min and very deep, and oxygen saturation is 95%. Pupils are sluggish, blood pressure (BP) is 160/90 mm Hg, and pulse is 72 beats/min. The girl's skin is cool, but she has been lying on the ground for at least half an hour.

Help arrives, and they apply a cervical collar, secure the patient to a backboard, and get her in the unit.

The closest trauma center is half an hour away by helicopter, so Dan and Tom call for the life flight crew to meet them on the scene. Because the patient is unresponsive, Dan and Tom decide to insert an advanced airway and administer 100% supplemental oxygen to her. They place two large-bore IV lines and administer normal saline. They are careful not to overload this patient with fluid because of the potential for a head injury. The electrocardiogram (ECG) monitor now shows a sinus bradycardia, respiration is 56 breaths/min, and BP is now 168/88 mm Hg. Life flight then takes over and flies the patient to the regional trauma center.

Dan and Tom later find out that the patient survives. She had a Le Fort III fracture and has some neurologic defects from the closed head injury, from which it will take several months to years to recover.

1. Chief complaint:

_____

_____

2. Vital signs:

_____

_____

3. Pertinent negatives:

_____

_____

4. Why is it important to get this patient to the regional trauma center?

_____

_____

5. Why is it so important to keep this patient's airway clear of blood?

_____

_____

6. What are the patient's serial vital signs telling the paramedics?

_____

_____

Ambulance Calls

The following case scenarios provide an opportunity to explore the concerns associated with patient management and paramedic care. Read each scenario, and then answer each question.

1. While enjoying a weekend off at a ski resort, you happen to see a young woman trip over the steps at the lodge and fall. As you rush to her assistance, you see blood coming from her mouth, and closer inspection reveals that she has knocked out one of her lower teeth entirely. Which steps should you take?

a. _____

b. _____

c. _____

d. _____

e. _____

2. You volunteer to accompany the young lady to the nearest hospital, some 2 hours away by road. Just as you are pulling away from the ski resort in a friend's car, the resort manager comes running after you, waving for you to stop. "I have someone else here who needs to go to the hospital," he says. Behind him, two ski instructors are leading a young man along. The patient had been involved in a fistfight and now has two black eyes. A thorough examination of an injured eye includes assessment of which visible ocular structures and ocular functions?

a. _____

b. _____

c. _____

d. _____

e. _____

f. _____

g. _____

h. _____

3. A 12-year-old boy lost control of his bicycle as he was riding down a long, steep hill into town. At the base of the hill, his front wheel struck the curb, and he was catapulted from the bicycle straight through the show window of the local wedding dress shop. When you arrive, you find him bleeding from multiple lacerations. The most profuse bleeding seems to be coming from a large laceration on the left side of his neck.

a. What are the principal dangers associated with the laceration of the neck?

_____

b. What should be done to the wound immediately?

_____

True/False

If you believe the statement to be more true than false, write the letter "T" in the space provided. If you believe the statement to be more false than true, write the letter "F."

_____   1. There are 22 facial bones that form the structure of the face without contributing to the cranial vault.

_____   2. Floaters are specks the patient describes in his or her field of vision.

_____   3. UV rays do not cause superficial burns to the eyes.

_____   4. Double vision usually points to trauma involving the extraocular muscles, such as an orbit fracture.

_____   5. Although painless to the patient, a ruptured tympanic membrane will not heal.

_____   6. Nasal fractures are often complicated by the presence of epistaxis.

_____   7. A Le Fort I fracture has a pyramidal shape and involves the nasal bone and inferior maxilla.

_____   8. The patient who has sustained an orbital fracture may report symptoms of diplopia.

_____   9. The avulsed tooth can be reimplanted successfully even if it has been out of the mouth for over a day.

_____   10. Bruising and swelling are the first clues to a maxillofacial fracture.

_____   11. To maintain an airway, it is acceptable to use blind nasotracheal intubation when there are signs of facial fractures.

_____   12. Blunt eye trauma can lead to retinal detachment, which is common in sports injuries.

_____   13. It is not necessary to cover both of the patient's eyes to prevent sympathetic eye movement.

_____   14. The area above the angle of the mandible is referred to as zone III.

_____ **15.** It may be difficult to determine the extent of bleeding in the mouth as a result of the patient swallowing the blood.

_____ **16.** You should always apply an occlusive dressing to an open neck wound to prevent an air embolism.

_____ **17.** Coughing up blood is known as dysphagia.

_____ **18.** Hoarseness or voice changes may indicate laryngeal fracture.

_____ **19.** A perforated tympanic membrane can occur from direct blows to the ear or pressure injuries.

_____ **20.** If part of the patient's external ear has been avulsed in a fight, you should save the piece in a container of ice.

Short Answer

Complete this section with short written answers using the space provided.

1. Injuries to the face may be quite frightening to look at, but they do not by themselves ordinarily pose an immediate threat to life. However, facial injuries may be associated with other conditions or injuries that can threaten life or limb. List two potentially serious or life-threatening conditions that may be associated with maxillofacial trauma.

   a. _____

   b. _____

2. In examining a trauma patient, which findings would lead you to suspect maxillofacial fracture? List five signs of maxillofacial fracture.

   a. _____

   b. _____

   c. _____

   d. _____

   e. _____

Fill in the Table

Fill in the missing parts of the table.

1. Summary of maxillofacial fractures

Injury	Signs and Symptoms
Multiple facial bone fractures	• Massive facial swelling • _____ • _____ • Anterior or _____ epistaxis
Zygomatic and orbital fractures	• Loss of sensation below the _____ • Flattening of the _____ • _____ of upward gaze
Nasal fractures	• Crepitus and instability • Swelling, tenderness, _____ • Anterior or _____ epistaxis
Maxillary (Le Fort) fractures	• Mobility of the _____ • Dental _____ • Facial swelling
Mandibular fractures	• Dental malocclusion • _____ instability

2. Signs and symptoms of injuries to the anterior part of the neck

Injury	Signs and Symptoms
Laryngeal fracture, tracheal transection	• Labored breathing or reduced _____ • Stridor • Hoarseness, voice changes • _____ (coughing up blood) • Subcutaneous emphysema • Swelling, edema • Structural irregularity
Vascular injury	• _____ bleeding • Signs of shock • Hematoma, swelling, edema • _____ deficits
Esophageal perforation	• _____ (difficulty swallowing) • _____ • _____ (suggests aspiration of blood)
Neurologic impairment	• Signs of a stroke (suggests air embolism or _____) • _____ or paresthesia • _____ nerve deficit • Signs of _____ shock

Head and Spine Trauma

Ow, my bottom really hurts!

That crew needs to hear the chief's 'Patient Discomfort and Pressure Sore' lecture during quality assessment.

© Jones & Bartlett Learning.

Matching

Part I

Match each of the terms in the right column to the appropriate definition in the left column.

_____ 1. Fracture generally resulting from the extension of a linear fracture into the base of the skull; usually occurs after a diffuse impact to the head (as in a fall or motor vehicle crash) and can be difficult to diagnose, even with radiography.

_____ 2. Upward movement of the toe(s) in response to stimulation to the sole of the foot. Under normal circumstances, the toe(s) move downward.

_____ 3. A long, slender extension of a neuron (nerve cell) that conducts electrical impulses away from the neuronal soma.

_____ 4. An increase in mean arterial pressure to compensate for decreased cerebral perfusion pressure; compensatory physiologic response that occurs in an effort to shunt blood to the brain; manifests clinically as hypertension.

_____ 5. A late, life-threatening complication of spinal cord injury in which stimulation of the sympathetic nervous system below the level of injury generates a massive, uninhibited, uncompensated cardiovascular response; also known as autonomic hyperreflexia.

_____ 6. A gradually increasing rate and depth of respirations followed by a gradual decrease with intermittent periods of apnea; associated with brainstem insult.

_____ 7. The largest portion of the brain; responsible for higher functions, such as reasoning; divided into right and left hemispheres, or halves.

_____ 8. Fluid produced in the ventricles of the brain that flows in the subarachnoid space and bathes the meninges.

_____ 9. The pressure of blood flow through the brain; the difference between the mean arterial pressure and intracranial pressure.

_____ 10. Excessive fluid in the brain; swelling of the brain.

_____ 11. The middle membrane of the three meninges that enclose the brain and spinal cord.

_____ 12. Loss of memory of events that occurred after an injury.

_____ 13. A condition that occurs with flexion injuries or fractures, resulting in the displacement of bone fragments into the anterior portion of the spinal cord. Findings include paralysis below the level of the insult and loss of pain, temperature, and touch perception.

A. Anterior cord syndrome

B. Anterograde (posttraumatic) amnesia

C. Arachnoid

D. Autonomic dysreflexia

E. Autoregulation

F. Axon

G. Babinski reflex

H. Basilar skull fracture

I. Battle sign

J. Biot (ataxic) respirations

K. Brainstem

L. Brown-Séquard syndrome

M. Cauda equina

_____ **14.** The midbrain, pons, and medulla, collectively.

_____ **15.** Irregular pattern, rate, and depth of respirations with intermittent periods of apnea; results from increased intracranial pressure.

_____ **16.** Bruising over the mastoid bone behind the ear often seen after a basilar skull fracture; also called retroauricular ecchymosis.

_____ **17.** The largest portion of the cerebrum; regulates voluntary skeletal movement and a person's level of awareness; a part of consciousness.

_____ **18.** A focal brain injury in which brain tissue is bruised and damaged in a defined area.

_____ **19.** Injury that occurs when the brain is jarred around in the skull; a mild diffuse brain injury that does not result in structural damage or permanent neurologic impairment.

_____ **20.** The brain region essential in coordinating muscle movements in the body; also called the athlete's brain.

_____ **21.** A condition associated with penetrating trauma and characterized by hemisection of the spinal cord and complete damage to all spinal tracts on the involved side.

_____ **22.** The location where the spinal cord separates; composed of nerve roots.

_____ **23.** A neurologic condition caused by compression of the bundle of nerve roots located at the end of the spinal cord.

_____ **24.** A condition resulting from hyperextension injuries to the cervical area that damage the dorsal column of the spinal cord; characterized by hemorrhage or edema. Findings include greater loss of function in the upper extremities, with variable sensory loss of pain and temperature.

_____ **25.** Deep, rapid respirations; similar to Kussmaul respirations, but without an acetone breath odor; commonly seen after brainstem injury.

N. Cauda equina syndrome

O. Central cord syndrome

P. Central neurogenic hyperventilation

Q. Cerebellum

R. Cerebral concussion

S. Cerebral contusion

T. Cerebral cortex

U. Cerebral edema

V. Cerebral perfusion pressure (CPP)

W. cerebrospinal fluid (CSF)

X. Cerebrum

Y. Cheyne-Stokes respirations

Part II

Match each of the terms in the right column to the appropriate definition in the left column.

_____ **1.** A specific, grossly observable brain injury.

_____ **2.** A type of injury that results from forward movement of the head, typically as the result of rapid deceleration, such as in a car crash, or with a direct blow to the occiput.

_____ **3.** The joint on which each vertebra articulates with adjacent vertebrae.

_____ **4.** An accumulation of blood between the skull and dura.

_____ **5.** The outermost layer of the three meninges that enclose the brain and spinal cord; the toughest meningeal layer.

_____ **6.** Hypertension (with a widening pulse pressure), bradycardia, and irregular respirations; the classic findings associated with increased intracranial pressure.

_____ **7.** Minimum cerebral perfusion pressure required to adequately perfuse the brain; 60 mm Hg in the adult.

_____ **8.** The bones that encase and protect the brain; the parietal, temporal, frontal, occipital, sphenoid, and ethmoid bones; also called the cranium or skull.

_____ **9.** Dual impacting of the brain into the skull, first at the point of impact and then on the opposite side of impact, as the brain rebounds.

_____ **10.** Total disruption of all spinal cord tracts, with permanent loss of all cord-mediated functions below the level of injury.

_____ **11.** Bleeding within the brain tissue (parenchyma) itself; also called an intraparenchymal hematoma.

A. Complete spinal cord injury

B. Coup-contrecoup injury

C. Cranial vault

D. Critical minimum threshold

E. Cushing triad

F. Decerebrate (extensor) posturing

G. Decorticate (flexor) posturing

H. Depressed skull fracture

I. Dermatome

J. Diffuse axonal injury (DAI)

K. Diffuse brain injury

_____ **12.** Spinal cord injury in which there is some degree of cord-mediated function; initial dysfunction may be temporary, and there may be potential for recovery.

_____ **13.** A high body temperature.

_____ **14.** Extension of a limb or other body part beyond its usual range of motion.

_____ **15.** Hyperacute pain to touch.

_____ **16.** Any injury that affects the entire brain.

_____ **17.** Diffuse brain injury that is caused by stretching, shearing, or tearing of nerve fibers with consequent axonal damage.

_____ **18.** An area of the body innervated by sensor components of spinal nerves.

_____ **19.** Fracture caused by high-energy direct trauma applied to a small surface area of the skull with a blunt object (such as a baseball bat striking the head); commonly accompanied by bone fragments driven into the brain, causing further injury.

_____ **20.** Abnormal posture characterized by flexion of the arms and extension of the legs; indicates pressure on the brainstem.

_____ **21.** A process in which tissue is forced out of its normal position, such as when the brain is forced from the cranial vault, either through the foramen magnum or over the tentorium.

_____ **22.** A general term that includes both head injuries and traumatic brain injuries.

_____ **23.** A traumatic insult to the head that may result in injury to soft tissues of the scalp and bony structures of the head and skull, not including the face.

_____ **24.** The most classic distraction injury, which occurs when a person is hanged by the neck. Bending and fractures occur at the C1 to C2 region, which quickly tear the spinal cord.

_____ **25.** The portion of the brain that is important in voluntary motor actions and personality traits.

_____ **26.** Abnormal posture characterized by extension of the arms and legs; indicates pressure on the brainstem.

L. Dura mater

M. Epidural hematoma

N. Facet joint

O. Flexion injury

P. Focal brain injury

Q. Frontal lobe

R. Hangman's fracture

S. Head injury

T. Head trauma

U. Herniation

V. Hyperesthesia

W. Hyperextension

X. Hyperpyrexia

Y. Incomplete spinal cord injury

Z. Intracerebral hematoma

Part III

Match each of the items in the left column to the appropriate injury in the right column. (Note: Some of the injury types can be applied more than once.)

_____ **1.** A 15-year-old skateboarder has hit the side of his head after a fall. After an initial bout of unconsciousness, he regains consciousness, only to lapse again about an hour later. His mother cannot wake him up again.

_____ **2.** A football player comes off the field after a helmet-to-helmet hit. He is a little disoriented and cannot remember the play. The coach says he just "got his bell rung." The player shows no other signs later in the evening or the next day.

_____ **3.** The other football player also comes off the field. He is very confused. He loses consciousness in the locker room for about 3 minutes. He is confused for the next 2 days.

_____ **4.** A 40-year-old woman is scrubbing the floor. As she rises, she hits the back of her head on the sink. At the time, she gets a slight headache. Later in the evening, her speech becomes slightly slurred.

_____ **5.** A 12-year-old girl is hit on the head with a baseball bat by her brother. She is knocked out but wakes back up to tell her mother what happened. Her mother decides to have her checked out. On the way to the doctor's office, the girl appears to go to sleep. When they arrive, the mother cannot wake her.

A. Cerebral concussion

B. Cerebral contusion

C. Epidural hematoma

D. Subdural hematoma

E. Intracerebral hematoma

_____ 6. The patient was the driver of a vehicle that was struck from the left side by another car. The door on the driver's side is dented. The patient is conscious, but witnesses say that he was "out cold" for a few minutes immediately after the collision. He complains of a headache and the feeling of pins and needles in his left hip and left leg. His skull is tender to palpation in the area just superior to the left ear. While he is under your care, his level of consciousness deteriorates until he is unconscious altogether, and his respirations become very slow.

_____ 7. The patient was a participant in a barroom brawl. This patient was "knocked out cold" for a few minutes. Now he seems alert, but he cannot remember what happened. He complains of a little dizziness. His vital signs are normal.

_____ 8. The patient was a front-seat passenger in a car that careened into a utility pole. He is confused and sleepy when you find him. His speech is slurred, and there is weakness of the right leg. He becomes increasingly more lethargic while under your care and vomits twice. The left pupil seems to be getting larger than the right.

_____ 9. The patient was an unrestrained front-seat passenger in a car involved in a head-on collision with another car. He apparently struck his head on the windshield because the windshield in front of the patient is cracked. The patient is found unconscious. His left pupil is larger than the right. His pulse is 56 beats/min, and his blood pressure is 190/90 mm Hg. Respirations are irregular.

_____ 10. You are called to a 70-year-old woman with a terrible headache. She hit her head on the cupboard about 2 hours ago. She initially had a severe headache at the site of the injury, but now it has moved to a larger area of her head. She is responsive only to questions and begins to vomit while you are taking care of her. She rapidly becomes unresponsive and begins to have a seizure.

F. Subarachnoid hemorrhage

Multiple Choice

Read each item carefully, and then select the best response.

_____ 1. The majority of all skull fractures are:

    A. open skull fractures.

    B. basilar skull fractures.

    C. depressed skull fractures.

    D. linear skull fractures.

_____ 2. The oculomotor nerve is the _____ cranial nerve.

    A. first

    B. second

    C. third

    D. fourth

_____ 3. The brain consumes _____ of the body's total oxygen.

    A. 10%

    B. 20%

    C. 30%

    D. 40%

_____ 4. Normally, the brain occupies about 80% of the space within the cranium. The remaining space is taken up by:

    A. muscle and fat.

    B. blood and CSF.

    C. water and glucose.

    D. lymph fluid.

_____ **5.** What is the reticular activating system (RAS) responsible for?

    A. Blood pressure

    B. Respiration

    C. Heart rate

    D. Consciousness

_____ **6.** When a patient has a basilar skull fracture, which of the following signs or symptoms would you LEAST expect to see?

    A. Raccoon eyes

    B. Battle sign

    C. Blowout fracture of the eye

    D. Draining of blood and CSF from the ear

_____ **7.** What is the minimum cerebral perfusion pressure in an adult that is required to perfuse the brain adequately?

    A. 15 mm Hg

    B. 30 mm Hg

    C. 45 mm Hg

    D. 60 mm Hg

_____ **8.** You are treating a patient who has starred the windshield in a car crash. The patient reports that he cannot remember what happened before the collision. This is called:

    A. anterograde amnesia.

    B. retrograde amnesia.

    C. amnesia.

    D. focal brain injury.

_____ **9.** After you drop off a patient whom you treated for a fall down the stairs, the doctor tells you she had bleeding into the brain tissue. What is the medical term for this condition?

    A. Epidural hematoma

    B. Intracerebral hematoma

    C. Subarachnoid hemorrhage

    D. Subdural hematoma

_____ **10.** What is the MOST important sign or symptom in evaluating a patient with a brain injury?

    A. Bleeding from the ears

    B. Pupil size and how the pupils react to light

    C. Level of consciousness

    D. Mechanism of injury

_____ **11.** Which of the following is NOT considered a sign or symptom of second-impact syndrome?

    A. Loss of eye movements

    B. A stunned appearance

    C. Coma

    D. Constricted pupils

_____ **12.** What is the MOST important step in managing any type of head injury?

    A. Maintaining airway and breathing

    B. Performing spinal immobilization

    C. Assessing where the bleeding is in the brain

    D. Establishing an IV line

_____ **13.** Which portion of the spine contains the most bones of the vertebral column?

    A. Cervical

    B. Thoracic

    C. Lumbar

    D. Sacral

_____ **14.** How many pairs of spinal nerves are there?
- **A.** 12
- **B.** 33
- **C.** 31
- **D.** 5

_____ **15.** The _____ plexus innervates the diaphragm.
- **A.** cervical
- **B.** sacral
- **C.** lumbar
- **D.** brachial

_____ **16.** Which of the following is NOT associated with high-risk mechanisms of injury (MOIs) for spinal injuries?
- **A.** Penetrating trauma near the spine
- **B.** Fall from two times the patient's height
- **C.** Unrestrained in a rollover crash
- **D.** Diving injury

_____ **17.** What is the initial step of assessment in a suspected spinal injury?
- **A.** Ensuring scene safety
- **B.** Clearing the airway
- **C.** Checking for a pulse
- **D.** Activating the trauma system

_____ **18.** What is the primary goal when immobilizing a patient with a spinal injury?
- **A.** Determining whether the patient will be paralyzed
- **B.** Determining where the exact injury is
- **C.** Preventing further injuries to the patient
- **D.** Securing the airway of the patient

_____ **19.** Which of the following is NOT done prior to applying a cervical collar to a patient?
- **A.** Determine the need for the collar.
- **B.** Perform manual stabilization of the head.
- **C.** Assess the extremities for distal pulse, motor, and sensory (PMS) functions.
- **D.** Check the patient's ability to move the neck.

_____ **20.** In which of the following situations should you NOT perform a rapid extrication?
- **A.** The patient's legs are tingling.
- **B.** The patient's condition requires immediate transport.
- **C.** The vehicle or scene is unsafe.
- **D.** You are unable to manage the airway.

_____ **21.** How many rescuers does it take to properly remove a helmet from a patient?
- **A.** One
- **B.** Two
- **C.** Three
- **D.** Never remove the helmet.

_____ **22.** The nerve root located at T4 is responsible for which dermatome area?
- **A.** Umbilicus
- **B.** Back of the leg
- **C.** Apex of axilla
- **D.** Nipple line

Labeling

Label the following diagrams with the correct terms.

1. Sections of the cervical, thoracic, and lumbar spine

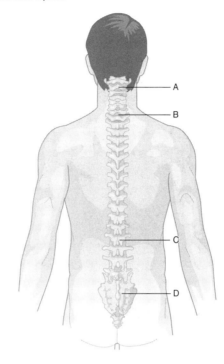

A. _____

B. _____

C. _____

D. _____

2. The meninges

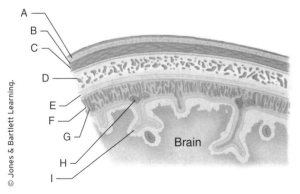

A. _____

B. _____

C. _____

D. _____

E. _____

F. _____

G. _____

H. _____

I. _____

3. Major regions of the brain

DIENCEPHALON

CEREBRUM

A

B

C

D

E

BRAIN STEM

CEREBELLUM

I

H

G

F

© Jones & Bartlett Learning.

A. _____

B. _____

C. _____

D. _____

E. _____

F. _____

G. _____

H. _____

I. _____

Fill in the Blank
Read each item carefully, and then complete the statement by filling in the missing word(s).

1. The _____ body, the anterior weight-bearing structure, is made of bone that supports and stabilizes the body.

2. The vertebral components include the _____, _____, and spinous processes.

3. The _____ is responsible for higher functions and is the largest portion of the brain.

4. The brainstem contains the midbrain, _____, and the _____.

5. The second layer of the meninges, which is a delicate, transparent membrane, is called the _____.

6. A(n) _____-_____ injury happens when the brain sloshes forward and hits the front of the skull and then recoils and hits the back part of the skull.

7. Increased intracranial pressure (ICP) can produce signs of _____, bradycardia, and irregular respirations. This set of findings is known as _____ _____.

8. A(n) _____ hematoma is the collection of blood between the dura mater and the skull.

9. Because of clenched teeth, the paramedic may have to perform _____ _____ _____ to intubate the patient with head injury safely.

10. Unlike patients who experience shock, the patient with a head injury can develop a very high _____ _____.

11. The components of the vertebral body are the spinous process, _____, and the _____.

12. The two vertebrae in the cervical area that allow for the rotational movement of the skull are _____ and _____.

13. The two components of the central nervous system are the _____ and the _____ _____.

14. The three components of the brainstem are the _____, _____, and _____.

15. The spinal cord attaches to the brain through the _____ _____, which is a hole in the base of the skull.

16. The nerves can also be injured at the _____ level, which is outside the spinal cord.

17. _____ spinal cord injury is total disruption of all tracts of the spinal cord, with all cord-mediated functions below the level of transaction being lost permanently.

18. The signs and symptoms of _____ _____ are hypotension and bradycardia, accompanied by warm, dry, flushed skin.

19. In most adults, the _____ cord extends from the base of the skull to L2; here it separates into the _____ equina.

20. During an assessment of the feet of a patient, when you stimulate the bottom of the feet, normally the toes move _____; with a positive Babinski reflex, the toes move _____.

Identify

Read the following case studies, and then list the chief complaint, vital signs, and pertinent negatives.

Part I

Tom and Janet, two off-duty paramedics, are leaving the midnight show at the local movie theater when they witness a collision between a car with two occupants and an 18-wheel tractor trailer flying down the highway. It is 0230 hours, and it looked like the car misjudged the speed of the truck when making a right-hand turn onto the main boulevard. The small car was struck on the left-side driver's door, spinning the vehicle and rolling it a couple times before it stopped by a telephone pole in the upright position. Tom begins a search around the crash site as he calls on his cell phone for the police, EMS, and the fire department for an engine and rescue. Janet begins to deal with traffic and then starts to check out the patients in the car.

Janet quickly recognizes the male driver is pinned behind the wheel and will require extrication. The female front-seat occupant probably did not have her seatbelt on as she struck the windshield and was thrown out the side door to the ground.

The woman is on her back with her arms drawn up to her chest, and her feet seem to be rigid and slightly turned in. A primary survey shows minor bleeding from the scalp but no life-threatening bleeding. The girl is a U on the AVPU scale, and Tom determines she is a 7 on the Glasgow Coma Scale (GCS). Her respirations are 34 breaths/min and very deep, and oxygen saturation is 98%. Pupils are sluggish, blood pressure (BP) is 160/90 mm Hg, and her pulse is 64 beats/min. The woman's skin is cool.

Help arrives. Fire personnel take over extrication of the male patient, while paramedics begin care for the female patient. The paramedics apply a cervical collar to the female patient, secure her to scoop stretcher, and load her into their ambulance.

The closest trauma center is 15 minutes away by helicopter, so the paramedics call for the life flight crew to meet them in a landing zone near the scene. Because the patient is unresponsive (and the paramedics know they should consider intubating a patient with a GCS score of less than 8), they decide to insert an advanced airway and administer 100% supplemental oxygen to the patient. They place two large-bore IV lines and administer normal saline. The paramedics are careful not to overload this patient with fluid because of the rising intracranial pressure (ICP). The ECG monitor now shows a sinus bradycardia. Respirations are 56 breaths/min, and the BP is now 168/88 mm Hg. An air ambulance then takes over and flies the patient to the regional trauma center. Ultimately, the patient makes it but has some neurologic defects, from which it will take several months to years to recover.

Answer the following questions regarding the female patient.

1. Chief complaint:

_____

_____

2. Vital signs:

_____

_____

3. Pertinent negatives:

_____

_____

4. Why is it important to get this patient to the regional trauma center?

_____

_____

5. What does the patient's position on the ground tell the paramedics?

_____

_____

6. What do the patient's serial vital signs tell the paramedics?

_____

_____

Part II

Your unit is called to a two-vehicle collision. It is a dark morning, and it is misting outside. The patient is a young woman with long hair who is trapped in a vehicle that has landed on its wheels after rolling two or three times. Her hair is trapped between the roof of the car and the headrest, and you are unable to get inside because of the damage of the collision. You find that the patient responds to a few of your questions, but the only thing she can remember is her first name. You need the Jaws of Life to get her out. After the car is cut apart, you can finally get in the car to perform manual stabilization. A cervical collar is applied, and you and your partners—with some help from a firefighter—do a rapid extrication, being very careful to move the patient in straight lines onto the backboard.

En route to the hospital, you perform a rapid trauma assessment, which reveals no bleeding from anywhere. The patient is very cold, and you learn that the crash happened about an hour before anyone found the two cars. She has a BP of 100/62 mm Hg and a pulse of 124 beats/min. Her oxygen saturation is 96% before applying supplemental oxygen via nonrebreathing mask at 15 L/min. Her rate of breathing is 26 breaths/min and somewhat shallow. Lungs are clear. You are unable to find a pulse in either of the feet. She is unable to move her legs, and she does not respond to you when you touch or pinch her feet, knees, or hips. The monitor shows sinus tachycardia with no ectopy. You start two large-bore IV lines with warm normal saline and use active rewarming, turning the heat on high in the unit to help bring the patient's body temperature back up. Her serial vital signs remain largely unchanged except for the oxygen saturation, which has increased to 98%. After a 500-mL bolus of fluid, her BP has come up slightly to 108/64 mm Hg. The next day, you learn the patient had a broken L2 vertebra and is paralyzed from there down.

1. Chief complaint:

_____

_____

2. Vital signs:

_____

_____

3. Pertinent negatives:

_____

_____

Complete the Patient Care Report (PCR)

Read the incident scenario in the preceding Identify, Part II, exercise, and then complete the following PCR for the patient.

EMS Patient Care Report (PCR)					
Date:	**Incident No.:**	**Nature of Call:**		**Location:**	
Dispatched:	**En Route:**	**At Scene:**	**Transport:**	**At Hospital:**	**In Service:**
Patient Information					
Age: **Sex:** **Weight (in kg [lb]):**		**Allergies:** **Medications:** **Past Medical History:** **Chief Complaint:**			
Vital Signs					
Time:	**BP:**	**Pulse:**	**Respirations:**		**SpO$_2$:**
Time:	**BP:**	**Pulse:**	**Respirations:**		**SpO$_2$:**
Time:	**BP:**	**Pulse:**	**Respirations:**		**SpO$_2$:**
EMS Treatment **(circle all that apply)**					
Oxygen @ _____ L/min via (circle one): NC NRM Bag-mask device		**Assisted Ventilation**	**Airway Adjunct**		**CPR**
Defibrillation	**Bleeding Control**	**Bandaging**	**Splinting**		**Other:**
Narrative					

Ambulance Calls

The following case scenarios provide an opportunity to explore the concerns associated with patient management and paramedic care. Read each scenario, and then answer each question.

1. In the old cowboy movies, one of the standard ways of preventing the bad guys from making their getaway was to tie a rope securely between two trees on either side of the road, at a height about 8 or 9 feet off the ground. When the bad guys came galloping down the road, the rope would catch them across the chest or neck and throw them from their horses.

    Imagine, then, that you are the Dodge City paramedic, called to attend a bad guy who has just been thrown from his horse after riding precipitously into a rope stretched across the road. You find the bad guy lying on the road and moaning. His voice is quite hoarse as he replies to your questions about what happened, and he seems very short of breath. On examination, you find a prominent bruise over the anterior neck. The patient's face and neck appear bloated, and the skin there has a crinkly feel to it.

    a. Which serious injury or injuries do you have to consider in this patient, given the mechanism of injury and the findings on examination?

    _____

    _____

    b. List the steps you would take in treating this patient.

    (1)_____

    (2)_____

    (3)_____

2. A 15-year-old boy was shot in the abdomen during a gang dispute. You find him lying supine on the sidewalk. He is conscious, alert, and crying out, "I can't move my legs! I can't move my legs!" You find an entrance wound just to the left of the umbilicus. You cannot find an exit wound. On examination, sensation is absent from the toes up to the bottom of the ribs. The patient cannot move either leg, but he has normal strength in both hands.

    a. At approximately which level of the spinal cord has this patient probably been injured?

    _____

    b. Suppose that your examination also revealed a systolic blood pressure of 80 mm Hg. What could you conclude from that finding?

    _____

3. A 34-year-old man has been injured in a road incident in which his head apparently struck the windshield with some force. When you first reach the scene, the patient is unconscious. He is breathing 8 breaths/min, inhaling approximately 500 mL of air with each breath.

    a. What is his minute volume? _____

    b. Is that volume greater or less than normal? _____

    c. Therefore, you can conclude that the patient's arterial P_{CO_2} will tend to _____ (increase or decrease?), so his pH will _____ (increase or decrease?). The net effect will be an acid–base disorder called a _____ (respiratory or metabolic?) _____ (acidosis or alkalosis?). The way you can help correct that abnormality is to _____.

    d. One reason to try to correct hypoventilation in a patient with a head injury is that hypoventilation may, through its effects on acid–base balance, worsen cerebral edema and thereby accelerate the increase in ICP. How would you know if this patient is developing an increase in ICP? List five signs of increasing ICP.

    (1)_____

    (2)_____

(3)_____

(4)_____

(5)_____

   e. Here are the findings of your initial neurologic assessment of the patient:
- He opens his eyes only when pinched, not when spoken to.
- He pulls his whole arm and shoulder away when you pinch his hand.
- He makes garbled sounds that you cannot understand.

   (1) What is his AVPU? _____

   (2) What is his score on the GCS? _____

4. Score each of the patients described in the following scenarios according to the AVPU scale and the GCS.

   a. The patient is found unconscious. He opens his eyes in response to a loud voice. He does not follow commands, but he pulls his hand away when pinched and makes a few garbled noises that you cannot understand.

   AVPU scale _____   GCS score _____

   b. The patient is found apparently unconscious, but he opens his eyes at the sound of your voice. He can follow simple commands, but he is a bit confused and cannot tell you what month it is or what day of the week it is.

   AVPU scale _____   GCS score _____

   c. The patient is found unconscious. He does not open his eyes when pinched or try to pull away from the painful stimulus; instead, his arms flex spasmodically across his chest while his legs go into hyperextension. He makes no sound.

   AVPU scale _____   GCS score _____

   d. The patient is found conscious. He gives you a coherent account of what happened to him, his name, and the day of the week, and he can follow simple commands.

   AVPU scale _____   GCS score _____

5. You are called to attend to a patient who was injured in an altercation that took place in a downtown drinking establishment. In the course of the dispute, someone broke a whiskey bottle over the patient's head. You find the patient conscious, bleeding profusely from his scalp, and in a distinctly unfriendly frame of mind, which he manifests by hurling tables and chairs in all directions while screaming uncomplimentary names at his assailants. List the steps you would take in treating this patient.

   a. _____

   b. _____

   c. _____

   d. _____

True/False

If you believe the statement to be more true than false, write the letter "T" in the space provided. If you believe the statement to be more false than true, write the letter "F."

_____ **1.** The cranial vault consists of 10 bones.

_____ **2.** The cerebral perfusion pressure (CPP) is the pressure of blood flow through the brain.

_____ **3.** The reticular activating system is responsible for maintenance of hearing and reading skills.

_____ **4.** According to the "90-90-9 rule" a single drop of the SpO_2 below 90% increases the chance of a brain injured patient's death.

_____ **5.** The frontal lobe of the brain is responsible for personality traits.

_____   **6.** The vagus nerve originates from the pons.

_____   **7.** CSF is manufactured in the ventricles of the brain.

_____   **8.** Motor vehicle crashes are among the most common causes of head injury.

_____   **9.** The body's response to a decrease of cerebral perfusion pressure is to increase mean arterial pressure.

_____   **10.** Decerebrate posturing is seen when the patient pulls the arms into the core of the body.

_____   **11.** Subarachnoid hematoma will usually present with a sudden and severe headache.

_____   **12.** The outermost of the meninges is the dura mater.

_____   **13.** There are 32 pairs of spinal nerves that emerge from the spinal cord.

_____   **14.** The vagus nerve is part of the parasympathetic nervous system.

_____   **15.** A flexion injury is usually caused by a rapid deceleration or a direct blow to the occipital region.

_____   **16.** Most fractures sustained in a vertical compression are classified as unstable.

_____   **17.** In central cord syndrome, the patient will demonstrate a greater loss of function in the lower extremities than in the upper extremities.

_____   **18.** The diaphragm is innervated by the phrenic nerve between C3 and C5.

_____   **19.** When there is an absent pulse in a patient with a spinal cord injury, it is acceptable not to start cardiopulmonary resuscitation (CPR) because of the region of the injury.

_____   **20.** A normal neurologic exam can immediately rule out a spinal cord injury.

_____   **21.** The preferred method of immobilizing a person to a long backboard is the two-person log-roll method.

_____   **22.** You should assess the pulse, motor, and sensory (PMS) functions in each extremity before and after placing the patient on a long backboard.

_____   **23.** A rapid extrication technique should be used for every patient who is in a seated position in a car crash.

_____   **24.** It is acceptable to release manual stabilization of the neck while you are measuring for a cervical collar. Make sure, however, to let your patient know not to move the head.

Short Answer

Complete this section with short written answers using the space provided.

1. When a patient has sustained a potential injury to the spinal cord, it does not pay to wait until there are symptoms and signs of spinal cord damage. By then, it may be too late to prevent permanent disability. The only sure way to prevent such disability is to anticipate spinal injury under the appropriate circumstances and handle the patient in a way that will protect his or her spinal cord from damage. List eight high-risk MOIs that strongly suggest spine injury.

a. _____

b. _____

c. _____

d. _____

e. _____

f. _____

g. _____

h. _____

Fill in the Table

Fill in the missing parts of the tables.

1. Signs and symptoms of head trauma

_____, contusions, or _____ to the scalp
Soft area or _____ noted on palpation of the scalp
Visible skull _____ or _____
_____ sign or _____ eyes
CSF rhinorrhea or _____
Traumatic Brain Injury
Pupillary abnormalities
• _____ pupil size
• Sluggish or _____ pupils
A period of unresponsiveness
Confusion or disorientation
Repeatedly asks the same questions (perseveration)
Amnesia (_____ and/or _____)
Combativeness or other abnormal behavior
Numbness or tingling in the _____
Loss of sensation and/or motor function
Focal _____ deficits
Seizures
_____ triad: hypertension, _____, and irregular or erratic respirations
Dizziness
Visual disturbances, blurred vision, or double vision (_____)
Seeing "stars" (flashes of light)
Nausea or vomiting
Posturing (_____ and/or _____)

2. Dermatomes

Nerve Root	Anatomic Location	Nerve Root	Anatomic Location
C2	_____	T10	Umbilicus
C3	_____	L1	_____ line
C5	Lateral side of _____	L2	Mid-anterior thigh
C6	Thumb and medial index finger (6-shooter)	L3	Medial aspect of the _____
C7	_____ finger	L5	_____
C8	_____ finger	S1–S3	Back of _____
T2	_____	S4–S5	_____ area
T4	_____ line		

Chest Trauma

I'm looking for engorged jugular veins.

I could help you with the 45° semi-Fowler's position, but maybe you should check his blue lips instead.

© Jones & Bartlett Learning.

Matching

Part I

Match each of the items in the right column to the appropriate description in the left column.

_____ 1. Blunt force injury to the heart that results in capillary damage, interstitial bleeding, and cellular damage in the area.

A. Atelectasis

_____ 2. A prominence of the jugular veins due to increased volume or increased pressure within the central venous system or the thoracic cavity.

B. Cardiac tamponade

_____ 3. The collection of blood within the normally closed pleural space.

C. Clavicle

_____ 4. A collection of blood and air in the pleural cavity.

D. Commotio cordis

_____ 5. An injury that involves two or more adjacent ribs fractured in two or more places, allowing the segment between the fractures to move independently of the rest of the thoracic cage.

E. Crepitus

_____ 6. Alveolar collapse that prevents use of that portion of the lungs for ventilation and oxygenation.

F. Exophthalmos

_____ 7. A condition in which the atria and right ventricle are collapsed by a collection of blood or other fluid within the pericardial sac, resulting in diminished cardiac output.

G. Flail chest

_____ 8. An S-shaped bone, also called the collarbone, that articulates medially with the sternum and laterally with the shoulder.

H. Hemopneumothorax

_____ 9. An event in which an often-fatal cardiac dysrhythmia is produced by a sudden blow to the thoracic cavity.

I. Hemothorax

_____ 10. A grating sensation made when two pieces of broken bone rub together or subcutaneous emphysema is palpated.

J. Jugular venous distention (JVD)

_____ 11. A pattern of injuries seen after a severe force is applied to the thorax, forcing blood from the great vessels and back into the head and neck.

K. Myocardial contusion

_____ 12. Dissection or rupture of the aorta.

L. Myocardial rupture

_____ 13. The collection of blood within the sclera of the eye, presenting as a bright red patch of blood over the sclera but not involving the cornea.

M. Needle decompression

_____ 14. The superior aspect of the thoracic cavity; this ring-like opening is created by the first vertebral vertebra, the first rib, the clavicles, and the manubrium.

N. Open pneumothorax

_____ 15. A life-threatening collection of air within the pleural space; the volume and pressure both collapse the involved lung and cause a shift of the mediastinal structures to the opposite side.

O. Pericardial sac

_____ 16. A procedure in which a needle or angiocatheter is introduced into the pericardial sac to relieve cardiac tamponade.

P. Pericardiocentesis

_____ **17.** The collection of air within the normally closed pleural space.

_____ **18.** Injury to the lung parenchyma that results in capillary hemorrhage into the tissue.

_____ **19.** Protrusion of the eyes from the normal position within the socket.

_____ **20.** A physical finding of air within the subcutaneous tissue.

_____ **21.** The potential space between the layers of the pericardium.

_____ **22.** The result of a defect in the chest wall that allows air to enter the thoracic space.

_____ **23.** A procedure in which a needle or angiocatheter is introduced into the pleural space in an attempt to relieve a tension pneumothorax; also referred to as needle thoracentesis.

_____ **24.** An acute traumatic perforation of the ventricles, atria, intraventricular septum, intra-atrial septum, chordae, papillary muscles, or valves.

_____ **25.** A drop in the systolic blood pressure of 10 mm Hg more than during inspiration; commonly seen in patients with cardiac tamponade or severe asthma.

Q. Pneumothorax

R. Pulmonary contusion

S. Pulsus paradoxus

T. Subconjunctival hematoma

U. Subcutaneous emphysema

V. Tension pneumothorax

W. Thoracic inlet

X. Traumatic asphyxia

Y. Traumatic aortic disruption

Part II

Certain signs identify specific lung injuries. Match the types of lung injuries to the signs.

_____ **1.** Hemoptysis, lack of tracheal deviation, and dullness noted on the side affected during percussion.

_____ **2.** Jugular vein distention, and tracheal deviation and absence of breath sounds on affected side.

_____ **3.** Diminished breath sounds heard on auscultation, a finding that is best heard anteriorly if the patient is in the supine position or in the apices if the patient is upright.

_____ **4.** A sucking chest wound or bubbling wound may be noted.

_____ **5.** Evidence of underlying injury may include contusions, tenderness, crepitus, or paradoxical motion. Auscultation may reveal wheezes or crackles (formerly known as rales).

A. Simple pneumothorax

B. Open pneumothorax

C. Tension pneumothorax

D. Massive hemothorax

E. Pulmonary contusion

Multiple Choice

Read each item carefully, and then select the best response.

_____ **1.** While riding his bicycle fast down a hill, a 16-year-old boy falls and sustains an injury to the chest. While palpating the chest, you feel what you believe to be the fracture of a number of adjacent ribs and observe that the patient is having paradoxical respirations. What you are feeling and observing is likely which type of injury?

A. Flail chest

B. Subcutaneous emphysema

C. Commotio cordis

D. Pulmonary contusion

_____ **2.** When a knife wound to the chest wall allows air to enter the thoracic space, what is the condition called?

A. Pulmonary contusion

B. Tension pneumothorax

C. Open pneumothorax

D. Myocardial contusion

_____ **3.** While standing by with an ambulance at a college baseball game, you see a player get hit with a line drive to the chest and suddenly fall to the ground. You immediately go to the player's side and find he is in cardiac arrest. You attach the automated external defibrillator (AED), and after the first defibrillation, the patient's pulse returns, and his eyes open. Which of the following is the condition you MOST likely observed?

    A. Myocardial rupture

    B. Commotio cordis

    C. Pulmonary contusion

    D. Diaphragmatic rupture

_____ **4.** Jugular vein distention is measured when the patient is in which position?

    A. Sitting upright (Fowler position)

    B. Lying supine

    C. Sitting at a 45° angle (semi-Fowler position)

    D. Prone position

_____ **5.** On arrival at the scene of a motor vehicle crash, you find a man who owns up to not wearing a seat belt. During your assessment, you observe significant bruising. You suspect the patient has a pericardial tamponade. Which of the following is NOT a sign of Beck triad?

    A. Hypotension

    B. Jugular vein distention

    C. Muffled heart tones

    D. Hyperresonant chest sounds

_____ **6.** In which age group are the ribs MOST pliable?

    A. Children

    B. Older adults

    C. Young adults past puberty

    D. Middle-aged persons

_____ **7.** Injuries to the great vessels, as well as cardiac tamponade, are much more likely to occur with which of the following types of injuries?

    A. Blunt trauma

    B. High-energy penetrating trauma

    C. Low-speed deceleration injury

    D. Posterior blunt force

_____ **8.** Where are breath sounds MOST likely to be diminished with an open pneumothorax?

    A. On both sides

    B. Over the unaffected side

    C. Over the affected side

    D. On neither side

_____ **9.** While performing the assessment of a patient involved in a high-speed motor vehicle crash, you observe decreased breath sounds and, upon palpation of the chest, note hyperresonance. You immediately suspect which of the following conditions?

    A. Simple pneumothorax

    B. Tension pneumothorax

    C. Hemothorax

    D. Open pneumothorax

_____ **10.** A critical patient has sustained a chest injury during a fall from a height of approximately 15 to 20 feet. Your assessment reveals a tension pneumothorax, and you determine an immediate needle decompression must be performed. After preparing the site, where should you insert the needle?

    A. Below the third rib midclavicular

    B. Below the third rib midaxillary

    C. Above the third rib midaxillary

    D. Above the third rib midclavicular

Labeling

Label the following diagram with the correct terms.

1. The thorax

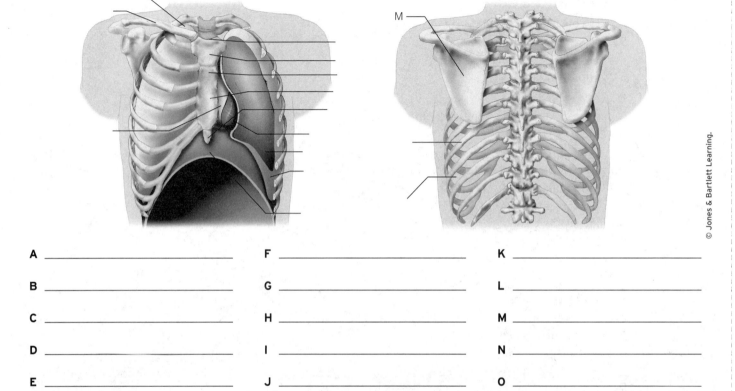

Anterior   Posterior

© Jones & Bartlett Learning.

A _____	F _____	K _____
B _____	G _____	L _____
C _____	H _____	M _____
D _____	I _____	N _____
E _____	J _____	O _____

Fill in the Table

Fill in the possible injuries for each of the following situations.

Many, if not most, serious chest injuries cannot be specifically identified in the field. An understanding of the mechanism of injury (MOI), however, should enable you to anticipate the injuries that might be present in any given case and thereby to assess the potential urgency of the situation. For each of the following MOIs or associated injuries, indicate the serious chest injury or injuries that are likely to be present. The MOI, or easily detected injuries, may give clues to the presence of injuries that are harder to find.

If you find:	The patient may have:
1. Steering wheel imprint on anterior chest	
2. Caved-in door on driver's side	
3. Fall from a height	
4. Bullet entrance wound in fifth left intercostal space	
5. Fracture of ribs 5–7 in a young man	
6. Fracture of first and second ribs	

Identify

Read the following case study, and then list the chief complaint, physical findings, and signs of Beck triad.

1. A 35-year-old man was involved in a motor vehicle crash. The patient is quickly extricated from the vehicle. You are the first paramedic to evaluate the patient. He is verbal, and when asked about pain and other symptoms, he states, "My chest hurts." During your assessment, you observe bruising on the lower chest, diaphoresis, cyanosis, dyspnea, and jugular vein distention. While assessing the vital signs, you identify equal bilateral breath sounds, tachycardia, weak peripheral pulses, hypotension, and muffled heart tones. An electrocardiogram (ECG) displays electrical alternans.

   a. Chief complaint:

   _____

   _____

   b. Physical findings:

   _____

   _____

   c. Signs of Beck triad:

   _____

   _____

   d. Do you suspect this patient has a pericardial tamponade or a tension pneumothorax?

   _____

   _____

Read the following trauma scenario, and then list the physical findings that indicate pulmonary contusion. Also describe the Spalding effect, inertial effects, and implosion in this scenario.

2. You respond to an assault of a 16-year-old boy. The patient has been struck in the chest with a baseball bat. Upon your arrival, he is conscious. You immediately perform a primary survey. The airway is open, and the patient is breathing with only mild distress. Crackles are heard upon auscultation. The pulse identifies a sinus tachycardia, and other vital signs are within normal limits. An ECG shows ischemic changes. There are no other signs of hypovolemia. You apply supplemental oxygen and initiate an IV line while en route to the hospital.

   You suspect this patient has sustained a pulmonary contusion. You believe that the pressure waves generated by the blunt trauma disrupted the capillary-alveolar membrane. The pressure created by the trauma compressed the gases within the lung. The tissues accelerated and decelerated at different rates, causing a tear.

   a. Physical findings:

   _____

   _____

   b. Spalding effect:

   _____

   _____

   c. Inertial effects:

   _____

   _____

d. Implosion:

_____

_____

e. Would you run the IV infusion wide open for this patient?

_____

_____

Ambulance Calls

The following case scenarios provide an opportunity to explore the concerns associated with patient management and paramedic care. Read each scenario, and then answer each question.

1. A 26-year-old woman was an unrestrained front-seat passenger in a car that was involved in a head-on collision. You find her lying unresponsive on the front seat, her face covered with blood. The dashboard on her side is dented in, and the windshield in front of her is smashed.

   a. List four things that might jeopardize the airway in this patient.

   (1)_____

   (2)_____

   (3)_____

   (4)_____

   b. Specify precisely what you would check in assessing the patient's breathing in the primary survey.

   (1) LOOK for:

   (a) _____

   (b) _____

   (c) _____

   (d) _____

   (2) LISTEN for:

   (a) _____

   (b) _____

   (c) _____

   (3) FEEL for:

   (a) _____

   (b) _____

   (c) _____

c. Which steps would you take at this point to ensure adequate breathing?

(1)_____

(2)_____

d. Specify precisely what you would check in assessing the patient's circulation in the primary survey.

(1)_____

(2)_____

(3)_____

(4)_____

(5)_____

2. A 22-year-old man was shot at close range by a "friend" wielding a shotgun. You find the patient slumped in a chair and in considerable respiratory distress. There is a ragged 2-inch hole in his left anterior chest, and the left chest does not seem to move with respirations.

a. This patient has a(n):

(1) simple pneumothorax.

(2) tension pneumothorax.

(3) open pneumothorax.

(4) spontaneous pneumothorax.

b. Which steps would you take to manage this situation?

(1)_____

(2)_____

(3)_____

(4)_____

(5)_____

3. A 71-year-old woman was crossing the street when she was struck by a car and thrown to the ground. She is complaining of severe pain in her right chest (she points to the exact spot, over the fifth right rib in the anterior axillary line). She says the pain is much worse when she coughs or takes a deep breath. On examination, she is conscious and alert and leaning toward her right side. Her skin is warm and moist. There is no cyanosis. Her pulse is 88 beats/min and regular; respirations are 24 breaths/min and shallow. Blood pressure is 160/90 mm Hg. The neck veins are flat. There is no tracheal deviation. There is extreme tenderness over the right fifth rib in the anterior axillary line. Breath sounds are diminished over the right chest, which sounds somewhat hollow to percussion. The rest of the exam seems to be within normal limits.

a. This patient probably has:

_____

b. What is the principal danger associated with the type of injury or injuries the patient has suffered?

_____

c. Which treatment is necessary in the field?

(1)_____

(2)_____

(3)_____

d. As you are transporting this patient to the hospital (a 20-minute drive from the collision scene), she suddenly becomes very restless and agitated and complains that she cannot breathe. Her skin becomes cold and sweaty, and her pulse gets very weak. Her neck veins seem to bulge out.

(1) What do you think has happened?

_____

_____

_____

(2) Which measures will you take?

_____

_____

_____

4. You are called to the scene of a two-car collision. A convertible going south on the interstate apparently jumped the median divider and plowed head-on into a station wagon traveling in the northbound lane. The driver of the convertible is lying unresponsive in the road. Your primary survey reveals gurgling respirations; broken teeth; flat neck veins; asymmetric chest movement; cold, sweaty skin; weak, rapid pulse; poor capillary refill; and brisk bleeding from wounds on the scalp and neck. You are 10 minutes from a regional trauma center. List in order the steps you would take in this case.

a. _____

b. _____

c. _____

d. _____

e. _____

f. _____

g. _____

5. A passenger was in a car that was struck from the right side by a truck running a red light. The right-hand front door of the car is rammed in, deforming the passenger compartment of the car. The patient, a middle-aged woman, is conscious and in considerable distress. Her skin is cold and moist. Her neck veins are distended. Her chest moves only minimally on respiration, and you have difficulty hearing breath sounds on the right. You cannot really assess the percussion note because of all the noise at the scene. The patient's pulse is 120 beats/min and weak, and her respirations are 36 breaths/min and shallow.

a. Which steps would you take at the scene?

(1)_____

(2)_____

(3)_____

(4)_____

b. Which steps would you take during transport?

(1)_____

(2)_____

(3)_____

6. A passenger car has been involved in a head-on collision with a pickup truck. When you arrive at the scene, you find the driver of the passenger car propped up against a tree, where he had been placed by bystanders who pulled him from the wreckage. The patient has numerous cuts on his face and arms and is in severe respiratory distress. He seems confused. His skin is cold, cyanotic, and sweaty, and his pulse is rapid and very weak. He can barely talk, but he manages to gasp, "Can't breathe..." You notice that the veins of his neck are bulging out. List in order the steps you would take in assessing and managing this patient.
Assessment:

a. _____

b. _____

(1)_____

c. _____

(1)_____

(2)_____

(3)_____

(4)_____

(5)_____

(6)_____

d. _____

(1)_____

(2)_____

(3)_____

e. _____

(1)_____

f. _____

(1)_____

g. _____

Management:

a. _____

b. _____

c. _____

d. _____

e. _____

f. _____

g. _____

h. _____

7. For each of the following patients, indicate what the MOST likely diagnosis is, and list the steps of prehospital management.

A. Tension pneumothorax

B. Massive hemothorax

C. Flail chest

D. Cardiac tamponade

E. Traumatic asphyxia

_____   **a.** A 20-year-old driver of a car that rammed a utility pole at high speed. He is in severe distress. His pulse is rapid and feeble, and every so often, you can hardly palpate a pulse at all. His neck veins are distended. There is a steering wheel imprint on his chest. The rib cage is stable. Breath sounds are equal bilaterally. It is too noisy to hear heart sounds. You are 30 minutes from the nearest hospital. Steps of management:

(1) _____

(2) _____

(3) _____

(4) _____

_____   **b.** A 23-year-old driver of a car that rammed a utility pole at high speed. His face, neck, and chest are cyanotic and look very bloated. His eyes are bloodshot and bulging. He is vomiting blood. Breathing is labored. His pulse is rapid and very weak. The chest looks caved-in. You are 5 minutes from a regional trauma center. Steps of management:

(1) _____

(2) _____

(3) _____

(4) _____

(5) _____

_____ c. A 70-year-old driver of a car that rammed a utility pole at high speed. He is conscious but in severe respiratory distress. The pulse is 92 beats/min, strong, and slightly irregular. Neck veins are flat. There are bruises on the anterior chest and point tenderness along the left sternal border and over the left fifth, sixth, seventh, and eighth ribs in the anterior axillary line. The chest seems to move asymmetrically on respiration. Breath sounds seem equal. It is too noisy to hear heart sounds. You are 10 minutes from the hospital. Steps of management:

(1) _____

(2) _____

(3) _____

(4) _____

(5) _____

(6) _____

_____ d. A 42-year-old front-seat passenger in a car that was struck from the right side by an ambulance that ran a red light. The patient is in severe respiratory distress. Her pulse is rapid and very weak. Her skin is cold and sweaty. The neck veins are distended. Breath sounds are decreased on the right side of the chest, which is hyperresonant to palpation. It is too noisy to hear heart sounds. You are 15 minutes from the nearest hospital. Steps of management:

(1) _____

(2) _____

(3) _____

(4) _____

(5) _____

(6) _____

(7) _____

(8) _____

_____ e. A 22-year-old man who was stabbed in the left chest. The patient is in severe distress. His pulse is rapid and very weak. His skin is cold and sweaty. His neck veins are flat. Breath sounds are decreased in the left chest, which is dull to percussion. It is too noisy to hear heart sounds. You are 15 minutes from the nearest hospital. Steps of management:

(1) _____

(2) _____

(3) _____

True/False

If you believe the statement to be more true than false, write the letter "T" in the space provided. If you believe the statement to be more false than true, write the letter "F."

_____ **1.** Children's ribs are pliable, so underlying structures may be injured even if the ribs are not fractured.

_____ **2.** In a traumatic asphyxia, the sudden compression of the chest causes pressure to be translated into the major veins of the head, neck, and kidneys.

_____ **3.** Cardiac tamponade is defined as fluid in the myocardium causing compression of the heart and decreasing cardiac output.

_____ **4.** Commotio cordis occurs when the thorax receives a direct blow during the critical portion of the heart's repolarization period, resulting in cardiac arrest.

_____ **5.** Atelectasis is alveolar collapse that prevents the use of a portion of the lung.

_____ **6.** Blunt disruptions of the diaphragm are usually associated with herniation of all or part of the liver into the right side of the chest.

_____ **7.** Esophageal injuries are not usually serious injuries.

_____ **8.** Jugular vein distention is usually an early sign of tension pneumothorax.

_____ **9.** Hypotension, as a late finding, should not be considered to either confirm or exclude the possibility of a tension pneumothorax.

_____ **10.** One physical finding of tension pneumothorax is distended neck veins.

Short Answer

Complete this section with short written answers using the space provided.

A 22-year-old man was shot in the right chest with a handgun at a range of 10 feet. There is an entrance wound in the right midclavicular line about 2 fingerbreadths below the right nipple. A slightly larger exit wound is visible 3 inches (7.5 cm) to the right of the vertebral column just below the lowest rib. Which organs are most likely to have been in the path of the bullet?

_____

_____

_____

I can't be having a heart attack, I'm a Baby Boomer!

© Jones & Bartlett Learning.

Abdominal and Genitourinary Trauma

Matching

Part I

Match each of the items in the right column with the appropriate definition in the left column.

_____ **1.** Crampy, aching pain deep within the body, the source of which is usually difficult to pinpoint; common with genitourinary problems.

_____ **2.** The area in the abdomen containing the aorta, vena cava, pancreas, kidneys, ureters, and portions of the duodenum and large intestine.

_____ **3.** Localized pain, usually felt deeply, that represents irritation or injury to tissue, causing activation of peripheral nerve tracts.

_____ **4.** Displacement of an organ outside the body.

_____ **5.** The presence of blood in the urine.

_____ **6.** The presence of extravasated blood in the peritoneal cavity.

_____ **7.** Left shoulder pain that may indicate a ruptured spleen.

_____ **8.** A membranous double fold of tissue in the abdomen that attaches various organs to the body wall.

_____ **9.** Pertaining to the area around the umbilicus.

_____ **10.** Inflammation of the peritoneum, the protective membrane that lines the abdominal and pelvic cavities.

_____ **11.** The area in the abdomen encased in the peritoneum. It consists of an upper and a lower part. The upper portion contains the diaphragm, liver, spleen, stomach, gallbladder, and transverse colon. The lower portion contains the small bowel, sigmoid colon, parts of the descending and ascending colon, and, in women, the internal reproductive organs.

_____ **12.** A membrane in the abdomen encasing the liver, spleen, diaphragm, stomach, and transverse colon.

A. Evisceration

B. Hematuria

C. Hemoperitoneum

D. Kehr sign

E. Mesentery

F. Peritoneal cavity

G. Peritoneum

H. Peritonitis

I. Periumbilical

J. Retroperitoneal space

K. Somatic pain

L. Visceral pain

Part II

Match each of the items in the left column to the appropriate injuries in the right column.

For each of the patients described here, given the mechanism of injury (MOI) and the clinical findings, indicate which injury from the right-hand column he or she is most likely to have experienced. (Note: A patient may have sustained more than one of the injuries listed.)

_____ 1. A 15-year-old girl was kicked in the left side by a horse. She is conscious and alert. Her pulse is rapid. She has a bruise over the left 10th rib in the anterior axillary line and has severe tenderness at that point.

A. Diaphragm injury

_____ 2. A 50-year-old man was a passenger in a car that slammed into a wall. He was wearing a lap seat belt. He complains of shortness of breath and abdominal pain. He winces when he coughs. His vital signs are as follows: pulse, 92 beats/min and regular; respirations, 36 breaths/min and shallow; and blood pressure, 120/80 mm Hg.

B. Ruptured spleen

_____ 3. An 18-year-old man was shot in the right upper quadrant by his girlfriend, who wielded a .38 special at a distance of about 10 feet. The patient is conscious. He has cold, sweaty skin and a weak, rapid pulse. There is an entrance wound in the right upper quadrant, about 2 fingerbreadths below the costal margin in the midclavicular line. The exit wound is near the left buttock.

C. Liver laceration

_____ 4. A 60-year-old man was struck by a car as he was crossing the street. The patient presents with gross hematuria; suprapubic pain and tenderness; difficulty voiding; and abdominal distention, guarding, and rebound tenderness.

D. Torn or ruptured bladder

_____ 5. A 42-year-old construction worker is extricated from underneath a pile of concrete blocks that caved in on top of him. He is unresponsive, with cold and clammy skin. His pulse is very weak. There are no bruises on the chest, which moves symmetrically with respiration. The abdomen is not rigid, but there seems to be a fullness in the center of the lower quadrant. The pelvis is unstable.

E. Retroperitoneal injuries

_____ 6. Your team is assessing a conscious, alert 18-year-old man who was involved in a high-speed car crash against a bridge abutment. The patient was unrestrained. The patient has an odor of ethyl alcohol; he is currently complaint-free. While you are evaluating the patient, you note ecchymosis of the flanks.

F. Cullen sign

_____ 7. It's another weekend night and another stabbing. On arrival, you have a conscious, alert male patient. He is lying on the ground with what appears to be exposed abdominal contents.

G. Evisceration

_____ 8. A patient is struck by falling debris. He was struck on the lower left quadrant and is found to be in profound shock. His lower left quadrant has point tenderness and is rigid.

_____ 9. A patient is a victim of blunt trauma; he is anxious and short of breath. He appears to have associated thoracic, abdominal, head, and extremity injuries.

_____ 10. A woman fell from a height while hiking. You are assessing the patient and recognize that she has Kehr sign.

Multiple Choice

Read each item carefully, and then select the best response.

_____ 1. The physical examination conducted as a part of the secondary assessment of abdominal injuries includes all of the following, EXCEPT:

    A. inspection.

    B. palpation.

    C. percussion.

    D. determination of baseline vital signs.

_____ **2.** A ruptured kidney will usually present with:
   A. flank pain.
   B. pain on inspiration in abdomen.
   C. gross hematuria.
   D. All of the above

_____ **3.** All of the following are considered hollow organs or structures of the abdomen, EXCEPT the _____, which is considered part of the genitourinary system.
   A. esophagus
   B. stomach
   C. bladder
   D. gallbladder

_____ **4.** Hollow organs are less likely to be injured, unless:
   A. they are empty.
   B. the MOI is a motor vehicle crash.
   C. they are full.
   D. the patient is a pregnant woman.

_____ **5.** The largest organ in the abdominal cavity and the most vascular is the:
   A. large intestine.
   B. pancreas.
   C. spleen.
   D. liver.

_____ **6.** Because of the nature of abdominal trauma in patients, which of the following should be required in your management plan?
   A. Obtaining a 12-lead ECG
   B. Securing the cervical spine
   C. Consulting with medical control on analgesia
   D. Establishing IV access for administration of fluids

_____ **7.** Injuries to the retroperitoneal space may include injuries to all of the following, EXCEPT the:
   A. pancreas.
   B. kidneys.
   C. vascular structures.
   D. liver.

_____ **8.** Crushing injuries may be caused by:
   A. crushing of abdominal contents by the abdominal wall and the spinal column.
   B. the dashboard of a car.
   C. the hood of the car.
   D. All of the above

_____ **9.** In penetrating trauma, it is helpful to:
   A. identify the type of weapon used.
   B. explore the wound to detect the path of destruction.
   C. cleanse the wound site to prevent life-threatening infection.
   D. remove all exposed foreign bodies.

_____ **10.** The primary survey for abdominal injuries should include all of the following, EXCEPT:
   A. road rash.
   B. bruising.
   C. swelling.
   D. epistaxis.

Labeling

Label the following diagrams with the correct terms.

1. Organs in the peritoneum

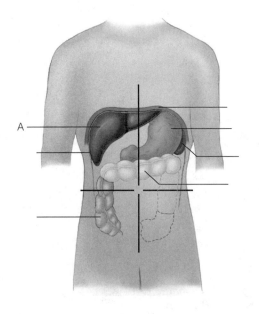

A. _____

B. _____

C. _____

D. _____

E. _____

F. _____

G. _____

2. Organs in the retroperitoneal space

A. _____

B. _____

C. _____

D. _____

E. _____

F. _____

G. _____

H. _____

3. Organs in the pelvis

A. _____

B. _____

C. _____

D. _____

E. _____

Fill in the Blank

Read each item carefully, and then complete the statement by filling in the missing word(s).

1. A(n) _____ is externalization of _____ organs through a wound in the abdominal wall.

2. Retroperitoneal bleeding can lead to ecchymosis of the flanks, commonly referred to as _____ _____

_____.

3. Retroperitoneal bleeding can lead to ecchymosis around the umbilicus, commonly referred to as _____

_____.

4. An injury to the _____ can cause signs and symptoms of ventilatory _____..

5. The _____ is relatively well protected due to its location in the _____.

6. The stomach is an intraperitoneal _____ organ that lies in the left upper quadrant and epigastric region.

7. The intestines are most commonly injured from _____ trauma, although they can be injured from severe ____ trauma

as well.

8. The spillage of toxins into the abdominal cavity due to trauma is called _____ and can be a potentially life-

threatening infection.

Identify
Read the following case studies, and then list the chief complaint, vital signs, and pertinent negatives.

1. You receive a Priority 1 response for a conscious and alert 54-year-old man involved in a domestic violence incident. When you arrive, you are advised that the scene is safe and secured by law enforcement. The patient denies any complaint. You notice that the patient's shirt is soaked with blood, and the police have placed a kitchen knife in an evidence bag. The patient is not very cooperative, and he appears ashen, diaphoretic, and slightly short of breath. After several minutes of prodding, the patient agrees to remove his shirt. The patient denies any previous medical history. You observe a half-inch laceration above his umbilicus. The wound is not actively bleeding. The patient denies chest pain or other injuries. His vital signs are as follows: pulse is 120 beats/min and regular; skin is ashen, cool, and diaphoretic; oxygen saturation is 90%; blood pressure (BP) is 86/60 mm Hg; and sinus tachycardia is found on the electrocardiogram (ECG).

   a. Chief complaint:

   _____

   _____

   b. Vital signs:

   _____

   _____

   c. Pertinent negatives:

   _____

   _____

2. Your unit is standing by at the local arena for an indoor motocross event. This high-speed motorcycle race features numerous elevated jumps and turns. The riders are well protected by helmets and specialized outerwear. While you are watching, you observe a rider crash into a retaining wall. He initially appears unresponsive. As you approach, the patient is alert and speaking clearly. He attempts to stand and get back on his motorcycle. You quickly notice that bystanders are pointing to the patient's abdomen; when you follow their signals, you see what appears to be a small protrusion of abdominal contents from the patient's left upper quadrant. It's obvious that the patient has an evisceration. You quickly assess the ABCs and immobilize the patient. He has the following vital signs: pulse is 100 beats/min and irregular; skin is pale, warm, and dry; oxygen saturation is 97% on room air; and BP is 160/90 mm Hg. After quickly treating the patient and initiating rapid transport, you become suspicious because of the patient's vital signs. The patient states he has a history of atrial fibrillation and hypertension. He currently denies chest pain.

   a. Chief complaint:

   _____

   _____

   b. Vital signs:

   _____

   _____

   c. Pertinent negatives:

   _____

   _____

Ambulance Calls

The following case scenarios provide an opportunity to explore the concerns associated with patient management and paramedic care. Read each scenario, and then answer each question.

1. You are called to the scene of an interstate collision in which an apparently intoxicated 25-year-old driver plowed his car into a bridge abutment at high speed. The front end of his vehicle is accordioned against the bridge. As you approach the disabled vehicle, your keen powers of observation enable you to perceive that the patient is conscious (he is screaming obscenities at a police officer). Describe the steps in evaluating this patient for possible abdominal injuries. In particular, which issues will you be looking for?

   a. _____

   b. _____

   c. _____

   d. _____

2. A 20-year-old man was the unrestrained driver of a car that was struck on the passenger side by another vehicle. The crash caused the empty bucket seat beside the driver to be jammed into his right side. On your arrival at the collision, you find the patient conscious but anxious and restless. His skin is ashen, cool, and diaphoretic. The patient has a delayed capillary refill greater than 2 seconds. His vital signs are a pulse of 140 beats/min and thready, respirations of 40 breaths/min and shallow, and BP of 72/40 mm Hg. There is a bruise over the right lower ribs. A large portion of the small bowel is eviscerated through an avulsion in the right side of the abdomen. The right elbow appears to be fractured. List the injuries and your priorities in managing this case.

   Injuries:

   a. _____

   b. _____

   c. _____

   d. _____

   Priorities:

   a. _____

   b. _____

   c. _____

   d. _____

   e. _____

   f. _____

   g. _____

3. During the usual Saturday night festivities at the local Knife & Gun Club, a 16-year-old boy is stabbed with a hunting knife in the left lower quadrant of the abdomen. When you arrive, you find him lying on the ground moaning. The knife is still embedded up to its hilt in the patient's abdomen. The patient's skin is pale, warm, and moist. Vital signs are a pulse of 100 beats/min, respirations of 32 breaths/min, and BP of 100/80 mm Hg. List the steps in managing this case.

a. _____

b. _____

c. _____

d. _____

e. _____

True/False

If you believe the statement to be more true than false, write the letter "T" in the space provided. If you believe the statement to be more false than true, write the letter "F."

_____ **1.** Hollow organs are less likely to cause life-threatening injuries.

_____ **2.** Contusions of the testicles or scrotal sac result in painful hematomas.

_____ **3.** Cullen sign is best described as ecchymosis around the umbilicus.

_____ **4.** Treatment of impaled abdominal objects includes removal of the object to allow for proper immobilization and transport of the patient.

_____ **5.** Delay in recognizing intra-abdominal or pelvic injury leads to early death from hemorrhage.

_____ **6.** The diaphragm plays a large role in the mechanical process of breathing.

_____ **7.** Visceral pain comes from organs inside the body that are affected by injury or illness.

_____ **8.** Severe injuries to the testicles are rare.

_____ **9.** Bladder injury should be suspected in any patient with trauma to the lower abdomen or pelvis.

_____ **10.** A saddle-type injury is likely to cause damage to the kidneys in a female patient.

Fill in the Table

Fill in the missing parts of the table.

1. Organs of the abdomen and their location.

Organ	Location: Peritoneal Cavity, Retroperitoneal Space, Pelvis (Fill in One of the Three Locations Below)
1. Liver	1.
2. Spleen	2.
3. Stomach	3.
4. Duodenum	4.
5. Kidney	5.
6. Aorta	6.
7. Uterus	7.
8. Rectum	8.
9. Bladder	9.

Short Answer

Complete this section with short written answers using the space provided.

1. Which of the abdominal organs is most likely to be injured in association with each of the following injuries?

    a. Rapid deceleration in a motor vehicle crash or a fall from a height: liver, _____, intestines, and spleen

    b. Right-sided chest trauma as well as abdominal trauma: _____

    c. Fracture of the pelvis: _____

    d. Stab wound to the right upper quadrant: _____

CHAPTER 37

Orthopaedic Trauma

Some ranges of motion are pretty clear without your checking them.

© Jones & Bartlett Learning.

Matching

Part I

Match the orthopaedic trauma term on the right with its best definition on the left.

_____ **1.** Compression of the ulnar nerve at the tunnel along the outer edge of the elbow, causing numbness, tingling, and possible partial loss of function of the little finger and medial aspect of the ring finger.

_____ **2.** A condition that arises after a body part that has been compressed for a significant period is released, leading to the entry of potassium and other metabolic toxins into the systemic circulation.

_____ **3.** A grating sensation felt when moving the ends of a broken bone.

_____ **4.** A fracture in which the bone is broken into two or more completely separate pieces.

_____ **5.** An increase in tissue pressure in a closed fascial space or compartment that compromises the circulation to the nerves and muscles within the involved compartment.

_____ **6.** Musculoskeletal injuries that commonly occur together.

_____ **7.** Inflammation of the joints.

_____ **8.** The part of the skeleton comprising the upper and lower extremities.

_____ **9.** The presence of an abnormal angle or bend in an extremity.

_____ **10.** Pain, paralysis, paresthesias, pulselessness, pallor, and pressure.

_____ **11.** The displacement of a bone from its normal position within a joint.

_____ **12.** An increase in the distance between the two sides of a joint.

_____ **13.** The loss of blood to a part of the body.

_____ **14.** A fracture in which the broken region of the bone is pushed deeper into the body than the remaining intact bone.

_____ **15.** The formation of a blood clot within the larger veins of an extremity, typically following a period of prolonged stabilization.

_____ **16.** A common incomplete fracture in children in which the cortex of the bone fractures from an excessive compression force; also called a torus fracture.

_____ **17.** A fracture of the head of the fifth metacarpal that usually results from striking an object with a clenched fist.

_____ **18.** The part of the skeleton comprising the skull, spinal column, and rib cage.

A. Six Ps of musculoskeletal assessment

B. Angulation

C. Appendicular skeleton

D. Arthritis

E. Associated fractures

F. Avascular necrosis

G. Avulsion fracture

H. Axial skeleton

I. Boxer's fracture

J. Buckle fracture

K. Buddy splinting

L. Bursitis

M. Cancellous bone

N. Carpal tunnel syndrome

O. Closed fracture

P. Comminuted fracture

Q. Compartment syndrome

R. Complete fracture

_____ 19. A fracture that occurs when a piece of bone is torn free at the site of attachment of a tendon or ligament.

_____ 20. Tissue death resulting from the loss of blood supply.

_____ 21. A fracture in which the bone is broken into three or more pieces.

_____ 22. A fracture in which the skin is not broken.

_____ 23. Compression of the median nerve at the wrist where it passes through the carpal canal, causing numbness and tingling in the hand and possible pain.

_____ 24. Trabecular or spongy bone.

_____ 25. Inflammation of a bursa.

_____ 26. Securing an injured digit to an adjacent uninjured one to allow the intact digit to act as a splint.

S. Crepitus

T. Crush syndrome

U. Cubital tunnel syndrome

V. Deep vein thrombosis

W. Depression fracture

X. Devascularization

Y. Diastasis

Z. Dislocation

Part II

Match the orthopaedic trauma term on the right with its best definition on the left.

_____ 1. A fracture that runs parallel to the long axis of a bone.

_____ 2. A force that is directed from the side toward the midline of the body.

_____ 3. A fracture that occurs in the region between the lesser and greater trochanters.

_____ 4. An injury that results from a force that is applied to one region of the body but leads to an injury in another area.

_____ 5. A fracture in which the bone does not fully break.

_____ 6. A painful disorder characterized by the crystallization of uric acid within a joint.

_____ 7. The process by which the kidneys filter the blood, removing excess wastes and fluids.

_____ 8. The socket in the scapula in which the head of the humerus rotates.

_____ 9. A break or rupture in the bone.

_____ 10. A break in the diaphysis of the femur.

_____ 11. A fracture that results from multiple compressive loads.

_____ 12. A strong, fibrous membrane that covers, supports, and separates muscles.

_____ 13. To bend the foot or hand backward.

_____ 14. An injury that results from a force that tries to increase the length of a body part or separate one body part from another.

_____ 15. A break in which the ends of the fractured bone move out of their normal positions.

_____ 16. The subluxation of the radial head that often results from pulling on an outstretched arm.

_____ 17. A break in which the bone remains aligned in its normal position.

_____ 18. The loss of the nerve supply, blood supply, or both to a region of the body, typically distal to a site of injury; characterized by alterations in sensation.

_____ 19. Muscle pain.

_____ 20. An avulsion fracture of the extensor tendon of the distal phalanx caused by jamming a finger into an object.

_____ 21. A broken bone in which the cortices of one bone become wedged into another bone, as could be the case in a fall from a significant height.

_____ 22. High levels of uric acid in the blood.

_____ 23. An abnormally elevated serum phosphate; often associated with decreased calcium. Normal phosphate levels are between 0.81 and 1.45 mmol/L.

_____ 24. An abnormally elevated level of potassium in the blood.

_____ 25. A type of fracture occurring most frequently in children in which there is incomplete breakage of the bone.

_____ 26. A complete dislocation.

A. Displaced fracture

B. Distraction injury

C. Dorsiflex

D. Fascia

E. Fatigue fracture

F. Femoral shaft fracture

G. Fracture

H. Glenoid fossa

I. Glomerular filtration

J. Gout

K. Greenstick fracture

L. Hyperkalemia

M. Hyperphosphatemia

N. Hyperuricemia

O. Impacted fracture

P. Incomplete fracture

Q. Indirect injury

R. Intertrochanteric fracture

S. Lateral compression

T. Linear fracture

U. Luxation

V. Mallet finger

W. Myalgia

X. Neurovascular compromise

Y. Nondisplaced fracture

Z. Nursemaid's elbow

Part III

Match the orthopaedic trauma term on the right with its best definition on the left.

_____ 1. The wrist bone that is found just beyond the most distal portion of the radius.

_____ 2. An inflammatory disorder that affects the entire body and leads to degeneration and deformation of joints.

_____ 3. The destruction of muscle tissue leading to a release of potassium and myoglobin.

_____ 4. The arc of movement of an extremity at a joint in a particular direction.

_____ 5. Obstruction of a pulmonary artery or arteries by solid, liquid, or gaseous material swept through the right side of the heart into the lungs.

_____ 6. A type of disorder in which multiple nerves become dysfunctional.

_____ 7. The tenderness that is sharply localized at the site of the injury, found by gently palpating along the bone with the tip of one finger.

_____ 8. The large bone that arises in the area of the last nine vertebrae and sweeps around to form a complete ring.

_____ 9. Stretching or tearing of a muscle by excessive stretching or overuse.

_____ 10. A fracture of the pelvis that results from landing on the peroneal region.

_____ 11. An injury, including a stretch or a tear, to the ligaments of a joint that commonly leads to pain and swelling.

_____ 12. A break in a bone that appears like a spring on a radiograph.

_____ 13. Any break in a bone in which the overlying skin has been damaged.

_____ 14. A life-threatening fracture of the pelvis caused by a force that displaces one or both sides of the pelvis laterally and posteriorly.

_____ 15. The proximal bony projection of the ulna at the elbow; the part of the ulna that constitutes the "funny bone."

_____ 16. A fracture that travels diagonally from one side of the bone to the other.

_____ 17. The region at the base of the thumb where the scaphoid may be palpated.

_____ 18. The dorsal deformity of the forearm that results from a Colles fracture.

_____ 19. Inflammation of a joint based on a bacterial or fungal infection.

_____ 20. A bone that is broken in more than one place.

_____ 21. The shoulder girdle.

_____ 22. A fracture that occurs in an area of abnormally weakened bone.

_____ 23. An abnormal sensation such as burning, numbness, or tingling.

_____ 24. The overlap of a bone that occurs from the muscle spasm that follows a fracture, leading to a decrease in the length of the bone.

_____ 25. A condition characterized by decreased bone density and increased susceptibility to fractures.

_____ 26. The degeneration of a joint surface caused by wear and tear that lead to pain and stiffness.

A. Oblique fracture

B. Olecranon

C. Open-book pelvic fracture

D. Open fracture

E. Osteoarthritis (OA)

F. Osteoporosis

G. Overriding

H. Paresthesia

I. Pathologic fracture

J. Pectoral girdle

K. Pelvic girdle

L. Point tenderness

M. Polyneuropathy

N. Pulmonary embolism

O. Range of motion

P. Rhabdomyolysis

Q. Rheumatoid arthritis (RA)

R. Scaphoid

S. Segmental fracture

T. Septic arthritis

U. Silver fork deformity

V. Anatomic snuffbox

W. Spiral fracture

X. Sprain

Y. Straddle fracture

Z. Strain

Part IV

Match the musculoskeletal injury on the left with the complication or other injury that is most likely to be associated with it on the right.

_____ 1. Pelvic fracture

_____ 2. Calcaneal fracture

_____ 3. Humeral shaft fracture

_____ 4. Posterior dislocation of the clavicle

_____ 5. Elbow fracture

_____ 6. Posterior dislocation of the hip

_____ 7. Open fracture

_____ 8. Patellar fracture

A. Fracture of the lumbar spine

B. Volkmann ischemic contracture

C. Fracture dislocation of the ipsilateral hip

D. Compartment syndrome

E. Deceleration injuries

F. Possible damage to underlying structures (eg, subclavian artery)

G. Infection

H. Ruptured bladder

Multiple Choice

Read each item carefully, and then select the best response.

_____ 1. Which of the following is considered one of the most common reasons that patients seek medical attention?

   A. Trauma

   B. Musculoskeletal injuries

   C. Dislocations

   D. Fractures

_____ 2. Which of the following is considered one of the functions of the musculoskeletal system?

   A. Providing support to the soft tissues

   B. Allowing the body to maintain an erect position

   C. Protecting internal organs

   D. All of the above

_____ 3. A fall on an outstretched hand is a mechanism that produces a characteristic _____ deformity.

   A. twisting.

   B. silver fork.

   C. crushing.

   D. glove.

_____ 4. Stress fractures are often referred to as _____ fractures.

   A. fatigue

   B. greenstick

   C. comminuted

   D. oblique

_____ 5. Crepitus is BEST described as a:

   A. loss of distal sensation.

   B. sure sign of dislocation.

   C. sign that occurs with fractures.

   D. grating sensation with fractures.

_____ 6. Which of the following statements MOST accurately describes an Achilles tendon rupture?

   A. It is rarely seen in adults.

   B. It often accompanies arthritis.

   C. It occurs with tendonitis.

   D. It can be identified with the Thompson test.

_____ 7. Assessing extremity injuries should include all of the following, EXCEPT:

   A. scene size-up.

   B. auscultation.

   C. inspection.

   D. examination.

_____ 8. Which of the following is the MOST common result of splinting fractured extremities?

   A. Increased pain

   B. Delay in transport

   C. Increased bleeding and nerve damage

   D. Reduced risk of further injury and less discomfort

_____ 9. Which of the following statements MOST accurately describes compartment syndrome?

   A. It can be one of the most devastating consequences of a musculoskeletal injury.

   B. It occurs as a result of loosely applied bandages.

   C. It does not occur with open fractures.

   D. It generally is not a painful injury.

_____ **10.** Pelvic fractures occur infrequently; however, they are:

    A. never fatal.

    B. responsible for a relatively high percentage of deaths.

    C. not to be splinted in the prehospital setting.

    D. rarely painful, and as a result, they are often misdiagnosed.

Labeling

Label the following diagram with the correct terms.

1. Types of fractures

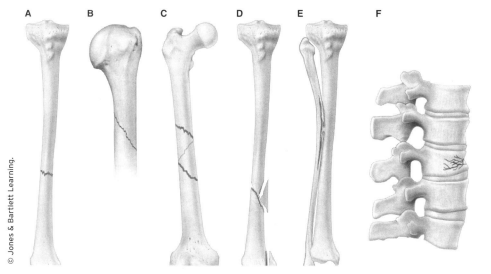

A. _____

B. _____

C. _____

D. _____

E. _____

F. _____

Fill in the Blank

Read each item carefully, and then complete the statement by filling in the missing word(s).

1. Vocabulary

    a. Within a limb, groups of muscles are surrounded by an inelastic membrane called _____.

    b. Inflammation of the joints is called _____.

    c. The process by which toxins and waste products are removed from circulating blood is called _____.

    d. The _____, also called the carpal navicular, is located just distal to the radius.

    e. A(n) _____ fracture is a fracture of the neck of the fifth metacarpal.

    f. A(n) _____ finger occurs when a finger is jammed into an object, such as a basketball.

    g. The kneecap is also called the _____.

    h. The _____ test can be performed in the field to identify an Achilles tendon rupture.

    i. The shoulder girdle is also called the _____ _____.

2. To detect a fracture, you have to know what a fractured extremity looks and feels like. Fill in the following signs and symptoms of fractures. (Some letters in the words have been provided as hints.)

    a. Unnatural shape: _____ _____ F _____ _____ _____ _____ _____

    b. Reduced length: _____ _____ _____ R _____ _____ _____ _____ _____

c. Fracture of the small finger: ____ ____ ____ E ____ ____ F ____ ____ ____ ____ ____ ____ ____

d. Numbness or tingling: ____ ____ R ____ ____ T ____ ____ ____ ____ ____ ____

e. Grating: ____ ____ ____ ____ ____ T ____ ____

f. Devastating consequence of musculoskeletal injuries: D ____ ____ ____ ____ ____ ____ ____ ____ ____

g. Protecting from movement: ____ ____ ____ R ____ ____ ____ ____

h. Hurts to touch it: ____ ____ ____ ____ ____ ____ ____ ____ ____ ____ ____ E ____ ____

i. Patient with a fracture may report this: Heard a S ____ ____ ____

j. Seen in open fracture: ____ X ____ ____ ____ ____ ____ ____ O ____ ____ ____ N ____ ____

Identify

Read the following case studies, and then list the chief complaint, vital signs, and pertinent negatives.

1. It is a snowy night in the Big Apple, and most people have decided to stay indoors. You are dispatched to the scene where a 48-year-old man slipped on the ice and snow while working late on Wall Street. As you turn the corner to the scene, you notice that law enforcement is already on scene. You mentally note to yourself that the scene is safe.

   Your patient states that he slipped and fell on the icy sidewalk. He complains of right ankle pain. The patient further states that he tried to catch himself and landed on his left wrist. He complains of severe wrist pain. You notice that the wrist is deformed, and the patient appears to be supporting it against his chest with his right arm.

   By questioning the patient, you discover that he has a previous medical history of angina, atrial fibrillation, and hypertension. He also takes one 81-mg aspirin tablet per day and an antihypertensive medication. He denies loss of consciousness and any head or neck pain. The patient denies any respiratory distress and any current chest discomfort. He denies any medical condition that may have caused him to fall. He adamantly states that he simply slipped on ice and fell. After quickly assessing the patient, you decide to move him into the warm ambulance for further treatment and evaluation.

   The patient's baseline vital signs reveal a pulse of 116 beats/min and irregular, respirations of 16 breaths/min and nonlabored, oxygen saturation on room air at 98%, and blood pressure (BP) of 150/90 mm Hg. His electrocardiogram (ECG) shows a rapid atrial fibrillation. Pupils are equal, round, and reactive to light and accommodation (PERRLA). Normal capillary refill of < 2 seconds. Skin is, warm, dry, and a normal color.

   a. Chief complaint:

   _____

   _____

   b. Vital signs:

   _____

   _____

   c. Pertinent negatives:

   _____

   _____

2. A 48-year-old woman was injured while waiting in line for a popular clothing store to open during the annual President's Day sale. This is the one day of the year when all the designer handbags are on sale. Unfortunately, at "crunch" time, the woman tripped on the curb in the parking lot and fell to the ground. Luckily, she wasn't trampled by the hordes of bargain shoppers as the doors opened. She did catch herself with her two outstretched arms. Besides her injured pride, she complains of bilateral wrist injuries and is found in extreme pain.

When you approach this patient, she is sitting in a chair with ice packs already applied and mall security providing first aid. You notice that both her wrists appear bruised and deformed. Her initial mental status is conscious and alert. Her skin is slightly ashen and diaphoretic, and she has positive distal motor and neurologic sensations in both hands. She denies other injuries. Her capillary refill is > 2 seconds, and she has bilateral radial pulses that appear to be equal.

Her blood pressure is obtainable only by palpation at 86 mm Hg. Her oxygen saturation is 96% on ambient air. She denies taking any medications or having allergies.

a. Chief complaint:

b. Vital signs:

c. Pertinent negatives:

3. You believe that this is just another medical evacuation. As you take off from the hospital's rooftop pad and head toward the scene, you pay attention to the radio as the patient information, landing zone description, coordinates, and weather are relayed through your headset. You have a 25-minute estimate time of arrival (ETA) and request any vital signs and relevant patient information. After several minutes, you begin to realize that this call is anything but routine. The flight dispatcher describes a farm mishap in which a tractor rolled on top of and is now pinning a 64-year-old man. The flight dispatcher advises that the ground crew is requesting medicated facilitated intubation immediately on your arrival. Once again, you request vital signs as you prepare the medications. Prior to your arrival, the patient is unresponsive, with a Glasgow Coma Scale (GCS) score < 8, severe respiratory distress, bilateral open femoral fractures, and a possible dislocated or fractured hip or pelvis. Further transmissions indicate a delayed capillary refill, sinus tachycardia, pulse of 128 beats/min, and BP of 64 mm Hg by palpation. The ground medics are attempting IV access while rescue crews are attempting to extricate the patient.

a. Chief complaint:

b. Vital signs:

c. Pertinent negatives:

Complete the Patient Care Report (PCR)

Reread the first incident scenario in the preceding Identify exercise, and then complete the following PCR for the patient.

EMS Patient Care Report (PCR)					
Date:	**Incident No.:**	**Nature of Call:**		**Location:**	
Dispatched:	**En Route:**	**At Scene:**	**Transport:**	**At Hospital:**	**In Service:**

Patient Information	
Age:	**Allergies:**
Sex:	**Medications:**
Weight (in kg [lb]):	**Past Medical History:**
	Chief Complaint:

Vital Signs				
Time:	**BP:**	**Pulse:**	**Respirations:**	**SpO$_2$:**
Time:	**BP:**	**Pulse:**	**Respirations:**	**SpO$_2$:**
Time:	**BP:**	**Pulse:**	**Respirations:**	**SpO$_2$:**

EMS Treatment (circle all that apply)				
Oxygen @ _____ L/min via (circle one): NC NRM Bag-mask device	**Assisted Ventilation**	**Airway Adjunct**		**CPR**
Defibrillation	**Bleeding Control**	**Bandaging**	**Splinting**	**Other:**

Narrative

Ambulance Calls

The following case scenarios provide an opportunity to explore the concerns associated with patient management and paramedic care. Read each scenario, and then answer each question.

1. Some injuries frequently come in pairs because they share a common mechanism of injury. When you find one of such a pair, you should be alert for the presence of the other. For each of the following cases, indicate which other injury or injuries you would look for in particular, given the injury already detected.

   a. A young man jumped from a second-story window to escape a fire. He complains of severe pain in the left heel, which is quite bruised and swollen. Which other injury or injuries might you expect to find in this patient?

   _____

   _____

   b. A 50-year-old woman was the front-seat passenger in a car that was hit head-on by an oncoming vehicle. Her right knee is bruised and swollen. Which other injury or injuries might you expect to find in this patient?

   _____

   _____

   c. A 60-year-old man fell sideways onto his outstretched hand. There is ecchymosis and tenderness at the base of his thumb. Which other injury or injuries might you expect to find in this patient?

   _____

   _____

   d. A construction worker has been extricated from under a pile of concrete blocks that fell on top of him, pinning him in a prone position, when part of a building collapsed. He has bruising over the left shoulder blade, and he cannot move the shoulder on that side. Which other injury or injuries might you expect to find in this patient?

   _____

   _____

2. For each of the following patients, list the most likely field diagnosis, answer any questions asked about the patient, and describe how you would manage the case.

   a. A 14-year-old boy fell from his skateboard onto his extended right elbow. The elbow is massively swollen and ecchymotic. The right hand is cool and pale, and the patient cannot feel a pinprick over the dorsum of the hand in the web space between the thumb and index finger.

   (1) What is the most likely field diagnosis?

   _____

   _____

   (2) Is there any particular danger in this case? If so, what is the danger?

   _____

   _____

   (3) How would you manage this case?

   _____

   _____

b. The mother of the boy just described fell over her son's skateboard as she was rushing to his assistance, and her outstretched left hand took the brunt of the impact as she hit the ground. As she walks toward the ambulance, she is gripping the dorsum of her left wrist with her right hand and holding the left wrist against her abdomen. When you inspect the left wrist from the side, it has a peculiar curve, rather like that of a dinner fork.

(1) What is the most likely field diagnosis?

_____

_____

(2) Is there any particular danger in this case? If so, what is the danger?

_____

_____

(3) How would you manage this case?

_____

_____

c. A front-seat passenger in a car that hit a tree is found with his right hip flexed, adducted, and internally rotated. The right leg looks shorter than the left leg. There are no other obvious injuries, and baseline vital signs are normal.

(1) What is the most likely field diagnosis?

_____

_____

(2) Is there any particular danger in this case? If so, what is the danger?

_____

_____

(3) How would you manage this case?

_____

_____

d. The driver of the vehicle in the preceding crash is unresponsive behind the wheel. His skin is cold and sweaty. When you are extricating him from the vehicle, you notice that his hips are unstable.

(1) What is the most likely field diagnosis?

_____

_____

(2) Is there any particular danger in this case? If so, what is the danger?

_____

_____

(3) What would your primary survey of this patient involve? How would you manage this case?

_____

_____

_____

_____

_____

e. As your 250-lb partner leaps from the ambulance to attend to the patients of a car crash, his ankle buckles underneath him. "Ow," he says, "that is rather painful." He manages to complete his work at the scene by hopping around on one foot, but by the time he gets back to the station, his ankle is quite swollen and hurts a lot. Aside from the swelling, there is no obvious deformity and no ecchymosis.

(1) What is the most likely field diagnosis?

_____

_____

(2) Is there any particular danger in this case? If so, what is the danger?

_____

_____

(3) How would you manage this case?

_____

_____

f. You are watching the championship football game pitting your local high school team against last year's regional champions. Your team's quarterback, who is about 5 feet 6 inches tall and weighs perhaps 150 pounds, is looking to pass when he gets sacked and buried under a horde of 225-pound defensive linemen from the other team. When the linemen unpile, your quarterback is very slow in getting up. Of course, you race over to offer your assistance. After peeling off the boy's shirt, shoulder pads, and other gear, you notice that his chest is not symmetric. There seems to be a hollow area just to the left of the sternum, at the base of the neck, and that spot is very tender. The boy, meanwhile, is quite pale, and he gasps, "I'm choking."

(1) What is the most likely field diagnosis?

_____

_____

(2) Is there any particular danger in this case? If so, what is the danger?

_____

_____

(3) How would you manage this case?

_____

_____

g. A 25-year-old man was struck by a car while crossing the street. The bumper caught him in the middle of his shin. His lower leg is severely angulated and bleeding from an open wound. He complains of severe pain in his leg and of "pins and needles" in his foot.

(1) What is the most likely field diagnosis?

_____

_____

(2) Is there any particular danger in this case? If so, what is the danger?

_____

_____

(3) How would you manage this case?

_____

_____

h. Another 25-year-old man was shot in the thigh at close range. The left thigh is swollen compared to the right, and the left leg as a whole looks shorter than the right leg. The left dorsalis pedis pulse seems weaker than that on the right side.

(1) What is the most likely field diagnosis?

_____

_____

(2) Is there any particular danger in this case? If so, what is the danger?

_____

_____

(3) How would you manage this case?

_____

_____

(4) If your management of this case included a splint, why did you use a splint? List three reasons for splinting an injured extremity.

(a) _____

(b) _____

(c) _____

i. You are spending a weekend on the ski slopes. While you are sailing down a particularly challenging hill, you see a skier stopped in the middle of the slope, admiring the view. Seconds later, about five other skiers come careening down the slope and, one after another, pile into the stationary skier. When the pile is unraveled, the skier at the bottom is found to have a severely deformed right knee, which seems to be swelling before your eyes.

(1) What is the most likely field diagnosis?

_____

_____

(2) Is there any particular danger in this case? If so, what is the danger?

_____

_____

(3) How would you manage this case?

_____

_____

3. You are called to the scene of a hit-and-run collision. A 45-year-old man is lying unresponsive in the street, surrounded by a crowd of highly agitated people. No one actually saw how the crash happened. At first glance, you can see that the man's right thigh is angulated, and the trouser leg on that side is soaked in blood.

a. Arrange the following steps in his management in the correct sequence. One step will be performed twice.

_____ Start an IV line.

_____ Take the vital signs.

_____ Cut away the trouser leg.

_____ Determine whether the patient is breathing (he is).

_____ Secure the patient to a backboard or scoop stretcher.

_____ Put manual pressure on the bleeding site.

_____ Open the airway.

_____ Start transport.

_____ Move the patient to a backboard or scoop stretcher.

_____ Check for a carotid pulse (pulse is present).

_____ Check for a dorsalis pedis pulse on the right side.

_____ Do the AVPU "mental status" check.

_____ Check for an open or tension pneumothorax.

_____ Put a pressure dressing over the open wound on the leg.

b. Have any steps been omitted? If so, which step(s)?

_____

4. A 56-year-old woman was struck by a car as she was crossing the street. You find her lying in the street, near the curb; her left leg is severely angulated and bleeding. She is conscious. There is no tenderness to palpation over the chest or spine (you don't want to remove her shirt in the middle of the street to inspect the chest). Her skin is warm. Pulse is 108 beats/min and regular, respirations are 28 breaths/min, and BP is 132/90 mm Hg. There is an open fracture of the left tibia. The dorsalis pedis pulses are equal, and sensation to pinprick is intact in both feet.

a. Which steps would you take at the scene?

(1)_____

(2)_____

(3)_____

(4)_____

b. Which steps would you take during transport?

(1)_____

(2)_____

(3)_____

True/False

If you believe the statement to be more true than false, write the letter "T" in the space provided. If you believe the statement to be more false than true, write the letter "F."

_____ **1.** Severely angulated fractures should be straightened before they are splinted.

_____ **2.** An air splint is also known as a pneumatic splint.

_____ **3.** There is no need to straighten or manipulate a fracture involving joints unless there is no distal pulse.

_____ **4.** A femoral shaft fracture places the patient at risk for fat emboli.

_____ **5.** Fingers or toes should be left out of the splint so that distal circulation can be monitored.

_____ **6.** A patient who sustained multitrauma is in unstable condition. One should splint the whole axial skeleton as a unit, on a long backboard or scoop stretcher, rather than take time to splint individual fractures.

_____ **7.** Vacuum splints consist of a sealed mattress that is filled with air and small plastic beads.

Fill in the Table

Fill in the missing parts of the table.

Potential Blood Loss From Fracture Sites	
Fracture Site	**Potential Blood Loss (mL)**
Pelvis	
Femur	
Humerus	
Tibia or fibula	
Ankle	
Elbow	
Radius or ulna	

Short Answer

Complete this section with short written answers using the space provided.

1. Fractures of the forearm or lower leg may be complicated by compartment syndrome when significant bleeding and swelling occur within one of the tight muscular compartments of the injured limb. Compartment syndrome, by cutting off the blood supply, can jeopardize the whole limb, so it is important to recognize the symptoms and signs that suggest that this condition may be developing. List six symptoms and signs of compartment syndrome.

   a. _____

   b. _____

   c. _____

   d. _____

   e. _____

   f. _____

2. Review the case of the man injured on the ski slope, which is repeated here. List the steps you would take in examining him. Looking for the signs of compartment syndrome is, in fact, only part of the assessment of an injured extremity.

   You are spending a weekend on the ski slopes. While you are sailing down a particularly challenging hill, you see a skier stopped in the middle of the slope, admiring the view. Seconds later, about five other skiers come careening down the slope and, one after another, pile into the stationary skier. When the pile is unraveled, the skier at the bottom is found to have a severely deformed right knee, which seems to be swelling before your eyes.

   a.

   _____

   _____

   b.

   _____

   _____

   c.

   _____

   _____

3. The equipment you should grab and take with you when you rush to the side of a severely injured patient should include the following items:

   a. _____

   b. _____

   c. _____

   d. _____

   e. _____

   f. _____

   g. _____

© Jones & Bartlett Learning.

Speech bubbles in image: "Means of determining core temperatures include rectal and tympanic measurements." / "Your medical director will decide which to use." / "WILDERNESS MEDICINE"

Environmental Emergencies

Matching

Part I

Match each of the terms in the right column to the appropriate definition in the left column.

_____ **1.** A condition due to prolonged exertion in hot environments coupled with excessive hypotonic fluid intake that leads to nausea, vomiting, and, in severe cases, mental status changes and seizures.

_____ **2.** The conversion of a liquid to a gas.

_____ **3.** Medical conditions caused or exacerbated by the weather, terrain, or unique atmospheric conditions, such as high altitude or underwater.

_____ **4.** The injecting of venom via a bite or sting.

_____ **5.** Mechanism by which body heat is picked up and carried away by moving air currents.

_____ **6.** Transfer of heat to a solid object or a liquid by direct contact.

_____ **7.** Secretion of large amounts of urine in response to cold exposure and the consequent shunting of blood volume to the body core.

_____ **8.** A serious heat illness that usually occurs during heat waves and is most likely to strike very old, very young, or bedridden people.

_____ **9.** The heat energy produced at rest from normal body metabolic reactions, determined mostly by the liver and skeletal muscles.

_____ **10.** Injury resulting from pressure disequilibrium across body surfaces.

_____ **11.** A measurement of ambient pressure; the weight of air at sea level, equivalent in pressure to 33 feet of seawater (fsw).

_____ **12.** Inability to coordinate the muscles; often used to describe a staggering gait.

_____ **13.** A condition in which lung tissue is damaged, characterized by hypoxemia, low lung volume, and pulmonary edema.

_____ **14.** An altitude illness characterized by headache plus at least one of the following: fatigue or weakness, gastrointestinal symptoms (nausea, vomiting or anorexia), dizziness or light-headedness, or difficulty sleeping.

_____ **15.** Continued fall in core temperature after a victim of hypothermia has been removed from a cold environment, due at least in part to the return of cold blood from the body surface to the body core.

_____ **16.** Conditions caused by the effects from hypobaric (low atmospheric pressure) hypoxia on the central nervous system and pulmonary systems as a result of nonacclimated people ascending to altitude; range from acute mountain sickness to high-altitude cerebral edema and high-altitude pulmonary edema.

A. Acute lung injury

B. Acute mountain sickness (AMS)

C. Afterdrop

D. Altitude illness

E. Arterial gas embolism (AGE)

F. Ataxia

G. Atmosphere absolute (ATA)

H. Barotrauma

I. Basal metabolic rate (BMR)

J. Boyle's law

K. Breath-hold diving

L. Chilblains

M. Classic heatstroke

N. Cold diuresis

O. Conduction

P. Convection

_____ **17.** A type of frostbite in which the affected part looks white, yellow-white, or mottled blue-white and is hard, cold, and without sensation.

_____ **18.** A broad range of signs and symptoms caused by nitrogen bubbles in blood and tissues coming out of solution on ascent.

_____ **19.** A term for decompression sickness (DCS) and air gas embolism (AGE).

_____ **20.** Each gas in a mixture exerts the same partial pressure that it would exert if it were alone in the same volume, and the total pressure of a mixture of gases is the sum of the partial pressures of all the gases in a mixture.

_____ **21.** The resultant gaseous emboli from the forcing of gas into the vasculature from barotrauma.

_____ **22.** Itchy, red and purple, swollen lesions that occur primarily on the extremities, due to longer exposure to temperatures just above freezing or sudden rewarming after exposure to cold.

_____ **23.** Also called free diving; a type of diving that does not require any equipment, except sometimes a snorkel.

_____ **24.** At a constant temperature, the volume of a gas is inversely proportional to its pressure (if you double the pressure on a gas, you halve its volume); written as $PV = K$, where P = pressure, V = volume, and K = a constant.

_____ **25.** The temperature in the part of the body comprising the heart, lungs, brain, and abdominal viscera.

_____ **26.** The process of experiencing respiratory impairment from submersion or immersion in liquid.

Q. Core body temperature (CBT)

R. Dalton's law

S. Decompression illness (DCI)

T. Decompression sickness (DCS)

U. Deep frostbite

V. Drowning

W. Envenomation

X. Environmental emergencies

Y. Evaporation

Z. Exercise-associated hyponatremia (EAH)

Part II

Match each of the terms in the right column to the appropriate definition in the left column.

_____ **1.** A condition that can result from common anesthesia medications (notably succinylcholine) and that presents with hyperthermia, muscular rigidity, altered mental status, and a hyperdynamic state.

_____ **2.** A potentially fatal condition resulting from a brown recluse spider bite that begins with a painful, inflamed vesicle that may progress to a gangrenous sloughing of the skin.

_____ **3.** Severe constriction of the larynx in response to allergy, noxious stimuli, or illness.

_____ **4.** Low oxygen levels in the arterial blood.

_____ **5.** Condition in which the core body temperature is significantly below normal.

_____ **6.** The amount of gas dissolved in a liquid is directly proportional to the partial pressure of the gas above the liquid.

_____ **7.** An orthostatic or near-syncopal episode that typically occurs in nonacclimated people who may be under heat stress.

_____ **8.** The least common and most deadly heat illness, caused by a severe disturbance in thermoregulation, usually characterized by a core temperature of more than 104°F (40°C) and altered mental status.

_____ **9.** The increase in core body temperature due to inadequate thermolysis.

_____ **10.** A clinical syndrome characterized by volume depletion and heat stress that is thought to be a milder form of heat illness and on a continuum leading to heatstroke.

_____ **11.** Acute and involuntary muscle pains, usually in the lower extremities, the abdomen, or both that occur because of profuse sweating and subsequent sodium losses in sweat.

_____ **12.** Permanent cell death.

A. Exertional heatstroke

B. Feet of seawater (fsw)

C. Frostbite

D. Frostnip

E. Gangrene

F. Heat cramps

G. Heat exhaustion

H. Heat illness

I. Heatstroke

J. Heat syncope

K. Henry's law

L. High-altitude cerebral edema (HACE)

_____ **13.** Early frostbite, characterized by numbness and pallor without significant tissue damage.

_____ **14.** Localized damage to tissues resulting from prolonged exposure to extreme cold.

_____ **15.** An indirect measure of pressure under water, equal to one atmosphere absolute (ATA).

_____ **16.** A serious type of heatstroke usually affecting young and fit people exercising in hot and humid conditions.

_____ **17.** A fall in blood pressure that occurs when moving from a recumbent to a sitting or standing position.

_____ **18.** Painful swallowing.

_____ **19.** A state resembling alcohol intoxication produced by nitrogen gas dissolved in the blood at high ambient pressure; also called rapture of the deep.

_____ **20.** A condition caused by antipsychotic and even common antiemetic medications that presents with hyperthermia, muscular rigidity, altered mental status, and a hyperdynamic state.

_____ **21.** Portion of the brain that regulates a multitude of body functions, including core temperature.

_____ **22.** Unusually elevated body temperature.

_____ **23.** Carbon dioxide in the blood.

_____ **24.** Processes that balance the supply and demand of the body's needs.

_____ **25.** An altitude illness characterized by at least two of the following: dyspnea at rest, cough, weakness or decreased exercise performance, or chest tightness or congestion. Also, at least two of the following signs: central cyanosis, audible crackles or wheezing in at least one lung field, tachypnea, or tachycardia.

_____ **26.** An altitude illness in which there is a change in mental status and/or ataxia in a person with acute mountain sickness or the presence of mental status changes and ataxia in a person without acute mountain sickness.

M. High-altitude pulmonary edema (HAPE)

N. Homeostasis

O. Hypercapnia

P. Hyperthermia

Q. Hypothalamus

R. Hypothermia

S. Hypoxemia

T. Laryngospasm

U. Loxoscelism

V. Malignant hyperthermia

W. Neuroleptic malignant syndrome (NMS)

X. Nitrogen narcosis

Y. Odynophagia

Z. Orthostatic hypotension

Part III

Place the letters HP next to the factors that increase heat production and the letters HL next to the factors that interfere with heat loss (dissipation).

_____ **1.** High ambient temperature

_____ **2.** Physical exertion

_____ **3.** Heavy or tight clothing

_____ **4.** Diabetic peripheral neuropathies

_____ **5.** Hyperthyroidism

_____ **6.** Response to infection

_____ **7.** Alcoholism

_____ **8.** Overdosing on such drugs as cocaine, caffeine, or Ecstasy

_____ **9.** Impaired vasodilation

_____ **10.** Agitated and tremulous state (such as from Parkinson disease or drug withdrawal)

Multiple Choice

Read each item carefully, and then select the best response.

_____ **1.** Heat syncope is seen in nonacclimated people who may be under heat stress and typically occurs in all of the following situations, EXCEPT:

    A. after standing suddenly.

    B. at mass outdoor gatherings.

    C. after prolonged standing.

    D. after swimming on a very hot day.

_____ 2. The major contributors to the basal metabolic rate (BMR), the heat energy produced at rest from normal body metabolic reactions, are the:

  A. spleen and lungs.

  B. kidneys and heart.

  C. liver and skeletal muscles.

  D. kidneys and gallbladder.

_____ 3. The loss of heat that takes place when moving air picks up heat and carries it away is:

  A. evaporation.

  B. convection.

  C. radiation.

  D. conduction.

_____ 4. A call to the scene of an outdoor high school track meet is for a 15-year-old student who was running the mile race. It is a humid day with the temperature in the 90s. The patient presents with muscle pain in the lower extremities and abdomen. Based on these symptoms, what is the MOST likely problem?

  A. Heat cramps

  B. Heat exhaustion

  C. Heatstroke

  D. Heat syncope

_____ 5. You are called to an apartment building on a hot July afternoon for a bedridden 78-year-old woman. Upon entering the apartment, you notice that it is extremely hot, and the patient is very warm with dry skin. The SAMPLE history identifies that the patient has heart failure and is taking beta-blockers and diuretics. Her blood glucose is normal. You should suspect:

  A. exertional heatstroke.

  B. malignant hyperthermia.

  C. neuroleptic malignant syndrome.

  D. classic heatstroke.

_____ 6. All of the following factors increase heat loss, EXCEPT:

  A. vasoconstriction.

  B. wet clothes.

  C. alcohol.

  D. diabetic neuropathies.

_____ 7. Which unique finding might be observed on an electrocardiogram (ECG) of a patient with a low core body temperature?

  A. Alternans

  B. Osborn waves

  C. Spiked waves

  D. Inverted T waves

_____ 8. You are called to a local boat dock for a patient returning from a scuba dive. His dive computer shows the maximum depth was 120 feet. The patient is reported by his buddy to have demonstrated inappropriate behavior while getting ready to ascend. The ascent was controlled with a safety stop for a few minutes at around 20 feet. Back in the dive boat, the patient complains of tingling in his lips and legs. He has no other reported symptoms. You most likely suspect that the patient may have a mild case of:

  A. arterial gas embolism.

  B. nitrogen narcosis.

  C. pulmonary overpressurization syndrome.

  D. barotitis externa.

_____   **9.** You are dispatched to the pool at a private residence for an unresponsive teenager. Upon arrival, you are told that the patient was competing with a friend to see who could hold his breath underwater for the longest amount of time. He was swimming underwater, and while coming to the surface, he went limp and was pulled from the water. You find the patient is breathing, and you administer supplemental oxygen and continue with an assessment. What do you expect is the patient's problem?

    A. Decompression sickness

    B. Barotrauma

    C. Shallow-water blackout

    D. Bends

_____   **10.** Deep frostbite usually involves the hands or feet, and the extremity may initially exhibit all of the following colors, EXCEPT:

    A. white.

    B. yellow-white.

    C. mottled blue-white.

    D. red.

Labeling

Label the following diagrams with the correct terms.

1. Dangerous snakes

A. _____

B. _____

C. _____

© SuperStock/Alamy.

Courtesy of Luther C. Goldman/U.S. Fish & Wildlife Service.

D. _____

Fill in the Blank

Read each item carefully, and then complete the statement by filling in the missing word(s).

1. The core temperature of the human body at any given moment represents a balance between the heat produced by the body and the heat shed by the body.

   a. List the potential sources of body heat and the mechanisms by which body heat can be dissipated.

Sources of Body Heat	Ways of Shedding Heat
1.	1.
2.	2.
3.	3.
4.	

   b. The body's mechanisms for dissipating excess heat have certain limitations. First, all of the mechanisms depend on _____ _____ to shunt blood from the core to the body surface. Furthermore, to be effective, three of the body's cooling mechanisms require a temperature gradient between the body and the outside. None of these three mechanisms—_____, _____, or _____—can work if the outside temperature is not at least a few degrees cooler than the body core. Finally, one of the body's cooling mechanisms is dependent on the ambient humidity. When the humidity is high, that mechanism—namely, _____ _____ _____—is ineffective in lowering the core temperature.

   c. A hatless hiker standing still on a mountaintop on a windless day loses heat from his head by _____. A breeze picks up. Now the hiker loses heat by _____ as well.

   d. A white-water enthusiast who capsizes his canoe in a swift-running river loses body heat by _____.

   e. A soldier on maneuvers in the desert in ambient temperatures of more than 37.7°C (100°F) can shed heat only by _____ _____ _____.

Identify

Read the following case study, and then list the chief complaint, vital signs, and pertinent negatives.

1. You are riding on Squad 5 and are dispatched to an incident in which a person fell through the ice at a local pond. Upon arrival, you find an 18-year-old man who is shivering with a blanket wrapped around him. It is reported that a Good Samaritan threw a rope and helped the patient get to shore. When you question the patient, he says that he was trying to walk home and didn't realize he had gotten lost. There is a smell of alcohol on the patient's breath. You immediately place the patient in your squad and turn the heat on high. The patient's wet clothes are removed, and he is wrapped in a number of blankets. He is placed on supplemental oxygen and a cardiac monitor. The ECG rhythm is regular, with no ectopy, but you do observe Osborn waves. You establish an IV line using warm crystalloid solution. The patient is transferred to the regional trauma center, which is located 15 minutes away. You continue to monitor the patient and perform a reassessment en route. You take serial vital signs every 5 minutes.

   a. Chief complaint:

   _____

   _____

   b. Vital signs:

   _____

   _____

   c. Pertinent negatives:

   _____

   _____

   d. Which three pieces of information not included in this scenario would be helpful to know?

   (1)_____

   (2)_____

   (3)_____

   e. Based on this scenario, which of the following four methods of heat loss is most responsible for the greatest amount of heat lost by this patient?
      A. Radiation
      B. Conduction
      C. Convection
      D. Evaporation

   f. You determine the patient is moderately hypothermic. How much IV fluid should you infuse initially?

   _____

Complete the Patient Care Report (PCR)

Reread the incident scenario in the preceding Identify exercise, and then complete the following PCR for the patient.

EMS Patient Care Report (PCR)					
Date:	**Incident No.:**	**Nature of Call:**		**Location:**	
Dispatched:	**En Route:**	**At Scene:**	**Transport:**	**At Hospital:**	**In Service:**
Patient Information					
Age: **Sex:** **Weight (in kg [lb]):**			**Allergies:** **Medications:** **Past Medical History:** **Chief Complaint:**		
Vital Signs					
Time:	**BP:**	**Pulse:**	**Respirations:**		**SpO$_2$:**
Time:	**BP:**	**Pulse:**	**Respirations:**		**SpO$_2$:**
Time:	**BP:**	**Pulse:**	**Respirations:**		**SpO$_2$:**
EMS Treatment **(circle all that apply)**					
Oxygen @ _____ L/min via (circle one): NC NRM Bag-mask device		**Assisted Ventilation**	**Airway Adjunct**		**CPR**
Defibrillation	**Bleeding Control**	**Bandaging**	**Splinting**		**Other:**
Narrative					

Ambulance Calls

The following case scenarios provide an opportunity to explore the concerns associated with patient management and paramedic care. Read each scenario, and then answer each question.

1. At the morning briefing, you are told that you will be doing a standby at an outdoor festival at a local college campus. These assignments are usually boring, but you will make the best of it. It is a very hot and humid day in late spring, and except for a few scrapes and blisters, you have few requests for service. The concert has been going for about an hour when you are called to a person who has passed out. When you arrive, you find an unresponsive man approximately 20 years old. His friends tell you that he had been standing listening to the concert and suddenly fell. As you are assessing the patient, he starts to regain consciousness. You can tell he has been drinking. You ask how many beers he had, and he tells you he drank two. In your mind, you at least double that number. You load the patient into the ambulance and turn up the air conditioner. The assessment indicates dehydration.

   a. What is the probable cause of the syncopal episode, and what may be some contributing underlying causes?

   _____

   _____

   _____

   b. How would you manage this patient?

   _____

   _____

   _____

   c. If the patient does not recover and stabilize quickly, what may be another presenting problem to consider?

   _____

   _____

2. You are called to the local high school playing field on a hot, sticky August afternoon to deal with a "casualty" of preseason football training—a 16-year-old fullback who "became crazy" during practice. You see him over near the goalposts, where several of his teammates are trying to restrain him. "None of my boys ever messed around with drugs before," the coach tells you, "and I sure never would have pegged Chuck as a junkie. But I don't know how else to explain his behavior. He's been touchy all afternoon, and he just started acting crazy."

   You find the fullback to be agitated and combative. He seems completely disoriented. His skin is warm and sweaty. His vital signs are as follows: Pulse is 120 beats/min and bounding, respirations are 30 breaths/min and shallow, blood pressure (BP) is 150/90 mm Hg, and oral temperature is 41.7°C (107°F). His pupils are widely dilated and react only sluggishly to light.

   a. This patient most likely has:

   _____

   _____

   b. List the steps in managing this case.

   (1)_____

   (2)_____

   (3)_____

   (4)_____

   (5)_____

   (6)_____

   (7)_____

3. The following day, it is even hotter, but mercifully, the humidity has dropped considerably. You are called to the very same playing field for another casualty of preseason football training—this time, a 14-year-old running back. You find him lying at midfield, writhing in pain. "I swear I didn't clip him," one of the other players is insisting. "I didn't even get near him. He just fell down by himself."

   "Sure, sure," says the coach, who is trying to massage the cramps out of the boy's legs. When you ask the boy what his problem is, he just moans and says, "My legs, my legs."

   On examination, the patient's skin is cool and sweaty. His pulse is 100 beats/min and regular, respirations are 30 breaths/min and shallow, BP is 110/70 mm Hg, and oral temperature is 37°C (98.6°F). There are no signs of injury to the extremities.

  a. This patient most likely has:

_____

_____

  b. List the steps in managing this case.

    (1)_____

    (2)_____

    (3)_____

    (4)_____

4. "As long as you folks are already here," says the coach, "maybe you could take a look at our quarterback. I think he's coming down with something, and I have to decide whether to send him home."

   You find the quarterback sitting on the bench looking quite miserable. He says that his girlfriend has mononucleosis, and he thinks he may be coming down with it as well because he feels very tired and achy. On examination, he is sweating profusely, and his skin feels clammy. His pulse is 110 beats/min and somewhat weak, respirations are 28 breaths/min and shallow, BP is 100/60 mm Hg, and oral temperature is 39.4°C (103°F).

  a. This patient most likely has:

_____

_____

  b. List the steps in managing this case.

    (1)_____

    (2)_____

    (3)_____

    (4)_____

    (5)_____

  c. Which advice should you give the football coach?

_____

_____

5. On the very same day, you are called to a local supermarket for a "sick baby." You arrive to find a nearly hysterical woman who looks scarcely out of her teens holding a comatose baby. "I just left her in the car for a minute while I ran in to buy a couple of things," she says, although you note three full shopping bags in the woman's cart. The baby, a 6-month-old, is unresponsive (AVPU = U). The pulse is 180 beats/min, respirations are 60 breaths/min, and BP is 100/80 mm Hg. The baby's rectal temperature is 43.3°C (110°F).

a. This patient most likely has:

_____

_____

b. List the steps in managing this case.

(1)_____

(2)_____

(3)_____

(4)_____

(5)_____

(6)_____

(7)_____

6. You are enjoying a week off at a mountain ski resort. On your first morning there, the manager of the resort asks for volunteers to join a search-and-rescue party that is going out to look for three skiers who failed to return to the lodge the previous night. You, of course, volunteer, and you set off with a team on skis to comb the slopes. You are all carrying two-way radios so that you can summon a snowmobile to help transport the lost skiers if you find them. Eventually, you locate two of the skiers, about 15 miles from the ski lodge, dug into a makeshift shelter in the snow (and unaware that only about 50 m away, beyond a stand of trees, is an empty cabin). Both skiers are alert.

a. The first skier tells you that he lost all sensation in his left leg sometime during the night. On examination, the leg is white, cold, and very hard. This patient most likely has:

_____

_____

b. Describe how you would manage this patient.

(1)_____

(2)_____

(3)_____

(4)_____

(5)_____

c. The second skier says, "I think I've got the same problem in my left foot." On examination, the foot has a waxy, white appearance. The skin feels very stiff, but there is "give" underneath when you press down hard on the skin. This patient most likely has:

_____

_____

d. How would you manage this patient?

(1)_____

(2)_____

(3)_____

(4)_____

(5)_____

e. Not long after those two skiers have been evacuated on stretchers by snowmobile, you find the third skier. He is sitting up against a tree, unresponsive. Apparently, he did not realize that he had come within 100 m of the main road. His skin is very cold. You cannot detect any pulse. The patient's pupils are dilated and unreactive. He does seem to be breathing, although only about once or twice a minute. You radio for a paramedic-staffed ambulance to meet you at the road. This patient most likely has:

_____

_____

f. Describe the management of this patient both until the ambulance comes and en route to the hospital.

(1)_____

(2)_____

(3)_____

(4)_____

(5)_____

(6)_____

(7)_____

(8)_____

7. You and your crew are at the local lake on a chilly November afternoon, covering an annual speedboat race that invariably produces a few minor casualties (mostly from indigestion among the picnicking spectators). While making a hairpin turn at high speed, one of the speedboats capsizes. After what seems like a very long time, you see the boat's driver bob to the surface of the water (he is wearing a life jacket) and begin swimming for shore. Describe the actions you should take in this situation.

a.　_____

b.　_____

c.　_____

d.　_____

e.　_____

f.　_____

g.　_____

h.　_____

8. During the first spell of bitterly cold weather of the season, you are called to the downtown bus terminal for a "man down." When you reach the scene, a police officer waves you over. "Sorry to bother you folks with this," he says. "He's just a vagrant who's been sleeping in the place for a few days, and probably all he needs is a night in the lockup to sober up." You find the patient, being restrained by another police officer, over in a corner. His speech is slurred, and he staggers when he tries to walk. His breath smells of wine. His skin is pale and cold.

a. List at least three diagnoses you must consider in this case.

(1)_____

(2)_____

(3)_____

b. In view of the diagnostic possibilities, describe how you would manage this case.

(1)_____

(2)_____

(3)_____

(4)_____

(5)_____

(6)_____

(7)_____

9. You decide to take a week's vacation to do some climbing in the Canadian Rockies. Of course, you are carrying a medical kit because it's hard for you to accept the idea that you are really on vacation. On your first day out, one of your buddies starts complaining of a headache—"probably because I didn't sleep really well last night," he says. You're a little concerned that he might be suffering from the altitude, but he shrugs it off and insists that you all keep going.

a. At that point, how could you check whether your friend has a serious case of acute altitude sickness?

_____

_____

b. As things turn out, you decide to continue climbing. About an hour later, you feel a tug on the rope and look back to see your friend really dragging. He seems out of breath. Now you're really concerned. List four signs or symptoms that would suggest your friend may have high-altitude pulmonary edema.

(1)_____

(2)_____

(3)_____

(4)_____

c. Assuming that you do find signs of high-altitude pulmonary edema (HAPE), which steps should you take to treat your friend?

(1)_____

(2)_____

(3)_____

10. When your next vacation comes up, you decide you won't make the same mistake twice: no more mountains where emergencies will spoil your relaxation. Instead, you sign up for a cruise to the West Indies—a week of sun and sand and steel drum bands. On the ship with you is a group of scuba enthusiasts who don't miss any opportunity to explore the local coral reefs each time you anchor.

One fine afternoon, as you are sunning yourself on deck with a rum swizzle in hand, you hear a commotion off to the starboard side of the ship. You leap from your chair and peer over the rail to see some of the diving crowd in a state of agitation in the rubber raft from which they've been diving. One of their number is lying motionless in the raft, and another two are just emerging from the water and climbing into the raft to join them. The captain, having spotted the situation, has already lowered a winch to bring up the raft and everyone in it.

As soon as the divers are back aboard the ship, you race to the side of the diver who is unresponsive. His friends tell you that he was the least experienced of their group. He had surfaced first, and a minute or so after being pulled onto the raft, he complained of chest pain, and his voice had sounded funny. Then, he just blacked out.

a. What do you think has happened to this diver?

_____

_____

b. Which steps should you take to manage this situation?

(1)_____

(2)_____

(3)_____

(4)_____

(5)_____

(6)_____

c. About an hour later, while you are monitoring the condition of the diver pending more definitive treatment, you hear one of his friends who was in the water with him saying to another member of the group, "Gee, my back is sure killing me. I must have pulled a muscle when I did my backflip off the raft. The hell of it is that I can't pee, either." You perk up your ears when you hear that because this bit of information makes you suspect that the speaker has:

_____

_____

True/False

If you believe the statement to be more true than false, write the letter "T" in the space provided. If you believe the statement to be more false than true, write the letter "F."

_____ **1.** A superficial frostbitten extremity is best warmed in front of a campfire or heater.

_____ **2.** With deep frostbite, the extremity feels cold and rock hard.

_____ **3.** If rescue circumstances require it, a patient with deep frostbite may walk on a frostbitten leg as long as the leg is not rewarmed in the field.

_____ **4.** Elapidae is the same family of snakes that includes mambas, cobras, and sea snakes.

_____ **5.** A frostbitten extremity will be excruciatingly painful until it is rewarmed.

_____ **6.** Injuries from the cold most often affects the tips of the ears, nose, fingers, and toes.

_____ **7.** Heat exhaustion is a clinical syndrome thought to represent a milder form of heat illness on a continuum leading to heatstroke.

_____ **8.** Classic heatstroke is less apt to affect older patients with chronic illnesses.

_____ **9.** Patients with heatstroke usually have dilated pupils.

_____ **10.** Radiation accounts for more than 65% of heat loss in a cooler setting.

Short Answer

Complete this section with short written answers using the space provided.

1. The body's normal response to entering a hot environment can place considerable stress on a person who has a limited cardiovascular reserve. Explain why.

_____

_____

_____

2. Anyone can succumb to a heat wave, but some people are more vulnerable than others. List five factors that increase a person's risk of experiencing significant heat illness in response to heat stress.

a. _____

b. _____

c. _____

d. _____

e. _____

3. Paramedics, like other public safety personnel, do not have the luxury of postponing heavy exertion until weather conditions are favorable. Instead, they must do their job whatever the weather, which means they may be exposed to a significant risk of heat illness during periods of high temperature.

a. List five measures you can take to reduce your risk of becoming ill from the heat.

(1)_____

(2)_____

(3)_____

(4)_____

(5)_____

b. If you do start to experience early symptoms of heat illness, you must stop your activities immediately. To do so, you must be able to recognize the warning symptoms of heat illness when they occur. List four warning symptoms of heat illness.

(1)_____

(2)_____

(3)_____

(4)_____

4. People wouldn't experience cold injury if they simply heeded the advice of their mothers. Mothers always know, even without taking a paramedic course, how to keep warm on cold days. Following are several statements you have probably heard at least once from your mother. Each statement reflects an intuitive knowledge of the ways in which the body generates and loses heat. For each statement, explain why your mother was right.

a. "Don't go out without a hat and scarf; it's freezing out there." Mother was right because:

_____

_____

b. "Stop rolling around in the snow. You'll get a death of a chill." Mother was right because:

_____

_____

c. "Get out of those wet clothes this minute." Mother was right because:

_____

_____

d. "Those skates are much too tight. Your toes will fall off." Mother was right because:

_____

_____

e. "Make sure you wear your windbreaker. It's blowing a gale out there." Mother was right because:

_____

_____

f. "Eat. Eat. You have to have something to keep you going in this weather." Mother was right because:

_____

_____

5. The body has only a limited repertoire of defenses against the cold. List three ways the body can defend itself against a drop in core temperature.

a. _____

b. _____

c. _____

6. Although anyone can experience cold injury, certain factors predispose a person to experience ill effects from the cold.

a. List five factors that predispose a person to experience frostbite when exposed to freezing conditions.

(1)_____

(2)_____

(3)_____

(4)_____

(5)_____

b. List four factors that predispose a person to experience hypothermia.

(1)_____

(2)_____

(3)_____

(4)_____

7. The stories that many of us learned as children contain many cautionary tales about cold exposure.

a. When the three little kittens lost their mittens, they became most vulnerable to:

_____

b. Sitting on an ice-cold tuffet on a winter day, Little Miss Muffet was losing heat from her body by:

_____

c. Who is at greater risk of experiencing hypothermia—Jack Sprat (who ate no fat) or his wife (who ate no lean)?

_____

d. Before venturing outside to try out his new ice skates, little Jack Horner retreated to a corner and ate his Christmas pie. Was that a good idea? Why or why not?

_____

e. Swinging about in the treetop is Baby in his cradle. When the wind blows, the cradle will rock. Furthermore, when the wind blows, Baby will lose heat from his body by the process called:

_____

Fill in the Table

Fill in the missing parts of the table.

1. Factors that predispose to cold illness

Increase Heat Loss	Impair Thermoregulatory Mechanism	Decrease Heat Production
_____	Dehydration	_____
Wet clothes	Parkinson disease or dementia	Age (very young or very old)
_____	_____	_____
Impaired judgment from drugs/alcohol	Anorexia nervosa	_____
_____	Central nervous system (CNS) bleeding or ischemia, spinal cord injury with neurogenic shock	Inability to shiver and immobility
Diabetic peripheral neuropathies	_____	
	Drugs interfering with vasoconstriction	

SHOCK AND RESUSCITATION

Responding to the Field Code

Here is a list of the clinics in your area. But first we need to take you to the hospital to make sure you are okay.

© Jones & Bartlett Learning.

Paramedics should take every opportunity to educate their patients.

Matching

Match each of the terms in the right column to the appropriate definition in the left column.

_____ **1.** In cardiopulmonary resuscitation (CPR), when two rescuers perform ventilations and compressions individually; ventilations are not timed and do not require waiting for the other rescuer to pause.

A. Active compression-decompression CPR

_____ **2.** A defibrillator that can analyze the patient's heart rhythm and determine whether a defibrillating shock is needed to terminate ventricular fibrillation (VF) or ventricular tachycardia (VT).

B. Asynchronous

_____ **3.** The code team member who has the responsibility for managing the rescuers or team members during a cardiac arrest, as well as choreographing the effort of the group.

C. Automated external defibrillator (AED)

_____ **4.** A member of the resuscitation team trying to revive the patient.

D. Automatic transport ventilator (ATV)

_____ **5.** The use of an unsynchronized direct current electric shock to terminate VF or VT.

E. Code team leader

_____ **6.** A mode available on automated external defibrillators, allowing the paramedic to interpret the cardiac rhythm and determine whether defibrillation is indicated (rather than the monitor making the determination).

F. Code team member

_____ **7.** The return of spontaneous heartbeat and blood pressure during the resuscitation of a patient in cardiac arrest.

G. Compression fraction

_____ **8.** A mnemonic used to describe the objectives of a community-based program to improve the survival of patients in out-of-hospital cardiac arrest: Specific, Measurable, Attainable and Achievable, Realistic and Relevant, and Timely.

H. Defibrillation

_____ **9.** An indication of how well the team is minimizing pauses in CPR; it is calculated by dividing the amount of time compressions are delivered by the amount of time compressions are indicated.

I. Manual defibrillation

_____ **10.** A portable mechanical ventilator attached to a control box that allows the variables of ventilation (such as rate and tidal volume) to be set.

J. Return of spontaneous circulation (ROSC)

_____ **11.** A procedure intended to lower body temperature in patients who are in a coma after return of spontaneous circulation; ideally performed in the hospital setting; formerly called therapeutic hypothermia.

K. SMART

_____ **12.** A manual technique that involves compressing the chest and then actively pulling it back up to its neutral position or beyond (decompression); may increase the amount of blood that returns to the heart and, thus, the amount of blood ejected from the heart during the compression phase.

L. Targeted temperature management (TTM)

Multiple Choice

Read each item carefully, and then select the best response.

_____ **1.** Which of the following is NOT considered a link in the chain of survival?

    A. Recognition and activation of the emergency response system

    B. Immediate high-quality CPR

    C. Early clotbuster therapy in the field

    D. Rapid defibrillation

_____ **2.** For which types of incidents does simulation training provide valuable preparation?

    A. High-frequency, low-risk incidents

    B. Low-frequency, high-risk incidents

    C. Low-frequency, low-risk incidents

    D. High-frequency, high-risk incidents

_____ **3.** With the issuance of the 2005, 2010, and 2015 ECC Guidelines, there was a strong emphasis on:

    A. advanced airway procedures.

    B. choices of cardiac medications.

    C. increasing the ventilation rates.

    D. high-quality compressions.

_____ **4.** When placing an advanced airway during resuscitation, the MOST important consideration would be:

    A. not to take any longer than 30 seconds.

    B. not to interrupt chest compressions for more than 10 seconds.

    C. to hyperventilate the patient as soon as possible.

    D. to insert the largest tube that will fit the patient.

_____ **5.** High-quality CPR, in the adult patient, consists of each of the following, EXCEPT:

    A. compressions at a rate of 100 to 120 per minute.

    B. allowing complete chest recoil after each compression.

    C. avoiding excessive ventilations.

    D. compression depth of 1½ inches on the adult patient.

_____ **6.** For the purposes of the ECC Guidelines, an infant is:

    A. age 1 year to adolescence.

    B. age 1 month to 1 year.

    C. within the first few hours after birth.

    D. within the first month after birth.

_____ **7.** When there are two health care providers doing CPR, the infant compression-to-ventilation ratio should be:

    A. 30:2.

    B. 15:1.

    C. 15:2.

    D. 30:1.

_____ **8.** When a pediatric patient needs to be defibrillated with an AED, it is acceptable to:

    A. use the pediatric dose-attenuator system.

    B. use a manual defibrillator.

    C. use the standard adult pads if that is all that is available.

    D. All of the above

_____ **9.** You are treating an adult patient who has overdosed from a narcotic. The patient is in respiratory arrest, and your partner is obtaining the naloxone (Narcan). What is the rate of ventilations that should be given to the patient prior to inserting an advanced airway?

    A. 1 breath every 5 to 6 seconds

    B. 2 breaths every 30 compressions

    C. 1 breath every 3 seconds

    D. 2 breaths every 3 seconds

_____ **10.** Of the following treatments for the patient with ROSC, which would NOT be appropriate?

  A. Normalize the blood pressure (BP) with dopamine (Intropin) or norepinephrine infusion to at least 100 mm Hg systolic.

  B. Elevate the patient's head to 30° if the BP allows.

  C. Stabilize the cardiac rhythm with an antidysrhythmic.

  D. Begin TTM if the patient is alert.

Labeling

Label the following diagrams with the correct terms.

1. CPR devices

A

B

C

A. _____

B. _____

C. _____

2. Resuscitation pyramid

A. _____

B. _____

C. _____

D. _____

E. _____

Fill in the Blank

Read each item carefully, and then complete the statement by filling in the missing word(s).

1. The _____ is an adjunct to adult CPR that provides both continuous chest compressions and ventilations.

2. If a(n) _____ _____ is in place, then the compressions and ventilations become asynchronous.

3. The _____ _____ _____ is marketed as the ResQPOD in the United States.

4. If an advanced airway is inserted, you should switch to _____ compressions of 100 to 120 per minute and

ventilate every _____ seconds.

5. For _____ or _____, do not deliver shocks.

6. Drug therapy for pulseless electrical activity (PEA) or asystole includes the _____ (epinephrine).

Identify

Read the following case study, and then list the chief complaint, vital signs, and pertinent negatives.

1. You are riding on Medic 480 and are dispatched along with a basic life support (BLS) unit to a person who is unresponsive in the shopping mall restroom. Upon arrival, you find a bystander and a security guard doing CPR on a 58-year-old man. When you question the patient's spouse, she says that he was complaining of pressure in his chest and indigestion before he went into the bathroom. She stated that he was only in there for a couple of moments when the bystander who started chest compressions had his son come out to get her and call 9-1-1. The security guard arrived soon thereafter with the AED. You immediately rotate the compressor, who is starting to get tired, and determine that the initial rhythm is not a shockable rhythm. As the other unit arrives, you begin to choreograph the resuscitation, making sure the patient is receiving high-quality chest compressions with as few interruptions as possible. Your partner is placing an intraosseous (IO) line in the leg so that the first epinephrine can be administered. At this point, the emergency medical technician (EMT) doing the ventilations reports that bag-valve mask ventilation is working just fine. After 2 minutes (of five cycles of compressions and ventilations), you note a rhythm change to VF, so the defibrillator is charged, and a shock is administered. After the shock is administered, the chest compressions are started immediately. Within moments, you note that the monitor is now showing a "normal"-looking electrocardiogram (ECG), so you stop the compressions and note that the patient has a strong carotid pulse. Because the patient is not yet breathing on his own, you decide to intubate and start your region's ROSC protocol. The wife, who has been observing all of the care, is very happy when the pulse returns. Further history reveals that the patient has been having these periods of chest discomfort for the past few weeks. He has no allergies and takes only vitamins each day. He has never had previous problems with his heart, head, or lungs, although his father did die from heart problems at a young age. En route to the hospital, a 12-lead ECG is taken, and the patient's BP is 108 mm Hg systolic, and his pulse rate is 96 beats/min and regular.

　　After delivering the patient right to the coronary catheterization lab for post–successful resuscitative measures, you note that the success of this resuscitation was definitely due to the bystander's immediate actions!

a. Chief complaint:

_____

_____

b. Vital signs:

_____

_____

c. Pertinent negatives:

_____

_____

d. What medication would most likely be administered to this patient?

_____

_____

e. Based on this scenario, what are the links in the chain of survival for this patient and all victims of sudden cardiac arrest?

(1)_____

(2)_____

(3)_____

(4)_____

(5)_____

Complete the Patient Care Report (PCR)

Reread the incident scenario in the preceding Identify exercise, and then complete the following PCR for the patient.

EMS Patient Care Report (PCR)					
Date:	Incident No.:		Nature of Call:		Location:
Dispatched:	En Route:	At Scene:	Transport:	At Hospital:	In Service:
Patient Information					
Age: Sex: Weight (in kg [lb]):			Allergies: Medications: Past Medical History: Chief Complaint:		
Vital Signs					
Time:	BP:		Pulse:	Respirations:	SpO$_2$:
Time:	BP:		Pulse:	Respirations:	SpO$_2$:
Time:	BP:		Pulse:	Respirations:	SpO$_2$:
EMS Treatment (circle all that apply)					
Oxygen @ _____ L/min via (circle one): NC NRM Bag-mask device		Assisted Ventilation		Airway Adjunct	CPR
Defibrillation	Bleeding Control		Bandaging	Splinting	Other:
Narrative					

Ambulance Calls

The following case scenarios provide an opportunity to explore the concerns associated with patient management and paramedic care. Read each scenario, and then answer each question.

1. At morning briefing, you are interrupted by a call for a possible cardiac arrest. The police have just arrived on the scene, and the supervisor is also en route to the call. As you arrive, you are met by a neighbor who states, "Mr. Jones was out shoveling snow when he suddenly collapsed. He was told by his heart doctor to leave the heavy work for his grandson!" Apparently, the grandson found him, carried him into the garage, called 9-1-1, and began hands-only CPR. As you and your partner are bringing in your equipment, you think to yourself, *The good news is CPR was started . . . The bad news is that he has a cardiac history.* Just then, a backup unit pulls up, as does the supervisor's truck. That means there are two medics (including you), two EMTs, a supervisor, and a police officer, and you will need to assign tasks so that this code runs with the speed and precision of a NASCAR pit stop.

   a. What is the highest priority during the entire code?

   _____

   _____

   _____

   b. If your role is that of the code team leader, what are your responsibilities?

   (1)_____

   (2)_____

   (3)_____

   (4)_____

   (5)_____

   (6)_____

   (7)_____

   (8)_____

   (9)_____

   c. If you need to assign roles to the code team members, what do they include?

   (1)_____

   (2)_____

   (3)_____

   (4)_____

2. Based on the scenario just described, if the grandson had come home to find his grandfather on the floor in the kitchen in cardiac arrest, and there was an unknown downtime before calling 9-1-1, the results could be entirely different. On your arrival at the scene this time, the grandson was not doing hands-only CPR because he missed that day when it was taught in high school.

   a. What are the criteria for NOT starting resuscitation?

   _____

   _____

   _____

b. With regard to the success of this resuscitation, what is the significance of chest compressions not being started prior to your arrival on the scene?

_____

_____

_____

3. Later that day, you and your partner respond to a private home where, on entering the living room, you note there is a hospital bed set up in the corner of the room. The daughter has called 9-1-1 because she thinks her father, who has been suffering for a long time, has passed away. She leads you to the bathroom, where you can hear the son counting "19 and 20 and 21 and ..." as he provides chest compressions to his father on the floor of the small bathroom. The daughter states, "We just didn't know what to do. Dad wouldn't have wanted all this." You and your partner quickly move the patient, who weighs about 100 pounds, out into the living room, where there is more room.

a. List the conditions (termination rules) when it would be appropriate to stop the resuscitation in consult with medical control.

(1)_____

(2)_____

(3)_____

(4)_____

b. From the scenario described, what might lead you to ask if the patient was in a hospice program or has a do not resuscitate (DNR) order?

(1)_____

(2)_____

(3)_____

(4)_____

True/False

If you believe the statement to be more true than false, write the letter "T" in the space provided. If you believe the statement to be more false than true, write the letter "F."

_____ **1.** A possible cause of PEA is hypovolemia.

_____ **2.** A clue to the patient in cardiac arrest due to cardiac tamponade may be jugular venous distention.

_____ **3.** Beyond managing a cardiac arrest, if you suspect a tension pneumothorax, you should do a needle decompression on the affected side.

_____ **4.** Putrefaction is a discoloration of the skin caused by pooling of blood.

_____ **5.** If the patient has torsades de pointes, the paramedic should consider administering magnesium.

_____ **6.** Once you start CPR in the field, you should not stop until 15 minutes have gone by.

_____ **7.** An impedance threshold device (ITD) selectively prevents excess air from rushing into the chest during resuscitation.

_____ **8.** Once ROSC occurs, the ITD can be used to assist in the patient's ventilations.

_____ **9.** The two-hands encircling method should be used by a single rescuer doing infant CPR.

_____ **10.** In an adult who is unresponsive, where you suspect a foreign body airway obstruction, CPR chest compressions are used to attempt to clear the obstruction.

Short Answer

Complete this section with short written answers using the space provided.

1. The 2015 Institute of Medicine (Health and Medicine Division of the National Academies of Science, Engineering, and Medicine) report entitled *Strategies to Improve Cardiac Arrest Survival: A Time to Act* included key recommendations. List five of the recommendations:

   a. _____

   b. _____

   c. _____

   d. _____

   e. _____

2. The chapter describes a plan for prehospital response to a cardiac arrest with a five-person team. This is just an example of a "best practice" that could be practiced in your community, but it certainly is not the only way to manage a cardiac arrest; each community has different responders and resources. List the roles of the five-person team, and describe what they are responsible for.

   a. _____

   _____

   _____

   _____

   _____

   b. _____

   _____

   _____

   _____

   c. _____

   _____

   _____

   _____

   _____

d. _____

_____

_____

_____

_____

e. _____

_____

_____

_____

_____

Fill in the Table

Fill in the missing parts of the table.

Procedure	Key Elements of CPR for Adults, Children, and Infants		
	Age 9 to Adult	Age 1–8 Years	Younger Than 1 Year[a]
Circulation			
Recognition	Unresponsive with no breathing or only agonal (gasping) respirations		
Pulse check	_____	_____	Brachial artery
Compression location	In the center of the chest (lower half of the sternum)	In the center of the chest (lower half of the sternum)	_____
Hand placement	Heel of both hands	_____	Two-fingers or two-thumb encircling-hands technique
Compression depth	At least 2 in. (5 cm); not to exceed 2.4 in. (6 cm)	At least one-third of anterior-posterior diameter of chest; approximately 2 in. (5 cm)	_____
Compression rate	_____		
Chest wall recoil	Allow full chest recoil in between compressions. No _____! Rotate rescuers delivering compressions every 2 min		
Interruptions	Limit interruptions in delivery of chest compressions to less than 10 s		
Compression-to-ventilation ratio (until an advanced airway is inserted)	_____	_____ (one rescuer); (two professional rescuers)	_____
Airway			
Airway positioning	Head tilt-chin lift maneuver; jaw-thrust maneuver if _____ is suspected		
Breathing			
Untrained rescuer	Compressions only		
Ventilations without advanced airway	2 breaths with a duration of _____ each, with enough volume to produce _____[b]		

Key Elements of CPR for Adults, Children, and Infants			
Procedure	Age 9 to Adult	Age 1-8 Years	Younger Than 1 Year[a]
Ventilations with advanced airway	1 breath every 6 s (10/min) _____ with chest compressions; duration of 1 s each, with enough volume to produce chest rise	*Age 1 month to the onset of puberty:* 1 breath every 6-8 s (8-10 breaths/min); chest compressions delivered continuously at a rate of at least 100/min with no pauses for ventilations; duration of 1 s each, with enough volume to produce visible chest rise	
Rescue breathing	1 breath every _____ (10-12 breaths/min)	1 breath every _____ (12-20 breaths/min)	1 breath every _____ (12-20 breaths/min)
Defibrillation			
Device	Adult AED	Use _____ unit if available; if unavailable, then use adult unit	Use _____ if available; if unavailable, use unit with pediatric dose-attenuator; if neither is available, then use adult unit
Procedure	Attach AED as soon as it is available. If two rescuers are available, then one should immediately begin CPR while the second retrieves and applies the AED. Minimize CPR interruptions. Resume CPR immediately after shock, beginning with _____.		
Airway Obstruction			
Foreign body obstruction	Responsive: _____	Responsive: _____	Responsive: _____
	Unresponsive: _____ [c]		

Abbreviations: AED, automated external defibrillator; CPR, cardiopulmonary resuscitation.

[a]Excluding newborns, in whom arrest is usually the result of asphyxiation and requires the rescue ventilations.

[b]Pause compressions to deliver ventilations.

[c]Look in the mouth for objects before delivering breaths in a patient with a known airway obstruction.

Data from: Kleinman ME, Brennan EE, Goldberger ZD, et al. Part 5: Adult basic life support and cardiopulmonary resuscitation quality: 2015 American Heart Association Guidelines Update for Cardiopulmonary Resuscitation and Emergency Cardiovascular Care. Circulation. 2015;132(suppl 2):S414–S435; Atkins DL, Berger S, Duff JP, et al. Part 11: Pediatric basic life support and cardiopulmonary resuscitation quality: 2015 American Heart Association Guidelines Update for Cardiopulmonary Resuscitation and Emergency Cardiovascular Care. *Circulation*. 2015;132(suppl 2):S519–S525.

Management and Resuscitation of the Critical Patient

Some people, when they think they're up to their ears in alligators, forget to look out for a swamp.

© Jones & Bartlett Learning.

Matching

Part I

Match each of the terms in the right column to the appropriate definition in the left column.

_____ **1.** Sense organs that monitor the levels of oxygen and carbon dioxide and the pH of cerebrospinal fluid and blood and provide feedback to the respiratory centers to modify the rate and depth of breathing based on the body's needs at any given time.

A. Aerobic metabolism

_____ **2.** A condition that consists of cardiogenic shock and obstructive shock (Weil–Shubin classification).

B. Afterload

_____ **3.** Failure of the heart and blood vessels; shock.

C. Anaerobic metabolism

_____ **4.** A condition caused by loss of 40% or more of the functioning myocardium; the heart is no longer able to circulate sufficient blood to maintain adequate oxygen delivery.

D. Anaphylactic shock

_____ **5.** The volume of blood pumped through the circulatory system in 1 minute.

E. Anchoring bias

_____ **6.** The blood pressure required to sustain organ perfusion; roughly 60 mm Hg in the average person.

F. Angioedema

_____ **7.** The point at which shock has progressed to a terminal stage, resulting in death.

G. Baroreceptors

_____ **8.** Pattern recognition and pattern matching, based on your own past experiences.

H. Capacitance vessels

_____ **9.** A condition that occurs when the circulating blood volume is inadequate to deliver adequate oxygen and nutrients to the body.

I. Cardiac output

_____ **10.** A condition that occurs when the level of tissue perfusion decreases below that needed to maintain normal cellular functions; also called shock.

J. Cardiogenic shock

_____ **11.** A patient who is in premorbid condition, has experienced major trauma, or is in the peri-arrest period.

K. Cardiovascular collapse

_____ **12.** A type of bias that occurs with the tendency to gather and rely on information that confirms your existing views and to avoid or downplay information that does not conform to your preexisting hypothesis or field diagnosis.

L. Central shock

_____ **13.** The early stage of shock, in which the body can still compensate for blood loss. The systolic blood pressure and brain perfusion are maintained.

M. Chemoreceptors

_____ **14.** The smallest venules.

N. Compensated shock

_____ **15.** Receptors in the blood vessels, kidneys, brain, and heart that respond to changes in pressure in the heart or main arteries to help maintain homeostasis.

O. Confirmation bias

_____ **16.** Recurrent large areas of subcutaneous edema of sudden onset, usually disappearing within 24 hours, which is seen mainly in young women, frequently as a result of an allergy to food or drugs.

_____ **17.** A type of bias in which an initial reference point distorts your estimates.

_____ **18.** A principle that states the movement and use of oxygen in the body are dependent on an adequate concentration of inspired oxygen, appropriate movement of oxygen across the alveolar–capillary membrane into the arterial bloodstream, adequate number of red blood cells to carry the oxygen, proper tissue perfusion, and efficient offloading of oxygen at the tissue level.

_____ **19.** A condition that occurs when there is widespread dilation of the resistance vessels, the capacitance vessels, or both.

_____ **20.** A process in which molecules move from an area of higher concentration to an area of lower concentration.

_____ **21.** The process of weighing the probability of one disease versus other diseases by comparing clinical findings that could account for a patient's illness; also refers to the list of possible conditions considered based on the patient's signs and symptoms.

_____ **22.** The late stage of shock, when blood pressure is falling.

_____ **23.** A severe hypersensitivity reaction that involves bronchoconstriction and cardiovascular collapse.

_____ **24.** Metabolism that takes place in the absence of oxygen.

_____ **25.** The pressure in the aorta against which the left ventricle must pump blood.

_____ **26.** Metabolism that can proceed only in the presence of oxygen.

P. Critical patient

Q. Decompensated shock

R. Differential diagnosis

S. Diffusion

T. Distributive shock

U. Fick principle

V. Hypoperfusion

W. Hypovolemic shock

X. Intuition

Y. Irreversible shock

Z. Mean arterial pressure (MAP)

Part II

Match each of the terms in the right column to the appropriate definition in the left column.

_____ **1.** The initial stretching of the cardiac muscle prior to contraction. It is related to the chamber volume of blood just prior to the contraction.

_____ **2.** A condition that consists of hypovolemic shock and distributive shock (Weil–Shubin classification).

_____ **3.** The period either just before or just after cardiac arrest when the patient is critical and care must be taken to prevent progression or regression into cardiac arrest.

_____ **4.** The delivery of oxygen and nutrients to the cells, organs, and tissues of the body.

_____ **5.** A drop in systolic blood pressure when moving a patient from a sitting to a standing position.

_____ **6.** The one diagnosis from a differential list used to base the patient's treatment plan.

_____ **7.** The amount of time that specific tissues of the body are deprived of oxygen, typically as a result of an injury or arterial occlusion.

_____ **8.** The resistance to blood flow within all of the blood vessels except the pulmonary vessels.

_____ **9.** The amount of blood that the left ventricle ejects into the aorta per contraction.

_____ **10.** The local neurologic condition that occurs after a spinal injury produces motor and sensory losses (which may not be permanent).

_____ **11.** Shock that occurs when there is a block to blood flow in the heart or great vessels, causing an insufficient blood supply to the body's tissues.

_____ **12.** Shock that occurs as a result of fluid loss contained within the body, such as in dehydration, burn injury, crush injury, and anaphylaxis.

A. Multiple-organ dysfunction syndrome (MODS)

B. Myocardial contractility

C. Neurogenic shock

D. Nonhemorrhagic shock

E. Obstructive shock

F. Orthostatic hypotension

G. Perfusion

H. Peri-arrest period

I. Peripheral shock

J. Preload

K. Premorbid condition

L. Psychogenic shock

_____ 13. Circulatory failure caused by paralysis of the nerves that control the size of the blood vessels, leading to widespread dilation; seen in patients with spinal cord injuries.

_____ 14. The ability of the heart to contract.

_____ 15. A circular muscular wall of capillaries that constricts and dilates, acting as a gate to increase or decrease blood flow.

_____ 16. A progressive condition usually characterized by combined failure of several organs, such as the lungs, liver, and kidneys, along with some clotting mechanisms, which occurs after severe illness or injury.

_____ 17. An abnormal state associated with inadequate oxygen and nutrient delivery to the metabolic apparatus of the cell; also called hypoperfusion.

_____ 18. Shock caused by severe infection, usually a bacterial infection.

_____ 19. Developing a sensitivity to a substance that initially caused no allergic reaction.

_____ 20. The smallest arterioles.

_____ 21. The difference between the systolic blood pressure and the diastolic blood pressure.

_____ 22. A sudden reaction of the nervous system that produces a temporary, generalized vascular dilation, resulting in syncope (vasovagal syncope).

_____ 23. A condition preceding the onset of disease.

M. Pulse pressure

N. Resistance vessels

O. Sensitization

P. Septic shock

Q. Shock

R. Sphincter

S. Spinal shock

T. Stroke volume

U. Systemic vascular resistance

V. Warm ischemic time

W. Working diagnosis

Multiple Choice

Read each item carefully, and then select the best response.

_____ 1. The short list of potential causes of the patient's presenting condition is called the:
A. definitive diagnosis.
B. presenting problem.
C. differential diagnosis.
D. disposition.

_____ 2. Conditions that come before the onset of disease are called:
A. peri-arrest conditions.
B. premorbid conditions.
C. risk factors.
D. congenital defects.

_____ 3. With a patient who has a chief complaint of altered mental status, a starting point for the differential diagnosis can be remembered using the acronym:
A. SAMPLE.
B. M-T-SHIP.
C. OPQRST.
D. AVPU.

_____ 4. Intuition has a definite role in the assessment of critical patients by experienced providers. Intuition can:
A. forewarn you of what may happen next.
B. lead you to make treatment errors.
C. be difficult to teach.
D. All of the above

_____ 5. A tendency to gather and rely on information that confirms your existing assessment views is called a(n):
A. personal bias.
B. confirmation bias.
C. relieved decision.
D. anchoring bias.

_____ 6. The amount of circulation of blood within an organ or tissue in adequate amounts to meet the cells' current needs for oxygen, nutrients, and waste removal is referred to as:

   A. stroke volume.

   B. contractility.

   C. preload.

   D. perfusion.

_____ 7. The initial stretching of the cardiac muscle prior to contraction is called the:

   A. cardiac output.

   B. preload.

   C. afterload.

   D. stroke volume.

_____ 8. Your patient has a blood pressure of 110/70 mm Hg. What is his mean arterial pressure?

   A. 40

   B. 56

   C. 83

   D. 92

_____ 9. Stimulation of the sympathetic nervous system can cause the pupils to _____ and the heart rate to _____.

   A. dilate; increase

   B. dilate; decrease

   C. constrict; increase

   D. constrict; decrease

_____ 10. Stimulation of the parasympathetic nervous system can cause the gastrointestinal tract to:

   A. decrease motility.

   B. shut down.

   C. increase salivation.

   D. All of the above

_____ 11. Of the following, which is NOT considered an essential element of the Fick principle?

   A. Proper tissue perfusion

   B. Adequate number of white blood cells to carry oxygen

   C. Adequate concentration of inspired oxygen

   D. Efficient offloading of oxygen at the tissue level

_____ 12. The perfusion triangle includes each of the following, EXCEPT:

   A. the blood volume.

   B. the heart.

   C. insulin release by the pancreas.

   D. the blood vessels.

_____ 13. A progressive condition characterized by the combined failure of two or more organs or organ systems that were initially unharmed by the patient's initial illness is called:

   A. cardiovascular collapse.

   B. compensated shock.

   C. decompensated shock.

   D. multiple-organ dysfunction syndrome.

_____ 14. Your patient has sustained a serious internal injury. He is agitated, anxious, and restless. He complains of nausea and thirst and has a normal blood pressure. What phase of shock is he MOST likely in?

   A. Irreversible shock

   B. Compensated shock

   C. Decompensated shock

   D. Terminal shock

_____ **15.** Pediatric patients are unique, as compared to adults, in that they can often compensate even when they have lost up to _____ of their blood volume.

A. 15%

B. 25%

C. 35%

D. 45%

Labeling

Label the following diagram with the correct terms.

1. Relationship between the organism and the cells

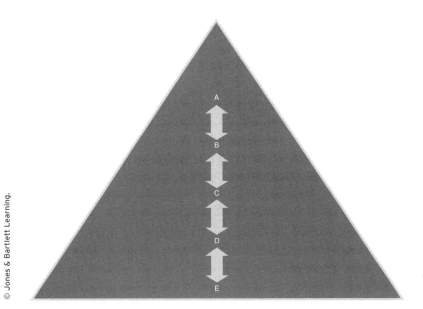

A. _____

B. _____

C. _____

D. _____

E. _____

© Jones & Bartlett Learning.

Fill in the Blank

Read each item carefully, and then complete the statement by filling in the missing word(s).

1. When the paramedic allows his or her initial reference point to distort an estimate while conducting the assessment, this is known as a(n) _____ bias.

2. To protect vital organs, the body attempts to _____ by _____ blood flow from organs that are more tolerant of low flow to vital organs that cannot tolerate hypoperfusion.

3. Blood flow through capillary beds is regulated by the capillary _____, circular muscular walls that constrict and dilate to increase or decrease flow.

4. Along with the baroreceptors are _____, which measure subtle shifts in the amount of carbon dioxide in the arterial blood.

5. The switch from _____ metabolism to _____ metabolism is a critical point that begins to produce lactic acidosis from this inefficient form of metabolism.

6. Effects of norepinephrine are primarily _____ and _____ in nature and center on vasoconstriction and

   _____ (increasing/decreasing) peripheral vascular resistance.

7. A reduction in _____ blood flow produces acute tubular _____, which in turn leads to _____ (urine

   output of less than 20 mL/h).

8. The last phase of shock, when this condition has progressed to a terminal stage, is _____ shock.

9. In cases of suspected _____ _____, you must recognize the need for expeditious transport for

   pericardiocentesis at the emergency department (ED).

10. _____ shock occurs when the heart is unable to circulate sufficient blood to maintain adequate peripheral oxygen

    delivery.

Identify

In the following case study, list the chief complaint, vital signs, and pertinent negatives.

You are called to the home of a 74-year-old man who is experiencing chest pain. Upon arrival, you begin your chest pain protocol. John, the patient, is experiencing tightness in his chest and left arm. You place John on high-flow supplemental oxygen and obtain a 12-lead electrocardiogram (ECG). You determine that John's heart is in a sinus bradycardia with a rate of 52 beats/min. Both his lungs have some crackles at their bases, he is breathing 24 breaths/min, and his room air saturation is SpO_2 92%. He is slightly confused, but he comes around with the oxygen and is able to answer all your questions. His pupils are equal, round, and reactive to light and accommodation (PERRLA). You are unable to feel a pulse in his wrist. His blood pressure (BP) is 80/56 mm Hg, and he is diaphoretic. You determine that the rate and strength of John's heart are causing the problem. You realize that John could be in cardiogenic shock. You start an IV line and a low-dose dopamine (Intropin) drip. You feel that John is a top priority and head to the most appropriate hospital as quickly as possible.

1. Chief complaint:

   _____

   _____

2. Vital signs:

   _____

   _____

3. Pertinent negatives:

   _____

   _____

Complete the Patient Care Report (PCR)

Reread the case study in the preceding Identify exercise, and then complete the following PCR for the patient.

EMS Patient Care Report (PCR)			
Date:	Incident No.:	Nature of Call:	Location:

Dispatched:	En Route:	At Scene:	Transport:	At Hospital:	In Service:

Patient Information	
Age: Sex: Weight (in kg [lb]):	Allergies: Medications: Past Medical History: Chief Complaint:

Vital Signs				
Time:	BP:	Pulse:	Respirations:	SpO$_2$:
Time:	BP:	Pulse:	Respirations:	SpO$_2$:
Time:	BP:	Pulse:	Respirations:	SpO$_2$:

EMS Treatment (circle all that apply)			
Oxygen @ _____ L/min via (circle one): NC NRM Bag-mask device	Assisted Ventilation	Airway Adjunct	CPR
Defibrillation	Bleeding Control	Bandaging	Splinting	Other:

Narrative

Ambulance Calls

The following case scenarios provide an opportunity to explore the concerns associated with patient management and paramedic care. Read each scenario, and then answer each question.

1. A 45-year old woman was struck by a motorcycle as she attempted to cross the street. You find her lying by the side of the road, reporting severe pain in her abdomen where the motorcycle hit her. To assess her state of perfusion, how will you assess the following?

   a. Her peripheral perfusion:

   _____

   b. The perfusion to her vital organs:

   _____

2. You are called to a downtown concert venue in which firearms may have been deployed. You find a man lying on the floor, unresponsive, with obvious bleeding on his leg. In the correct sequence, list the steps you will take in treating this patient who you suspect may be in shock.

   a. _____

   b. _____

   c. _____

   d. _____

   e. _____

   f. _____

3. A bomb exploded at a bus stop, injuring a number of bystanders. There was flying debris, including pieces of metal torn from the "backpack bomb." The first patient you come upon has multiple wounds, including a deep gash on the right side of the neck and a laceration that has partially severed the left leg near the groin. The leg laceration is gushing blood; it is too proximal to benefit from a tourniquet. Pulse is around 100 beats/min and somewhat weak; respirations are 30 breaths/min, and you suspect that the patient is already in shock.

   a. What steps would you take at the scene?

   (1)_____

   (2)_____

   (3)_____

   (4)_____

   b. What steps would you take during transport?

   (1)_____

   (2)_____

   (3)_____

4. A second patient from the bombing incident, an 18-year-old male, was injured by flying debris, which made a clean 10-inch incision straight across his abdomen. He is responsive and in moderate distress. This patient is a picture of shock. His pulse is 104 beats/min and regular, respirations are 28 breaths/min and slightly labored, and BP is 104/70 mm Hg. You see the patient's intestines outside his abdomen.

   a. What steps would you take at the scene?

      (1)_____

      (2)_____

      (3)_____

   b. What steps would you take during transport?

      (1)_____

      (2)_____

      (3)_____

5. A third patient from the car bombing incident is a 20-year-old female in considerable respiratory distress. There is a 2-inch-wide hole in her right chest through which you can hear air being sucked on inhalation. Her skin is warm. Her pulse is 108 beats/min and regular, respirations are 30 breaths/min and gasping, and BP is 112/64 mm Hg.

   a. What steps would you take at the scene?

      (1)_____

      (2)_____

      (3)_____

   b. What steps would you take during transport?

      (1)_____

      (2)_____

      (3)_____

6. A 55-year-old female was the driver of a car that crashed into a bridge abutment in the early hours of the morning. The patient is responsive but very restless. She is sweating profusely. Her chest is stable (it's too dark to see whether there are bruises). She can move all her extremities. Her pulse is 88 beats/min, respirations are 28 breaths/min, and BP is 100/68 mm Hg.

   a. What steps would you take at the scene?

      (1)_____

      (2)_____

      (3)_____

      (4)_____

      (5)_____

b. What steps would you take during transport?

(1)_____

(2)_____

(3)_____

(4)_____

True/False

If you believe the statement to be more true than false, write the letter "T" in the space provided. If you believe the statement to be more false than true, write the letter "F."

_____   **1.** The patient with obstructive shock may have jugular vein distention.

_____   **2.** Cardiogenic shock can lead to warm skin and hypertension.

_____   **3.** Severe bacterial infection can lead to septic shock.

_____   **4.** Simple fainting is also called psychogenic shock.

_____   **5.** The capacitance vessels are the small arterioles.

_____   **6.** When a patient is in "cold shock," he or she may benefit from epinephrine.

_____   **7.** Neurogenic shock usually results from spinal cord injury.

_____   **8.** Sensitization means developing a heightened reaction to a substance.

_____   **9.** A recurrent large area of subcutaneous edema of sudden onset, usually disappearing within 24 hours and mainly seen in young women, is called angioedema.

_____   **10.** Poor vessel function, a cause of shock, can be caused by infection and/or drug abuse.

Short Answer

Complete this section with short written answers using the space provided.

1. List what each of the following could indicate using the acronym M-T-SHIP:

M._____

T._____

S._____

H._____

I._____

P._____

2. Karl Weick's "five-step process" for communicating intuitive decisions and obtaining feedback from team members includes:

a._____

b._____

c._____

d._____

e._____

Fill in the Table

Fill in the missing parts of the tables.

1. The "H and T" questions of cardiac arrest

Reversible Causes of Cardiac Arrest	Questions to Ask Your Team
Hypovolemia	Does this patient have any evidence of internal or external bleeding or fluid loss?
	How well is the patient oxygenating?
_____	Could there have been a respiratory event that led to this cardiac arrest?
Hydrogen ion (acidosis)	Is there any reason for metabolic or respiratory acidosis in this patient?
	Does this patient undergo renal dialysis?
_____	Might the electrolytes be altered (ie, is the patient on a liquid diet)?
Hypothermia	Does the patient feel cold to touch? If so, obtain the core body temperature.
_____	Does the patient have diabetes? What is the blood glucose level?
Tension pneumothorax	Does the patient have bilateral breath sounds?
	Is the patient becoming difficult to ventilate?
	Consider the need for chest decompression.
	Is there penetrating trauma to the patient's heart?
_____	Consider the need for pericardiocentesis or ultrasound (in the emergency department).
Toxins	Consider substance abuse (ie, narcotics or opiates). Consider naloxone (Narcan) intravenously/intramuscularly/intranasally.
	Does the patient have a history of blood clots?
	Does the patient smoke and/or take birth control?
_____	Has the patient had a recent long-bone immobilization?
Thrombosis (coronary)	Does the patient have a large acute myocardial infarction developing?
	Is this patient a candidate for percutaneous coronary intervention (PCI)?
_____	Is there a mechanism of injury for life-threatening trauma?

2. Compensated versus decompensated shock

Compensated Shock	Decompensated Shock
• Agitation, anxiety, restlessness	• Altered mental status (verbal to unresponsive)[a]
• _____	• _____
• Weak, rapid (thready) pulse	• _____
• Clammy (cool, moist) skin	• Thready or absent peripheral pulses
• _____	• Ashen, mottled, or cyanotic skin
• _____	• _____
• Nausea, vomiting	• Diminished urine output (oliguria)
• Delayed capillary refill in infants and children	• _____
• _____	
• _____	

[a]Mental status changes are late indicators.

3. Types of shock

Types of Shock	Examples of Potential Causes	Signs and Symptoms	Assessment and Treatment
_____	Inadequate heart function Disease of muscle tissue Impaired electrical system Disease or injury	Chest pain Irregular pulse Weak pulse Low BP Cyanosis (lips, under nails) Cool, clammy, mottled, or flushed skin Anxiety Rales Pulmonary edema Hepatomegaly	_____ _____

_____	Mechanical obstruction of the cardiac muscle causing a decrease in cardiac output
	1. Tension pneumothorax
	2. Cardiac tamponade
		Dependent on cause:
		• Dyspnea
		• Rapid, weak pulse
		• Rapid, shallow breaths
		• Decreased lung compliance
		• Unilateral, decreased, or absent breath sounds
		• Decreased BP
		• JVD
		• Subcutaneous emphysema
		• Cyanosis
		• Tracheal deviation toward affected side
		• Beck triad (cardiac tamponade):
		  – JVD
		  – Narrowing pulse pressure
		  – Muffled heart tones
			_____
			_____
			_____
			_____

_____	Severe bacterial infection	Warm, unstable skin temperatures Tachycardia Low blood pressure	_____ _____ _____
_____	Cervical or thoracic spinal cord injury, which causes widespread blood vessel dilation	Bradycardia (slow pulse) or normal pulse Low BP Signs of neck injury	_____ _____
_____	Extreme life-threatening allergic reaction	Develop within seconds Mild itching or rash Burning skin Vascular dilation Generalized edema Coma Rapid death	_____ _____ _____ _____

	Temporary, generalized vascular dilation Anxiety, bad news, sight of injury or blood, prospect of medical treatment, severe pain, illness, tiredness	Rapid pulse Normal or low BP	
	Blood or fluid loss	Rapid, weak pulse Low BP Change in mental status Cyanosis (lips, nail beds) Cool, clammy skin Increased respiratory rate	
	Severe chest injury, airway obstruction	Rapid, weak pulse Low BP Change in mental status Cyanosis (lips, nail beds) Cool, clammy skin Increased respiratory rate	

Abbreviations: BP, blood pressure; CPAP/BPAP, continuous positive airway pressure/bilevel positive airway pressure; IM, intramuscularly; JVD, jugular venous distention; KVO, keep vein open.

SPECIAL PATIENT POPULATIONS

Obstetrics

Puerperal fevers declined significantly with the novel introduction of physicians washing their hands between patients.

PARAMEDICS HAVE NO EXCUSE!

EMT 101

SLAM

© Jones & Bartlett Learning.

Matching

Part I

Match each of the items in the left column to the appropriate term in the right column.

_____ **1.** The developing, unborn infant inside the uterus.

_____ **2.** A situation in which a fetus is large, usually defined as weighing more than 4,500 g (almost 9 pounds); also known as "large for gestational age."

_____ **3.** An incision in the perineal skin made to prevent tearing during childbirth.

_____ **4.** Intentional expulsion of the fetus.

_____ **5.** Thinning and shortening of the cervix; a normal process that occurs as the uterus contracts.

_____ **6.** A disease of the liver that occurs only during pregnancy, in which hormones affect the gallbladder by slowing down or blocking the normal bile flow from the liver; the most common symptom is profuse, painful itching, particularly of the hands and feet.

_____ **7.** The interior of the cervix.

_____ **8.** A situation in which the head of the fetus is larger than the woman's pelvis; in most cases, cesarean section is required for such a delivery.

_____ **9.** A delivery in which the buttocks come out first.

_____ **10.** A plug of mucus, sometimes mixed with blood, that is expelled from the dilating cervix and discharged from the vagina.

_____ **11.** The fluid-filled, baglike membrane in which the fetus develops.

_____ **12.** An extremely rare, life-threatening condition that occurs when amniotic fluid and fetal cells enter the pregnant woman's pulmonary and circulatory system through the placenta via the umbilical veins, causing an exaggerated allergic response from the woman's body.

_____ **13.** A watery fluid that provides the fetus with a weightless environment in which to develop.

_____ **14.** A premature separation of the placenta from the wall of the uterus.

_____ **15.** Expulsion of the fetus, from any cause, before 20 weeks' gestation.

_____ **16.** A scoring system for assessing the status of a newborn that assigns a number value to each of five areas of assessment.

_____ **17.** The term for an oocyte once it has been fertilized and multiplies into cells.

_____ **18.** A hormone produced by the anterior pituitary gland that is important in the menstrual cycle.

A. Abortion

B. Abruptio placenta

C. Amniotic fluid

D. Amniotic fluid embolism

E. Amniotic sac

F. Apgar scoring system

G. Blastocyst

H. Bloody show

I. Breech presentation

J. Cephalopelvic disproportion

K. Cervical canal

L. Cholestasis

M. Chronic hypertension

N. Complete abortion

O. Corpus luteum

P. Crowning

Q. Cytomegalovirus (CMV)

R. Eclampsia

_____ **19.** The stage of labor that begins with the onset of regular labor pains (crampy abdominal pains) during which the uterus contracts and the cervix effaces.

_____ **20.** An egg that attaches outside the uterus, typically in a fallopian tube.

_____ **21.** Seizures that result from severe hypertension in a pregnant woman.

_____ **22.** A herpesvirus that can produce symptoms of prolonged high fever, chills, headache, malaise, extreme fatigue, and an enlarged spleen.

_____ **23.** The appearance of the newborn's body part (usually the head) at the vaginal opening at the beginning of labor.

_____ **24.** The remains of a follicle after an oocyte has been released; secretes progesterone.

_____ **25.** Expulsion of all products of conception from the uterus.

_____ **26.** A blood pressure that is equal to or greater than 140/90 mm Hg and exists prior to pregnancy, occurs before the 20th week of pregnancy, or persists postpartum.

S. Ectopic pregnancy

T. Effacement

U. Elective abortion

V. Episiotomy

W. Fetal macrosomia

X. Fetus

Y. First stage of labor

Z. Follicle-stimulating hormone (FSH)

Part II

Match each of the items in the left column to the appropriate term in the right column.

_____ **1.** A dark green-black material in the amniotic fluid that indicates fetal distress, and that can be aspirated into the fetus's lungs during delivery; the fetus's first bowel movement.

_____ **2.** The vaginal discharge of blood and mucus that occurs following delivery of a newborn; it usually lasts several days and then gradually decreases over the weeks following delivery.

_____ **3.** In pregnancy, a feeling of relief of pressure in the upper abdomen; a premonitory sign of labor.

_____ **4.** The mechanism by which the fetus and the placenta are expelled from the uterus.

_____ **5.** A protein that plays a key role in the menstrual cycle by triggering release of follicle-stimulating hormone.

_____ **6.** The outer protective layer of tissue in the uterus.

_____ **7.** The number of live births a woman has had.

_____ **8.** A mature oocyte.

_____ **9.** A situation in which the umbilical cord is wrapped around the fetus's neck; cord compression may occur during labor, causing the fetal heart rate to slow and resulting in fetal distress.

_____ **10.** The middle layer of tissue in the uterus.

_____ **11.** A situation in which the umbilical cord comes out of the vagina before the newborn.

_____ **12.** The state of the pregnant woman before birth.

_____ **13.** A condition of late pregnancy that involves gradual onset of hypertension, headache, visual changes, and swelling of the hands and feet; also called pregnancy-induced hypertension or toxemia of pregnancy.

_____ **14.** The period of time after a woman has given birth.

_____ **15.** A condition in which the placenta develops over and covers the cervix.

_____ **16.** A situation in which a fetus has died during the first 20 weeks of gestation, but has remained in utero.

_____ **17.** The tissue attached to the uterine wall that nourishes the fetus through the umbilical cord.

_____ **18.** Expulsion of the fetus that results in some products of conception remaining in the uterus.

A. Gestational hypertension

B. Gestational period

C. Gravidity

D. Habitual abortion

E. Human immunodeficiency virus (HIV)

F. Hydramnios

G. Hyperemesis gravidarum

H. Imminent abortion

I. Incomplete abortion

J. Inhibin

K. Labor

L. Lightening

M. Lochia

N. Meconium

O. Missed abortion

P. Myometrium

Q. Nuchal cord

R. Ovum

_____ **19.** A spontaneous abortion that cannot be prevented.

_____ **20.** A condition of persistent nausea and vomiting during pregnancy.

_____ **21.** A condition in which there is too much amniotic fluid; also known as polyhydramnios.

_____ **22.** The time that it takes for the fetus to develop in utero, normally 38 weeks.

_____ **23.** The total number of times a woman has been pregnant, including the current pregnancy.

_____ **24.** Three or more consecutive pregnancies that end in miscarriage.

_____ **25.** An infection that causes acquired immune deficiency syndrome (AIDS).

_____ **26.** High blood pressure that develops after 20th week of pregnancy in women with previously normal blood pressures, and that resolves spontaneously in the postpartum period; formerly known as pregnancy-induced hypertension.

S. Parity

T. Perimetrium

U. Placenta

V. Placenta previa

W. Postpartum

X. Preeclampsia

Y. Prenatal

Z. Prolapsed umbilical cord

Part III

Match each of the items in the left column to the appropriate term in the right column.

_____ **1.** A potentially fatal complication of childbirth in which the placenta fails to detach properly and results in the uterus turning inside out.

_____ **2.** The interior of the body of the uterus.

_____ **3.** The conduit connecting the pregnant woman to the fetus via the placenta; it contains two arteries and one vein.

_____ **4.** A delivery in which the fetus lies crosswise in the uterus; one hand may protrude through the vagina.

_____ **5.** Expulsion of the fetus that occurs naturally; also called miscarriage.

_____ **6.** A complication of delivery in where there is difficulty delivering the shoulders of a newborn; the shoulder cannot get past the woman's symphysis pubis.

_____ **7.** A life-threatening emergency in which the uterus becomes infected following any type of abortion.

_____ **8.** The stage of labor in which the newborn's head enters the birth canal, during which contractions become more intense and more frequent.

_____ **9.** Expulsion of the fetus that is attempting to take place but has not occurred yet; usually occurs in the first trimester.

_____ **10.** The stage of labor in which the placenta is expelled.

_____ **11.** Low blood pressure resulting from compression of the inferior vena cava by the weight of the pregnant uterus when the woman is supine.

_____ **12.** A protein found on the red blood cells of most people; when a woman without this protein is impregnated by a man with this protein, the woman's body can create antibodies against the protein that attack future pregnancies.

_____ **13.** An infection caused by a parasite that pregnant women may get from handling or eating contaminated food or exposure from handling cat litter; the fetus can become infected.

_____ **14.** An infection that occurs in neonates as a result of organisms passing through the placenta from the woman to the fetus; includes toxoplasmosis, other agents, rubella, cytomegalovirus, and herpes simplex.

A. Rh factor

B. Second stage of labor

C. Septic abortion

D. Shoulder dystocia

E. Spontaneous abortion

F. Supine hypotensive syndrome

G. Third stage of labor

H. Threatened abortion

I. TORCH syndrome

J. Toxoplasmosis

K. Transverse presentation

L. Umbilical cord

M. Uterine cavity

N. Uterine inversion

Multiple Choice

Read each item carefully, and then select the best response.

_____ 1. An abortion that occurs naturally and affects 10% to 25% of all pregnancies is called a(n):

   A. spontaneous abortion.

   B. septic abortion.

   C. threatened abortion.

   D. incomplete abortion.

_____ 2. What is the condition in which the placenta is implanted low in the uterus and, as it grows, it partially obscures the cervical canal?

   A. Abruptio placenta

   B. Molar pregnancy

   C. Pseudocyesis

   D. Placenta previa

_____ 3. Which of the following terms describes a woman who has had two or more pregnancies, irrespective of the outcome?

   A. Multigravida

   B. Primipara

   C. Multipara

   D. Parity

_____ 4. When the baby's head enters the birth canal, the _____ stage of labor begins.

   A. fourth

   B. third

   C. second

   D. first

_____ 5. The Apgar scoring system is an evaluation tool for the newborn's vital functions and is recommended to be taken at which intervals after birth?

   A. 2 minutes and 10 minutes

   B. 1 minute and 5 minutes

   C. 5 minutes and 10 minutes

   D. 1 minute and 2 minutes

_____ 6. _____ of blood loss, or more, after delivery is considered postpartum hemorrhage.

   A. 1,000 mL

   B. 150 mL

   C. 750 mL

   D. 500 mL

_____ 7. Which of the following medications can be used to control postpartum hemorrhage in the prehospital setting?

   A. Oxytocin

   B. Terbutaline

   C. Magnesium sulfate

   D. Diphenhydramine

_____ 8. An infection that occurs in neonates as a result of organisms passing through the placenta from woman to fetus is referred to as:

   A. RSV.

   B. toxoplasmosis.

   C. hemolytic disease.

   D. Down syndrome.

_____ **9.** The normal gestational period for an infant to develop in the uterus is how many weeks?

    A. 30

    B. 32

    C. 38

    D. 42

_____ **10.** A pregnant woman's heart rate gradually increases during pregnancy by an average of how many beats/min by term?

    A. 15 to 20 beats/min

    B. 5 to 10 beats/min

    C. 20 to 25 beats/min

    D. 15 to 30 beats/min

Labeling

Label the following diagram with the correct terms.

1. Structures of the pregnant uterus

© Jones & Bartlett Learning.

A. _____

B. _____

C. _____

D. _____

E. _____

Fill in the Blank

Read each item carefully, and then complete the statement by filling in the missing word(s).

1. The _____ is a membranous bag that encloses the fetus in watery fluid.

2. The workload of the heart _____ significantly during both gestation and labor.

3. As maternal oxygen demand _____, the respiratory physiology changes.

4. _____ is the most serious of the hypertension disorders that occur during pregnancy.

5. _____ _____ develops after the 20th week of pregnancy in women with a normal blood pressure.

6. Some women experience recurrent miscarriages or _____ _____.

7. _____ _____ refers to a premature partial or incomplete separation of a normally implanted placenta from the uterus.

8. The _____ _____ of labor begins with the onset of labor.

9. In a(n) _____ presentation, the fetus lies crosswise in the uterus and may wave at the paramedic with one hand protruding from the vagina.

10. _____ _____ is a drug used in pregnancy as the principal management for eclampsia.

Identify

After reading the following case study, list the chief complaint, vital signs, and pertinent findings.

You are called to a private residence for a report of a pregnant patient who has vaginal bleeding. The patient is lying in bed. When you ask what is wrong, she tells you, "I am bleeding from my vagina." You see blood on the sheets. You and your partner start a primary survey. You then take the vital signs, and your partner obtains a SAMPLE history. The patient is 35 years old and states that she started to bleed about half an hour ago. Upon questioning, she tells you there is no pain, the blood was bright red, this is her third pregnancy, and she is in her eighth month. Both the previous pregnancies were full term and delivered by cesarean section. She states that she had strong contractions, but they have decreased. She feels weak and asks if she can have a drink of water. She has no allergies, is taking vitamin supplements per doctor's orders, has no significant past medical history, and had a light breakfast of toast and juice about 2 hours ago. Your partner reports the pulse to be 110 beats/min and thready, respirations are 24 breaths/min, blood pressure (BP) is 100/70 mm Hg, SpO_2 is 94%, and the patient is pale and diaphoretic. The patient tells you that the BP reading you just measured is lower than the pressure the doctor measured last week at her checkup appointment. You put the patient on 100% supplemental oxygen using a nonrebreathing mask, place a loose trauma pad over the vagina, prepare for immediate transport, start a large-bore IV line in the ambulance, contact medical control to discuss the use of magnesium sulfate (some emergency medical services [EMS] systems may use this medication in this kind of case), and notify the hospital so that personnel there can be properly prepared upon your arrival. You arrive at the receiving facility in 15 minutes and are told to go immediately to the delivery room. Later that evening while delivering another patient to the same hospital, you are informed that the mother delivered, and although the baby's birth weight is low, both the mother and the baby are expected to be fine.

1. Chief complaint:

_____

_____

2. Vital signs:

_____

_____

3. Pertinent findings:

_____

_____

Complete the Patient Care Report (PCR)

Reread the incident scenario in the preceding Identify exercise and then complete the following PCR for the patient.

EMS Patient Care Report (PCR)			
Date:	Incident No.:	Nature of Call:	Location:
Dispatched:	En Route:	At Scene:	Transport:	At Hospital:	In Service:

Patient Information	
Age:	Allergies:
Sex:	Medications:
Weight (in kg [lb]):	Past Medical History:
	Chief Complaint:

Vital Signs

Time:	BP:	Pulse:	Respirations:	SpO$_2$:
Time:	BP:	Pulse:	Respirations:	SpO$_2$:
Time:	BP:	Pulse:	Respirations:	SpO$_2$:

EMS Treatment
(circle all that apply)

Oxygen @ _____ L/min via (circle one): NC NRM Bag-mask device	Assisted Ventilation	Airway Adjunct	CPR
Defibrillation	Bleeding Control	Bandaging	Splinting	Other:

Narrative

Ambulance Calls

The following case scenarios provide an opportunity to explore the concerns associated with patient management and paramedic care. Read each scenario, and then answer each question.

1. A 22-year-old woman calls for an ambulance because of vaginal bleeding. She states that she is "about 3 months pregnant" and that the bleeding started yesterday, when she thinks she passed some tissue. She has used about 10 sanitary napkins since then. On examination, her skin feels cool and wet. Her pulse is 120 beats/min and weak, and her BP is 90/60 mm Hg.

   a. This woman is likely experiencing a(n) _____ abortion.

     A. threatened

     B. imminent

     C. incomplete

     D. missed

     E. septic

   b. List the steps in the prehospital management of this patient.

     (1)_____

     (2)_____

     (3)_____

     (4)_____

     (5)_____

     (6)_____

     (7)_____

2. A 32-year-old woman calls for an ambulance because she is "feeling poorly." She states that she is "about 6 months along" in a pregnancy. She has not had any prenatal care. She had some vaginal bleeding "early on," but it lasted only a few days and then stopped. Now, for several days, the patient has felt vaguely unwell. She has had a brownish vaginal discharge that smells rank, and "things are very quiet in there." On physical examination, the patient does not appear to be in any distress. Her pulse is 74 beats/min and regular, respirations are 18 breaths/min and unlabored, and BP is 120/80 mm Hg. On abdominal examination, you can feel the uterine fundus just above the pelvic brim; it feels quite hard. You are not able to hear fetal heart tones, but the room is noisy, so you are not sure what to make of that finding.

   a. This woman is likely experiencing a(n) _____ abortion.

     A. threatened

     B. imminent

     C. incomplete

     D. missed

     E. septic

   b. Describe the prehospital management required for this patient.

     _____

     _____

3. A 20-year-old primigravida calls for an ambulance because of vaginal bleeding. She states that she is in her fourth month of pregnancy and has been fine up to now, but this morning she noticed some bleeding. She denies abdominal pain or cramping. On physical examination, there are no abnormal findings.

   a. This woman is likely experiencing a(n) _____ abortion.

     A. threatened

     B. imminent

     C. incomplete

     D. missed

     E. septic

b. Describe the prehospital management required for this patient.

_____

_____

4. You are called to a suburban home for a "sick girl." The patient is a 16-year-old girl with a high fever. She insists on giving you her history privately, without her parents in the room. After her parents exit, the girl tells you that she had gone that morning to "some hole in the wall" to have an abortion. A few hours after she got home, she started to feel sick, and she has been having a bad-smelling, bloody vaginal discharge ever since. On examination, she looks very ill. Her pulse is 120 beats/min and weak, respirations are 28 breaths/min and shallow, BP is 80/60 mm Hg, and oral temperature is 40°C (104°F).

a. This patient is likely experiencing a(n) _____ abortion.
- **A.** threatened
- **B.** imminent
- **C.** incomplete
- **D.** missed
- **E.** septic

b. List the steps in the prehospital management of this patient.

(1)_____

(2)_____

(3)_____

(4)_____

(5)_____

(6)_____

5. You are called to the home of a weeping 26-year-old woman in the 15th week of pregnancy. "It's happening again," she sobs, "I just know it's happening again." She tells you that she has had three miscarriages in the past and that this morning she started having severe abdominal cramps and bleeding, "just like all the other times." She has used six sanitary napkins since the bleeding started about 3 hours ago. On physical examination, she is very distraught. Her pulse is 110 beats/min and regular, respirations are 24 breaths/min and unlabored, BP is 110/70 mm Hg, and she is febrile. On palpating the abdomen, you can feel the uterine contractions.

a. This woman is likely experiencing a(n) _____ abortion.
- **A.** threatened
- **B.** imminent
- **C.** incomplete
- **D.** missed
- **E.** septic

b. List the steps in the prehospital management of this patient.

(1)_____

(2)_____

(3)_____

(4)_____

(5)_____

6. You are called to the home of a 36-year-old grand multipara whose chief complaint is bleeding. She is in her 11th pregnancy and "due any day now." She states that the bleeding, a bright red blood, started a few hours ago without any warning. She has not had any cramps or other symptoms, and "the baby is still kicking like a soccer player." On physical examination, the woman looks a little pale and apprehensive. Her pulse is 124 beats/min and regular, respirations are 28 breaths/min and unlabored, and BP is 100/68 mm Hg; she is afebrile. On gentle palpation, you find the abdomen soft. The fundus is at the level of the xiphoid, and fetal heart tones are audible. The fetal heart rate is 140 beats/min.

a. List three possible causes of this woman's bleeding.

(1)_____

(2)_____

(3)_____

b. Of those three causes, which do you think is the most likely cause in her case?

_____

c. Which signs led you to this diagnosis?

(1)_____

(2)_____

(3)_____

(4)_____

d. List the steps you will take in managing this patient.

(1)_____

(2)_____

(3)_____

(4)_____

(5)_____

(6)_____

7. You are called to see a 28-year-old woman in her 35th week of pregnancy after she had a "fainting spell." The patient's husband greets you at the door and tells you, "We were just sitting there talking—Agnes was lying in bed, and I was sitting in the chair—and suddenly I look over, and I see that she's out cold. Not sleeping, just out." The patient has meanwhile regained consciousness. She says she feels rather dizzy and has a slight headache but otherwise feels well. She denies vaginal bleeding. On physical examination, her pulse is 104 beats/min and regular, her respirations are 24 breaths/min and unlabored, and her BP is 90/60 mm Hg. You have her roll onto her side and recheck her vital signs a few minutes later; her pulse is now 88 beats/min and her BP is 120/72 mm Hg. Her fundus is nearly at the level of the xiphoid, and fetal heart tones are present at a rate of 160 beats/min.

a. This woman is likely experiencing

   A. an inevitable abortion.
   B. preeclampsia.
   C. eclampsia.
   D. abruptio placenta.
   E. supine hypotensive syndrome.

b. List the steps in the prehospital care of this patient.

(1)_____

(2)_____

(3)_____

(4)_____

(5)_____

8. You are called to a downtown department store, where an obviously pregnant woman has fallen and twisted her ankle. You find her surrounded by a knot of agitated people, none of them more agitated than the store manager. As you are checking the woman's pedal pulses, you notice that both ankles are swollen—not just the one she injured. You decide you had better get a set of vital signs because you vaguely remember learning that vital signs should be measured in every patient, especially every pregnant patient. In this woman, you find the pulse is 110 beats/min and regular, respirations are 20 breaths/min and unlabored, and BP is 150/90 mm Hg. As you are taking the radial pulse, you notice that the patient's hands seem puffy. It is too noisy in the store to even bother trying to listen for fetal heart tones, but the woman tells you that the baby is "kicking away."
   a. This woman is likely experiencing:
   A. an inevitable abortion.
   B. preeclampsia.
   C. eclampsia.
   D. abruptio placenta.
   E. supine hypotensive syndrome.

   b. List the steps in the prehospital care of this patient.

   (1)_____

   (2)_____

   (3)_____

   c. En route to the hospital, you find yourself locked in a traffic jam on the freeway. Meanwhile, your patient starts complaining of cramping abdominal pains. "I've never had a baby before," she says, "but I think these are labor pains." While you look helplessly at the line of cars stretching endlessly in front of and behind the ambulance, the woman's eyes suddenly roll back, and she has a grand mal seizure. Which steps will you take now?

   (1)_____

   (2)_____

   (3)_____

   (4)_____

   (5)_____

9. A 26-year-old woman in her 30th week of pregnancy was the driver of a car that skidded off the road and plowed head-on into a tree. The woman was wearing a shoulder/lap seat belt. Sitting in the passenger seat of the same car was a woman in her 28th week of pregnancy (they were returning together from a natural childbirth class), also wearing a seat

belt. En route to the call, you try to review in your mind the injuries you will need to look for in particular because you remember that pregnancy makes a woman more vulnerable to trauma.

a. List five anatomic or physiologic changes of pregnancy that affect a woman's susceptibility or response to trauma.

(1)_____

(2)_____

(3)_____

(4)_____

(5)_____

b. On reaching the scene of the accident, you find the driver of the car conscious, still sitting behind the wheel of the car. She complains of thirst. On physical examination, her skin is cool and moist. Her pulse is 120 beats/min and regular, respirations are 24 breaths/min and shallow, and BP is 110/68 mm Hg. There is a steering wheel bruise on the upper abdomen. The abdomen is not particularly tender, and it is not rigid. The conditions are too noisy to try to hear fetal heart tones. List the steps in managing this patient.

(1)_____

(2)_____

(3)_____

(4)_____

(5)_____

(6)_____

(7)_____

c. The front-seat passenger is also fully conscious. She complains of "whiplash" but otherwise feels well. "At least the baby's okay," she says. "I can feel him moving around." On physical examination, her skin is warm and moist. Her pulse is 100 beats/min and regular, respirations are 20 breaths/min and unlabored, and her BP is 124/70 mm Hg. You do not find any evidence of injury. Can you conclude that there has been no injury to the fetus? Explain the reason for your answer.

_____

_____

_____

_____

10. For each of the following cases, indicate one of the following:

T There is time to transport the woman to the hospital for delivery.

D You will have to assist in emergency delivery in the field.

For each case that you decide requires prehospital delivery, indicate which, if any, complications you must anticipate.

_____ **a.** A 20-year-old nullipara (gravida 1, para 0) in her first pregnancy. She says her water broke about 6 hours ago. Now her contractions are about 2 minutes apart, and she feels a need to move her bowels. You are 20 minutes from the hospital. Which, if any, complications may occur?

_____

_____

_____ **b.** A 32-year-old multipara (gravida 10, para 8) who has been in labor about 5 hours. Her contractions are 3 minutes apart. She says she thinks the baby's coming. You are 10 minutes from the hospital. What, if any, complications may occur?

_____

_____

_____ **c.** A 25-year-old nullipara (gravida 1, para 0) who has been in labor for 9 hours. Her contractions are 4 to 5 minutes apart. You are 20 minutes from the hospital. Which, if any, complications may occur?

_____

_____

_____ **d.** A 30-year-old multipara (gravida 4, para 3) who has been in labor for 6 hours. She had two of her three children by cesarean section. Her contractions are 2 minutes apart, and she is crowning. You are 5 minutes from the hospital. Which, if any, complications may occur?

_____

_____

_____ **e.** A 28-year-old nullipara (gravida 1, para 0) whose contractions started 24 hours ago. They do not come at regular intervals, and they have not gotten much more intense since they started. You are 25 minutes from the hospital. Which, if any, complications may occur?

_____

_____

_____ **f.** A 24-year-old multipara (gravida 3, para 2) who announces, as you enter her apartment, "Hurry, the twins are coming any minute!" She says she has been in labor "quite a while," and you time her contractions as coming less than 2 minutes apart. You are 20 minutes from the hospital. Which, if any, complications may occur?

_____

_____

11. You are assisting in the delivery of a baby in the lingerie section of a downtown department store.
   a. The baby's head delivers spontaneously, and you notice that it is covered with a membrane. What should you do?

_____

_____

   b. You deal with that problem successfully. The next thing you notice is that the umbilical cord is wound tightly around the baby's neck. What should you do about that?

_____

_____

   c. List the steps in carrying out the remainder of the delivery (second and third stages).

   (1)_____

   (2)_____

(3)_____

(4)_____

(5)_____

(6)_____

(7)_____

(8)_____

(9)_____

12. During another one of your weekends off at the ski lodge, when you are cheerfully snowed in, one of the other guests arrives in the lounge and asks, "Does anyone here know anything about delivering a baby? My wife seems to be in labor." You shrivel up into a corner of your chair, hoping someone else will come forward, but there do not seem to be any obstetricians among the skiers. So, with a sigh, you stand up and follow the distraught husband to his room. There you find a woman in active labor, already crowning. Inspecting the presenting part, you note that it looks awfully smooth, and it has a sort of crack running down the middle.

a. What are you dealing with?

_____

_____

b. Describe how you will manage this case.

(1)_____

_____

(2)_____

_____

(3)_____

_____

(4)_____

_____

(5)_____

_____

(6)_____

_____

(7)_____

_____

13. The day after you get back to work, your very first call is another "possible OB." The patient is a 24-year-old woman in her first pregnancy whose labor started about 10 hours earlier. "This wasn't supposed to happen for another month and a half," she tells you. The contractions are now about 2 minutes apart. When you inspect her to see whether she is crowning, you see a short length of umbilical cord protruding from her vagina. Describe how you will manage this case.

a. _____

b. _____

c. _____

d. _____

e. _____

f. _____

14. You are called to the home of a 30-year-old gravida 6, para 5, who has gone into labor. "It's twins," she announces as soon as you come in the door. "I'm carrying twins, and they're coming at any moment. I can feel it." And indeed, when you examine the woman, you find that she is crowning.
   a. Describe the special measures necessary in this case.

   (1)_____

   (2)_____

   b. After delivery of the placenta, the mother continues bleeding quite briskly from her vagina. Did this woman have any risk factors for postpartum hemorrhage? If so, what were they?

   _____

   _____

   c. List three other risk factors for postpartum hemorrhage.

   (1)_____

   (2)_____

   (3)_____

   d. Describe how you will manage this situation.

   (1)_____

   (2)_____

   (3)_____

   (4)_____

   (5)_____

   (6)_____

True/False

If you believe the statement to be more true than false, write the letter "T" in the space provided. If you believe the statement to be more false than true, write the letter "F."

_____   1. If you are transporting a woman in labor, and she begins crowning when you are only a minute or two from the hospital, you should instruct her to cross her legs until you reach the emergency department (ED).

_____   2. If the fetal heart rate is less than 120 beats/min, the fetus is in danger.

_____   3. A woman should be discouraged from sitting up or squatting for delivery of her baby because those positions are counter to natural physiology and increase the demand on the mother's energy.

_____   4. If the baby is coming fast, it is more important to control the delivery than it is to drape the mother with sterile towels.

_____   5. If the cut ends of the umbilical cord are oozing blood, you should unclamp them and reapply the clamps more tightly.

_____   6. If the placenta has not delivered within 20 minutes of the baby's delivery, you should exert gentle traction on the umbilical cord while you vigorously massage the uterus.

_____   7. With the exception of buttocks breech, all other abnormal presentations must be delivered in the hospital.

Short Answer

Complete this section with short written answers using the space provided.

1. List the three abnormalities typically found in a child born with fetal alcohol syndrome.

a. _____

b. _____

c. _____

Fill in the Table

Fill in the missing parts of the following tables.

1. Fill in the amount of time needed for the three stages of labor for a nullipara and for a multipara.

The Stages of Labor: Nullipara Versus Multipara		
Stages of Labor	**Nullipara**	**Multipara**
First stage		
Second stage		
Third stage		

2. Fill in the missing information in distinguishing false labor from true labor.

False Labor Versus True Labor		
Parameter	**True Labor**	**False Labor**
Contractions		Irregularly spaced
Interval between contractions	Gradually shortens	
Intensity of contractions		Stays the same
Effects of analgesics	Do not abolish the pain	
Cervical changes		No changes

Don't milk the umbilical cord.

Neonatal Care

Matching

Part I

Match each of the definitions in the left column to the appropriate term in the right column.

_____ 1. A fissure or hole in the palate (roof of the mouth) that forms a communicating pathway between the mouth and nasal cavities.

_____ 2. An abnormal defect or fissure in the upper lip that failed to close during development; often associated with cleft palate.

_____ 3. A narrowing or blockage of the nasal airway by membranous or bony tissue; a congenital condition, meaning it is present at birth.

_____ 4. Blue discoloration of the skin due to the presence of deoxygenated hemoglobin in blood vessels near the skin surface.

_____ 5. An injury of childbirth affecting the spinal nerves C8 to T1 of the brachial plexus.

_____ 6. An event where one part of the intestine folds into another part of the intestines, leading to a blockage.

_____ 7. A congenital condition in which part of the bowel is narrow.

_____ 8. A congenital condition in which part of the bowel does not develop.

_____ 9. Marked hypertrophy and hyperplasia of the two (circular and longitudinal) muscular layers of the pylorus.

_____ 10. A hole in the atrial septal wall that allows oxygenated and deoxygenated blood to mix; patients with this hole have a higher incidence of stroke.

_____ 11. Condition of severely deficient supply of oxygen to the body, leading to end-organ damage.

_____ 12. Scale used to assess the status of a newborn 1 and 5 minutes after birth (range 0 to 10).

_____ 13. Oxygen administered via oxygen tube and a cupped hand on the patient's face.

_____ 14. A decrease in the amount of oxygen delivered to the extremities; the hands and feet turn blue because of narrowing of small arterioles toward the end of the arms and legs.

_____ 15. Pinching or narrowing of the aorta that obstructs blood flow from the heart to the systemic circulation.

_____ 16. An opening in the septum of the heart that closes after birth.

A. Acrocyanosis

B. Apgar score

C. Asphyxia

D. Atrial septal defect

E. Central cyanosis

F. Choanal atresia

G. Cleft lip

H. Cleft palate

I. Coarctation of the aorta

J. Congenital heart disease (CHC)

K. Diaphragmatic hernia

L. Erb palsy

M. Fetal transition

N. Foramen ovale

O. Free-flow oxygen

P. Gestation

_____ **17.** The process through which the fluid in the fetal lungs is replaced with air, the ductus arteriosus constricts, and the newborn begins adequate oxygenation of its own blood.

_____ **18.** Lack of movement at the shoulder due to nerve injury resulting from the stretching of the cervical nerve roots during delivery of the newborn's head during birth; usually transient, but can be permanent.

_____ **19.** Passage of loops of bowel with or without other abdominal organs, through a developmental defect in the diaphragm muscle; occurs as the bowel from the abdomen "herniates" upward through the diaphragm into the chest (thoracic) cavity.

_____ **20.** The most common birth defect; associated with hypoxia in the newborn period requiring intervention during the first months of life.

_____ **21.** Damage to cells in the central nervous system (the brain and spinal cord) from inadequate oxygen.

_____ **22.** Low or poor muscle tone (floppiness).

_____ **23.** Underdevelopment of the aorta, aortic valve, left ventricle, and mitral valve; this defect involves the entire left side of the heart.

_____ **24.** Period of time from conception to birth. For humans, the full period is normally 9 months (or 40 weeks).

Q. Hypoplastic left heart syndrome

R. Hypotonia

S. Hypoxic-ischemic encephalopathy

T. Infantile hypertrophic pyloric stenosis (IHPS)

U. Intestinal atresia

V. Intestinal stenosis

W. Intussusception

X. Klumpke paralysis

Part II

Match each of the definitions in the left column to the appropriate term in the right column.

_____ **1.** A situation in which the ductus arteriosus does not transition after birth to become the ligamentum arteriosum; the connection between the pulmonary artery and the aorta remains, allowing some oxygenated blood to move back into the heart rather than all of it moving out of the aorta and into the systemic circulation.

_____ **2.** Decreased volume of amniotic fluid during a pregnancy; a risk factor associated with abnormalities of the urinary tract, postmaturity, and intrauterine growth retardation.

_____ **3.** An infant within the first few hours after birth.

_____ **4.** A congenital anomaly of rotation of the midgut, in which the small bowel is found predominantly on the right side of the abdomen; results in increased incidence of intestinal volvulus.

_____ **5.** The pulse oximetry value obtained during neonatal resuscitation, which evaluates the oxygenation status of blood from the brachiocephalic artery, prior to the ductus arteriosus.

_____ **6.** Any pregnancy that lasts more than 42 weeks.

_____ **7.** An excessive amount of amniotic fluid; may cause preterm labor.

_____ **8.** Abnormally high red blood cell count.

_____ **9.** Abnormal location of the placenta in the lower part of the uterus, near or over the cervix.

_____ **10.** Seizure activity that involves more than one site, is asynchronous, and is usually migratory.

_____ **11.** An infant during the first month after birth.

_____ **12.** A cardiac anomaly that consists of four defects: a ventricular septal defect, pulmonary stenosis, right ventricular hypertrophy, and an overriding aorta.

_____ **13.** Describes a newborn delivered at 38 to 42 weeks' gestation.

A. Malrotation

B. Meconium

C. Multifocal seizure

D. Neonate

E. Newborn

F. Oligohydramnios

G. Patent ductus arteriosus

H. Persistent pulmonary hypertension

I. Pierre Robin sequence

J. Placenta previa

K. Polycythemia

L. Polyhydramnios

M. Postterm

_____ **14.** An infant whose size and weight are considerably less than the average for infants of the same age.

_____ **15.** A condition in which asphyxia continues after primary apnea, and the infant responds with a period of gasping respirations, falling pulse rate, and falling blood pressure.

_____ **16.** A disease of the eye that affects premature infants, thought to be caused by disorganized growth of retinal detachment; can lead to blindness in serious cases.

_____ **17.** Describes an infant delivered at less than 37 completed weeks' gestation.

_____ **18.** Underdeveloped; the condition of an infant born too soon; refers to infants delivered before 37 weeks from the first day of the last menstrual period.

_____ **19.** Delayed transition from fetal to neonatal circulation.

_____ **20.** A condition present at birth marked by a small lower jaw; the tongue tends to fall back and downward, and there is a cleft soft palate.

_____ **21.** A dark green fecal material that accumulates in the fetal intestines and is discharged around the time of birth.

_____ **22.** Narrowing of the pulmonary valve.

_____ **23.** Elevated blood pressure in the pulmonary arteries from constriction; causes problems with the blood flow in the lungs, and makes the heart work harder.

_____ **24.** The condition in which the umbilical cord presents itself outside of the uterus while the fetus is still inside; an obstetric emergency during pregnancy or labor that acutely endangers the life of the fetus.

_____ **25.** First pregnancy.

_____ **26.** Apnea caused by oxygen deprivation; usually corrected with stimulation, such as drying or slapping the newborn's feet.

N. Preductal oxygen saturation

O. Premature

P. Preterm

Q. Primary apnea

R. Primigravida

S. Prolapsed cord

T. Pulmonary hypertension

U. Pulmonary stenosis

V. Retinopathy of prematurity

W. Secondary apnea

X. Small for gestational age

Y. Term

Z. Tetralogy of Fallot

Multiple Choice

Read each item carefully, and then select the best response.

_____ **1.** As the baby is delivered, a rapid series of events must occur to enable the baby to breathe; this process is called fetal:

A. transportation.

B. transposition.

C. transmission.

D. transition.

_____ **2.** A newborn delivered at less than 37 completed weeks of gestation is considered:

A. preterm.

B. term.

C. postterm.

D. None of the above

_____ **3.** The Apgar score—named after Dr. Virginia Apgar, who developed this measure in 1953—helps record the condition of the newborn based on five signs. The Apgar score is typically recorded at _____ minutes after birth.

A. 2 and 10

B. 5 and 10

C. 1 and 5

D. 1 and 3

_____ **4.** Fewer than 1% of deliveries involve bradycardia that requires treatment with chest compressions or emergency medications. The most common etiology for bradycardia in a newborn is:

    A. fetal alcohol syndrome.

    B. maternal drug abuse.

    C. hypoxia.

    D. prolapsed cord.

_____ **5.** Infants do not normally pass stool before birth, but if they do and then inhale the meconium-stained amniotic fluid either in utero or at delivery, their airways may become plugged, and hypoxia may ensue. This, in turn, can lead to:

    A. atelectasis.

    B. pneumonitis.

    C. pneumothorax.

    D. All of the above

_____ **6.** Tetralogy of Fallot is a combination of four heart defects. These infants are born with each of the following, EXCEPT:

    A. hypoplastic left heart.

    B. ventricular septal defect.

    C. overriding aorta.

    D. pulmonary stenosis.

_____ **7.** Shock, hypoperfusion, sepsis, and cold stress may be indicators of which factor for hypoglycemia in a newborn?

    A. Prematurity

    B. Severe anemia

    C. Genetic disorders

    D. Disturbed oxidative metabolism

_____ **8.** A diagnosis of diaphragmatic hernia is suspected clinically in a newborn with:

    A. apnea.

    B. heart sounds shifted to the left.

    C. scaphoid abdomen.

    D. All of the above

_____ **9.** Primary apnea is often characterized by a short period of hypoxia and:

    A. rapid breathing, followed by apnea, and bradycardia.

    B. slow breathing, followed by apnea, and bradycardia.

    C. a lengthy period of apnea.

    D. a lengthy period of bradycardia.

_____ **10.** The lungs of a premature infant are weak, so the paramedic should use:

    A. the maximum allowable ventilatory pressure to expand lung tissue.

    B. mechanical devices to administer positive-pressure ventilation (PPV).

    C. small puffs from the paramedic's cheek with a pocket mask to ventilate.

    D. sufficient pressure to result in visible but not excessive chest rise.

Fill in the Blank

Read each item carefully, and then complete the statement by filling in the missing word(s).

1. Fetal circulation has three major blood flow deviations from that of an adult. These _____ occur at the ductus venosus, _____ _____, and ductus arteriosus.

2. Many newborns become centrally pink but have blue hands and feet. This is called _____.

3. Room air is preferred when resuscitating _____ infants, and the addition of supplemental oxygen may not be necessary.

4. The _____ _____ sequence is a series of developmental anomalies including a small chin and posteriorly positioned tongue.

5. In a newborn, it is important to provide the correct timing for ventilation at a rate of _____ to _____ breaths/min because breaths delivered at a higher rate can lead to _____, air trapping, or _____.

6. Oral airways are rarely used for neonates, but they can be lifesaving if airway _____ leads to respiratory failure. Bilateral _____ _____ can be rapidly fatal but usually responds to placement of an oral airway.

7. Gastric _____ using a(n) _____ tube is indicated for prolonged bag-mask ventilation, if abdominal distention is impeding ventilation, or in the presence of a(n) _____ hernia.

8. Jitteriness is often confused with a(n) _____. Jitteriness is characteristically a disorder of the _____ and is rarely seen at a later age.

9. _____ is a congenital anomaly of rotation of the midgut.

10. Antiemetics should not be administered in the field. The infant may be dehydrated, however, and may need fluid _____. Dry mucous membranes, tachycardia, or a sunken _____ are clues that the patient needs hydration.

11. The _____ is the most frequently fractured bone in the newborn during even normal childbirth.

12. The most common cause of acute diarrhea in children is _____ _____.

Identify

In the following case studies, identify the appropriate resuscitation steps.

1. You are dispatched to the scene of a call for an infant with a seizure. The mother states that her baby daughter was "jerking her left arm and kicking her right leg for about a minute." At this point, the child is resting, and you note no irregularities during your primary survey.

    a. List five types of seizures that occur in infants.

    (1)_____

    (2)_____

    (3)_____

    (4)_____

    (5)_____

    b. Based on the mother's description, which type of seizure did her child most likely have?

    _____

2. After assisting in the delivery of a full-term newborn boy, you bulb suction the infant's mouth and nose and dry and stimulate the baby.

  a. After 30 seconds, the baby is centrally cyanotic of the trunk and mucous membranes. Which treatment would you now initiate?

   (1)_____

   (2)_____

  b. After 30 seconds of adequate ventilation by PPV with 100% supplemental oxygen via a bag-mask device, the infant's pulse rate is less than 60 beats/min. Which treatment would you now initiate?

   (1)_____

   (2)_____

   (3)_____

Ambulance Calls

The following case scenarios provide an opportunity to explore the concerns associated with patient management and paramedic care. Read each scenario, and then answer each question.

1. You are called to attend a 38-year-old woman who is in active labor at home. She has not had any prenatal care. She tells you that "this baby is a month late according to my calendar and is sure a long time in coming." Her contractions started about 10 hours ago and are now 2 minutes apart. Her "bag of waters" broke 10 minutes before your arrival, and you notice greenish stains on the bedclothes. The woman says she feels as if she has to move her bowels.

  a. Because birth is imminent, your partner sets up for delivery while you prepare for newborn resuscitation. List the categories of equipment that may be needed:

   (1)_____

   (2)_____

   (3)_____

   (4)_____

   (5)_____

   (6)_____

  b. You immediately set up for delivery—and none too soon! You scarcely have your gloves on before the baby is crowning, and a moment later, the head is delivered. It is covered with a thick, greenish substance. List the steps you would take at this point.

   (1)_____

   (2)_____

  c. The delivery went quickly. The infant is centrally blue and pale, has a pulse rate of 80, gives no response to flicking the bottom of the feet, and is limp, with slow and irregular respirations. Based on the information in the Apgar scoring table in your textbook, what is the Apgar score at this point, and how did you arrive at the score?

   A _____

   P _____

   G _____

   A _____

   R _____

   Total score at 1 minute = _____

d. What are the steps in the neonatal resuscitation pyramid that you will need to quickly follow with this newborn?

(1)_____

(2)_____

(3)_____

(4)_____

(5)_____

2. You are called to a movie theater where a 23-year-old woman who is gravida 4, para 3, went into active labor while watching *Return of the Spider Monster*. You find the patient in a cold, drafty ladies' room, sitting on the floor, panting. "I'm only in my seventh month," she says. "This can't be happening." As she makes that statement, the baby's head delivers spontaneously. You scramble to the floor to control the rest of the delivery. Within seconds, you find yourself holding a very red, wrinkled little baby.

a. List in sequence the steps you would take at this point.

(1)_____

(2)_____

(3)_____

(4)_____

b. At which point would you clamp and cut the baby's umbilical cord? (Explain the reasoning behind your answer.)

_____

_____

_____

c. Which steps can you take to prevent the baby from becoming hypothermic?

(1)_____

(2)_____

(3)_____

(4)_____

(5)_____

3. You are called to a downtown apartment for a "sick woman." You arrive to find a teenage girl sitting on the toilet, having given birth only seconds before. The placenta has not yet delivered. You quickly remove the newborn from the toilet.

a. List the steps you would take at this point.

(1)_____

(2)_____

(3)_____

(4)_____

(5)_____

b. What would be the indications for starting artificial ventilation on this baby?

(1)_____

(2)_____

(3)_____

c. As it turns out, the baby has one of those indications, so you start artificial ventilation with a bag-mask device and 100% supplemental oxygen. After a minute, you reassess the baby and find that its heart rate is 84 beats/min. What should you do now?

_____

_____

_____

d. After another minute or so, you reassess again. The baby's heart rate is now 56 beats/min. What should you do now?

_____

_____

_____

_____

e. Under which circumstance should you administer IV epinephrine to this baby?

_____

True/False

If you believe the statement to be more true than false, write the letter "T" in the space provided. If you believe the statement to be more false than true, write the letter "F."

_____ **1.** Jaundice that persists in a newborn beyond 2 to 3 weeks may indicate liver disease.

_____ **2.** Even slight meconium staining of the amniotic fluid indicates a need to intubate the newborn immediately after delivery.

_____ **3.** Administration of naloxone (Narcan) to a newborn who was just born of an addicted mother is routine clinical practice.

_____ **4.** The typical umbilical cord has two arteries and one vein.

_____ **5.** Infants may die of cold exposure at temperatures adults find comfortable.

_____ **6.** Most newborns who require resuscitation will need cardiopulmonary resuscitation (CPR).

_____ **7.** The umbilical vein is a large, thin-walled vessel usually found at the 4 o'clock position, as compared to the two thick-walled umbilical arteries usually found at 12 and 8 o'clock.

_____ **8.** Newborns weighing less than 5.5 pounds (2,500 g) are considered low birth weight.

_____ **9.** A normal number of stools per day for an infant is five to six, especially if the infant is breastfeeding, when infants often produce stool after every feeding.

_____ **10.** Meconium-stained amniotic fluid, which is present in 10% to 15% of deliveries, carries a high risk of morbidity.

Short Answer

Complete this section with short written answers using the space provided.

1. Neonatal IV access under the best circumstances can be difficult and stressful. An important alternative is catheterization of the umbilical vein. Detail the steps necessary to perform this task.

a. _____

_____

b. _____

_____

c. _____

_____

d. _____

_____

e. _____

_____

2. One of the most important skills that a paramedic must acquire and maintain is the ability to intubate neonates. Describe the steps necessary to properly intubate a neonate.

a. _____

b. _____

c. _____

d. _____

e. _____

Fill in the Table

1. Complete the following table by filling in the causes of neonatal seizures.

Causes of Neonatal Seizures
• Hypoxic-ischemic encephalopathy
• _____
• _____
• _____
• _____
• _____
• Development defects
• Hypocalcemia
• _____
• _____
• _____

Problem Solving

Practice your calculation skills by solving the following math problems using the Apgar score. The Apgar scoring table is provided in your textbook.

You have just assisted in the delivery of a full-term newborn.

1. At 1 minute, the baby is centrally blue and pale, and the pulse rate is 100 beats/min; the baby grimaces, has some extremity flexion, and has a slow and irregular respiratory effort. The Apgar score is _____.

2. At 5 minutes, the baby is pink with blue extremities, has a pulse rate of 120 beats/min, is actively crying with a strong effort, and has active motion. The Apgar score is _____.

Pediatric Emergencies

Matching

Part I

Match the following statements with the age group(s) most applicable to each. The statements may apply to more than one age group.

_____ **1.** Don't let your guard down regarding scene safety.

_____ **2.** They can be distracted by jangling keys and cooing noises.

_____ **3.** Give them appropriate choices and control whenever possible, and provide ongoing reassurance and encouragement.

_____ **4.** Assessment begins with observation of their interactions with the caregiver, vocalizations, and mobility, measured through the Pediatric Assessment Triangle.

_____ **5.** They should be examined on the parent's lap if stable.

_____ **6.** They can provide at least some of the history.

_____ **7.** They do not do very much other than eat, sleep, and cry.

_____ **8.** Tailor the physical exam to their age and developmental stage.

_____ **9.** Friends are key support figures, and this is a time of experimentation and risk-taking behaviors.

_____ **10.** Child abuse or maltreatment comes in many forms: physical abuse, sexual abuse, emotional abuse, and child neglect.

_____ **11.** They become much more analytic and capable of abstract thought. At this age, they can understand cause and effect.

_____ **12.** Use play and distraction techniques whenever possible.

_____ **13.** Make sure your hands and stethoscope are warm.

_____ **14.** Once secondary sexual characteristics have developed, they should be treated as an adult.

_____ **15.** They will be able to tell you what hurts and may have a story to share about the illness or injury.

A. Neonates and infants

B. Toddlers

C. Preschoolers

D. School-age children

E. Adolescents

Part II

Match the definitions in the left column with the most appropriate term in the right column.

_____ **1.** A condition seen in children younger than 2 years, characterized by dyspnea and wheezing.

_____ **2.** An unexpected sudden episode of color change, tone change, or apnea that requires mouth-to-mouth resuscitation or vigorous stimulation; formerly known as apparent life-threatening event (ALTE).

_____ **3.** A method of delivering oxygen by holding a face mask or similar device near an infant's or a child's face; used when a nonrebreathing mask is not tolerated.

_____ **4.** A group of congenital conditions that cause either accumulation of toxins or disorders of energy metabolism in the neonate; characterized by an infant's failure to thrive and by vague signs such as poor feeding.

_____ **5.** A condition in which the pituitary gland does not produce normal amounts of some or all of its hormones. It can be congenital; occur secondary to tumors, infection, or stroke; or develop after trauma or radiation therapy.

_____ **6.** A condition in which the heart muscle is unusually thick, forcing the heart to pump harder to get blood to leave.

_____ **7.** A short, low-pitched sound at the end of exhalation, present in children with moderate to severe hypoxia. It reflects poor gas exchange because of fluid in the lower airways and air sacs.

_____ **8.** A type of seizure characterized by manifestations that indicate involvement of both cerebral hemispheres.

_____ **9.** A tube that is surgically placed directly into the patient's stomach through the skin to provide nutrition or medications.

_____ **10.** An acute bacterial infection of the subglottic area of the upper airway that is complicated by copious thick, pus-filled secretions.

_____ **11.** Cyanosis of the extremities.

_____ **12.** A type of seizure characterized by a brief lapse of attention during which the patient may stare and not respond; formerly known as a petit mal seizure.

_____ **13.** The increased accumulation of cerebrospinal fluid within the ventricles of the brain.

_____ **14.** A bleeding disorder that is primarily hereditary, in which clotting does not occur or occurs insufficiently.

_____ **15.** Inflammation of the epiglottis.

_____ **16.** A condition in which the heart becomes weakened and enlarged, making it less efficient and causing a negative impact to the pulmonary, hepatic, and other systems.

_____ **17.** A genetic disease that primarily affects the respiratory and digestive systems.

_____ **18.** A type of child maltreatment in which a parent or guardian physically leaves a child, without regard for the child's health, safety, or welfare.

_____ **19.** Any improper or excessive action that injures or otherwise harms a child or infant.

_____ **20.** The community-based legal organization responsible for protection, rehabilitation, and prevention of child maltreatment and neglect; it has the legal authority to temporarily remove children from homes if there is reason to believe they are at risk for injury or neglect and to secure foster placement.

A. Abandonment

B. Absence seizures

C. Acrocyanosis

D. Bacterial tracheitis

E. Blow-by technique

F. Brief resolved unexplained event (BRUE)

G. Bronchiolitis

H. Bronchopulmonary dysplasia

I. Central venous catheter

J. Child abuse

K. Child protective services (CPS)

L. Complex febrile seizures

M. Complex partial seizures

N. Congenital adrenal hyperplasia (CAH)

O. Croup

P. Cystic fibrosis (CF)

Q. Dilated cardiomyopathy

R. Epiglottitis

S. Gastrostomy tube (G-tube)

T. Generalized seizures

_____ **21.** An unusual form of seizure that occurs in association with a rapid increase in body temperature.

_____ **22.** A spectrum of lung conditions found in premature neonates who require long periods of high-concentration oxygen and ventilator support, ranging from mild reactive airway to debilitating chronic lung disease.

_____ **23.** A catheter inserted into the vena cava to permit intermittent or continuous monitoring of central venous pressure and to facilitate obtaining blood samples for chemical analysis.

_____ **24.** A common disease of childhood due to upper airway obstruction and characterized by stridor, hoarseness, and a barking cough.

_____ **25.** Inadequate production of cortisol and aldosterone by the adrenal gland.

_____ **26.** A type of seizure characterized by alteration of consciousness with or without complex focal motor activity.

U. Grunting

V. Hemophilia

W. Hydrocephalus

X. Hypertrophic cardiomyopathy

Y. Hypopituitarism

Z. Inborn errors of metabolism (IEMs)

Part III

Match the definitions in the left column with the most appropriate term in the right column.

_____ **1.** The inadequate production or absence of the pituitary hormones, including adrenocorticotropic hormone, cortisol, thyroxine, luteinizing hormone, follicle-stimulating hormone, estrogen, testosterone, growth hormone, and antidiuretic hormone.

_____ **2.** An area where cartilage is transformed through calcification into a new area of bone.

_____ **3.** A stiff or painful neck; commonly associated with meningitis.

_____ **4.** Refusal or failure on the part of the caregiver to provide life necessities to a child.

_____ **5.** A type of seizure that involves focal motor jerking or sensory abnormality in a patient who remains conscious.

_____ **6.** A brief, self-limited, generalized seizure in a previously healthy child between ages 6 months and 6 years that is associated with the onset of or sudden increase in fever.

_____ **7.** A disease that causes red blood cells to be misshapen, resulting in a poor oxygen-carrying capability and potentially resulting in lodging of the red blood cells in blood vessels or the spleen.

_____ **8.** A pathologic state, usually in a febrile patient, resulting from the presence of invading microorganisms or their poisonous products in the bloodstream.

_____ **9.** A tube that is surgically placed directly into the patient's stomach through the skin to provide nutrition or medications.

_____ **10.** Hypertrophy (enlargement) of the pyloric sphincter of the stomach; ultimately leads to intestinal obstruction, often in infants.

_____ **11.** Pertaining to bruising of the skin.

_____ **12.** An inflammation of the lungs caused by bacterial, viral, or fungal infections or infections with other microorganisms.

_____ **13.** Inflammation of the myocardium.

_____ **14.** A condition of abnormal skin circulation, caused by vasoconstriction or inadequate perfusion.

_____ **15.** Inflammation of the meningeal coverings of the brain and spinal cord; usually caused by a virus or bacterium. The viral type is less severe than the bacterial type; the bacterial type can result in brain damage, hearing loss, learning disability, or death.

A. Intussusception

B. Malrotation with volvulus

C. Meckel diverticulum

D. Meningitis

E. Mottling

F. Myocarditis

G. Neglect

H. Nuchal rigidity

I. Ossification center

J. Panhypopituitarism

K. Partial seizures

L. Pediatric Assessment Triangle (PAT)

M. Pertussis

N. Petechial

O. Pneumonia

_____ **16.** One of the most common congenital malformations of the small intestines, which presents with painless rectal bleeding.

_____ **17.** A sign of respiratory distress characterized by skin pulling inward between and around the ribs and clavicles during inhalation.

_____ **18.** A virus that affects the upper and lower respiratory tracts. Disease (ie, pneumonia and bronchiolitis) is more prevalent in the lower respiratory tract.

_____ **19.** A clinical state of inadequate oxygenation, ventilation, or both.

_____ **20.** A clinical state characterized by increased respiratory rate, effort, and work of breathing.

_____ **21.** A condition that occurs when there is a twisting of the bowel around its mesenteric attachment to the abdominal wall.

_____ **22.** Telescoping of the intestines into themselves.

_____ **23.** Characterized by small purple, nonblanching spots on the skin.

_____ **24.** An acute infectious disease characterized by a catarrhal stage, followed by a paroxysmal cough that ends in a whooping inspiration; also called whooping cough.

_____ **25.** An assessment tool that allows rapid formation of a general impression of the type and level of illness or injury in an infant or child without touching him or her; consists of assessing appearance, work of breathing, and circulation to the skin.

_____ **26.** A type of seizure that involves only one part of the brain.

P. Purpuric

Q. Pyloric stenosis

R. Respiratory arrest

S. Respiratory distress

T. Respiratory failure

U. Respiratory syncytial virus (RSV)

V. Retractions

W. Sepsis

X. Sickle cell disease

Y. Simple febrile seizures

Z. Simple partial seizures

Multiple Choice

Read each item carefully, and then select the best response.

_____ **1.** Although child abuse can generate a big emotional response from the emergency medical services (EMS) crew, your primary focus as a paramedic should be:

A. documenting the suspected abuse for further prosecution.

B. separating the patient from the suspected abuser.

C. the trauma assessment, management, and ensuring the safety of the child.

D. properly securing the crime scene for investigators.

_____ **2.** A child's developmental stage affects his or her response to injury. As a result:

A. being strapped to a backboard may be considered fun.

B. a paramedic could turn an activity as serious as immobilizing a child's spine on a backboard into a "game."

C. being immobilized on a backboard may be terrifying and anxiety provoking.

D. children should never be strapped or immobilized on a backboard.

_____ **3.** All of the following injury patterns may be more common in pediatric patients, EXCEPT:

A. blunt force trauma.

B. falls.

C. skull fractures.

D. joint dislocations.

_____ **4.** PAT is an acronym developed:

A. from a popular children's book to help soothe a sick or injured child.

B. to remember the proper methods of conducting a hands-on assessment of a child.

C. to stand for the technique of palpating a tender abdomen.

D. to stand for the Pediatric Assessment Triangle.

_____ **5.** One of the best ways to assess a pediatric patient's oxygenation status is to:

    A. evaluate the child's respiratory rate.

    B. evaluate the work of breathing.

    C. auscultate the lung.

    D. obtain the pulse.

_____ **6.** Abnormal positioning and retractions are physical signs of increased work of breathing that can easily be assessed without touching the patient. All of the following are signs of increased work of breathing, EXCEPT:

    A. the sniffing position.

    B. tripoding.

    C. retractions.

    D. All of the above are signs of increased work of breathing.

_____ **7.** Which of the following is a child with a serious mechanism of injury, who may need immediate transport to the emergency department (ED)?

    A. A child with an unstable or compromised airway from a motor vehicle crash

    B. A child with an isolated extremity fracture from a fall

    C. A conscious, alert child who crashed his or her bicycle while wearing a helmet that cracked

    D. A skateboarder with an obviously fractured wrist

_____ **8.** Paramedics may encounter children with special health care needs. These special needs may include:

    A. physical, developmental, and learning disabilities.

    B. tracheostomy tubes and artificial ventilators.

    C. gastrostomy tubes (G-tubes).

    D. All of the above

_____ **9.** The federally funded program that was created more than 25 years ago in an effort to reduce child disability and death caused by severe illness and injury is known as:

    A. the DOT curriculum.

    B. NHYSA.

    C. EMSC.

    D. TSA.

_____ **10.** Inserting an oral airway in a child is similar to inserting an airway in an adult, EXCEPT:

    A. you use a different method for determining the proper size.

    B. an oral airway should not be used in the presence of ingested caustics.

    C. an oral airway is inserted in a child in an inverted manner, then flipped over into the correct position.

    D. you must take care to avoid injuring the hard palate.

_____ **11.** When a parent or guardian physically leaves a child, without regard for the child's health or safety, this condition is referred to as:

    A. physical abuse.

    B. sexual abuse.

    C. abandonment.

    D. neglect.

_____ **12.** Which of the following is NOT a risk factor for child abuse?

    A. Child with disability

    B. Disorganized family structure

    C. Parent was abused

    D. Financial stability

_____ **13.** You are called to the scene of a 4-year-old child injured inside a residence. You enter the house and find the child and a parent. You assess the child and become suspicious about the injury. Your partner interviews the parent. Which of the following is a red flag for child abuse by a caregiver?

    A. The caregiver overreacts to the child's condition.

    B. The caregiver seems forthcoming about what happened.

    C. The caregiver is enraged about care being provided by EMS.

    D. The caregiver seems concerned.

_____ **14.** You have completed a call where there is a high suspicion of child abuse. When you write the patient care report, which type of information is helpful to include for child protective services when those personnel review the report?

    A. Subjective analysis of the situation

    B. Speculative view on what might be going on

    C. Conjecture and results of your investigation

    D. Verbatim comments in quotes

_____ **15.** You have been called to a residence where there is a 5-year-old boy who reportedly fell while running and hit his forehead. He has a bruise and an abrasion. While you do an assessment to determine if there are any additional injuries, you notice the boy has numerous bruises of different colors. Which location of bruises on the child would make you MOST suspicious of child abuse?

    A. Knees

    B. Arms

    C. Lower legs

    D. Back

Labeling

On the following diagram, indicate the technique for measuring the distance to insert a nasogastric (NG) or an orogastric (OG) tube.

A. _____

B. _____

C. _____

Fill in the Blank

Read each item carefully, and then complete the statement by filling in the missing word(s).

1. A nasopharyngeal airway is usually well _____ and is not as likely as the _____ airway to cause vomiting.

2. The _____ - _____ _____ can be used for a child with mild respiratory distress who will not tolerate a facial mask.

3. Bag-mask ventilation is always the first step in assisted _____, and it represents definitive _____ _____ for many patients.

4. Potential complications of pediatric intubation include damage to _____ and oral structures, _____ of gastric contents, and incorrect placement.

5. Because _____ can occur during intubation, the paramedic should apply a cardiac monitor and a(n) _____ _____.

6. The types of shock you may encounter are the same in adults and children: _____, _____, and _____.

7. A pediatric patient with _____ shock will often appear listless or lethargic and may have compensatory _____. The child may appear pale, _____, or cyanotic.

8. Further assessment of a pediatric patient in shock may identify signs of dehydration such as sunken eyes, dry _____ _____, poor skin _____, or _____ capillary refill, with cool extremities.

9. Complications associated with IO infusion may include _____ _____, growth plate injury, and bone inflammation caused by _____.

10. Cardiogenic shock is uncommon in the pediatric population but may be present in children with underlying _____ heart disease or _____ disturbances.

11. When you are confronted with a pediatric patient in _____ arrest, the most important consideration is to provide high-quality cardiopulmonary resuscitation (CPR). Attach a(n) _____ or defibrillator to determine the underlying cardiac rhythm.

12. Approximately 1,600 infants died of _____ in 2015. This condition is the leading cause of death among infants 1 to 12 months old.

Identify

After reading the following case studies, list the chief complaint, vital signs, and pertinent negatives.

1. It's about 0330 hours, and you are dispatched on a Priority 1 call for a 2-year-old child with difficulty breathing. As you approach the residence, you notice a family member frantically trying to wave you down. You think to yourself that this doesn't look good. You grab your pediatric gear and electrocardiogram (ECG) monitor and quickly enter the house. Once inside, you are told that the girl woke the whole household with a terrible barky cough. This child is now sitting on her mother's lap. The mother states that the child has been irritable for several days with symptoms consistent with an upper respiratory infection: coughing, runny nose, and sneezing. The child has audible stridor and a "seal-like" barking cough; she is conscious and alert. She has an oxygen saturation of 95% on ambient room air. She also has a normal capillary refill. When you attempt to take her blood pressure (BP), she begins to get agitated and clings to her mother.

   a. Chief complaint:

_____

_____

b. Vital signs:

_____

_____

c. Pertinent negatives:

_____

_____

2. Today is your shift on medivac duty. You are dispatched to intercept a ground ambulance about 25 minutes to the west. As you lift off, you discover that the patient is only 1 week old and was the survivor of a motor vehicle crash involving a fatality. You and your crew arrive on the scene several minutes before the ambulance arrives. The state police are on scene securing the landing zone. They advise you that the patient's mother was holding the baby; both were unrestrained in the vehicle and were ejected on impact. The mother suffered fatal injuries. You are thinking the worst and begin to set up your pediatric resuscitation equipment. When the ambulance arrives, you are quickly handed the neonatal trauma patient. The baby has oxygen in place, appears to be wrapped well, and is thoroughly secured with a vacuum splint conforming to his tiny body. The baby appears to be sleeping peacefully and has only a small forehead abrasion. You begin the primary survey during your flight to the trauma center. The assessment indicates an infant with no visible distress. The baby has an intact airway and is breathing at 30 breaths/min, he has an apical pulse rate at 150 beats/min, his skin color appears normal, and the skin is warm and dry. Lung sounds are clear and equal. Oxygen saturation is 96%. Remarkably, he does not appear to have any noticeable external bleeding. In fact, the assessment is totally unremarkable. After a "not so routine" mechanism of injury, the infant is safely delivered to the regional trauma center.

a. Chief complaint:

_____

_____

b. Vital signs:

_____

_____

c. Pertinent negatives:

_____

_____

3. While working in the advanced life support (ALS) "fly car," you are dispatched on a Priority 1 call for a mutual assist with a local basic life support (BLS) ambulance. The BLS team requests that you meet them while they begin the response to the local pediatric ED. They are treating a 2½-year-old girl in "status." You arrange a safe place to meet the ambulance and secure your vehicle. As you await the BLS crew's arrival, you prepare your pediatric ALS equipment and begin reviewing protocols. Once on the ambulance, you notice the small patient secured to the cot. The mother is in the front passenger's seat. The child has recently been sick with an upper respiratory infection and low-grade fever. The child suddenly appeared to go into convulsions after being given oral pediatric acetaminophen for an elevation in her fever. The BLS crew states that the patient was actively seizing on their arrival. They initiated high-flow supplemental oxygen with a pediatric nonrebreathing face mask, requested ALS assistance, and initiated transport. When you first encounter the child, she is postictal, with the following vital signs: ashen skin that is warm and dry and a rectal temperature of 100.3°F. The patient responds to pain. Her oxygen saturation is 98%. Pupils are sluggish but equal. The patient has equal bilateral breath sounds. The remainder of the exam is unremarkable. The

patient's mother denies any other medications, history, or allergies to medications. She further denies any recent injury or trauma to the child.

a. Chief complaint:

_____

_____

b. Vital signs:

_____

_____

c. Pertinent negatives:

_____

_____

Complete the Patient Care Report (PCR)

Reread the first incident scenario in the preceding "Identify" exercises, and then complete the following PCR for the patient.

EMS Patient Care Report (PCR)				
Date:	**Incident No.:**	**Nature of Call:**		**Location:**
Dispatched:	**En Route:**	**At Scene:**	**Transport:**	**At Hospital:** **In Service:**

Patient Information	
Age:	**Allergies:**
Sex:	**Medications:**
Weight (in kg [lb]):	**Past Medical History:**
	Chief Complaint:

Vital Signs				
Time:	**BP:**	**Pulse:**	**Respirations:**	**SpO₂:**
Time:	**BP:**	**Pulse:**	**Respirations:**	**SpO₂:**
Time:	**BP:**	**Pulse:**	**Respirations:**	**SpO₂:**

EMS Treatment (circle all that apply)				
Oxygen @ _____ L/min via (circle one): NC NRM Bag-mask device		**Assisted Ventilation**	**Airway Adjunct**	**CPR**
Defibrillation	**Bleeding Control**	**Bandaging**	**Splinting**	**Other:**

Narrative

Ambulance Calls

The following case scenarios provide an opportunity to explore the concerns associated with patient management and paramedic care. Read each scenario, and then answer each question.

1. You are called to the scene of a collision in which a 6-year-old child was struck by a car as he darted into the street in front of his home. The child is lying in the street surrounded by a small group of people, including his very distraught parents.

   a. Given the mechanism of injury (MOI), list at least three injuries you must look for in particular in this child.

   (1)_____

   (2)_____

   (3)_____

   b. As you are kneeling beside the injured child, carefully going through the steps of the primary survey, the child's father (who looks like a pro wrestler) charges over and starts shouting at you: "What the h— do you think you're doing with my kid? Stop messing around and take him to a *hospital*. Can't you see he's hurt bad? He's going to die here while you dingbats muck about." [The father's actual comments are less polite but are not quoted verbatim in this workbook.]

   (1) What are your feelings at this moment?

   _____

   _____

   (2) How will you deal with this situation?

   (a) _____

   (b) _____

   (c) _____

   (d) _____

   c. On checking the child's vital signs, you find the following: pulse is 120 beats/min and regular; respirations are 24 breaths/min and unlabored; BP is 90/60 mm Hg. Which of the following conclusions can be drawn from those vital signs?

   (1) The child is going into shock.

   (2) The child has increasing intracranial pressure.

   (3) The vital signs are normal for a child of that age.

   (4) There is probably significant intrathoracic injury.

   (5) There is probably significant intra-abdominal bleeding.

2. You are called around 0100 hours for a child who "can't breathe." A haggard father greets you at the door and tells you that his 2-year-old Tammy has had "a little cold" for a couple of days but otherwise seemed fine. ("It didn't slow her down a bit.") Tonight, however, she began coughing, and the cough kept getting worse. Indeed, even as you are walking toward the child's room, you can hear a loud barking noise. On reaching Tammy's room, you see a very agitated 2-year-old struggling in her mother's lap. Her nostrils are flaring with each inhalation, and there are retractions of her neck muscles. Her lips are bluish. She flails and has a fit of dry coughing as you start to come near. Eventually, you manage to measure a pulse of 160 beats/min and a respiratory rate of 52 breaths/min. When you try to auscultate the child's chest, however, she grabs your stethoscope and yanks it out of your ears.

   a. The vital signs are _____ (normal or abnormal?) for a child of this age.

   b. The most likely diagnosis is _____.

   c. Which steps will you take in managing this child?

      (1)_____

      (2)_____

      (3)_____

      (4)_____

      (5)_____

3. You are called for a 4-month-old infant in respiratory distress. His mother says that he has been "off his feed" for a couple of days and has been sneezing a lot. On examination, you notice that the baby seems to be breathing like a rabbit. The pulse is 180 beats/min, respirations are 60 breaths/min, and BP is 90/60 mm Hg. There is diffuse wheezing throughout the chest.

   a. The vital signs are _____ (normal or abnormal?) for a child of this age.

   b. The most likely diagnosis is _____.

   c. Which steps will you take in managing this child?

      (1)_____

      (2)_____

      (3)_____

      (4)_____

      (5)_____

      (6)_____

4. You are called for a 2½-year-old child having difficulty breathing. The mother says that she left little Bobby playing quietly in his room, and when she returned half an hour later, she found him in severe respiratory distress. She thinks he has had a slight respiratory infection, nothing serious: "You know, it's just one runny nose after another all winter with them. Each one gives it to the others, and I've got five little ones—so I can't always keep track of who has a runny nose."

You find Bobby in severe respiratory distress. He makes high-pitched squeaks when he tries to inhale, and his eyes look like they are popping out of his head. His lips are blue. You place the back of your hand on his forehead and note that the skin does not feel abnormally warm.

   a. The most likely diagnosis is _____.

   b. Which steps will you take in managing this child?

      (1)_____

      _____

      (2)_____

      _____

      (3)_____

      _____

      (4)_____

      _____

(5)_____

_____

(6)_____

_____

(7)_____

_____

5. You are called to see a 4-year-old child who is "very sick." His mother says that he was fine until a few hours ago, when he began complaining of a sore throat. Since then, he would not eat or drink anything, and he is very feverish. You find the child sitting very still, bolt upright in bed, with his chin thrust forward. He does not reply to your questions but only nods or shakes his head slightly. Saliva is dribbling out of the corners of his mouth. His skin feels very hot. His pulse is 140 beats/min, respirations are 40 breaths/min and quiet, and BP is 90/60 mm Hg. The chest is clear.

  a. The vital signs are _____ (normal or abnormal?) for a child of this age.

  b. The most likely diagnosis is _____.

  c. Which steps will you take in managing this child?

  (1)_____

  (2)_____

  (3)_____

  (4)_____

  (5)_____

  d. What is the special danger threatening this child?

  _____

  _____

6. You are called to a field about 6 miles outside of town where a 6-year-old child in the first-grade nature study class is having difficulty breathing. The teacher says that she noticed him lagging behind the others several times during the morning, and finally she found him sitting by himself under a tree, struggling to breathe. You find the child still sitting under the tree, but apparently dozing. It is difficult to wake him, and when he does open his eyes, he just stares at you blankly. When you ask him whether he has taken any medicine today, he just shakes his head and seems to doze again.

  On examination, the child's pulse is 160 beats/min and somewhat weak, respirations are 52 breaths/min and shallow, and BP is 90/60 mm Hg on exhalation and 50 mm Hg systolic during inhalation. The lips look bluish. There is retraction of the neck muscles. The chest does not seem to move with respiration, and it sounds like an empty barrel when you tap on it. You can hardly hear any breath sounds at all. On the child's wrist is a medical identification bracelet inscribed "asthmatic."

  a. List five signs that suggest this child is having a very serious asthmatic attack.

  (1)_____

  (2)_____

  (3)_____

  (4)_____

  (5)_____

b. List the steps you would take in managing this case.

(1)_____

(2)_____

(3)_____

(4)_____

(5)_____

(6)_____

7. The very same evening, you are called to see a child who is "short of breath." The child has been diagnosed with asthma in the past.

a. List five questions you would ask the child and his parents in taking the history.

(1)_____

(2)_____

(3)_____

(4)_____

(5)_____

b. Your protocol calls for administering albuterol for an acute asthmatic attack.

(1) What are the relevant *contraindications* to albuterol?

_____

_____

(2) What are the possible adverse *side effects* of albuterol?

_____

_____

(3) What is the correct *dosage*, and how is the drug administered?

_____

_____

8. You are called to a downtown apartment for a "very sick baby." A frightened-looking young mother greets you at the door and hurries you into the bedroom, where a baby is lying very still in its crib. You observe at once that the baby's color is grayish and that it is not breathing. When you touch the baby to open the airway, you can feel that the skin is cold. Describe what you will do from this point on.

_____

_____

_____

_____

9. You are called for a 2-year-old child who is "having a fit." En route to the call, you review in your mind the possible causes of seizures in children.

a. List five causes of seizures in children.

(1)_____

(2)_____

(3)_____

(4)_____

(5)_____

b. List five questions you should ask in taking the child's history.

(1)_____

(2)_____

(3)_____

(4)_____

(5)_____

c. List five things you would look for in particular in examining the child.

(1)_____

(2)_____

(3)_____

(4)_____

(5)_____

d. You learn that the child has never experienced a seizure before. On examining him, you find that he is no longer seizing but is still somewhat drowsy. His skin is very hot, so you take an axillary temperature and get a reading of 39°C (102.2°F). The pupils are equal and reactive, the neck is supple, and the chest is clear. Describe how you would manage this case.

(1)_____

(2)_____

10. You are summoned to a local high school where a 14-year-old girl is having a seizure. The school nurse tells you that the child has never experienced a seizure in school before. This seizure came on while the girl was in the auditorium watching a movie. The seizure lasted about 5 minutes. One of the teachers then carried the girl to the nurse's office. The nurse was in the middle of trying to contact the girl's mother when the child had another grand mal seizure. Now, as you are speaking with the nurse, you witness a third grand mal seizure that lasts about 6 minutes.

a. List the steps in treating this patient.

(1)_____

(2)_____

(3)_____

(4)_____

(5)_____

(6)_____

(7)_____

b. Which drug is used in the emergency treatment of repeated seizures, and what are its contraindications?

_____

_____

11. You are called to attend to a 10-month-old baby who sustained burns to the foot when he "stepped on a cigarette." Something about the story sounds "fishy" to you, and you find yourself on the alert for evidence that the child has been abused.

a. What's "fishy" about the story?

_____

_____

b. List 10 possible clues that might substantiate your suspicion that a child has been abused.

(1)_____

(2)_____

(3)_____

(4)_____

(5)_____

(6)_____

(7)_____

(8)_____

(9)_____

(10)_____

c. By the time you finish examining the child, you are privately convinced that the baby was deliberately burned and that, furthermore, he has been burned and beaten in the past. How should you manage this case?

(1)_____

(2)_____

(3)_____

(4)_____

(5)_____

d. Suppose the child's parent refuses to allow the child to be transported to the hospital? What should you do then?

(1)_____

(2)_____

(3)_____

12. You are called to treat an 18-month-old baby who fell off a second-floor balcony to the ground 5 meters (about 15 feet) below. On examination, you find the baby conscious but drowsy. Vital signs are a pulse of 80 beats/min and regular, respirations are 16 breaths/min, and BP is 100/70 mm Hg. There is a bruise on the left forehead. The pupils are equal and reactive to light. The point of maximal impulse (PMI) is in the midclavicular line. Breath sounds are equal bilaterally. The abdomen does not appear distended. The baby is moving all extremities. List the steps in the prehospital management of this case.

a. _____

b. _____

c. _____

d. _____

e. _____

f. _____

13. You are called to the scene of a smoky house fire just as one of the firefighters is emerging from the building carrying a baby. "He was in the thick of it," the firefighter tells you. "Out cold when I found him." The baby still seems very drowsy.
a. Should this infant be intubated? Why or why not?

_____

_____

b. List five indications for the immediate intubation of an infant or small child who has been in a fire.

(1)_____

(2)_____

(3)_____

(4)_____

(5)_____

14. You are all settled in to watch a football game on your day off when a neighbor comes running in, carrying her lethargic 2-year-old child. "Johnny's choking on peanuts!" she wails. "Did what?" you ask, not really wanting to know the answer.

"He's choking. Help, do something, he's turning blue!"
a. What is the recommended method to relieve a severe airway obstruction in a conscious child?

_____

_____

b. List the steps you would take to relieve the child's airway obstruction.

(1)_____

_____

(2)_____

_____

(3)_____

_____

(4)_____

_____

(5)_____

_____

(6)_____

_____

True/False

If you believe the statement to be more true than false, write the letter "T" in the space provided. If you believe the statement to be more false than true, write the letter "F."

_____   **1.** A child who is seriously ill or injured will always be agitated and showing clear signs of distress.

_____   **2.** A sunken anterior fontanel in an infant suggests meningitis or a head injury.

_____   **3.** Neonates and infants can easily communicate their needs when they are in pain.

_____   **4.** Grunting is a sign of respiratory distress in small children.

_____   **5.** An infant falling from a height is most likely to sustain injury to the head.

_____   **6.** RSV may be transmitted by direct contact with large droplets or indirect contact with contaminated hands.

_____   **7.** To insert an oropharyngeal airway (OPA) in a small child, introduce the airway tip-upward, and then rotate it 180° and slide it into place.

_____   **8.** Hypotension is an early response to blood loss in infants and small children.

_____   **9.** The first step in assembling the equipment for pediatric intubation is to check the cuff on the endotracheal (ET) tube you have selected.

_____   **10.** A straight blade is preferred for pediatric intubation.

_____   **11.** Adrenal insufficiency can lead to distributive shock.

_____   **12.** The narrowest point in an infant's airway is the opening between the vocal cords.

_____   **13.** Initial burn management begins with removal of burning clothing and support of the ABCs.

_____   **14.** Pediatric trauma victims must have a rigid cervical collar in place prior to transport.

_____   **15.** Sinus tachycardia, referring to a pulse rate higher than normal for age, is common in children.

Short Answer

Complete this section with short written answers using the space provided.

1. List six signs suggestive of hypovolemic shock in infants and small children.

a. _____

b. _____

c. _____

d. _____

e. _____

f. _____

2. Upon completing the primary survey of any seriously injured person, of any age, the paramedic must make a decision whether to transport at once or to proceed to the secondary assessment. List five indications for immediate transport ("load-and-go") of injured infants and children.

a. _____

b. _____

c. _____

d. _____

e. _____

Fill in the Table

Fill in the missing parts of the following tables.

1. In examining an injured infant or child, you must know exactly what you are looking for so that each second spent on the physical examination is well invested. In the following table, indicate what, in particular, you would be looking for as you examine each part of the body areas mentioned.

Pediatric Physical Examination	
Body Area	**What I Am Looking for in Particular**
Head	• _____ • _____ • _____
Neck	• _____ • _____
Chest	• _____ • _____ • _____
Abdomen	• _____ • _____
Extremities	• _____ • _____ • _____

2. In the following table, provide the normal respiratory rate for each pediatric age group.

Pediatric Respiratory Rates	
Age	**Respiratory Rate (breaths/min)**
Infant	
Toddler	
Preschool-age child	
School-age child	
Adolescent	

Data from: **American Heart Association (AHA). Vital signs in children. In: AHA.** *Pediatric Advanced Life Support.* **Dallas, TX: AHA; 2015.**

3. In the following table, provide the normal pulse rate for each pediatric age group.

Pediatric Pulse Rates	
Age	**Pulse Rate (beats/min) [Awake]**
Infant	
Toddler	
Preschool-age child	
School-age child	
Adolescent	

Data from: **American Heart Association (AHA). Vital signs in children. In: AHA.** *Pediatric Advanced Life Support.* **Dallas, TX: AHA; 2015.**

4. In the following table, provide the normal blood pressure for each pediatric age group.

Normal Blood Pressure for Age	
Age	**Minimal Systolic Blood Pressure (mm Hg)**
Infant	
Toddler	
Preschool-age child	
School-age child	
Adolescent	

Data from: American Heart Association (AHA). Vital signs in children. In: AHA. *Pediatric Advanced Life Support.* Dallas, TX: AHA; 2015.

5. In the following table, describe what the letters in the CHILD ABUSE mnemonic represent.

CHILD ABUSE Mnemonic	
Mnemonic	**What the Letter Represents**
C	
H	History consistent with injuries
I	
L	Lack of supervision
D	
A	Affect
B	
U	Unusual injury patterns
S	
E	Environmental clues

Problem Solving

Practice your calculation skills by solving the following math problems.

1. For children 1 to 10 years old, you would calculate the lower limit of acceptable blood pressure for age using the following formula:

$$\text{Minimal systolic blood pressure} = 70 + (2 \times \text{age in years})$$

a. You are evaluating a pediatric trauma patient. His age is 6 years. What would you estimate a normal systolic BP to be?

b. This patient is a 10-year-old asthmatic. What would you estimate a normal systolic BP to be?

c. On arrival, you have an unconscious pediatric patient. You estimate his age to be 5 or 6 years. What would normal BP be for a patient this age?

2. You would calculate the ET tube size for a child older than 2 years as follows:

$$4 + (\text{Age in years} \div 4) = \text{Uncuffed tube size (in mm)}$$

a. Calculate the appropriate ET tube size for a 6-year-old child.

b. Calculate the appropriate ET tube size for a 9-year-old child.

3. You have been called to the scene for a 4-year-old child who is unconscious and unresponsive after being shocked by sticking his finger into an electrical outlet. He is also pulseless and apneic.

a. The child weighs 40 pounds. Appropriate two-person BLS is in progress on your arrival. You attach the patient to your defibrillator/monitor and notice ventricular fibrillation (VF). Which energy setting would you use to administer defibrillations?

_____

_____

b. How much energy should be used on subsequent defibrillations?

_____

_____

4. You have been called to the scene for a 6-year-old girl who has severe anaphylaxis after ingesting peanuts at a ball game. The child is anxious, and she has an increased work of breathing and poor circulation. She weighs 60 pounds.

a. As the paramedic in charge, you decide that among all your other treatment priorities, this patient requires epinephrine. How will you administer this drug and at which dose?

_____

_____

b. This patient further requires the administration of diphenhydramine (Benadryl). How will you administer this drug and at which dose?

_____

_____

c. Fortunately, your patient is beginning to improve, but she is still wheezing. Which drug would you consider and at which dose?

_____

_____

© Jones & Bartlett Learning.

I hate asking about suicide—I feel like I'm giving the patient ideas.

If we can't deal with suicidality, who will?

Geriatric Emergencies

CHAPTER

44

Matching

Match each of definitions in the left column to the appropriate term in the right column.

_____ **1.** Inflammation of the joints.

_____ **2.** The assessment and treatment of disease in someone 65 years or older.

_____ **3.** A chronic deterioration of mental functions.

_____ **4.** A progressive organic condition in which neurons die, causing dementia.

_____ **5.** An ulcer that occurs when pressure is applied to the body tissue, resulting in a lack or perfusion and ultimately necrosis.

_____ **6.** An inflammatory disorder that affects the entire body and leads to degeneration and deformation of joints.

_____ **7.** A degenerative condition resulting in decreased mobility of vertebral joints and compression of neural elements.

_____ **8.** Swelling that presents around the sacral region of the spinal column.

_____ **9.** A disease state that results from the presence of microorganisms or their toxic products in the bloodstream.

_____ **10.** An acute confusional state characterized by global impairment of thinking, perception, judgment, and memory.

_____ **11.** Sadness from loss; grieving.

_____ **12.** A disease in bone mass and density.

_____ **13.** An acute inflammation in the skin caused by a bacterial infection.

_____ **14.** An organization that investigates cases involving abuse and neglect and provides case management services in some cases.

_____ **15.** Shingles; a contagious condition caused by the reactivation of the varicella virus or nerve roots.

_____ **16.** A tendency toward constancy or stability in the body's internal milieu.

_____ **17.** An organization that provides end-of-life care to patients with terminal illnesses and their families.

_____ **18.** The ability to perceive the position and movement of one's body or limbs.

_____ **19.** A formula used to determine the number of older people in a society as compared with the number of potential workers who are theoretically capable of providing resources to sustain the whole population. It is the number of older people (65 years and older) for every 100 adults (potential caregivers) between the ages of 18 and 64 years.

_____ **20.** The degeneration of a joint surface caused by wear and tear that leads to pain and stiffness.

A. Adult protective services (APS)

B. Alzheimer disease

C. Arthritis

D. Bereavement

E. Cellulitis

F. Delirium

G. Dementia

H. Geriatrics

I. Herpes zoster

J. Homeostasis

K. Hospice

L. Old-age dependency ratio

M. Osteoarthritis

N. Osteoporosis

O. Parkinson disease

P. Polypharmacy

Q. Presbycusis

R. Pressure ulcer

S. Proprioception

T. Rheumatoid arthritis (RA)

_____ **21.** A neurologic condition in which the portion of the brain responsible for production of dopamine has been damaged or overused, resulting in tremors.

_____ **22.** The use of multiple medications.

_____ **23.** Progressive hearing loss, particularly in the high frequencies, along with lessened ability to discriminate between a particular sound and background noise.

U. Sacral edema

V. Sepsis

W. Spondylosis

Multiple Choice

Read each item carefully, and then select the best response.

_____ **1.** Geriatrics is the assessment and treatment of disease in someone _____ years or older.

    A. 55

    B. 65

    C. 75

    D. None of the above

_____ **2.** A 35-year-old is aging just as fast as an 85-year-old, but the older person exhibits the cumulative results of a _____ process.

    A. longer

    B. shorter

    C. degenerative

    D. cumulative

_____ **3.** In older adults, cardiac output during exercise may _____ by as much as 30% to 40%.

    A. increase

    B. strengthen

    C. decline

    D. weaken

_____ **4.** Musculoskeletal changes, such as _____, may also affect pulmonary function by limiting lung volume and maximal inspiratory pressure.

    A. kyphosis

    B. osteoporosis

    C. decreased bone mass

    D. arthritis

_____ **5.** Incontinence is not a normal part of aging and can lead to:

    A. skin irritation.

    B. skin breakdown.

    C. urinary tract infections.

    D. All of the above

_____ **6.** _____ enables us to maintain postural stability by using a variety of receptors in the joints and information provided by the eyes. As these mechanisms fail with age, people become less steady on their feet, and the tendency to fall increases markedly.

    A. Balance

    B. Posture

    C. Proprioception

    D. Homeostasis

_____ **7.** Older adults are much more vulnerable to the following temperature stresses, EXCEPT:

    A. heat exhaustion.

    B. hypothermia.

    C. the absence of a febrile response to illness.

    D. hormonal temperature effects.

_____ **8.** Chronic obstructive pulmonary disease (COPD) includes all of the following, EXCEPT:

    A. chronic asthma.

    B. chronic bronchitis.

    C. emphysema.

    D. diuretic intolerant edema.

_____ **9.** The extent of bone loss that a person undergoes is influenced by numerous factors, including:

    A. genetics, smoking, and level of activity.

    B. age, sex, and genetics.

    C. age, skin condition, and diet.

    D. smoking, age, and skin condition.

_____ **10.** Some patients fear that mentioning a symptom will lead to a diagnosis or treatment that will jeopardize their independence. "If I mention those pains in my stomach," the older person may reason:

    A. "They'll put me in that nursing home to die."

    B. "My kids will think I'm going to die, and they'll start fighting over the money."

    C. "They'll put me in the hospital, and I can't afford another hospitalization and more prescriptions."

    D. "They'll put me in the hospital, and I may never come out of that place again."

Labeling

Label the components of the gastrointestinal (GI) system, and place an asterisk (*) next to the primary location(s) for GI bleeding.

1. Upper GI system

A. _____

B. _____

C. _____

D. _____

E. _____

F. _____

G. _____

H. _____

I. _____

J. _____

2. Lower GI system

A. _____

B. _____

C. _____

D. _____

E. _____

F. _____

G. _____

H. _____

I. _____

J. _____

Fill in the Blank

Read each item carefully, and then complete the statement by filling in the missing word(s).

1. _____ adults constitute an ever-increasing proportion of patients in the health care system, particularly the _____ care sector.

2. There is a widespread tendency to attribute genuine disease symptoms to "_____ _____ _____" and fail to provide proper treatment.

3. Some changes in _____ performance are probably not a direct consequence of _____, but rather reflect the _____ effect of sedentary lifestyle.

4. A person's _____ capacity also undergoes significant _____ with age, largely due to decreases in the elasticity of the lungs and in the size and strength of the respiratory muscles.

5. As a person ages, the kidneys shrink in size. This decline in weight results from a loss of functioning _____ _____, which translates into a smaller effective _____ surface.

6. The decrease in _____ may lead to malnutrition. Other changes in the mouth include a reduction in the volume of _____, with a resulting _____ of the mouth.

7. Narrowing of the _____ disks and _____ _____ of the vertebrae contribute to a decrease in _____ as a person ages, along with changes in posture.

8. A hearing-related impairment noted in the older adult population is _____ _____. Onset of symptoms

usually occurs in early middle age, with symptoms presenting in _____ that last several _____ at a time.

9. _____ and loss of _____ of the skin are the most visible signs of aging. Wrinkling occurs because the skin

becomes thinner, _____, less elastic, and more _____.

10. Heart attack or myocardial infarction is the major cause of _____ and _____ in people older than 65 years,

and its potential for mortality increases significantly after a person reaches _____ years.

Identify

In the following case studies, list the chief complaint, vital signs, and pertinent negatives.

1. On arrival to the Adult Day Care Center, you discover an 84-year-old woman who has "fallen." She normally walks with the assistance of a cane or walker. She is lying on a deeply carpeted floor and is conscious, alert, and complaining of right-sided midthigh pain. The fall was reportedly not witnessed. Her aide was assisting another client when the fall occurred. Your patient does not have a good recollection of what happened. She denies chest pain, shortness of breath, dizziness, nausea, or vomiting. She also denies tripping and falling. The area appears clear of obstacles, rugs, or other obvious trip hazards. Your physical exam is as previously indicated. You notice some inward rotation and shortening of the extremity. Her pulse is 84 beats/min and very irregular. Her oxygen saturation is 88% on room air. Her blood pressure (BP) is 106/86 mm Hg. The patient's skin turgor is poor. Pupils are equal, round, regular in size, and reactive to light and accommodation (PERRLA). An electrocardiogram (ECG) shows a sinus rhythm with frequent premature ventricular contractions (PVCs) and short runs of ventricular tachycardia (VT) (with a pulse).

   a. Chief complaint:

   _____

   _____

   b. Vital signs:

   _____

   _____

   c. Pertinent negatives:

   _____

   _____

2. It's early afternoon on a clear and warm spring day. You are dispatched to the parking lot of a local supermarket for a reported motor vehicle crash. On arrival, you discover an elderly man who is 92 years old. He is the driver of a vehicle that struck several parked cars. Bystanders state that the patient appears to be either sleeping or unconscious. You find the patient to be conscious but not alert to person, place, time, or purpose. The police identify his home phone number and call it. A pleasant-sounding elderly woman answers and states that her husband left home over an hour ago to pick up some groceries. She states that he has a problem with "sugar" and wonders if he has his hearing aids in place. As you begin examining the patient and taking his history, it becomes obvious that he is not wearing hearing aids. There is minimally detectable damage to the vehicle as well as the vehicles that were struck. The patient was found not to be wearing his seat belt. He does have a medical identification bracelet on, and it indicates extensive cardiac and diabetic history. Vital signs indicate a blood glucose level of 66 mg/dL. His pulse rate is 92 beats/min and regular, and BP is 160/72 mm Hg. His skin is warm and moist, his capillary refill is normal, and he has an oxygen saturation of 96% on room air. The patient is able to maintain his own airway and gag reflex. He was initially assisted

with oral glucose by the emergency medical responders (EMRs) at the scene. He is becoming increasingly alert and oriented and denies any injury.

a. Chief complaint:

_____

_____

b. Vital signs:

_____

_____

c. Pertinent negatives:

_____

_____

Complete the Patient Care Report (PCR)

Read the first incident scenario in the preceding Identify exercises and then complete the following PCR for the patient.

EMS Patient Care Report (PCR)					
Date:	**Incident No.:**	**Nature of Call:**		**Location:**	
Dispatched:	**En Route:**	**At Scene:**	**Transport:**	**At Hospital:**	**In Service:**
Patient Information					
Age:			**Allergies:**		
Sex:			**Medications:**		
Weight (in kg [lb]):			**Past Medical History:**		
			Chief Complaint:		
Vital Signs					
Time:	**BP:**	**Pulse:**	**Respirations:**		**SpO$_2$:**
Time:	**BP:**	**Pulse:**	**Respirations:**		**SpO$_2$:**
Time:	**BP:**	**Pulse:**	**Respirations:**		**SpO$_2$:**
EMS Treatment (circle all that apply)					
Oxygen @ _____ L/min via (circle one): NC NRM Bag-mask device		**Assisted Ventilation**	**Airway Adjunct**		**CPR**
Defibrillation	**Bleeding Control**	**Bandaging**	**Splinting**		**Other:**
Narrative					

Ambulance Calls

The following case scenarios provide an opportunity to explore the concerns associated with patient management and paramedic care. Read each scenario, and then answer each question.

1. One way to try to ensure that you don't miss anything important in the patient's history is to ask some general screening questions, irrespective of the patient's chief complaint. Suppose an 80-year-old woman has called for an ambulance because she feels "tired and weak." List 10 general screening questions you would ask to assess the status of her major organ systems.

   a. _____

   b. _____

   c. _____

   d. _____

   e. _____

   f. _____

   g. _____

   h. _____

   i. _____

   j. _____

2. You are called to the apartment of a 78-year-old woman who fell down.
   a. List six questions you would ask in taking the history of the present illness for an older patient who sustained trauma.

      (1)_____

      (2)_____

      (3)_____

      (4)_____

      (5)_____

      (6)_____

   b. List the information you should obtain about the patient's past (other) medical history.

      (1)_____

      (2)_____

      (3)_____

      (4)_____

   c. List six things that your environmental assessment should include:

      (1)_____

      (2)_____

      (3)_____

(4)_____

(5)_____

(6)_____

    d. While conducting the physical examination, you will of course be alert for signs or symptoms of those injuries to which older people are particularly vulnerable. List three injuries to which older adult patients are more susceptible.

        (1)_____

        (2)_____

        (3)_____

3. You are called to a shopping center where an older adult man tripped on a potted plant and fell, sustaining a minor laceration to his arm. As you are applying a dressing to the laceration, you notice that he seems very listless and depressed. List six factors of a "social assessment" you should consider.

    a. _____

    b. _____

    c. _____

    d. _____

    e. _____

    f. _____

True/False

The public (and also, regrettably, health care professionals) holds many widespread misconceptions about older adults and the process of aging that result in inaccurate stereotypes of older adults. If you believe the statement to be more true than false, write the letter "T" in the space provided. If you believe the statement to be more false than true, write the letter "F."

_____ **1.** The rate of aging is the same in a 35-year-old as it is in an 85-year-old.

_____ **2.** As the brain gets smaller and lighter, it loses its reserve capacity to store information.

_____ **3.** Older adults are more likely than younger individuals to seek emergency care for minor, nonserious complaints.

_____ **4.** The pain mechanism is often slowed among the older adults, causing burn injuries.

_____ **5.** The possibility of hearing loss increases with age.

_____ **6.** Sweat gland activity increases, hindering the ability to sweat and to regulate heat.

_____ **7.** Tachypnea can be a sensitive indicator of acute illness in older people.

_____ **8.** The older adult is at a higher risk of developing peripheral vascular disease.

_____ **9.** The earliest stage of Alzheimer disease involves forgetting components of one's life history and difficulty writing letters.

_____ **10.** One clue to elder abuse is unexplained injuries that do not fit the stated cause.

Short Answer

Complete this section with short written answers using the space provided.

1. Patients older than 65 years account for one-third of all ambulance calls today. As the population continues to age, that percentage can be expected to increase. It is therefore important for paramedics to understand the special problems and challenges posed by caring for the elderly. List five characteristics of the older adults that make it particularly challenging to diagnose their problems correctly and provide them with appropriate care.

a. _____

b. _____

c. _____

d. _____

e. _____

2. The process of aging in our society is nearly always accompanied by social and psychological stresses that may have an enormous impact on health. List two potentially stressful changes that tend to occur in a person's life as he or she approaches the "golden age."

a. _____

b. _____

3. The normal aging process produces changes in nearly every organ system of the body. It is important to know what constitutes a *normal* age-related change so that such a change will not be mistaken for a sign of disease (and, conversely, so that signs of disease will not be disregarded as "just part of getting old"). For each of the following organ systems, list two changes in structure or function that occur as a normal consequence of aging.

a. Cardiovascular

(1) _____

(2) _____

b. Respiratory

(1) _____

(2) _____

c. Renal

(1) _____

(2) _____

d. Digestive

(1) _____

(2) _____

e. Musculoskeletal

(1) _____

(2) _____

f. Nervous

(1) _____

(2) _____

g. Homeostatic

(1) _____

(2) _____

4. In younger patients, the chief complaint often has considerable value in localizing the patient's underlying problem. A middle-aged man suffering an acute coronary syndrome, for example, will usually complain of pain or discomfort in his chest, whereas a young person with pneumonia usually will have a cough and a fever. Among the elderly, on the other hand, the response to serious illness tends to be less specific. List four responses to illness common among seriously ill elderly patients.

a. _____

b. _____

c. _____

d. _____

5. Obtaining an accurate history from an elderly patient requires considerable skill because there are a number of obstacles to history taking among older adults that do not exist when you talk with younger patients. List four obstacles to obtaining a medical history from an elderly person, and indicate what steps you can take to overcome each of them.

a. Obstacle:

_____

_____

What I can do to try to overcome the obstacle:

_____

_____

b. Obstacle:

_____

_____

What I can do to try to overcome the obstacle:

_____

_____

c. Obstacle:

_____

_____

What I can do to try to overcome the obstacle:

_____

_____

d. Obstacle:

_____

_____

What I can do to try to overcome the obstacle:

_____

_____

6. In a middle-aged patient, the clinical presentation of such conditions as acute myocardial infarction (AMI) or heart failure is usually straightforward. In an elderly person with the same problem, the clinical presentation may be much less clear-cut. List at least two signs or symptoms that are commonly part of the clinical presentation of AMI and of heart failure in the elderly.

Condition	Possible Signs and Symptoms in the Elderly
Acute myocardial infarction	
Heart failure	

7. One of the most common presenting symptoms among the elderly is an acute confusional state (delirium). Complete the list of conditions likely to present as delirium in the elderly, which are represented by the letters in the acronym DELIRIUMS that follows:

D: _____

E: _____

L: _____

I: _____

R: _____

I: _____

U: _____

M: _____

S: _____

Fill in the Table

Fill in the missing parts of the following tables.

1.

Causes of Falls in Older Adults	
Cause	Clues to Suggest This Cause
	Obvious environmental hazard at the scene, such as poor lighting, scatter rugs, uneven sidewalk, or ice or other slippery surface
	Sudden fall; patient found on the ground somewhat confused, often temporarily paralyzed and unable to get up; no premonitory symptoms
	Fall when getting up from a recumbent or sitting position (Check medications the patient is taking, and ask about occult blood loss, such as presence of black stools. Measure blood pressure in recumbent and sitting positions.)
	Marked bradycardia or tachydysrhythmias
	Other characteristic signs of stroke, such as hemiparesis, hemiplegia, or aphasia
	Patient felt something snap before falling

2.

Signs of Dehydration in Older Adults
Dry tongue
Dry mucous membranes
Confusion
Sunken eyes

Because you picked up on the discrepancy in that kid's history, the police got that guy out of the family's life.

Patients With Special Challenges

Matching

Part I

Match each of the terms in the right column to the appropriate definition in the left column.

_____ **1.** A type of hearing impairment due to problems with the middle ear bones' ability to conduct sounds from the outer ear to the inner ear.

_____ **2.** Medical treatment aimed at symptom relief and providing comfort for the patient.

_____ **3.** A plastic pouch or bag attached over a colostomy to collect stool.

_____ **4.** The surgical establishment of an opening between the colon and the surface of the body for the purpose of providing drainage of the bowel.

_____ **5.** A tube placed in the body to relieve pressure by drawing excess cerebrospinal fluid from the brain or spinal cord.

_____ **6.** The part of a tracheostomy tube that is used to stabilize the tube to the patient's neck.

_____ **7.** A surgically created connection between an artery and a vein, usually in the arm, for dialysis access.

_____ **8.** Having perforations, holes, or openings.

_____ **9.** An area that a device was not intended to be inserted into—for example, a tracheostomy tube inserted into an area other than the trachea.

_____ **10.** A form of abuse that may be verbal (such as ridicule, threats, blaming, or humiliation) or nonverbal (such as caregiver ignoring the victim or isolating the victim from others). The abuse causes a substantial change in the victim's behavior, emotional response, or cognitive function or may manifest as a variety of mental illnesses.

_____ **11.** A developmental condition in which damage is done to the brain. It presents during infancy as a delay in walking or crawling and can take on a spastic form in which muscles are in a nearly constant state of contraction.

_____ **12.** A disorder in which patients have difficulty interpreting speech and differentiating it from other sounds that are present.

_____ **13.** Excessive growth and division of abnormal cells within the body that can occur in many body systems, tissues, and organs and that can progress rapidly and cause death in a relatively short period.

A. Acute angle-closure glaucoma (AACG)

B. Apraxia

C. Auditory neuropathy

D. Autism

E. Autism spectrum disorder

F. Bariatrics

G. Cancer

H. Central auditory processing disorder (CAPD)

I. Cerebral palsy (CP)

J. Cerebrospinal fluid shunt (CSF shunt)

K. Colostomy

L. Colostomy bag

M. Comfort care

_____ **14.** The medical specialty dedicated to prevention and treatment of obesity.

_____ **15.** A group of complex disorders of brain development, characterized by difficulties in social interaction, repetitive behaviors, and verbal and nonverbal communication.

_____ **16.** A speech disorder caused by neuromuscular disturbance that causes speech to become slow and slurred.

_____ **17.** A genetic chromosomal defect that can occur during fetal development and that results in intellectual disability and certain physical characteristics, such as a round head with a flat occiput and slanted, wide-set eyes.

_____ **18.** Insufficient development of a portion of the brain, resulting in some level of dysfunction or impairment.

_____ **19.** A broad term that describes an infant or child's failure to reach a particular developmental milestone by the expected time.

_____ **20.** A genetic disorder of the endocrine system that makes it difficult for chloride to move through cells; primarily targets that respiratory and digestive systems.

_____ **21.** A developmental disorder characterized by impairments of social interaction; may include severe behavioral problems, repetitive motor activities, and impairments in verbal and nonverbal skills.

_____ **22.** A condition characterized by normal function of the structures of the ear without a corresponding stimulation of auditory centers of the brain; also called dyssynchrony.

_____ **23.** A neurologic impairment in which the brain is intermittently unable to carry out the command for speech or other tasks.

_____ **24.** Increased intraocular pressure that leads to ocular pain and decreased visual acuity. Sudden onset is a medical emergency.

_____ **25.** Medical treatment aimed at curing an illness.

_____ **26.** A psychological conditional in which stress or mental conflict is converted into physical complaints.

N. Conductive hearing loss

O. Conversion disorder

P. Curative care

Q. Cystic fibrosis (CF)

R. Developmental delay

S. Developmental disability

T. Down syndrome

U. Dysarthria

V. Emotional abuse

W. False lumen

X. Fenestrated

Y. Fistula

Z. Flange

Part II

Match each of the terms in the right column to the appropriate definition in the left column.

_____ **1.** A congenital condition characterized by failure of the optic nerve to completely develop, possibly resulting in optic nerve atrophy over time.

_____ **2.** An autoimmune disorder in which the extraocular muscles become weakened and are fatigued.

_____ **3.** A solid plug at the end of a tracheostomy.

_____ **4.** A condition in which a person's body mass index is greater than 30 kg/m^2.

_____ **5.** A developmental anomaly in which a portion of the spinal cord or meninges protrudes outside the spinal column or even outside the body, usually in the area of the lumbar spine; also called a spina bifida.

_____ **6.** A category of professional required by some states to report suspicions of child maltreatment. Prehospital professionals may be included.

_____ **7.** A type of disability in which difficulties with reading, spelling, or writing cause a person to fall behind expectations for a given age.

_____ **8.** A balloon that is inserted into the aorta and connected to a pump via a catheter. This therapy helps to increase the blood flow to the coronary arteries during diastole (inflation) and decrease afterload of blood from the left ventricle (deflation).

A. Hemodynamic monitoring

B. Heparinized solution

C. Hospice

D. Hydrocephalus

E. Ileus

F. Inner cannula

G. Intellectual disability

H. Intra-aortic balloon pump

_____ **9.** A medical condition in which there is an abnormal buildup of cerebrospinal fluid in the skull; this can be acquired (occurring after birth) or congenital (developing before birth).

I. Language-based learning disability

_____ **10.** An organization that provides end-of-life care to patients with terminal illnesses and their families.

J. Mandatory reporter

_____ **11.** A saline solution mixed with heparin, an anticoagulant used to prevent blood clots from forming.

K. Muscular dystrophy

_____ **12.** Monitoring and measurement of blood movement, volume, and pressure.

L. Myasthenia gravis

_____ **13.** Paralysis of the upper and lower extremities.

M. Myasthenic crisis

_____ **14.** The death of nerve fibers as a late consequence of polio. The syndrome is characterized by swallowing difficulties, weakness, fatigue, and breathing problems.

N. Myelomeningocele

_____ **15.** A viral infection that attacks and destroys motor axons. The disease can cause weakness, paralysis, and respiratory arrest. Because an effective vaccine has been developed, the incidence of the disease is now rare.

O. Obesity

_____ **16.** A form of abuse that involves an intentional act, such as throwing, striking, hitting, kicking, burning, or biting a vulnerable person.

P. Obturator

_____ **17.** A category of disorders that impact a person's ability to produce sounds that combine into spoken words.

Q. Ocular myasthenia gravis

_____ **18.** A complication of myasthenia gravis in which weakened respiratory muscles lead to respiratory failure.

R. Optic nerve hypoplasia

_____ **19.** A condition in which the body generates antibodies against its own acetylcholine receptors, causing muscle weakness, often in the face.

S. Outer cannula

_____ **20.** A broad term that describes a category of incurable genetic diseases that cause a slow, progressive degeneration of the muscle fibers.

T. Palliative care

_____ **21.** A primarily cognitive disorder that appears during childhood and is accompanied by lack of adaptive behaviors, such as the ability to live and function independently or interact successfully with others; generally defined as an intelligence quotient below 70; formerly called mental retardation.

U. Paraplegia

_____ **22.** The inner tube that is inserted into the outer cannula of a tracheostomy tube.

V. Phonologic process disorders

_____ **23.** Disruption or loss of normal gastrointestinal motility.

W. Physical abuse

_____ **24.** Paralysis of the lower extremities.

X. Poliomyelitis

_____ **25.** Medical care aimed at relief of pain and suffering in terminally ill patients.

Y. Postpolio syndrome

_____ **26.** The larger (outer) tube of a tracheostomy tube.

Z. Quadriplegia

Part III

Match each of the terms in the right column to the appropriate definition in the left column.

_____ **1.** A person legally authorized to make health care decisions on behalf of a patient who is incapable of making or communicating the decision on his or her own.

A. Retinopathy

_____ **2.** A developmental anomaly in which a portion of the spinal cord or meninges protrudes outside the spinal column or even outside the body, usually in the area of the lumbar spine (the lower third of the spine); also called myelomeningocele.

B. Semantic-pragmatic disorder

_____ **3.** A form of cerebral palsy in which all four limbs are affected.

C. Sensorineural hearing loss

_____ **4.** A chronic form of paralysis in which the affected muscles experience continued spasm.

D. Sexual abuse

_____ **5.** A surgically constructed opening for the urinary system.

_____ **6.** A device that converts energy or pressure into electrical signals.

_____ **7.** A plastic tube placed within the tracheostomy site (stoma).

_____ **8.** A sickness that a patient cannot be cured of. Death is imminent.

_____ **9.** A form of abuse that involves forcing a vulnerable person to perform or be involved in sexual acts, or to be involved in sexual activities, such as pornography, in return for something they need or want, such as money, food, or shelter.

_____ **10.** A form of abuse that involves a vulnerable person being forced into unwanted sexual acts, or into involvement in sexual activities such as pornography.

_____ **11.** A permanent lack of hearing caused by a lesion or damage of the inner ear.

_____ **12.** A condition characterized by delayed language developmental milestones, resulting in the person repeatedly using irrelevant phrases out of context, confusing word pairs, and having trouble following conversations.

_____ **13.** Any eye disorder in which the retina becomes diseased, leading to partial or total vision loss.

E. Sexual exploitation

F. Spastic paralysis

G. Spastic tetraplegia

H. Spina bifida

I. Surrogate decision maker

J. Terminal illness

K. Tracheostomy tube

L. Transducer

M. Urostomy

Multiple Choice

Read each item carefully, and then select the best response.

_____ **1.** Which of the following would be considered speech impairments?

     A. Articulation disorders

     B. Language disorders

     C. Fluency disorders

     D. All of the above

_____ **2.** Congenital causes of visual impairment would include each of the following, EXCEPT:

     A. fetal exposure to cytomegalovirus.

     B. cerebrovascular accident.

     C. retinopathy of prematurity.

     D. hydrocephalus.

_____ **3.** Bruises on the torso, _____, and buttocks are suggestive of abuse.

     A. ears

     B. proximal arms

     C. abdomen

     D. All of the above

_____ **4.** The different types of paralysis include all of the following, EXCEPT:

     A. spastic paralysis.

     B. quadriplegia.

     C. myasthenia gravis.

     D. paraplegia.

_____ **5.** Which of the following is NOT typically tunneled under the skin and into the vena cava?

     A. Hickman

     B. Port-a-Cath

     C. Vas-Cath/Permcath

     D. Broviac

_____ **6.** Patients with a terminal illness who receive continued medical care, hoping for a statistically improbable recovery, are receiving:

   A. comfort care.

   B. acute care.

   C. curative care.

   D. palliative care.

_____ **7.** Chemotherapy medications are notorious for causing:

   A. nausea and vomiting.

   B. loss of appetite.

   C. immune system compromise.

   D. All of the above

_____ **8.** A potentially devastating, nonprogressive neurologic disorder resulting from brain tissue injury during brain development is a condition called:

   A. epilepsy.

   B. cerebral palsy.

   C. cystic fibrosis.

   D. multiple sclerosis.

_____ **9.** Which of the following devices serves as a long-term replacement for an endotracheal (ET) tube in a patient who has a chronic condition?

   A. A ventricular assist device

   B. A tracheostomy tube

   C. An obturator

   D. A stoma

_____ **10.** You are treating a 62-year-old man who is complaining of chest pain for the past 35 minutes. You have decided to administer aspirin, nitroglycerin, and oxygen and to start an IV. The patient has been receiving treatments through a long-term vascular access device in his chest. If there are still distal IV sites available, why should the paramedic _avoid_ using the long-term device in the patient's chest?

   A. The device may be inserted directly into the vena cava.

   B. It may require a special needle to access the port.

   C. The device may be maintained with a high dose of heparin.

   D. All of the above

Labeling

Label the following diagrams with the correct terms.

   1. American Sign Language (ASL) signs for common terms related to illness or injury

© Jones & Bartlett Learning.

© Jones & Bartlett Learning.

A. _____

B. _____

C. _____

D. _____

E1. _____

E2. _____

F. _____

G. _____

H. _____

I. _____

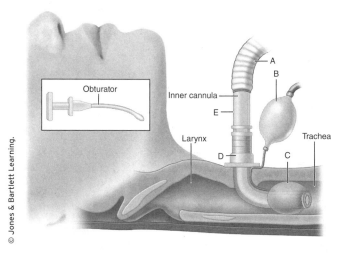

J. _____

2. Parts of the tracheostomy tube

Obturator

Inner cannula

Larynx

Trachea

A

B

E

D

C

A. _____

B. _____

C. _____

D. _____

E. _____

Fill in the Blank

Read each item carefully, and then complete the statement by filling in the missing word(s).

1. Hearing challenges are generally classified into two types: _____ and _____ deafness.

2. Hearing _____ may be _____ or acquired.

3. Speech impairment may be divided into disorders impacting _____, voice _____, fluency, and _____.

4. Autistic patients may present with a(n) _____-_____ disorder of speech.

5. Patients may receive a(n) _____ following _____ trauma or surgery.

6. The medical specialty of _____ has emerged in response to the widespread and profound incidence of adult and

   childhood _____.

7. Myelomeningocele, also known as _____ _____, is a birth defect caused by improper development of the

   _____ _____ tube consisting of the brain and spinal cord.

8. Infants and young children may be diagnosed with _____ _____ (_____), a genetic disorder that

   is characterized by increased production of mucus in the lungs and digestive tract. This disorder is caused by a(n)

   _____ _____ gene, inherited from each parent.

9. Cerebral palsy generally produces _____ _____ muscle function or _____.

10. Spina bifida, also known as _____, is a birth defect caused by improper _____ of the fetal neural

    tube consisting of the brain and _____ cord.

Identify

Read the following case studies, and then list the chief complaint, the history of the present illness, and other medical history.

1. You have been called to the scene by distraught family members. The patient is becoming increasingly disoriented and appears unresponsive. The patient is exhibiting an irregular breathing pattern with periods of apnea. His blood pressure (BP) is about 70/palp, and his pulse is very fast and erratic. Some family members have what appears to be a valid prehospital do not resuscitate (DNR) order.

   a. Chief complaint:

   _____

   _____

   b. History of the present illness:

   _____

   _____

   c. Other medical history:

   _____

   _____

2. You are responding to a call to an adult group home for adults with disabilities. The nature of the call is for a patient with seizures. On arrival, you are met by staff members who have the patient's complete chart. The patient has a history of Down syndrome and a seizure disorder. The patient is on multiple medications and has been given rectal diazepam (Diastat).

   a. Chief complaint:

_____

_____

   b. History of the present illness:

_____

_____

   c. Other medical history:

_____

_____

3. Your patient has a chief complaint of fever. The patient's home health aide states that the patient's urine has been cloudy and that he's suddenly developed a fever of 101.3°F. He is conscious and alert, and his vitals are a BP of 110/70 mm Hg and a heart rate of 108 beats/min. He is always confined to a wheelchair. He communicates with a writing board. He is a quadriplegic and has a Foley catheter, tracheotomy, colostomy, and feeding tube. He is taking an antibiotic and a steroid medicine.

   a. Chief complaint:

_____

_____

   b. History of the present illness:

_____

_____

   c. Other medical history:

_____

_____

Complete the Patient Care Report (PCR)

Read incident scenario 3 in the preceding Identify exercises, and then complete the following PCR for the patient.

EMS Patient Care Report (PCR)					
Date:	Incident No.:	Nature of Call:		Location:	
Dispatched:	En Route:	At Scene:	Transport:	At Hospital:	In Service:

Patient Information	
Age:	Allergies:
Sex:	Medications:
Weight (in kg [lb]):	Past Medical History:
	Chief Complaint:

Vital Signs				
Time:	BP:	Pulse:	Respirations:	SpO$_2$:
Time:	BP:	Pulse:	Respirations:	SpO$_2$:
Time:	BP:	Pulse:	Respirations:	SpO$_2$:

EMS Treatment (circle all that apply)				
Oxygen @ _____ L/min via (circle one): NC NRM Bag-mask device		Assisted Ventilation	Airway Adjunct	CPR
Defibrillation	Bleeding Control	Bandaging	Splinting	Other:

Narrative

Ambulance Calls

The following case scenarios provide an opportunity to explore the concerns associated with patient management and paramedic care. Read each scenario, and then answer each question.

1. You receive an "alpha" response for a patient with chronic pain. On arrival, you note the wheelchair ramp in front of the apartment. Once inside, you recognize your patient. You have provided care for her in the past. She is 36 years old and is complaining of severe lower back pain and requesting transportation to the medical center. She is somewhat difficult to interact with and is not very polite. Despite that, you continue to be professional and initiate care. She has a history of spina bifida and is seated in her motorized wheelchair. She is covered in a blanket.

   a. What can you do to help alleviate her discomfort during transfer from her wheelchair to the cot?

   _____

   _____

   b. Based on your knowledge of spina bifida, what other medical issues may be present?

   _____

   _____

2. Tonight you are working a special event at the civic center. It's the concert of a popular country singer. The place is packed. Other than a couple of requests for ice packs and ear plugs, the event has been uneventful. Suddenly, security requests emergency medical services (EMS) to section 103 for a person having a seizure. Your patient is a 12-year-old girl with her mom. The patient has Down syndrome and a seizure disorder. The seizure is over by the time you arrive, but the patient appears postictal and has a large amount of saliva and snoring-type respirations.

   a. How would you go about treating the patient?

   _____

   _____

   b. What are the characteristic physical features of someone with Down syndrome?

   _____

   _____

True/False

If you believe the statement to be more true than false, write the letter "T" in the space provided. If you believe the statement to be more false than true, write the letter "F."

_____ 1. Whatever the source of the challenge, patients with special needs will require you to adapt your assessment and management to accommodate their needs.

_____ 2. A method of instilling a special solution through a catheter into the renal patient's abdomen is referred to as hemodialysis.

_____ 3. A phonologic process disorder impacts a person's ability to produce sounds that combine into spoken words.

_____ 4. Patients with nearsightedness have an impairment known as myopia.

_____ 5. It is not necessary to modify patient assessment techniques for the patient with a cognitive impairment.

_____ 6. Patients with mental impairments view all strangers, especially paramedics in uniform, in a friendly and calm manner.

_____ 7. Cystic fibrosis is a chronic dysfunction of the endocrine system that targets multiple body systems but primarily the respiratory and digestive systems.

_____ 8. Muscular dystrophy is an acquired muscular disease that causes degeneration of the muscle fibers. In many cases, the destroyed fibers are replaced by fat or connective tissue.

_____ **9.** Patients with myasthenia gravis have facial and throat muscles that could become so weak that the patient suffers an acute onset of respiratory failure.

_____ **10.** Patients with obesity may have a diminished respiratory reserve, causing hypoxia quickly.

_____ **11.** Speech is not possible unless expired air is allowed to pass around a tracheostomy tube and through the larynx.

Short Answer
Complete this section with short written answers using the space provided.

1. Many of the patients a paramedic encounters have hearing impairments. Sometimes this impairment is readily noticeable.

   a. What clues would indicate to you that your patient has a hearing impairment?

      (1) _____

      (2) _____

      (3) _____

   b. List five ways you can go about communicating with someone with a hearing impairment.

      (1) _____

      (2) _____

      (3) _____

      (4) _____

      (5) _____

2. Transporting obese patients can be particularly challenging for paramedic crews. List five strategies that would be helpful to the patient and the EMS providers.

   a. _____

   b. _____

   c. _____

   d. _____

   e. _____

3. You respond to a car crash. On arrival, you discover a frightened but apparently uninjured rear-seat passenger. Everyone else appears to be out of the car and walking around. You discover that the passenger has a visual impairment.

   a. What are some of the causes of visual impairments?

      (1) _____

      (2) _____

      (3) _____

b. What can paramedics do to alleviate some of the fears felt by patients with visual impairments?

(1) _____

(2) _____

(3) _____

(4) _____

Fill in the Table

Fill in the missing parts of the tables.

1. A list of the known causes of developmental disabilities is found in the following table. Fill in the missing parts of the table.

Known Causes of Development Disabilities
Genetic abnormality
Maternal trauma, hemorrhage, or infection during fetal development
Malnutrition
Neurologic insult, injury, or infection
Toxic exposure
Near drowning
Trauma or hypoxia during delivery

Data from: Facts about developmental disabilities. Centers for Disease Control and Prevention website. https://www.cdc.gov/ncbddd/developmentaldisabilities/facts.html. Updated July 9, 2015. Accessed May 4, 2017; Pivalizza P, Lalani SR. Intellectual disability in children: evaluation for a cause. UpToDate website. http://www.uptodate.com/contents/intellectual-disability-in-children-evaluation-for-a-cause. Updated May 26, 2016. Accessed May 4, 2017; and Pivalizza P, Lalani SR. Intellectual disability in children: definition, diagnosis, and assessment of needs. UpToDate website. http://www.uptodate.com/contents/intellectual-disability-in-children-definition-diagnosis-and-assessment-of-needs?source=see_link. Updated August 15, 2016. Accessed May 4, 2017.

2. Complete the list of causes of obesity.

Causes of and Contributing Factors to Obesity
Poor dietary choices
Hormonal changes
Low basal metabolic rate
Cessation/reduction of cigarette smoking

Data from: Dare S, Mackay DF, Pell JP. Relationship between smoking and obesity: a cross-sectional study of 499,504 middle-aged adults in the UK general population. *PLoS One.* 2015;10(4):e0123579. https://www.ncbi.nlm.nih.gov/pmc/articles/PMC4401671/. Accessed May 4, 2017.

Transport Operations

We forgot about the ice!

EMS   EMS

The size-up of the emergency scene is a critical process. . .

© Jones & Bartlett Learning.

Matching

Part I

Match each of the numbered items to the appropriate type of ambulance transport.

Your air ambulance transports to a regional trauma center. Your ground ambulance transports to a community hospital. Choose the correct transportation for your patient.

A. Air ambulance

G. Ground ambulance

_____ **1.** 50-year-old in cardiac arrest

_____ **2.** 8-year-old having an asthma attack

_____ **3.** 22-year-old thrown from a rollover crash

_____ **4.** 44-year-old with amputation of the left hand

_____ **5.** 26-year-old mountain climber who fell approximately 50 feet

_____ **6.** 24-year-old with a breech presentation delivery

_____ **7.** 56-year-old with an active upper gastrointestinal bleed

_____ **8.** 18-year-old with a broken femur from an all-terrain vehicle crash

_____ **9.** 2-year-old submersion victim who fell through ice at the local pond

_____ **10.** 34-year-old with a broken ankle from a football game

Part II

Match each of the definitions in the left column to the appropriate term in the right column.

_____ **1.** A sensation that when an operator depresses the brake pedal, the steering wheel is being pulled to the left or the right.

A. Aircraft transport

_____ **2.** A person who assists a driver in backing up an emergency vehicle to compensate for blind spots at the back of the vehicle.

B. Belt noise

_____ **3.** A sensation of looseness or sloppiness in a vehicle's steering.

C. Blind spot

_____ **4.** A safe distance maintained between your vehicle and other vehicles on any side of you.

D. Brake fade

_____ **5.** Federal standards that regulate the design and manufacturing guidelines of emergency medical vehicles.

E. Brake pull

_____ **6.** A finding that when the operator lets go of the steering wheel, a vehicle consistently wanders to the left or right.

F. Cleaning

_____ **7.** The process of removing dirt, dust, blood, or other visible contaminants from a surface.

G. Cushion of safety

_____ **8.** Driving with awareness and responsibility for other drivers on the roadways when you are operating an emergency vehicle in the emergency mode, and making sure that other drivers are aware of your approach.

H. Decontaminate

_____ 9. An extra-heavy-duty transport vehicle.

_____ 10. Standard van, forward-control integral cab-body.

_____ 11. Specialty van, forward-control integral cab-body.

_____ 12. The killing of pathogenic agents by using potent means of disinfection.

_____ 13. Medical or trauma evacuation of a patient by helicopter.

_____ 14. Fixed-wing aircraft and helicopters that have been modified for medical care; used to evacuate and transport patients with life-threatening injuries to treatment facilities.

_____ 15. A chirping or squealing sound, synchronous with engine speed.

_____ 16. To remove or neutralize radiation, chemical, or other hazardous material from clothing, equipment, vehicles, and personnel.

_____ 17. The killing of pathogenic agents by direct application of chemicals.

_____ 18. An area of the road that is blocked from your sight by your own vehicle or mirrors.

_____ 19. A sensation that an emergency vehicle has lost its power brakes.

_____ 20. A time of day or day or week in which the call volume is at its highest.

_____ 21. The placement of an emergency vehicle at a specific geographic location to cover larger areas of territory and reduce response times.

_____ 22. A drift that is persistent enough that an operator can feel a tug on the steering wheel.

_____ 23. A process, such as heating, that removes microbial contamination.

_____ 24. The staging of emergency vehicles to strategic locations within a service area to allow for coverage of emergency calls.

_____ 25. Conventional, truck-cab chassis with a modular body that can be transferred to a new chassis as needed.

_____ 26. A vibration, synchronous with road speed, that can be felt in the steering wheel.

_____ 27. A condition in which the tires of a vehicle may be lifted off the road surface as water "piles up" under them, making the vehicle feel as though it is floating.

_____ 28. A designated location for the landing of aircraft.

_____ 29. A common finding at low speeds when a vehicle has a bent wheel.

I. Disinfection
J. DOT KKK 1822
K. Drift
L. Due regard
M. Heavy-duty emergency vehicle
N. High-level disinfection

O. Hydroplaning
P. Landing zone

Q. Medevac
R. Peak load

S. Posting
T. Spotter
U. Steering play

V. Steering pull

W. Sterilization
X. Strategic deployment

Y. Type I emergency medical vehicle

Z. Type II emergency medical vehicle

AA. Type III emergency medical vehicle

BB. Wheel bounce
CC. Wheel wobble

Multiple Choice

Read each item carefully, and then select the best response.

_____ 1. The design and manufacturing specifications outlined in KKK 1822 federal guidelines are developed by the:

   A. American Heart Association.

   B. General Services Administration.

   C. Bureau of Transport.

   D. National Fire Protection Association.

_____ 2. Which of the following should be done at the beginning of each shift?

   A. Change the oil in the ambulance.

   B. Complete an ambulance equipment/supply checklist.

   C. Wash the ambulance.

   D. Repair the equipment tagged as faulty.

_____ 3. When leaving the scene, what should you tell family members who are following you to the hospital?

   A. Drive as fast as you can with your flashers on.

   B. Follow the ambulance with your flashers on.

   C. Drive normally, and do not follow the ambulance.

   D. Don't come until the doctor has called you.

_____ **4.** What can happen to the grass on the side of the road if you park the ambulance on it?

    A. Nothing.

    B. It can catch fire.

    C. It can die from the fumes of the ambulance.

    D. It can clog up the underside of the ambulance and cause the ambulance to stop running.

_____ **5.** What should you use when backing up an ambulance?

    A. The mirrors

    B. The guidance system that beeps when you are about to run into something

    C. The mirrors and a spotter

    D. Never back up an ambulance; always park so that you can leave without backing up.

_____ **6.** All of the following are considered advantages of using an air ambulance, EXCEPT:

    A. they can provide access to remote areas.

    B. they are used when rapid transport is needed.

    C. they can carry many caregivers.

    D. specialized equipment or skills are needed.

_____ **7.** What size should the standard landing zone be for a typical helicopter?

    A. 50 × 50 feet

    B. 75 × 75 feet

    C. 100 × 100 feet

    D. 100 × 100 yards

_____ **8.** What type of light should you use to mark a landing zone?

    A. A headlight facing downward, in each corner of the zone

    B. A strobe light in the center of the zone

    C. A spotlight shining straight up in the center of the zone

    D. Blue flares in the center of the zone

_____ **9.** When should you approach the helicopter after it has landed?

    A. Only after the blades have come to a complete stop

    B. As soon as it touches down

    C. When the pilot or crew on the helicopter signal for you to approach

    D. Never approach; let the crew come to you.

_____ **10.** Which of the following is NOT a key factor in staffing your ambulances?

    A. Unit cost of each run

    B. Taxpayer subsidies

    C. Response times

    D. The types of calls you will respond to

_____ **11.** You had a very busy overtime shift and have not gotten any rest in the last 24 hours. You are feeling exhausted and still have 6 more hours to go. What should you do?

    A. Admit to yourself and your partner you are fatigued.

    B. Do not drive the ambulance.

    C. Ask your supervisor to place your unit out of service for a while.

    D. All of the above are appropriate.

_____ **12.** If you are driving the ambulance to the hospital and notice that you are being tailgated very closely by another vehicle, what should you do?

    A. Get out and confront the driver.

    B. Notify your dispatcher to alert the police.

    C. Speed up to attempt to lose the tailgater.

    D. Slam on your brakes to try to scare the other driver.

Labeling

Label the following diagrams with the correct terms.

1. Locations of the landing zone
   A. Where to post guard
   B. Pilot's blind area
   C. Pilot's area of vision

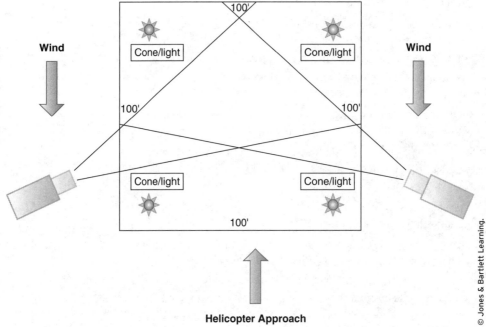

A. _____

B. _____

C. _____

2. Helicopter hand signals

A. _____   D. _____

B. _____   E. _____

C. _____   F. _____

Fill in the Blank

Assume you have been called to the scene of a road crash. Among the equipment listed here, mark an X beside that which you would grab to take along on your first dash from the ambulance to the patient. If any equipment you need has been left off the list, add it at the end, and explain why you need it.

One sure way to *waste* time at the scene of a collision (or at any call) is to make a dozen trips back and forth to the ambulance to fetch equipment and supplies that you left behind. Well-organized paramedics take with them everything needed for the primary survey and first stages of management.

_____ Long-leg air splint   _____ Stethoscope

_____ Drug box   _____ Flashlight

_____ Portable suction unit   _____ Triangular bandages

_____ Oxygen cylinder   _____ Chemical cold packs

_____ OB kit   _____ Cervical collar

_____ Pocket mask   _____ Traction splint

_____ Oropharyngeal airways   _____ Nonrebreathing mask

_____ Intravenous fluid bags   _____ Long backboard/straps

_____ Dressing materials   _____ Oral thermometer

_____ Large-bore IV cannulas   _____ Fire extinguisher

_____ Head immobilizer   _____ Bed pan

_____ Self-adhering roller bandage _____ Heavy-duty scissors

_____ Selection of board splints   _____ Emesis basin

_____ Wheeled cot stretcher   _____ Handheld radio

_____ ECG monitor   _____ Adhesive bandages

_____ Contact lens remover

Other equipment that might be needed:

_____

_____

Identify

Read the following case study, and then list the chief complaint, vital signs, and pertinent negatives.

Walt and Dave respond to a two-vehicle crash. Their patient is a 41-year-old woman who tried to avoid a car that crossed the centerline on the highway. The sports utility vehicle (SUV) she was driving rolled twice and landed on its wheels. The back portion was struck by the oncoming car. Walt is able to gain access through a back door and performs manual stabilization. Dave begins an assessment on the patient. She is conscious and alert and remembers the entire collision. She is complaining of pain in her left shoulder area. The trauma assessment shows a deformity of the left collarbone and bruising beginning around the seat belt marks. Because of the collarbone, a cervical collar won't fit, and so Dave and Walt immobilize the woman on a backboard, pad the neck and head with towels, and then tape them down. Walt first applies supplemental oxygen because the SpO_2 is 94%, then begins baseline vital signs on the woman. He finds that her breathing is 22 breaths/min and shallow with decreased lung sounds on the left. Her pulse is 114 beats/min, and blood pressure (BP) is 132/84 mm Hg. The heart monitor shows sinus tachycardia with a few premature ventricular contractions (PVCs) every few minutes. The patient can feel her arms and legs and is rating her pain in the shoulder at a 9/10. Her pupils are equal, round, and reactive to light and accommodation (PERRLA). Skin is warm, but to help with shock, Dave turns the heat on in the unit and places a blanket over her. Walt starts an IV line, and they monitor her heart and breathing on the way to the trauma center. Walt does a secondary assessment and a physical exam that turns up a few small scrapes and bruises to her legs. He gets a SAMPLE history just as they pull into the regional trauma center.

a. Chief complaint:

_____

_____

b. Vital signs:

_____

_____

c. Pertinent negatives:

_____

_____

Complete the Patient Care Report (PCR)

Reread the case study in the preceding Identify exercise, and then complete the following PCR for the patient.

EMS Patient Care Report (PCR)					
Date:	Incident No.:		Nature of Call:		Location:
Dispatched:	En Route:	At Scene:	Transport:	At Hospital:	In Service:
Patient Information					
Age:			Allergies:		
Sex:			Medications:		
Weight (in kg [lb]):			Past Medical History:		
			Chief Complaint:		
Vital Signs					
Time:	BP:		Pulse:	Respirations:	SpO$_2$:
Time:	BP:		Pulse:	Respirations:	SpO$_2$:
Time:	BP:		Pulse:	Respirations:	SpO$_2$:
EMS Treatment (circle all that apply)					
Oxygen @ _____ L/min via (circle one): NC NRM Bag-mask device		Assisted Ventilation	Airway Adjunct		CPR
Defibrillation	Bleeding Control	Bandaging	Splinting		Other:
Narrative					

Ambulance Calls

The following case scenarios provide an opportunity to explore the concerns associated with patient management and paramedic care. Read each scenario, and then answer each question.

1. Unit 2 has been dispatched to a new subdivision for a man who fell off a second-story roof. When Cory and Bill arrive, they find a 22-year-old man unconscious and lying on a large pile of dirt. Cory and Bill don't really like each other much, and neither one is willing to concede to the other. They both sprint to the patient to try to be the "lead" medic on the scene. Neither one of them has bothered to take any equipment. The patient is lying on his back. Cory finally performs C-spine stabilization while Bill starts a secondary assessment, including a trauma assessment, but that is kind of hard because he has no equipment. Bill sends a worker from the scene to get his orange airway bag out of the squad. After the airway bag arrives, oxygen is applied, and Bill does his assessment. The patient doesn't seem to have any broken bones, but he is still out cold. One of the workers is trying to tell Cory what happened, but Cory won't listen. He lets the worker know that they are "here" now, and they will handle any medical problems. After about 15 minutes of being on scene, Bill finally has to go get a rigid cervical collar, scoop stretcher, and cot because the construction workers can't seem to find them even with Bill yelling at them. After they get the patient in the unit, they take vital signs, and they both try to grab the airway bag so that they can intubate. After a few seconds of arguing, they decide to do rock, paper, scissors to pick who gets to intubate. Cory wins and succeeds in intubating, and Bill decides to start a couple of IV lines. Bill gives Cory a high five after he sticks a 14-gauge in the left AC. After they get ready to roll, there is a discussion and another rock, paper, scissors contest to decide who is going to drive. Thirty-four minutes after reaching the scene, they are on the road to the closest hospital. Because their patient is starting to posture, they decide to turn around and head for the trauma center, another 15 minutes away.

   a. What should Cory and Bill have done *prior* to arriving on the scene?

   _____

   _____

   b. List six moves Cory and Bill made that were unprofessional while on the scene.

   (1)_____

   (2)_____

   (3)_____

   (4)_____

   (5)_____

   (6)_____

   c. Discuss Cory and Bill's transport decision and what you would have done differently.

   _____

   _____

   _____

   _____

2. Jeff and Larry both show up just a few minutes late for their shift. Both of them were up late the night before watching the Monday night football game on TV. They both agree that because they are late and because they each have headaches, they will skip the morning check of the squad and go straight for the coffee and aspirin. Right away, they get a call for a woman who has fallen in front of the local grocery store. As they climb into the unit and take off, Jeff can hardly keep the squad on the road. It is doing a shimmy and shake down the road. When they arrive at the grocery store, the patient seems to be okay and doesn't want to go anywhere but home. She denies any pain and is alert. She states she just stepped off of the curb wrong and lost her balance. The store manager is the one who insisted on calling for an ambulance. Jeff turns off the squad when they decide this is a no-transport and grabs the paperwork for the patient to

sign off on. After getting that all cleared up, they jump back into the squad to leave, but it won't start. They miss two calls while waiting for a tow truck. After they get the squad back to the service station, they are really embarrassed to find they were out of gas, and the shimmy they felt earlier was because of low pressure in a back tire. They finally make it back to the station around noon and are greeted by a very angry supervisor and a stressed-out crew number 2 who had to cover calls for Jeff and Larry.

a. Why should you check your emergency vehicle at the beginning of every shift?

_____

_____

b. What visual factors would you check before jumping in and running a call?

_____

_____

True/False

If you believe the statement to be more true than false, write the letter "T" in the space provided. If you believe the statement to be more false than true, write the letter "F."

_____ **1.** The standards for ambulances are determined by the Food and Drug Administration (FDA).

_____ **2.** Original guidelines called for ambulances to be painted orange and white.

_____ **3.** The DOT KKK 1822 standards developed the three main types of ambulances.

_____ **4.** The defibrillator and pulse oximeter do not need to be tested.

_____ **5.** Brake fade is tested before driving the ambulance.

_____ **6.** The Commission on Accreditation of Ambulance Services (CAAS) recommends that urban response time should be less than 8 minutes.

_____ **7.** One of the system status management (SSM) goals is to have a paramedic in every unit.

_____ **8.** It is the responsibility of every EMS agency to ensure that personnel are given emergency vehicle operation courses after they are hired.

_____ **9.** Due regard states that if you have your lights and sirens on, you have the right of way and can break the traffic laws.

_____ **10.** Patient cost is a disadvantage of using an air ambulance.

Short Answer

Complete this section with short written answers using the space provided.

When you are dispatched to an emergency, you must decide which route will be used to arrive at the scene safely. There are a number of ways to accomplish this. List three:

1. _____

2. _____

3. _____

Fill in the Table

Fill in the missing parts of the table.

Advantages and Disadvantages of Using Helicopter Transport	
Advantages	**Disadvantages**
• Reduced transport time	• _____
• _____	• Altitude limitations
• _____	• _____
	• Aircraft cabin size limitations
	• Terrain that poses landing challenges
	• _____
	• Patient condition that is not suited to helicopter transport
	• Restrictions on the number of responders
	• _____

Incident Management and Mass-Casualty Incidents

Matching

Part I

Match each of the terms in the right column to the appropriate description in the left column.

_____ **1.** A Department of Homeland Security system designed to enable federal, state, and local governments and private-sector and nongovernmental organizations to effectively and efficiently prepare for, prevent, respond to, and recover from domestic incidents, regardless of cause, size, or complexity, including acts of catastrophic terrorism.

_____ **2.** An agreement between neighboring emergency medical services (EMS) systems to respond to mass-casualty incidents or disasters in each other's region when local resources are insufficient to handle the response.

_____ **3.** Any situation with more than one patient but that will not overwhelm available resources.

_____ **4.** In incident command, the person who works with area medical examiners, coroners, and law enforcement agencies to coordinate the disposition of dead victims.

_____ **5.** A group of operations in a unified command system, whose three designated sector positions are triage, treatment, and transport.

_____ **6.** A type of patient sorting used to rapidly categorize patients; the focus is on speed in locating all patients and determining an initial priority as their condition warrants.

_____ **7.** In incident command, the component that ultimately produces a plan to resolve any incident.

_____ **8.** In incident command, the section that is responsible for managing the tactical operations, including standard triage, treatment, and transport of patients.

_____ **9.** An ongoing or uncontained incident in which rescuers will have to search for patients and then triage or treat them. The situation may produce more patients. Examples include school shootings, tornadoes, a hazardous materials release, and rising floodwaters.

_____ **10.** A contained incident in which patients are found in one focal location, and the situation is not expected to produce more patients than are initially present.

_____ **11.** In incident command, the position that oversees the incident, establishes the objectives and priorities, and from there develops a response plan.

_____ **12.** A process that confronts responses to critical incidents and defuses them.

A. Closed incident

B. Command

C. Critical incident stress management (CISM)

D. Demobilization

E. Disaster

F. Extrication task force leader

G. Finance section chief

H. Freelancing

I. Hospital surge capacity

J. Incident action plan (IAP)

K. Incident commander (IC)

L. Incident command system (ICS)

_____ **13.** The process of directing responders to return to their facilities when work at a disaster of mass-casualty incident has finished, at least for the particular responders.

_____ **14.** A situation declared by a locale, county, state, or the federal government for the purposes of providing additional resources and funds to those in need.

_____ **15.** In incident command, the person appointed to determine the type of equipment and resources needed for a situation involving extrication or special rescue; also called the rescue task force leader.

_____ **16.** An emergency situation that can place a great demand on the equipment or personnel of the EMS system or has the potential to overwhelm available resources.

_____ **17.** In incident command, the section that helps procure and stockpile equipment and supplies during an incident.

_____ **18.** In incident command, the person who relays information, concerns, and requests among responding agencies.

_____ **19.** There is a minor adaptation for infants and children (including those with special needs) who cannot ambulate on their own.

_____ **20.** An area designated by the incident commander, or a designee, in which public information officers from multiple agencies disseminate information about the incident.

_____ **21.** In incident command, the position in an incident responsible for accounting of all expenditures.

_____ **22.** When individual units or different organizations make independent and often inefficient decisions about the next appropriate action.

_____ **23.** The capabilities of a receiving hospital to handle a large number of unexpected emergency patients, such as those seen in a mass-casualty incident.

_____ **24.** A system implemented to manage disasters and mass-casualty incidents in which section chiefs, including operations, finance, logistics, and planning, report to the incident commander.

_____ **25.** The overall leader of the incident command system to whom commanders or leaders of the incident command system divisions report.

_____ **26.** An oral or written plan stating general objectives reflecting the overall strategy for managing an incident.

M. Joint information center (JIC)

N. JumpSTART triage

O. Liaison officer (LNO)

P. Logistics section

Q. Mass-casualty incident (MCI)

R. Medical incident command

S. Morgue unit leader

T. Multiple-casualty incident

U. Mutual aid response

V. National Incident Management System (NIMS)

W. Open incident

X. Operations section

Y. Planning section

Z. Primary triage

Part II

Match each of the terms in the right column to the appropriate description in the left column.

_____ **1.** Simple Triage And Rapid Treatment; a patient-sorting process that uses a limited assessment of the patient's ability to walk, respiratory status, hemodynamic status, and neurologic status.

_____ **2.** In incident command, the person who locates an area to stage equipment and personnel and tracks unit arrival and deployment from the staging area.

_____ **3.** In incident command, the subordinate positions under the commander's direction to which the workload is distributed; the supervisor-to-worker ratio.

_____ **4.** A command system in which one person is in charge, generally used with small incidents that involve only one responding agency or one jurisdiction.

_____ **5.** In incident command, the person who keeps the public informed and relates any information to the press.

_____ **6.** In incident command, the person who establishes an area that provides protection for responders from the elements and the situation.

A. Public information officer (PIO)

B. Rehabilitation group leader

C. Rescue task force leader

D. Safety officer

E. Secondary triage

F. Single command system

_____ **7.** A command system used in larger incidents in which there is a multiagency or multijurisdictional response to coordinate decision making and cooperation among the agencies.

_____ **8.** The person in charge of prioritizing patients, whose primary duty is to ensure that every patient receives initial triage.

_____ **9.** To sort patients based on the severity of their conditions and prioritize them for care accordingly.

_____ **10.** In incident command, the person responsible for locating, setting up, and supervising the treatment area.

_____ **11.** In incident command, the person who coordinates transportation and distribution of patients to appropriate receiving hospitals.

_____ **12.** A type of patient sorting used in the treatment sector that involves retriage of patients.

_____ **13.** In incident command, the person who gives the "go ahead" to plan or who may stop an operation when rescuer safety is an issue.

_____ **14.** In incident command, the person appointed to determine the type of equipment and resources needed for a situation involving extrication or special rescue; also called the extrication task force leader.

_____ **15.** In incident command, when an incident commander turns over command to someone with more experience in a critical area.

_____ **16.** The end of the incident command structure when an incident draws to a close.

G. Span of control

H. Staging area manager

I. START triage

J. Termination of command

K. Transfer of command

L. Transportation unit leader

M. Treatment unit leader

N. Triage

O. Triage unit leader

P. Unified command system

Multiple Choice

Read each item carefully, and then select the best response.

_____ **1.** The incident command system (ICS) is designed to control duplication of effort and:
- **A.** triaging.
- **B.** application of triage tags.
- **C.** freelancing.
- **D.** communication coding.

_____ **2.** A large hazardous materials incident would require what kind of command system?
- **A.** Single command system
- **B.** Unified command system
- **C.** Rescue command system
- **D.** Medical command system

_____ **3.** When sizing up the scene of a multiple-casualty incident (MCI), in addition to asking yourself "What do I have?" what other question is a part of the scene size-up?
- **A.** Why were we dispatched?
- **B.** What is the best response route?
- **C.** What resources do I need?
- **D.** How many police are responding?

_____ **4.** What is the triage unit leader ultimately responsible for?
- **A.** Triage of every patient
- **B.** Movement of patients to a treatment sector
- **C.** Counting and prioritizing all patients
- **D.** Transportation to the hospitals

_____ **5.** Where should the rehabilitation area be located?
- **A.** As close as possible to the treatment area
- **B.** Next to the media area
- **C.** Outside
- **D.** Away from the scene and the media

6. What does the *D* stand for in the IDME mnemonic that applies to triage?

   A. Delayed

   B. Dead

   C. Don't move

   D. Decompensated shock

7. Which of the following is NOT a special consideration during triage?

   A. A hysterical and disruptive patient

   B. An injured rescue worker

   C. Death of a friend

   D. Hazardous material exposure

8. What color triage tag would you give a patient at an MCI who is breathing 4 breaths/min after you have opened the person's airway?

   A. Green

   B. Yellow

   C. Red

   D. Black

9. When arriving on a scene to begin triage, what is a good thing to yell to the patients?

   A. If you can walk, move across the street to the oak tree.

   B. Stay where you are, and we will move all of you.

   C. Everyone just lie still, and raise your hand if you think you are okay.

   D. Run for your lives! Clear the area as fast as you can.

10. What is your number-one priority at the scene of an MCI?

   A. Triage of patients

   B. Scene safety

   C. Treatment of patients

   D. Setting up the proper sectors

Labeling

Label the following diagrams with the correct terms.

1. Diagram of an MCI
   Label the following areas:
   A. Incident area
   B. Extrication area
   C. Triage area
   D. Treatment area

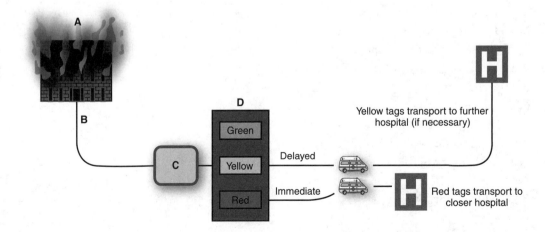

2. The JumpSTART pediatric MCI triage algorithm
Indicate if the following are deceased (black), immediate (red), or delayed (yellow).

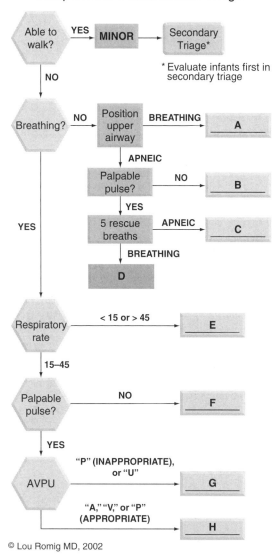

JumpSTART Pediatric MCI Triage©

© Lou Romig MD, 2002

© Lou Romig MD, 2002.

Fill in the Blank

Read each item carefully, and then complete the statement by filling in the missing word(s).

1. A(n) _____-_____ _____ refers to any situation with more than one patient but that will not overwhelm available resources.

2. One of the organizing principles of the _____ is limiting the _____ __ _____, the number expressed as a ratio of supervisors to responders.

3. The _____ section chief is responsible for documenting all expenditures at the incident that will need to be reimbursed.

4. The three officers that will help incident command (IC) the most are the _____, _____, and _____ officers.

5. _____ involves the decisions made and basic _____ done before an incident occurs.

6. The _____ unit leader coordinates and distributes patients to the appropriate hospitals.

7. Initial triage done in the field is known as _____, and then the _____ triage is done as the patients are

brought to the treatment sector.

8. The *R* in the START triage system stands for _____.

9. _____START was developed for pediatric patients involved in an MCI.

10. The _____ area manager is in charge of parking vehicles and collecting supplies to be used at the scene.

Identify

Read the following case study, and then list the chief complaint, vital signs, and pertinent negatives.

You have responded to a blast at a local fertilizer plant. Your patient is a 32-year-old man who is found outside the blast area. He is lying on his side because he has a piece of wood impaled in his left buttock. He is conscious and alert. The wood is sticking out about 6 inches, and there is not much blood. He is unable to move because of the wood. Your partner starts the primary survey and secondary assessment as you apply oxygen. The trauma assessment shows small nicks and cuts on the man's back and legs, but they are all secondary injuries that are not life threatening. He says he was knocked to the ground when the explosion occurred. You are taking no chances and place him in a rigid cervical collar even though you won't be able to lay him flat. He is breathing 20 breaths/min, with an oxygen saturation of 97% and clear lung sounds. Pulse is 98 beats/min and regular, and blood pressure (BP) is 136/88 mm Hg. The patient rates his pain at a 7/10. His skin is warm and dry. You stabilize the wood in place and place the patient on a backboard and then use pillows to help stabilize him from rolling off his right side. You get him in the unit, place him on the electrocardiogram (ECG) monitor (which shows normal sinus rhythm), and then start an IV line on him. You give him 5 mg of morphine for the pain because it is really starting to hurt since you moved him. You opt for the regional trauma center even though it is 7 minutes farther away than the community hospital.

1. Chief complaint:

_____

_____

2. Vital signs:

_____

_____

3. Pertinent negatives:

_____

_____

Ambulance Calls

The following case scenarios provide an opportunity to explore the concerns associated with patient management and paramedic care. Read each scenario, and then answer each question.

1. It is a hot, stuffy day in June in your community of 1,600 people. You are on a volunteer rescue squad in your home community and work for a critical care ground transport company in the city 25 miles away. It is your day off, and you are enjoying the weather, but there have been tornado watches issued for your area. Later in the afternoon, the weather begins to get a little more serious, and you switch on your radio to get the latest updates. At 1630, the sirens indicating a tornado in the area go off, so you head down to the basement with your kids and the dog. Your wife is at work at the local nursing home. Before you know it, it sounds as if a freight train has hit your home. After everything is quiet, you fight your way out of the basement only to see total devastation of what used to be your community. You check with your neighbors to see if they are okay and decide to leave your kids with them. Because your truck is nowhere to be found, you grab a bike lying in the street and head down to the fire department.

Okay, take a little break here to answer a few questions. Consider working in teams and comparing notes after you have answered your questions.

a. List 10 things you would like to have in your emergency kit to take with you.

(1)_____

(2)_____

(3)_____

(4)_____

(5)_____

(6)_____

(7)_____

(8)_____

(9)_____

(10)_____

b. There is a lot of damage in the area, and people are gathering in the streets. What are you going to tell them to do as you ride by on your bicycle?

_____

_____

c. What type of hazards can you expect during the 2-mile ride to the fire station?

_____

_____

2. You finally arrive at the fire department as the rest of your crew gathers; there are 24 emergency responders present. It has been estimated that at least 100 homes were destroyed plus the nursing home, which houses 75 patients. This really worries you because you know your wife was there when the storm hit. The firehouse and the high school two blocks away have not been touched by the twister. You have three ambulances and six fire trucks. Emergency management has two pickups, and the sheriff's office has three cars available. Word has gone out to the surrounding communities, asking for all the help you can get.

a. Who should take command of this situation, and where should you set up the command post?

_____

_____

b. What type of buildings can be used for an emergency center for the walking wounded and displaced victims of the storm?

_____

_____

3. This is going to be a long night. Power is out all over town. You quickly begin to break into teams to begin searching for patients. There are many injuries at the nursing home as a result of the large number of people who were unable to get underground. You are sent there to work in the treatment center, and you see around 60 people with injuries over the next 6 hours. Your wife has made it through okay with only minor cuts. She is classified as walking wounded and actually pitches in to help with the patients who are worse. It takes 24 hours for all the homes to be searched, and your town suffers three deaths caused by this tornado. Three days later, most of the power has been restored to the houses that are still standing, and things start to calm down around town. There will be cleanup going on for the next few months, and it will take a couple of years to put everything back together. You are thankful that all the agencies in your town, even though they are small, work well together and have prepared for this type of emergency.

   a. List some outside agencies in your area that will be able to help you in the first 3 hours of this disaster.

   _____

   _____

True/False

If you believe the statement to be more true than false, write the letter "T" in the space provided. If you believe the statement to be more false than true, write the letter "F."

_____   1. There will never be physicians on the scene of an MCI.

_____   2. The planning section solves problems as they arise at an MCI.

_____   3. Critical incident stress management should be available to responders, but its benefits are not evidence based.

_____   4. An open incident is contained, with patients found in one focal point.

_____   5. Command functions include triage and treatment functions.

_____   6. The safety officer has the power to stop all rescue functions.

_____   7. One function of the planning section is the development of an incident action plan.

_____   8. Face-to-face communications are the best because of infrastructure problems at the scene of an MCI.

_____   9. Yellow-tag patients are deemed immediate-priority patients because they have the best chance of survival.

_____   10. The second step in the START process is triage of the nonwalking patients.

Short Answer

Complete this section with short written answers using the space provided.

1. Discuss the first step of the START triage system.

   _____

   _____

2. Discuss the second step of the START triage system.

   _____

   _____

3. Why is the JumpSTART triage system needed for a pediatric patient?

   _____

   _____

4. Why should you participate in the critical incident stress management in the rehabilitation sector?

   _____

   _____

Fill in the Table

Fill in the missing parts of the table.

MCI Equipment and Supplies	
Airway control	PPE (gloves, face shield, HEPA or N95 mask)
	_____
	_____
	Rigid-tip Yankauer and flexible suction catheters
	Laryngeal mask airway, i-gel or King LT airway, ET tubes[a]
	_____
	Commercial tube holder, tape, syringes, stylet[a]
	ETCO$_2$ device
Breathing	_____
	Bag-mask device (adult and child), spare masks
	Oxygen delivery devices (nonrebreathing mask, cannula, extension tubing)
	_____
	_____
	Large-bore IV catheter for thoracic decompression[a]
Circulation	_____
	Sphygmomanometer, stethoscope
	Burn dressings, burn sheets, sterile water for irrigation
	_____
	Hemolytic dressings
	1,000-mL bags of normal saline, IV start kits, catheters[a]
Disability	_____
	Head beds, wide tape, backboard straps
	_____
Exposure	Space blanket to cover patients
	Scissors
Logistic/Command	Sector vests (triage, treatment, transport, staging, command, rescue)
	Pads of paper, pencils, pens, markers
	_____
	Assessment cards
	Tarps: red, yellow, green, black

[a]These items could be packaged in an advanced life support (ALS) kit.

Vehicle Extrication and Special Rescue

My partner's so petite that she slid right through the window to stabilize the patient.

© Jones & Bartlett Learning.

Matching

Part I

Match each of the definitions in the left column to the appropriate term in the right column.

_____ **1.** A rope rescue operation carried out on a mildly sloping surface (less than 45°) or on level ground. The ground is the rescuer's primary means of support, and the rope system is the secondary means of support.

A. Accountability system

_____ **2.** A type of window glazing that incorporates a sheeting material to keep the glass from breaking into shards. This kind of glass, often used for windshields, resists even deliberate breakage.

B. Alternative power vehicle

_____ **3.** An atmospheric concentration of any toxic, corrosive, or asphyxiant substance that poses an immediate threat to life or could cause irreversible or delayed adverse health effects. There are three general IDLH atmospheres: toxic, flammable, and oxygen deficient.

C. Awareness

_____ **4.** The area that directly surrounds an incident site and is considered immediately dangerous to life and health. All personnel working in the hot zone must wear all appropriate protective clothing and equipment. Entry requires approval by the incident commander (IC) or a designated sector officer. Complete backup, rescue, and decontamination teams must be in place at the perimeter before operations begin.

D. Belay

_____ **5.** A rope rescue operation in which the angle of the slope is greater than 45°. Rescuers depend on life safety rope rather than working from a fixed support surface, such as the ground.

E. Box crib

_____ **6.** A position used by a swift-water rescuer to avoid objects below the surface; the rescuer rolls into a faceup arched position, with the lower back higher than the feet (which are held together and face in the direction of travel—that is, feet first) and the arms at the sides.

F. Cold-protective response

_____ **7.** A collapse that occurs after the primary trench, excavation, or structural collapse.

G. Cold zone

_____ **8.** The process of locating a lost or overdue person and removing him or her from a hostile environment.

H. Complex access

_____ **9.** A cross between hill climbing and rock climbing used to ascend rocky surfaces and ridges.

I. Confined space

_____ **10.** The act of descending from a height on a fixed rope.

J. Cribbing

_____ **11.** A technique used to control a rope as it is fed out to climbers.

_____ **12.** The first level of rescue training provided to all responders; emphasizes recognizing hazards, securing the scene, and calling for appropriate assistance. There is no use of actual rescue skills.

_____ **13.** A vehicle powered by energy other than petroleum-based fuel, or a vehicle that relies on a combination of petroleum and another fuel or energy source for power.

_____ **14.** A method of accounting for all personnel at an emergency incident and ensuring only those with specific assignments are permitted to work within the various zones.

_____ **15.** Also known as a life vest, a water rescue device that allows the body to float.

_____ **16.** The act of preparing a patient for movement as a unit by means of a backboard or similar stabilization device.

_____ **17.** The technical rescue training level geared toward working in the warm zone of an incident. Training at this level allows responders to directly assist those conducting the rescue operation and to use certain rescue skills and procedures.

_____ **18.** Any tool or piece of equipment operated by human power.

_____ **19.** A circumstance in which a patient is unable to extricate himself or herself from an impediment, such as debris or soil.

_____ **20.** Use of specialized tools and advanced techniques to free a patient from the area or object in which he or she is trapped.

_____ **21.** A pallet-like framework used to shore up a heavy load.

_____ **22.** A phenomenon associated with cold-water immersion in which the body reflexively lowers its metabolic rate in an effort to preserve basic bodily functions.

_____ **23.** A safe area for agencies involved in a rescue operation; the incident commander, command post, EMS providers, and other necessary support functions should be located in the cold zone.

_____ **24.** Complicated entry requiring special tools, advanced training, and the use of force, such as breaking windows.

_____ **25.** A space that is not meant for continuous occupancy and to which access is limited or restricted, such as a manhole, well, or tank.

_____ **26.** A type of basic physical support, such as blocks or short lengths of wood, used to stabilize a vehicle during a rescue operation.

K. Disentanglement

L. Entrapment

M. Hand tool

N. High-angle operation

O. Hot zone

P. Immediately dangerous to life and health (IDLH)

Q. Laminated glass

R. Low-angle operation

S. Operations

T. Packaging

U. Personal flotation device (PFD)

V. Rappelling

W. Scrambling

X. Search and rescue (SAR)

Y. Secondary collapse

Z. Self-rescue position

Part II

Match each of the definitions in the left column to the appropriate term in the right column.

_____ **1.** A type of glass that is heat-treated so that it breaks into small, relatively dull pieces.

_____ **2.** The level of training necessary for a rescuer directly involved in a rescue operation; indicates a high level of competency in technical or hazardous materials rescue.

_____ **3.** A group of rescuers expertly trained in the various disciplines of technical rescue.

_____ **4.** A tapered shaft of wood or other material used to snug loose cribbing.

_____ **5.** The area located between the hot and cold zones at an incident. Decontamination stations are located in the warm zone.

A. Shim

B. Shoring

C. Simple access

D. Special weapons and tactics (SWAT) team

E. Spoil pile

_____ **6.** A vehicle design with no formal frame structure. The body and frame are one piece, which is considered to be the structural integrity of the vehicle.

_____ **7.** The process of coordinating different partner agencies to detect, respond to, and clear traffic incidents as quickly as possible to reduce the impacts of incidents on safety and congestion, while protecting the safety of on-scene responders and the traveling public.

_____ **8.** A complex rescue requiring specially trained personnel and sophisticated equipment and involving vehicle extrication; rescue from water, ice, or confined spaces; rescue following trench, structural, or other collapse; high-angle rescue; response to hazardous materials incidents; or wilderness search and rescue.

_____ **9.** A high-risk situation involving the potential for physical violence or armed combat typically involving law enforcement teams interacting with potentially dangerous criminal suspects.

_____ **10.** A system of specialized devices, such as airbags and seat belt pre-tensioners, used to restrain a driver or passenger in the protected passenger compartment of a motor vehicle during a crash.

_____ **11.** A slim, low-profile, wedgelike object used to snug loose cribbing under a load or to fill a void.

_____ **12.** A hydraulic, pneumatic, or wood system to support a trench wall or reinforce building components such as walls, floors, or ceilings to prevent collapse.

_____ **13.** Access easily achieved with the use of simple hand tools or application of force.

_____ **14.** A specialized law enforcement tactical unit.

_____ **15.** A specialized cribbing assembly of wood or plastic blocks arranged in a step configuration.

_____ **16.** The pile of dirt unearthed from an excavation. The pile may be unstable and prone to collapse.

F. Step chock

G. Supplemental restraint system

H. Tactical situation

I. Technical rescue incident (TRI)

J. Technical rescue team

K. Technician

L. Tempered glass

M. Traffic incident management (TIM)

N. Unibody construction

O. Warm zone

P. Wedge

Multiple Choice

Read each item carefully, and then select the best response.

_____ **1.** Which of the following is NOT considered a technical rescue incident?
- **A.** Trench collapse
- **B.** A fender-bender collision
- **C.** Water rescue
- **D.** Wilderness search and rescue

_____ **2.** What is the first priority in a rescue situation?
- **A.** Mobilizing the correct teams
- **B.** Following the golden rule of public service
- **C.** Protecting the patient during the rescue
- **D.** Ensuring rescuer safety

_____ **3.** Which of the following is NOT considered a step in a special rescue?
- **A.** Critique
- **B.** Access
- **C.** Disentanglement
- **D.** Removal

_____ **4.** You find the entry and rescue teams in the _____ zone(s).

    A. cold

    B. warm

    C. hot

    D. warm and hot

_____ **5.** Which of the following is NOT necessary to know when gathering information about a scene before you arrive?

    A. The road conditions en route to the incident

    B. The nature of the incident

    C. The location of the incident

    D. Hazards at the scene

_____ **6.** Who is in charge of having all of the utilities shut down at a scene?

    A. Dispatcher

    B. Incident command

    C. Police chief

    D. Fire chief

_____ **7.** Of the following means of powering a vehicle, which is NOT considered an alternative power source?

    A. LPG

    B. Diesel fuel

    C. Ethanol and flex

    D. Electric or hybrid

_____ **8.** On a vehicle, the "A" post is the post:

    A. between the front seat and back seat.

    B. between the middle seat and back seat.

    C. that holds in the windshield.

    D. that holds in the back window.

_____ **9.** When you need to stabilize a vehicle, you usually use the most basic physical support for vehicle stabilization, which is called:

    A. a step block.

    B. wedging.

    C. a "C block."

    D. cribbing.

_____ **10.** If you are unable to gain easy access by opening a door to the wrecked vehicle, what is the next best procedure?

    A. Break the windshield

    B. Displace the door

    C. Peel back the roof

    D. Break a side window

Labeling

Label the following diagrams with the correct terms.

1. Label the A, B, and C posts on the vehicle.

2. Label the following photos with the appropriate type of wood cribbing design.

A.

B. _____

C. _____

D. _____

Fill in the Blank

Read each item carefully, and then complete the statement by filling in the missing word(s).

1. A(n) _____ that has deployed during a crash presents no safety _____ for the rescuer.

2. Do not attempt to cut a steering wheel if the _____ _____ contains an undeployed airbag.

3. During a(n) _____ collision, the vehicle's _____ may be pushed down or backward.

4. A(n) _____ _____ is a structure that is not designed for continuous occupancy.

5. _____ _____ is a gas that is released when bacteria break down organic material without oxygen. It is

flammable, toxic, and colorless.

6. When dealing with an entrapment or trench collapse, the patient is dug out only after _____ has been put in place.

7. If you find yourself being swept away in fast water during a rescue, you should position yourself in the _____-

_____ _____.

8. The first thing to do when attempting to help a person during a water rescue is to _____ _____ to the person.

9. In North America, the most common _____ water rescue scenario involves people who have attempted to

_____ through floodwaters.

10. You respond to a rescue situation where the patient is down a slope that is less than 45°. This is known as a(n)

_____-_____ operation.

Identify

Read the following case study, and then list the chief complaint, vital signs, and pertinent negatives.

You are called to a vehicle that has rolled down a 75-foot embankment. The rappelling team responded and has secured your patient on a backboard and then placed him in a Stokes basket. They pull the basket up the embankment for you to start working on the patient. He was wearing his seat belt when he lost control of the car and rolled. The patient, Jim, is conscious but unable to answer any questions except for providing his first name. Your partner applies high-flow supplemental oxygen, and you begin a trauma assessment while your partner takes the baseline vitals. Jim has multiple cuts on his face and head, with some blood coming from his left ear. You find instability in the pelvic region and a deformed left arm and collarbone. Jim's blood pressure (BP) is 102/68 mm Hg, and pulse is thready in the wrist at a rate of 116 beats/min. His oxygen saturation is 96%, and his breathing is shallow at 24 breaths/min. Lung sounds are slightly diminished on the left side. Jim is cool to the touch and appears very pale. His pupils are equal, round, and regular in size, but they do not react very quickly to light. You know that Jim needs to be at a regional trauma center, and you call for air medical transport. After hooking up the heart monitor, you find that Jim is in sinus tachycardia. Your partner does a halo test on the blood coming from his ear, and it is negative. Jim begins to come around a little more but doesn't remember any of the crash. Your partner starts two large-bore IV lines with normal saline while you do a secondary assessment. You find some rigidity in the lower abdomen. After you give a quick report to the helicopter personnel, Jim is flown to the closest regional trauma center.

1. Chief complaint:

_____

_____

2. Vital signs:

_____

_____

3. Pertinent negatives:

_____

_____

Complete the Patient Care Report (PCR)

Read the case study in the preceding Identify exercise, and then complete the following PCR for the patient.

EMS Patient Care Report (PCR)					

Date:	Incident No.:		Nature of Call:		Location:

Dispatched:	En Route:	At Scene:	Transport:	At Hospital:	In Service:

Patient Information					

Age:		Allergies:			
Sex:		Medications:			
Weight (in kg [lb]):		Past Medical History:			
		Chief Complaint:			

Vital Signs					

Time:	BP:	Pulse:	Respirations:	SpO$_2$:
Time:	BP:	Pulse:	Respirations:	SpO$_2$:
Time:	BP:	Pulse:	Respirations:	SpO$_2$:

EMS Treatment (circle all that apply)				

Oxygen @ _____ L/min via (circle one): NC NRM Bag-mask device	Assisted Ventilation	Airway Adjunct	CPR
Defibrillation	Bleeding Control	Bandaging	Splinting	Other:

Narrative

Ambulance Calls

The following case scenario provides an opportunity to explore the concerns associated with patient management and paramedic care. Read the scenario, and then answer each question.

1. You and your crew (two other paramedics) are called to the scene of a highway crash just outside of town. Arriving at the scene, you see a late-model sedan "accordioned" against a utility pole. The windshield is shattered. The driver is unconscious, bleeding, and tightly pinned between the steering wheel and the seat. There are no passengers.

   a. List in order the steps you would take. Include details of how you would reach the patient.

   (1)_____

   _____

   (2)_____

   _____

   (3)_____

   _____

   (4)_____

   _____

   (5)_____

   _____

   (6)_____

   _____

   (7)_____

   _____

   (8)_____

   _____

   b. List the actions you would take after the patient has been transferred to the care of emergency department (ED) personnel.

   (1)_____

   (2)_____

True/False

If you believe the statement to be more true than false, write the letter "T" in the space provided. If you believe the statement to be more false than true, write the letter "F."

_____   **1.** In an extrication, the primary function of a paramedic is to direct the disentanglement of the patient from the wreckage.

_____   **2.** Initial access to the patient may be limited because of safety hazards or physical restrictions.

_____   **3.** Care of the car crash victim should start even before the patient is removed from the vehicle.

_____   **4.** The paramedic should treat all downed wires as if they are charged until the power company turns them off.

_____ **5.** To protect the scene and the rescuers, place a large emergency vehicle at an angle to provide a barrier against oncoming traffic.

_____ **6.** A disabled vehicle that is upright on four wheels still needs to be stabilized before anyone enters it to reach the injured inside.

_____ **7.** The windshield is another easy way to gain access.

_____ **8.** The most common tool used to remove tempered glass is a flat-head axe.

_____ **9.** Removal of the patient is referred to as disentanglement.

_____ **10.** The side and rear windows are typically made of safety glass.

Short Answer
Complete this section with short written answers using the space provided.

1. Discuss the three phases of training that you might receive in technical rescue.

    a. Awareness:

    _____

    _____

    b. Operations:

    _____

    _____

    c. Technician:

    _____

    _____

2. Discuss the four guidelines that are useful when working with a rescue team.

    a. _____

    _____

    b. _____

    _____

    c. _____

    _____

    d. _____

    _____

3. What gear is considered minimal for a water rescuer?

_____

_____

4. When breaking glass in an automobile, discuss the differences of the glass in the windows versus the windshield.

_____

_____

Fill in the Table

Fill in the missing parts of the table.

1. Write in the correct statement for the letters for the mnemonic "THREAT."

The Hartford Consensus: THREAT	
T	
H	
R	
E	
A	
T	

Hazardous Materials

Oh for Pete's sake, surely someone in your training must have told you that the hazardous materials cold zone has nothing to do with temperature!

© Jones & Bartlett Learning.

Matching

Part I

Match each of the items in the right column to the appropriate definition in the left column.

_____ **1.** A glass, plastic, or steel nonbulk storage container, ranging in volume from 5 to 15 gallons (19 to 600 L).

_____ **2.** A chemical asphyxiant that results in cellular respiratory failure; this gas ties up hemoglobin to the extent that oxygen in the blood becomes inaccessible to the cells.

_____ **3.** Computer-Aided Management of Emergency Operations; a tool to help predict downwind concentrations of hazardous materials based on the input of environmental factors into a computer model.

_____ **4.** A chemical asphyxiant used in many industrial processes; exposure can occur from by-products of combustion at structure fires.

_____ **5.** A class of chemicals with either high or low pH levels. Exposure can cause severe soft-tissue damage.

_____ **6.** Any vessel or receptacle that holds material, including storage vessels, pipelines, and packaging.

_____ **7.** A document carried by drivers of commercial vehicles that should provide specific information about what is carried on the vehicle.

_____ **8.** An organization, office, or person responsible for enforcing the requirements of a code or standard, or for approving equipment, materials, an installation, or a procedure.

_____ **9.** Any gas that displaces oxygen from the atmosphere; can be deadly if exposure occurs in a confined space.

_____ **10.** A type of decontamination that is done with large pads that the hazardous materials team uses to soak up liquid and remove it from the patient.

_____ **11.** Bulk packaging that is permanently attached to or forms a part of a motor vehicle or is not permanently attached to any motor vehicle, and that, because of its size, construction, or attachment to a motor vehicle, is loaded or unloaded without being removed from the motor vehicle.

_____ **12.** A substance that interferes with the use of oxygen at the cellular level.

_____ **13.** A resource available to emergency responders via telephone on a 24-hour basis.

A. Absorption

B. Asphyxiant

C. Authority having jurisdiction (AHJ)

D. Bill of lading

E. CAMEO

F. Carbon monoxide

G. Carboy

H. Cargo tank

I. Chemical asphyxiant

J. CHEMTREC (Chemical Transportation Emergency Center)

K. Container

L. Corrosives

M. Cyanide

_____ **14.** A portable, nonbulk, compressed gas container used to hold liquids and gases. Uninsulated compressed gas cylinders are used to store substances such as nitrogen, argon, helium, and oxygen. They have a range of sizes and internal pressures.

N. Cylinder

_____ **15.** Any substance that is toxic, poisonous, radioactive, flammable, or explosive and causes injury or death with exposure.

O. Decontamination corridor

_____ **16.** The minimum temperature at which a liquid or a solid releases sufficient vapor to form an ignitable mixture with air.

P. Dilution

_____ **17.** An expression of a fuel-air mixture, defined by upper and lower limits, that reflects an amount of flammable vapor mixed with a given volume of air.

Q. Disposal

_____ **18.** The removal or relocation of people who may be affected by an approaching release of a hazardous material.

R. Dose effect

_____ **19.** The process of removing the bulk of contaminants from a person without regard for containment. It is used in potentially life-threatening situations, without the formal establishment of a decontamination corridor.

S. Drum

_____ **20.** A mnemonic that stands for diarrhea, urination, miosis/muscle weakness, bradycardia/bronchospasm/bronchorrhea, emesis, lacrimation, seizures/salivation/ sweating, which are the signs and symptoms that can be produced by exposure to organophosphate and carbamate pesticides or other nerve-stimulating agents.

T. Dry bulk cargo tank

_____ **21.** A controlled area within the warm zone where decontamination takes place.

U. DUMBELS

_____ **22.** A type of decontamination method that uses copious amounts of water to flush the contaminant from the skin or eyes.

V. Emergency decontamination

_____ **23.** A type of decontamination in which as much clothing and equipment as possible is disposed of to reduce the magnitude of the problem.

W. Evacuation

_____ **24.** The principle that the longer a hazardous material is in contact with the body or the greater the concentration, the greater the effect will most likely be.

X. Flammable range

_____ **25.** A barrel-like nonbulk storage vessel used to store a wide variety of substances, including food-grade materials, corrosives, flammable liquids, and grease. Drums may be constructed of low-carbon steel, polyethylene, cardboard, stainless steel, nickel, or other materials.

Y. Flash point

_____ **26.** A tank designed to carry dry bulk goods such as powders, pellets, fertilizers, or grain. Such tanks are generally V-shaped with rounded sides that funnel toward the bottom.

Z. Hazardous material

Part II

Match each of the items in the right column to the appropriate definition in the left column.

_____ **1.** The concentration of a material in air that, on the basis of laboratory tests (inhalation route) is expected to kill a specified number of the group of test animals when administered over a specified period.

A. HAZWOPER

_____ **2.** A dose that would be lethal to 50% of the test population.

B. Ignition temperature

_____ **3.** A type of signage at least 3.9 inches (9.9 cm) on each side that is often required on all four sides of individual packages and boxes that are being transported.

C. Immediately dangerous to life and health (IDLH)

_____ **4.** A bulk container that serves as both a shipping and a storage vessel. Such tanks hold between 5,000 and 6,000 gallons (18,900 to 22,700 L) of product and can be pressurized or nonpressurized. Intermodal tanks may be shipped by all modes of transportation.

D. Intermodal tank

_____ **5.** An atmospheric concentration of any toxic, corrosive, or asphyxiant substance that poses an immediate threat to life or could cause irreversible or delayed adverse health effects or serious interference for a team member attempting to escape from the dangerous atmosphere. A respirator is mandatory when working in such an environment.

_____ **6.** An effect of a hazardous material on the body that is limited to the area of contact.

_____ **7.** The level of protection that firefighter turnout gear provides.

_____ **8.** A level of personal protective equipment that provides splash protection.

_____ **9.** Personal protective equipment that is one step less protective than Level A but provides for a high level of respiratory protection.

_____ **10.** The highest level of protection suit worn by hazardous materials personnel; may also be referred to as fully encapsulating because the suit covers everything, including the breathing apparatus.

_____ **11.** The federal Occupational Safety and Health Administration (OSHA) regulation that governs hazardous materials waste site and response training. Specifics can be found in Title 29, standard number 1910.120. Subsection (q) is specific to emergency response.

_____ **12.** The minimum temperature at which a fuel, when heated, will ignite in air and continue to burn; also called the autoignition temperature.

_____ **13.** A single dose that causes the death of a specified number of the group of test animals exposed by any route other than inhalation.

_____ **14.** An exposure that occurs with direct contact with the hazardous material.

_____ **15.** A type of signage at least 10.8 inches (27 cm) on each side that is often required to be on all four sides of transport vehicles identifying the hazardous contents of the vehicle.

_____ **16.** The minimum amount of gaseous fuel that must be present in the air for the air-fuel mixture to be flammable or explosive.

_____ **17.** The physical process of reducing or removing surface contaminants from large numbers of victims in potentially life-threatening situations in the fastest time possible.

_____ **18.** A vehicle that typically carries between 6,000 and 10,000 gallons (22,700 to 37,900 L) of a product such as gasoline or other flammable and combustible materials. The tank is nonpressurized.

_____ **19.** The maximum concentration of a chemical that a person may be exposed to under OSHA regulations.

_____ **20.** Any container other than a bulk storage container, such as drums, bags, compressed gas cylinders, and cryogenic containers; hold commonly used commercial and industrial chemicals, such as solvents, cleaners, and compounds.

_____ **21.** A type of decontamination that uses one chemical to change the hazardous material into two less harmful substances; rarely used by hazardous materials teams.

_____ **22.** The process of assessing the health status of hazardous materials team members before and after entry to a hazardous materials incident site.

_____ **23.** A tanker with a rounded or horseshoe-shaped tank capable of holding 6,000 to 7,000 gallons (22,700 to 26,500 L) of flammable liquid, mild corrosives, and poisons. The tank has a high internal working pressure.

E. Label

F. LD_{50}

G. Lethal concentration (LC)

H. Lethal dose (LD)

I. Level A ensemble

J. Level B ensemble

K. Level C ensemble

L. Level D ensemble

M. Local effect

N. Lower flammable limit (LFL)

O. Mass decontamination

P. MC-306/DOT 406 flammable liquid tanker

Q. MC-307/DOT 407 chemical hauler

R. MC-312/DOT 412 corrosive tanker

S. MC-331 pressure cargo tanker

T. MC-338 cryogenic tanker

U. Medical monitoring

V. Neutralization

W. Nonbulk storage vessel

_____ **24.** A tanker that often carries aggressive (highly reactive) acids such as concentrated sulfuric and nitric acid. It is characterized by several heavy-duty reinforcing rings around the tank and holds approximately 6,000 gallons (22,700 L) of product.

_____ **25.** A tanker that carries materials such as ammonia, propane, Freon, and butane. This type of tank is commonly constructed of steel and has rounded ends and a single open compartment inside. The liquid volume inside the tank varies, ranging from the 1,000-gallon (3,800-L) delivery truck to the full-size 11,000-gallon (41,600-L) cargo tank.

_____ **26.** A low-pressure tanker designed to maintain the low temperature required by the cryogens it carries. A boxlike structure containing the tank control valves is typically attached to the rear of the tanker.

X. Permissible exposure limit (PEL)

Y. Placard

Z. Primary contamination

Part III

Match each of the items in the right column to the appropriate definition in the left column.

_____ **1.** A property that indicates that a material can be dissolved in water.

_____ **2.** A property that indicates that a material will undergo a chemical reaction (eg, explosion) when mixed with water.

_____ **3.** For the purpose of this chapter, the pressure associated with liquids held inside any type of closed container.

_____ **4.** The weight of an airborne concentration (vapor or gas) as compared with an equal volume of dry air.

_____ **5.** A high-volume transportation device made up of several individual compressed gas cylinders banded together and affixed to a trailer. Tube trailers carry compressed gases, such as hydrogen, oxygen, helium, and methane. One trailer may carry several different gases in individual tubes.

_____ **6.** Hazardous chemical compounds that are released when a material decomposes under heat.

_____ **7.** The concentration at which direct or airborne contact with a material could result in possible and significant exposure from absorption through the skin, mucous membranes, and eyes.

_____ **8.** The concentration of a substance that a worker can be exposed to for up to 15 minutes by no more than four times per day with at least 1 hour between each exposure.

_____ **9.** The maximum amount of gaseous fuel that can be present in the air if the air-fuel mixture is to be flammable or explosive.

_____ **10.** The maximum concentration of hazardous material to which a worker should not be exposed, even for an instant.

_____ **11.** A cargo document kept by the conductor of a train, also referred to as a consist.

_____ **12.** An engineered method to control spilled or released product if the main containment vessel fails.

_____ **13.** Exposure to a hazardous material by contact with a contaminated person or object.

_____ **14.** A method of safeguarding oneself or others' position during an emergency or event; in the context of a hazardous material, for example, by remaining in a safe atmosphere, usually inside structures.

_____ **15.** A substance that is capable of dissolving other substances.

_____ **16.** The concentration of a substance that is supposed to be safe for exposure of no more than 8 hours per day and 40 hours per week.

A. Safety data sheet (SDS)

B. Secondary containment

C. Secondary contamination

D. Shelter-in-place

E. Solvent

F. Specific gravity

G. Systemic effect

H. Technical decontamination

I. Threshold limit value (TLV)

J. Threshold limit value/ceiling (TLV/C)

K. Threshold limit value/ short-term exposure limit (TLV-STEL)

L. Threshold limit value/skin

M. Toxic products of combustion

N. Tube trailer

O. Upper flammable limit (UFL)

P. Vapor density

_____ 17. A multistep process of carefully scrubbing and washing contaminants from a person or object, collecting runoff water, and collecting and properly handling all items.

Q. Vapor pressure

_____ 18. A physiologic effect on the entire body or one of the body's systems.

R. Water reactive

_____ 19. The measure that indicates whether a hazardous material will sink or float in water.

S. Water soluble

_____ 20. A document that provides a detailed product description and that is kept on site at workplaces for every potentially hazardous chemical at the workplace.

T. Waybill

Multiple Choice

Read each item carefully, and then select the best response.

_____ 1. You can learn a great deal from a pesticide label. Of the following, which would NOT be found on a label?
   A. The EPA registration number
   B. The UN Classification number
   C. The active ingredients
   D. The total amount of product in the container

_____ 2. A hazardous liquid, such as propane, is transported in which type of truck?
   A. The MC-331 pressure cargo tanker
   B. The MC-338 cryogenic tanker
   C. The MC-307/DOT 407 chemical hauler
   D. The MC-306/DOT 406 flammable liquid tanker

_____ 3. The threshold limit value (TLV) is the maximum concentration of a toxin that someone can be exposed to in _____ over a typical 30-year career.
   A. 1 hour
   B. 24 hours
   C. 1 year
   D. a 40-hour work week

_____ 4. Emergency decontamination should be performed:
   A. at each and every hazardous materials incident.
   B. only if a qualified decontamination team is responding.
   C. only after appropriate personal protective equipment (PPE) has been donned.
   D. after a series of containment pools have been set up.

_____ 5. To prepare an ambulance for the transportation of contaminated patients, paramedics should do all of the following, EXCEPT:
   A. remove all unnecessary equipment, including the stretcher mattress.
   B. use as much disposable equipment as necessary.
   C. wrap the patient in a plastic barrier.
   D. line the interior of the ambulance with plastic sheets.

_____ 6. A paramedic should have a working knowledge of hazardous materials spills and properly providing care for injured patients. This knowledge should include training to which of the following levels?
   A. Technician
   B. Awareness
   C. Operations
   D. EMS operations

_____ 7. The safety data sheet (SDS) for a product provides a considerable amount of useful information to emergency responders. Of the following, which is NOT provided on the SDS?
   A. The product identifier
   B. The hazard identification
   C. The cost of the product
   D. The emergency telephone number

_____ 8. Hazardous materials teams have many high-tech tools at their disposal. These tools include all of the following, EXCEPT:

    A. Computer-Aided Management of Emergency Operations (CAMEO).

    B. air-monitoring equipment.

    C. colorimetric devices.

    D. self-contained breathing apparatus (SCBA).

_____ 9. Which of the following steps must be performed by paramedics who discover that a routine-sounding call is a hazardous materials incident?

    A. Isolate the incident as much as possible using the guidelines in the _Emergency Response Guidebook_ (ERG).

    B. Remain in the hot zone to evacuate injured patients.

    C. Approach and position your unit downwind from the incident.

    D. Don Level A protection, and begin setting up the decontamination corridor.

_____ 10. Paramedics need to balance the risk/benefit of invasive procedures for hazardous materials patients because:

    A. IV lines may help contamination pass the skin barrier.

    B. splints would become contaminated and have to be incinerated.

    C. endotracheal (ET) tubes may cause upper airway obstruction as the plastic vaporizes.

    D. There is no known risk; paramedics need to perform patient care as normal.

Fill in the Blank

Read each item carefully, and then complete the statement by filling in the missing word(s).

1. With _____ _____, you will not use rescue skills.

2. When you first arrive at a call and recognize a hazardous materials incident, your most important job will be to

_____ _____ _____.

3. All emergency medical services (EMS) personnel should receive appropriate hazardous materials response training,

based on the needs and requirements of the _____ _____ _____ and the local EMS agency.

4. Responding paramedics must gather as much _____ as possible when calling for the hazardous materials team.

5. If you are responding to an incident that involves a(n) _____ setting in which _____ may be in use or

accidentally released, you should have a high index of suspicion of hazardous materials.

6. Other good sources of information for identifying hazardous materials include the _____ _____ _____,

which should be carried by the truck driver in the cab, and the _____ or "consist" that is carried by the conductor

of a train.

7. There are two basic types of contamination: _____ and _____.

8. _____ _____ is the direct exposure of a patient to a hazardous material.

9. _____ _____ takes place when a hazardous material is transferred to a person from another person or from

contaminated objects.

10. A(n) _____ _____ may be described as a reddening of the skin or formation of blisters. Some chemicals may

have a(n) _____ effect on your patient.

Identify

1. Respond to the following questions by basing your answers on the following *Emergency Response Guidebook* (*ERG*) information.

GUIDE 123   GASES - TOXIC AND/OR CORROSIVE   **ERG2004**

POTENTIAL HAZARDS

HEALTH
- **TOXIC; may be fatal if inhaled or absorbed through skin.**
- Vapors may be irritating.
- Contact with gas or liquefied gas may cause burns, severe injury and/or frostbite.
- Fire will produce irritating, corrosive and/or toxic gases.
- Runoff from fire control may cause pollution.

FIRE OR EXPLOSION
- Some may burn, but none ignite readily.
- Vapors from liquefied gas are initially heavier than air and spread along ground.
- Cylinders exposed to fire may vent and release toxic and/or corrosive gas through pressure relief devices.
- Containers may explode when heated.
- Ruptured cylinders may rocket.

PUBLIC SAFETY

- **CALL Emergency Response Telephone Number on Shipping Paper first. If Shipping Paper not available or no answer, refer to appropriate telephone number listed on the inside back cover.**
- As an immediate precautionary measure, isolate spill or leak area for at least 100 meters (330 feet) in all directions.
- Keep unauthorized personnel away.
- Stay upwind.
- Many gases are heavier than air and will spread along ground and collect in low or confined areas (sewers, basements, tanks).
- Keep out of low areas.
- Ventilate closed spaces before entering.

PROTECTIVE CLOTHING
- Wear positive pressure self-contained breathing apparatus (SCBA).
- Wear chemical protective clothing that is specifically recommended by the manufacturer. It may provide little or no thermal protection.
- Structural firefighters' protective clothing provides limited protection in fire situations ONLY; it is not effective in spill situations where direct contact with the substance is possible.

EVACUATION

Spill
- See the Table of Initial Isolation and Protective Action Distances for highlighted substances. For non-highlighted substances, increase, in the downwind direction, as necessary, the isolation distance shown under "PUBLIC SAFETY".

Fire
- If tank, rail car or tank truck is involved in a fire, ISOLATE for 800 meters (1/2 mile) in all directions; also, consider initial evacuation for 800 meters (1/2 mile) in all directions.

Page 194

a. How dangerous of a substance is this?

_____

_____

b. What type of PPE should you be wearing if you are working in the "inner circle"?

_____

_____

c. Based on the preceding information, what should you do regarding your location and staging area?

_____

_____

2. Identify the four levels of PPE for hazardous materials scenes. Label each photo with the corresponding PPE level (A-D), then indicate their uses.

_____

_____

Level A:

Level B:

Level C:

Level D:

Ambulance Calls

The following case scenarios provide an opportunity to explore the concerns associated with patient management and paramedic care. Read each scenario, and then answer each question.

1. You are called to the infirmary of a local factory to see an employee who was injured in an unspecified "industrial accident." The plant manager who escorts you in explains, "There was a nasty accident. The valve on the tank of toluene wouldn't close. Jon was splashed in his face. I hope he's OK. He seems to have some trouble breathing. Our hazardous materials team had to go in and get him, and it took a few minutes for them to suit up and go in."

   Before initiating patient contact, you take out your *ERG* and look up the chemical. The *ERG* lists guide number 130. You look up guide 130. Under Protective Clothing, it lists:
   - Wear positive-pressure self-contained breathing apparatus (SCBA).
   - Structural firefighters' protective clothing will provide only limited protection.
     Under Health, it states:
   - May cause toxic effects if inhaled or absorbed through skin.
   - Inhalation or contact with material may irritate or burn skin and eyes.
   - Fire will produce irritating, corrosive, and/or toxic gases.
   - Vapors may cause dizziness or suffocation.
   - Runoff from fire control or dilution water may cause pollution.
   a. Is the scene safe? List considerations for your own immediate safety and patient decontamination.

   (1)_____

   (2)_____

   (3)_____

2. You are called to the scene of a railway incident in which the last 5 cars of a 12-car freight train derailed and toppled onto a highway below, crushing motor vehicles beneath them. Before approaching the derailed freight cars and the injured motorists underneath them, you want to make sure those train cars were not carrying a hazardous cargo.
   a. List three potential sources of information regarding the nature of the train's cargo.

   (1)_____

   (2)_____

   (3)_____

   b. You manage to determine that one of the derailed cars was carrying liquid chlorine, and as a matter of fact, you can already smell chlorine in the air. List the precautions you should be taking (assume that you are in the first public safety vehicle to reach the scene).

   (1)_____

   (2)_____

   (3)_____

   (4)_____

True/False

If you believe the statement to be more true than false, write the letter "T" in the space provided. If you believe the statement to be more false than true, write the letter "F."

1. You are called to the scene of a transportation crash in which a truck carrying radioactive waste (UN Class 7) overturned and caught fire. When you arrive, firefighters have just extinguished the fire, but there is still a lot of smoke. The driver of the truck is pinned inside the crushed cabin. Indicate which of the following statements about handling this call are true and which are false.
   _____ a. The ambulance should be parked upwind from the wrecked truck.
   _____ b. The ambulance does not need to be prepared in a special fashion before the driver transports to the hospital.

_____ **c.** The *ERG* should provide evacuation distances.
_____ **d.** The SDSs are helpful in managing hazardous materials.
_____ **e.** The bill of lading describes the contents carried within a vehicle.

2. Indicate which of the following statements regarding hazardous materials incidents are true and which are false.
_____ **a.** If there are no unusual odors at the scene of a transportation crash, it is safe to assume that hazardous materials are not involved.
_____ **b.** EMS personnel at a hazardous materials incident may become contaminated with toxic materials by touching a patient who is contaminated.
_____ **c.** In decontaminating a patient exposed to hazardous materials, one should use a brush to scrub the skin briskly with strong soap and lots of water.
_____ **d.** When decontamination is carried out at the scene, it is unnecessary to notify the receiving hospital that you are bringing in a hazardous materials case.
_____ **e.** It is preferable that an ambulance team that was not involved in treating and decontaminating the patient be summoned to transport the patient to the hospital.

Short Answer
Complete this section with short written answers using the space provided.

1. The *Emergency Response Guidebook* (*ERG*) can provide responders with the following information:

a. _____

b. _____

c. _____

2. List other sources of information that may be useful to paramedics responding to a hazardous materials incident.

a. _____

b. _____

c. _____

d. _____

e. _____

3. Although it's axiomatic in EMS that you never know what you may find at a call until you reach the scene, there are nonetheless certain types of calls that should start red lights flashing in the back of your brain: ALERT! Possible hazardous materials call! Listed here are some calls to 9-1-1 during a busy month. Determine whether each case is apt to involve hazardous materials, and if so, indicate what sort of hazardous materials might be involved.

a. Two-car collision downtown

_____

b. Apartment-house fire

_____

c. Three municipal workers collapsed in a sewer

_____

d. Two police officers injured in a riot

_____

e. Fire in a garden supply store warehouse

_____

f. Semitrailer overturned on the interstate

_____

g. Two "men down" on the maintenance staff of the municipal swimming pool

_____

h. Freight train struck car on level crossing

_____

i. Fire in a furniture factory

_____

Terrorism Response

WE HAVE NOTHING TO FEAR BUT FEAR ITSELF!

You are in too close when you have: defecation...urination... miosis...bradycardia... emesis...lacrimation... and salivation.

SLAM

© Jones & Bartlett Learning.

Matching

Part I

Match each of the items in the right column to the appropriate definition in the left column.

_____ **1.** Terrorism that is carried out by native citizens against their own country.

_____ **2.** The means with which a terrorist will spread a disease—for example, by poisoning the water supply or aerosolizing the agent into the air or ventilation system of a building.

_____ **3.** An infected animal that spreads a disease to another animal.

_____ **4.** A bomb that is used as a radiologic dispersal device (RDD).

_____ **5.** A natural process in which a material that is unstable attempts to stabilize itself by changing its structure.

_____ **6.** A form of warfare in which a small group that is not part of the official military engages in combat that uses the element of surprise, such as raids and ambushes; sometimes used by terrorists to protect their training camps and bases of operation.

_____ **7.** A type of energy that is emitted from a strong radiologic source that is far faster and stronger than alpha and beta rays. These rays easily penetrate the human body and require several inches of either lead or concrete to prevent penetration; share key characteristics with x-rays.

_____ **8.** Early nerve agents that were developed by German scientists in the period after World War I and into World War II. There are three such agents: sarin, soman, and tabun.

_____ **9.** A threat level in which a terrorist event is suspected, but there is no specific information about its timing or location.

_____ **10.** A nerve agent antidote kit that contains a single injection of both atropine (2 mg) and 2-PAM chloride (pralidoxime chloride; 600 mg).

_____ **11.** An agent that affects the body's ability to use oxygen. It is a colorless gas that has an odor similar to almonds. The effects begin on the cellular level and are very rapidly seen at the organ system level.

_____ **12.** Contamination of a person that results from coming into contact with another contaminated person, as opposed to coming into contact with the original source of contamination.

_____ **13.** An act in which the public safety community generally has no prior knowledge of the time, location, or nature of the attack.

_____ **14.** The characteristic of being communicable from one person to another person.

A. Alpha radiation

B. Ammonium nitrate

C. Anthrax

D. Apocalyptic violence

E. Bacteria

F. Beta radiation

G. Botulinum

H. Buboes

I. Bubonic plague

J. Chlorine

K. Communicability

L. Contact hazard

M. Contagious

N. Covert

_____ **15.** A hazardous agent that gives off little or no vapors and typically enters the body through the skin; also called a skin hazard.

_____ **16.** A deadly bacterium (*Bacillus anthracis*) that lies dormant in a spore (protective shell); the germ is released from the spore when exposed to the optimal temperature and moisture. The route of entry is inhalational, cutaneous, or gastrointestinal (from consuming food that contains spores).

_____ **17.** A commonly used industrial-grade fertilizer that is not in itself dangerous to handle or transport but forms an extremely explosive compound when mixed with fuel and other components.

_____ **18.** A type of energy that is emitted from a strong radiologic source. It is the least harmful penetrating type of radiation and cannot travel fast or through most objects.

_____ **19.** A type of violence sought by some terrorists, such as violent religious groups and doomsday cults, in which they wish to bring about the end of the world.

_____ **20.** Microorganisms that reproduce by binary fission. These single-cell creatures reproduce rapidly. Some can form spores (encysted variants) when environmental conditions are harsh.

_____ **21.** The ease with which a disease spreads from one human to another human.

_____ **22.** The first chemical agent ever used in warfare. It has a distinct odor of bleach and creates a green haze when released as a gas. Initially, it produces upper airway irritation and a choking sensation.

_____ **23.** An epidemic that spread throughout Europe in the Middle Ages, causing over 25 million deaths, also called the Black Death; transmitted by infected fleas and characterized by acute malaise, fever, and the formation of tender, enlarged, inflamed lymph nodes that appear as lesions, called buboes.

_____ **24.** Enlarged lymph nodes (up to the size of tennis balls) that are characteristic of people infected with the bubonic plague.

_____ **25.** A very potent neurotoxin produced by bacteria; when introduced into the body, this neurotoxin affects the nervous system's ability to function and causes muscle paralysis.

_____ **26.** A type of energy that is emitted from a strong radiologic source. It is slightly more penetrating than alpha and requires a layer of clothing to stop it.

O. Cross-contamination

P. Cyanide

Q. Decay

R. Dirty bomb

S. Disease vector

T. Dissemination

U. Domestic terrorism

V. DuoDote

W. Elevated

X. G agents

Y. Gamma radiation

Z. Guerilla warfare

Part II

Match each of the items in the right column to the appropriate definition in the left column.

_____ **1.** An area in the lymphatic system where infection-fighting cells are housed.

_____ **2.** A blistering agent that has a rapid onset of symptoms and produces immediate, intense pain and discomfort on contact. Its military abbreviation is L.

_____ **3.** The amount of an agent or substance that will kill 50% of people who are exposed to this level.

_____ **4.** Energy that is emitted in the form of rays or particles.

_____ **5.** Terrorism that is carried out by those not of the host's country; also known as cross-border terrorism.

_____ **6.** Any container that is designed to disperse radioactive material.

_____ **7.** Any material that emits radiation.

_____ **8.** A strategically placed facility that has been preestablished for the mass distribution of antibiotics, antidotes, and vaccinations, along with other medications and supplies.

A. Imminent

B. Improvised explosive device (IED)

C. Incubation

D. International terrorism

E. Ionizing radiation

F. LD_{50}

G. Lewisite

H. Lymph node

_____ **9.** A lung infection, also known as plague pneumonia, that is the result of inhalation of plague bacteria.

_____ **10.** A blistering agent that has a rapid onset of symptoms and produces immediate, intense pain and discomfort on contact. Its military abbreviation is CX.

_____ **11.** Biologic agents that are the most deadly substances known to humans. They include botulinum toxin and ricin.

_____ **12.** A class of chemicals called organophosphates that function by blocking an essential enzyme in the nervous system, which causes the body's organs to become overstimulated and burn out.

_____ **13.** The US system for informing citizens of a potential terrorist threat; replaced the color-coded Homeland Security Advisory System.

_____ **14.** Bilateral pinpoint constricted pupils.

_____ **15.** A nerve agent antidote kit containing two auto-injector medications, atropine, and 2-PAM chloride (pralidoxime chloride).

_____ **16.** A passive circulatory system that transports a plasma-like liquid called lymph, a thin fluid that bathes the tissues of the body.

_____ **17.** A pulmonary agent that is a product of combustion, such as might be produced in a fire at a textile factory or house or at the site of metalwork or burning Freon; a very potent agent that has a delayed onset of symptoms, usually hours. Its military abbreviation is CG.

_____ **18.** The length of time that a chemical agent will stay on a surface before it evaporates.

_____ **19.** The source that is causing people to become sick or injured.

_____ **20.** The period between the person's exposure to the agent and the onset of symptoms.

_____ **21.** An explosive device built from unrestricted and often common equipment.

_____ **22.** A threat level in which a terrorist event is known to be impending or will occur very soon.

_____ **23.** A location to which responders move patients to allow for safe assessment and treatment; also known as a casualty collection point.

_____ **24.** A class of chemical found in many insecticides used in agriculture and in the home. Nerve agents fall into this class of chemicals.

_____ **25.** The emitting of an agent after exposure, for example, from a person's clothes that have been exposed to the agent.

_____ **26.** A type of energy that is emitted from a strong radiologic source. It is the fastest-moving and most powerful form of radiation. The particles easily penetrate lead and require several feet of concrete to stop them.

I. Lymphatic system

J. MARK 1

K. Miosis

L. National Terrorism Advisory System (NTAS)

M. Nerve agents

N. Neurotoxins

O. Neutron radiation

P. Off-gassing

Q. Organophosphates

R. Patient collection point

S. Patient generator

T. Persistency

U. Phosgene

V. Phosgene oxime

W. Pneumonic plague

X. Point of distribution (POD)

Y. Radioactive material

Z. Radiologic dispersal device (RDD)

Part III

Match each of the items in the right column to the appropriate definition in the left column.

_____ **1.** A nerve agent that is one of the G agents; 36 times more persistent than sarin and approximately half as lethal. It has a fruity smell and is unique because the components used to manufacture the agent are easy to acquire, and the agent is easy to manufacture. Its military abbreviation is GA.

_____ **2.** The monitoring, usually by local or state health departments, of patients presenting to emergency departments and alternative care facilities and the recording of emergency medical services (EMS) call volume and the use of over-the-counter medications.

_____ **3.** A vesicant that is generally considered very persistent. It is a yellow-brown oily substance that has the distinct smell of garlic or mustard and, when released, is quickly absorbed into the skin and/or mucous membranes and begins an irreversible process of damaging the cells. Its military abbreviation is H.

A. Ricin

B. Route of exposure

C. Sarin

_____ **4.** A terrorist who wears or carries a weapon, such as an explosive, and triggers its detonation, killing himself or herself in the process.

_____ **5.** A small, suitcase-sized nuclear weapon that is designed to destroy individual targets, such as important buildings, bridges, tunnels, or large ships.

_____ **6.** Generally healthy people who seek medical treatment because they are concerned that they are exhibiting symptoms associated with a particular illness or incident they recently learned about.

_____ **7.** The creation of a weapon from a biologic agent generally found in nature and that causes disease. The agent is cultivated, synthesized, and/or mutated to maximize the target population's exposure to the germ.

_____ **8.** Any agent designed to bring about mass death, casualties, and/or massive damage to property and infrastructure (bridges, tunnels, airports, and seaports).

_____ **9.** The length of time that a chemical agent will stay on a surface before it evaporates.

_____ **10.** A germ that requires a living host to multiply and survive.

_____ **11.** A nerve agent that is one of the G agents; twice as persistent as sarin and five times as lethal. It has a fruity odor as a result of the type of alcohol used in the agent and is both a contact and an inhalation hazard that can enter the body through skin absorption and through the respiratory tract. Its military abbreviation is GD.

_____ **12.** A highly contagious disease that may be spread in an aerosolized form as an act of warfare or terrorism. It is most contagious when blisters begin to form.

_____ **13.** An additional explosive device used by terrorists that is set to explode after the initial bomb.

_____ **14.** A nerve agent that is one of the G agents; a highly volatile colorless and odorless liquid that turns from liquid to gas within seconds to minutes at room temperature. Its military abbreviation is GB.

_____ **15.** The manner by which a toxic substance enters the body.

_____ **16.** A group of diseases that includes the Ebola, Rift Valley, and yellow fever viruses, among others. This group of viruses causes the blood in the body to seep out from the tissues and blood vessels.

_____ **17.** A blister agent. The primary route of entry is through the skin.

_____ **18.** An agent that enters the body through the respiratory tract.

_____ **19.** A nerve agent that is one of the G agents; over 100 times more lethal than sarin and extremely persistent. It is a clear, oily agent that has no odor and looks like baby oil.

_____ **20.** A violent act dangerous to human life, in violation of the criminal laws of the United States, to intimidate or coerce a government, the civilian population, or any segment thereof, in furtherance of political or social objectives.

_____ **21.** A neurotoxin derived from mash that is left from pressing oil from a castor bean; causes pulmonary edema and respiratory and circulatory failure, leading to death.

D. Secondary device

E. Smallpox

F. Soman

G. Special atomic demolition munition (SADM)

H. Suicide bomber

I. Sulfur mustard

J. Syndromic surveillance

K. Tabun

L. Terrorism

M. VX nerve agent

N. Vapor hazard

O. Vesicant

P. Viral hemorrhagic fever (VHFs)

Q. Virus

R. Volatility

S. Weapon of mass destruction (WMD)

T. Weaponization

U. Worried well

Multiple Choice

Read each item carefully, and then select the best response.

_____ **1.** A virus that has been added to the water supply is called a(n) _____ weapon.

    A. incendiary

    B. chemical

    C. biologic

    D. explosive

_____ 2. The Department of Homeland Security rates the current terrorist threats using the National Terrorism Advisory System (NTAS). What does the term "imminent" mean in the NTAS system?
- **A.** There is a general risk of terrorist attack warning.
- **B.** There is currently no specific information about a terrorist attack.
- **C.** There is currently no risk of a terrorist attack.
- **D.** The threat is believed to be impending or expected soon.

_____ 3. A vesicant may produce all of the following, EXCEPT:
- **A.** seizures.
- **B.** large blisters.
- **C.** stridor.
- **D.** irritated eyes.

_____ 4. How long does it take for a patient to begin experiencing the signs and symptoms of sulfur mustard after being exposed?
- **A.** Minutes
- **B.** 2 to 4 hours
- **C.** 4 to 6 hours
- **D.** 6 to 8 hours

_____ 5. Which of the following agents causes chest tightness, severe cough, and shortness of breath?
- **A.** Vesicant agent
- **B.** Pulmonary agent
- **C.** Nerve agent
- **D.** All of the above

_____ 6. What does the "S" stand for in the medical mnemonic SLUDGEM?
- **A.** Salivation
- **B.** Signs and symptoms
- **C.** Stridor
- **D.** Seizures

_____ 7. Which of the following statements correctly distinguishes a smallpox rash from other types of rashes?
- **A.** The lesions will be in various stages of healing.
- **B.** The lesions will all be identical in their development.
- **C.** The lesions will start on the chest.
- **D.** The lesions will be different sizes and shapes.

_____ 8. Which of the following is NOT a route of exposure for the bubonic plague?
- **A.** Infected fleas
- **B.** Infected rodents
- **C.** Waste from infected rodents
- **D.** Infected birds

_____ 9. What is the most deadly substance known to humans?
- **A.** Anthrax
- **B.** Smallpox
- **C.** Neurotoxin
- **D.** Vesicant

_____ 10. What is the LEAST harmful form of radiation?
- **A.** Alpha
- **B.** Beta
- **C.** Gamma
- **D.** X-rays

Labeling

Label the three types of energy emitted from a strong radiologic source.

1. Alpha, beta, and gamma radiation

A. _____

B._____

C. _____

Fill in the Blank

Read each item carefully, and then complete the statement by filling in the missing word(s).

1. _____ _____ _____ _____ is any agent designed to bring about mass death, casualties, and

massive damage to property.

2. Most of the terrorist acts are _____, meaning the public has no previous knowledge of the attack.

3. Additional explosives set at a site that are intended to injure responders are known as _____ devices.

4. _____ _____ _____ is how an agent most effectively enters the body.

5. _____ _____ are the most deadly chemicals developed.

6. G agents were developed by _____ scientists in the early to mid-1900s.

7. Bubonic plague infects the _____ system.

8. _____ is a deadly bacterium that lies dormant in a spore.

9. Ricin is made from _____ _____.

10. _____ _____ _____ are strategically placed stockpiles of antibiotics, vaccinations, and other

medications.

Identify

Read the following case study, and then list the chief complaint, vital signs, and pertinent negatives.

In your private vehicle, you respond to a vehicle crash about 2 miles from your home. Upon arriving at the scene, you see a truck that has rolled. The patient is outside of the truck, and bystanders are trying to help him. He is covered in white powder that has spilled from the truck. You walk up and take spinal precautions and start to assess the patient, knowing that your squad is about 3 minutes behind you. Jeff is 56 years old and is answering all your questions. You ask him what is in the truck because it is all over him, and now you have some on you also. He says it is some kind of chemical he was taking to a local plant. Jeff has some cuts on his arms. As your squad arrives, you yell at everyone to get back, and you call for the fire department. Unfortunately, you forgot the first rule of scene safety and didn't look around well enough before entering the scene. The chemical is raw organophosphate. You and Jeff get a wonderful water bath from the fire department before anyone can come and help you. Finally, you get Jeff in the squad and find that he is bradycardic with a heart rate of 50 beats/min, and his blood pressure (BP) is 98/66 mm Hg. He begins to lose consciousness, respirations are dropping quickly to 9 breaths/min, oxygen saturation is 88%, and he is drooling terribly. You realize that atropine is indicated in organophosphate poisoning. After starting an IV line, you give him 2 mg of atropine. You can give up to 5 mg, but you go with the lower dose because of his condition. You have your partner bagging him with 100% oxygen. After what seems like an eternity, he responds well with an increasing heart rate, BP, and respiratory rate. You run Priority 1 (Code 3) all the way to the hospital. You are also evaluated as soon as you get there to make sure you will be okay.

1. Chief complaint:

_____

_____

2. Vital signs:

_____

_____

3. Pertinent negatives:

_____

_____

Complete the Patient Care Report (PCR)

Reread the case study in the preceding Identify exercise, and then complete the following PCR for the patient.

EMS Patient Care Report (PCR)					
Date:	**Incident No.:**	**Nature of Call:**		**Location:**	
Dispatched:	**En Route:**	**At Scene:**	**Transport:**	**At Hospital:**	**In Service:**
Patient Information					
Age:		**Allergies:**			
Sex:		**Medications:**			
Weight (in kg [lb]):		**Past Medical History:**			
		Chief Complaint:			
Vital Signs					
Time:	**BP:**	**Pulse:**	**Respirations:**		**SpO$_2$:**
Time:	**BP:**	**Pulse:**	**Respirations:**		**SpO$_2$:**
Time:	**BP:**	**Pulse:**	**Respirations:**		**SpO$_2$:**
EMS Treatment (circle all that apply)					
Oxygen @ _____ L/min via (circle one): NC NRM Bag-mask device		**Assisted Ventilation**	**Airway Adjunct**		**CPR**
Defibrillation	**Bleeding Control**	**Bandaging**	**Splinting**		**Other:**
Narrative					

Ambulance Calls

The following case scenarios provide an opportunity to explore the concerns associated with patient management and paramedic care. Read each scenario, and then answer each question.

1. You are among the first ambulance personnel to reach the scene of a train derailment involving at least 60 casualties. Authorities on the scene think that this could be an act of terrorism.
    a. As you recall, there are five categories of terrorist incidents. They are:

    (1)_____

    (2)_____

    (3)_____

    (4)_____

    (5)_____

    b. You are directed to begin triage of the people trying to get clear of the wreckage. There seem to be a lot of people who are ambulatory, but you are located in a bean field with nothing around you to send the walking wounded toward. There is only one road close by, and it is jammed up with emergency vehicles. What can you do with the ambulatory people?

    _____

    _____

2. You respond to the local swimming pool right before it is scheduled to open. Dispatch says there are several kids coughing, and the lifeguards are having a hard time talking on the phone because of coughing spasms. As you arrive, you notice a green haze floating in the air around the pool house. There are about 50 kids standing around waiting for the pool to open.
    a. What is the cause of this green haze?

    _____

    _____

    b. Before you get out of the ambulance, what should you do?

    _____

    _____

    c. You have a total of seven kids who are coughing hard, and you have two lifeguards who are really struggling to breathe. After help arrives, you begin treatment on one of the lifeguards. What type of problems should you expect?

    _____

    _____

True/False

If you believe the statement to be more true than false, write the letter "T" in the space provided. If you believe the statement to be more false than true, write the letter "F."

_____   1. There are suits made for paramedics to shield them from radiation.

_____   2. Radiologic material can be found at hospitals, power plants, and colleges.

_____   3. Antibiotics will not help with bacteria.

_____   4. A virus can live and thrive outside the host body.

_____ **5.** The period of time between being exposed and showing signs and symptoms is known as the incubation period.

_____ **6.** Ebola is a type of hemorrhagic fever.

_____ **7.** Sarin is a vesicant.

_____ **8.** In addition to men, women and children have also acted as suicide bombers.

_____ **9.** The Oklahoma City Federal Building bombing was done by a domestic terrorist.

_____ **10.** The greatest threats to a paramedic during an attack involving weapons of mass destruction (WMDs) are contamination and cross-contamination.

Short Answer

Complete this section with short written answers using the space provided.

1. List five examples of potential high-value targets for terrorists.

a. _____

b. _____

c. _____

d. _____

e. _____

2. List four potential locations where sources of radiologic materials may be found.

a. _____

b. _____

c. _____

d. _____

Fill in the Table

Fill in the missing parts of the tables.

1. Nerve agents

Name	Code Name	Odor	Special Features	Onset of Symptoms	Volatility	Route of Exposure
_____ _____		Fruity	Easy to manufacture	Immediate	Low	Both contact and vapor hazard
_____ _____		None (if pure) or strong	Will off-gas while on victim's clothing	Immediate	High	Primarily respiratory vapor hazard; extremely lethal if skin contact is made
_____ _____		Fruity	Ages rapidly, making it difficult to treat	Immediate	Moderate	Contact with skin; minimal vapor hazard
_____ _____		None	Most lethal chemical agent; difficult to decontaminate	Immediate	Very low	Contact with skin; no vapor hazard (unless aerosolized)

Chapter 50

2. Chemical agents

Class	Military Designation	Odor	Lethality	Onset of Symptoms	Volatility	Primary Route of Exposure
_____	Mustard (H) _____ Lewisite (L) _____ Phosgene oxime (CX)		Causes large blisters to form on victims; may severely damage upper airway if vapors are inhaled; severe, intense pain and gray skin discoloration (L, CX)	_____ _____	Very low (H, L) Moderate (CX)	Primarily contact; with some vapor hazard
_____	Chlorine (CL) _____ Phosgene (CG)		Causes irritation; choking (CL); severe pulmonary edema (CG)	_____ _____	Very high	Vapor hazard
_____	Tabun (GA) _____ Sarin (GB) Soman (GD) VX agent (VX)		Most lethal chemical agents can kill within minutes; effects are reversible with antidotes	_____	Moderate (GA, GD) Very high (GB) Low (VX)	Vapor hazard (GB) Both vapor and contact hazard (GA, GD) Contact hazard (VX)
_____	Hydrogen cyanide (AC) _____ Cyanogen chloride (CK)		Highly lethal chemical gases; can kill within minutes; effects are reversible with antidotes	_____	Very high	Vapor hazard

3. Symptoms of persons exposed to nerve agents

Mnemonic: SLUDGEM	
S	Salivation
L	_____
U	Urination
D	_____
G	Gastrointestinal (GI) distress
E	_____
M	Miosis
Mnemonic: Killer Bs	
B	Bradycardia
B	_____
B	Bronchospasm

Disaster Response

CHAPTER 51

Matching

Match each of the terms in the right column to the appropriate description in the left column.

_____ **1.** Blasts from flowing or standing lava that can have a wide dispersal circumference, spewing ash and magma.

_____ **2.** A strategically placed facility that has been preestablished for the mass distribution of antibiotics, antidotes, and vaccinations, along with other medications and supplies.

_____ **3.** An illness or disease that affects a high proportion of the population over a broad or potentially worldwide geographic area.

_____ **4.** A situation in which a reservoir overflows its borders.

_____ **5.** Documents that preplan how you will access help from other areas when needed.

_____ **6.** A command system used in larger incidents in which there is a multiagency response or multijurisdictional response to coordinate decision making and cooperation among the agencies.

_____ **7.** Debris from satellites and other man-made objects that reenter the earth's atmosphere.

_____ **8.** A method of safeguarding oneself or others' position during an emergency event or event involving a hazardous material; includes measures such as remaining in a safe atmosphere, usually inside structures, or other simple measures such as shutting the windows, going to the cellar, or turning off the heating and air-conditioning systems.

_____ **9.** Depression that can affect people in long periods of bad weather, usually winter.

_____ **10.** Heavy canvas bags that can be hung from trees containing water in amounts from 40 to 100 gallons (151 to 379 L).

_____ **11.** A guideline to follow regarding the distance to place between oneself and a person who sneezes or coughs, to avoid exposure to germs.

_____ **12.** A system implemented to manage disasters and mass-casualty incidents in which section chiefs, including operations, finance, logistics, and planning, report to the incident commander.

_____ **13.** A team, usually staffed with physicians, nurses, and emergency medical services (EMS) providers, that performs minor surgical procedures and debridements in the field, taking some of the load from the hospital facility.

A. 6-feet rule

B. After-action report (AAR)

C. All-hazards approach

D. Ashfall

E. Casualty collection points

F. Cold stress

G. Continuity of operations plan (COOP)

H. Critical infrastructure

I. Directed area

J. Disaster

K. Disaster management

L. Dust suffocation

M. Emergency operations center (EOC)

_____ **14.** An illness or disease that affects or tends to affect a disproportionately large number of people within a specific population, community, or region at the same time.

_____ **15.** A central command and control facility, found at all government levels, responsible for strategic overview; tactical decisions are left to incident commanders.

_____ **16.** The external foundation in communities made up of structures and services critical in the day-to-day living activities of humans; energy sources, fuel, water, sewage removal, food, hospitals, and transportation systems.

_____ **17.** The detailed plan describing the functioning of the agency in situations that disrupt normal operations.

_____ **18.** A psychologic condition that can develop in people who are exposed to cold weather for long periods of time, even if sheltered.

_____ **19.** Areas where slightly injured or noninjured displaced people can be gathered together and transported by bus or truck for further treatment.

_____ **20.** The residue left behind from a volcanic eruption.

_____ **21.** A phenomenon that can occur during an earthquake, in which particles of dust and debris are loosened and released into the air, producing a toxic and hypoxic atmosphere.

_____ **22.** A planned, coordinated response to a disaster that involves cooperation of multiple responders and agencies and enables effective triage and provision of care according to triage decisions.

_____ **23.** A sudden, calamitous event, such as an accident or catastrophe, that causes great damage, loss, or destruction.

_____ **24.** An area away from the command post or emergency operations center, considered by engineering expertise to be a safe place to stage until directed otherwise.

_____ **25.** The act of conducting comprehensive preplanning that will apply to any disaster.

_____ **26.** The official internal report of the entire event, such as a disaster, which should contain the facts of the incident reflected in a chronologic, accurate manner.

N. Epidemic

O. Forward surgical team

P. Incident command system (ICS)

Q. Lister bags

R. Mutual aid agreements

S. Overtopping

T. Pandemic

U. Point of distribution (POD)

V. Pyroclastic explosions

W. Seasonal affective disorder (SAD)

X. Shelter-in-place

Y. Space junk

Z. Unified command system

Multiple Choice

Read each item carefully, and then select the best response.

_____ **1.** The critical infrastructure includes the food and hospitals as well as which of the following?
   A. Communications systems
   B. Electrical power grid
   C. Sewage removal
   D. All of the above

_____ **2.** Disaster response preplanning includes assessing each of the following, EXCEPT:
   A. geography of response areas.
   B. number of paramedics on each ambulance.
   C. immunizations of personnel.
   D. training standards.

_____ **3.** In planning for disasters, which nongovernmental organization should be included to assist with disaster relief?
   A. Homeland Security Agency
   B. The Red Cross
   C. Federal Emergency Management Agency (FEMA)
   D. National Highway and Traffic Safety Administration (NHTSA)

_____ **4.** When planning for sheltering, what will your plan need to consider?
   A. Adult supervision for children
   B. Access to automated teller machines (ATMs)
   C. Facilities for mass decontamination
   D. Housing for wild animals

_____ **5.** Which of the following is NOT considered a high priority for after a disaster event?
   A. Physical examination of personnel
   B. Stress reaction review
   C. Mobilization of personnel
   D. Finance and reimbursement

_____ **6.** Each of the following is considered a natural disaster, EXCEPT:
   A. flooding.
   B. a tanker crash.
   C. a pandemic.
   D. a landslide or avalanche.

_____ **7.** During an earthquake, the release of particles of debris into the air can cause:
   A. dust suffocation.
   B. a landslide.
   C. flooding.
   D. magma release.

_____ **8.** In which of the following incidents should you consider sheltering-in-place?
   A. An earthquake nearby
   B. A drought in the valley this season
   C. A sandstorm or dust storm
   D. Prolonged cold weather and power outages

_____ **9.** When people are exposed to cold weather for long periods of time, even though sheltered, they can develop a condition called:
   A. trench foot.
   B. frostbite.
   C. walking pneumonia.
   D. cold stress.

_____ **10.** Which of the following is NOT a man-made disaster?
   A. A hazardous materials incident
   B. A pandemic
   C. A civil disturbance
   D. An IT (cyber) disruption

Fill-in-the-Blank

Read each item carefully, and then complete the statement by filling in the missing word(s).

1. The act of conducting comprehensive _____ for all types of disasters is called a(n) _____-_____

approach.

2. EMS is normally accustomed to _____ _____ _____ that allow EMS agencies and fire departments in

neighboring jurisdictions to cover emergency calls.

3. The _____ supervisor must maintain a(n) _____ of all patients and the hospitals to which they are

transported.

4. You must keep the _____ updated on field conditions so that they can _____ their priorities, if necessary.

5. Consider a press _____ location and provide prompt _____ so that all the facts that you are allowed to

release about the incident can be communicated through the _____.

6. The _____-_____ _____ is your official internal report of the entire event.

7. You may need to help set up field hospitals and first-aid stations at _____ _____ _____.

8. EMS may be represented in the _____ _____ _____ or in the unified command center.

9. During a heat wave, small, more frequent meals are better than large ones. Eat foods that are _____ in fluids, such

as _____, fruits, and salads.

10. A(n) _____ is illness that affects a disproportionately large geographic area and number of people. A(n)

_____ is an extensive one.

Identify

Read the following case study, and then list the chief complaint, vital signs, and pertinent negatives.

You have responded to a structure fire involving a strip mall with eight stores in a row. The suspected arsonist had a grudge against the owner of the Software Plus store and pried open the rear door and started a fire with gasoline. It was around midnight, and all the stores were closed, so aside from the potential danger to the firefighters, there were no victims in the buildings. While you are standing by in the rehab sector, you are notified that the police found the suspected arsonist hiding in a nearby alleyway. They bring him to your EMS unit because most of the front of his clothing has been burned, and he is disoriented and in a lot of pain. Your patient is a 22-year-old man who at first inspection has burns to his hands, arms, and the front of his chest, and his beard has been mostly burned off. Apparently, the fire got out of control before he was able to exit the building, and the gasoline had splashed the front of his clothing. He is conscious and alert, but you note that he has a raspy voice and is in extreme pain. (He reports a 20 on the 10 scale!) He did remember the grade-school lesson to "stop, drop, and roll," managing to put the fire on his clothing out by rolling around in a puddle in the alley.

Your partner starts the primary survey and secondary assessment as you apply oxygen with a nonrebreathing mask. The rapid trauma exam shows only partial-thickness burns on the hands and arms, but his chest is a full-thickness burn. You are most concerned with the potential for a respiratory burn and know this patient will end up in a burn bed this morning. As you remove his watch and rings and give them to the officer, your partner gets some vital signs. He is breathing 24 breaths/min and shallow, with an oxygen saturation of 96% and clear lung sounds. Pulse is 110 beats/min and regular, and blood pressure (BP) is 108/68 mm Hg. His pupils are equal, round, and reactive to light and accommodation (PERRLA) and fortunately were not burned. The patient rates his pain at a 10/10. His skin, in the noninjured areas, is pale, cool, and moist. You remove his remaining clothing and have him lie down on a burn sheet that was placed on your stretcher. The patient denies taking any medications and denies any allergies. He says he is normally as healthy as a horse. You get him in the unit, place him on the heart monitor (which shows sinus tachycardia with no ectopic beats), and then start a large-bore IV line in a vein in an area that was not burned. You decide to administer plenty of fluids for the burns and fentanyl for pain due to his dropping BP. After consultation with medical control, the decision is to transport him to the local high school soccer field, where a landing zone has been set up for the regional medevac helicopter crew to pick him up and transport him to the regional burn center.

1. Chief complaint:

_____

_____

2. Vital signs:

_____

_____

3. Pertinent negatives:

_____

_____

Ambulance Calls

The following case scenario provides an opportunity to explore the concerns associated with patient management, paramedic care, and preparation for major incidents in your community. Read the scenario, and then answer each question.

1. It is a hot, stuffy day with high humidity in July in your community. You are on the medic unit today and state to your partner, "This makes 10 straight days of 90-degree temps." You have been running calls all morning, mostly patients with respiratory complaints. At 1500 hours, you get a call for the Fairwood Nursing Home for an unresponsive patient. On arrival, you find a five-floor facility that normally houses 200 patients. It is extremely hot inside the lobby. As you are led to room 105 by a nursing aide, your partner notices that there are a number of patients in a community room who look unconscious on the couch with the TV blasting. The aide tells you that the air conditioner has been broken all week, and the place only has two aides for each floor and one nurse in the office. Some doctors stop by in the mornings, but they are not there today. As you walk into the patient's room, you note it is a semiprivate room, and both occupants are restrained in a seated position in chairs. That sure makes it difficult for them to keep drinking fluids when they can't even get up out of their chairs. Further, they are wearing flannel nightgowns! The aide, who has been very talkative, says he thinks there are a lot of patients getting sicker; he certainly is not feeling well. He also states that the windows have never been opened. There is a large fan in the hallway, basically blowing hot air around the hallways.

As your partner begins to assess the patient in room 105, you decide to pick up the phone and discuss this situation with your supervisor, who promptly alerts dispatch to assign a group of ambulances, the police, the fire department (for ventilation), and the Special Operations Unit.

This story is based on an actual incident that occurred in the heat wave of 1978 in Queens, New York. It could happen in your community, too, if you live in a warmer climate.

a. List four problems and potential solutions to issues that occur during a heat wave.

(1) _____

_____

(2) _____

_____

(3) _____

_____

(4) _____

_____

b. What are five examples of the illnesses that you may be treating in a nursing home during a heat emergency similar to the one described in the scenario?

(1)_____

(2)_____

(3)_____

(4)_____

(5)_____

True/False

If you believe the statement to be more true than false, write the letter "T" in the space provided. If you believe the statement to be more false than true, write the letter "F."

_____   **1.** Woodland fires have a much higher death rate than structural fires.

_____   **2.** The trend of increasing frequency and severity of extreme weather is expected to continue in the foreseeable future.

_____   **3.** When it is very cold out, you should dress in loose clothing and multiple layers.

_____   **4.** A hurricane can occur anywhere, but they tend to happen in the northern states and inland regions.

_____   **5.** Tsunamis can come in a series.

_____   **6.** The biggest immediate danger from an earthquake is structural collapse.

_____   **7.** Cave-ins can release sewer and chemical gases.

_____   **8.** The media should not be a concern during a disaster.

_____   **9.** Your agency's designated infection control officer should be aware of each member's immunization status.

_____   **10.** If a crew is sent to another area, it may need to be self-sustaining for 48 to 72 hours.

Short Answer

Complete this section with short written answers using the space provided.

1. List the three phases of any plan of response to a disaster.

a. _____

b. _____

c. _____

2. List the considerations during a disaster.

_____

_____

_____

Fill-in-the-Table

Fill in the missing parts of the table.

1. Examples of natural and man-made disasters

Natural Disasters	Man-Made Disasters
Forest and brush fires	_____
_____	Construction failures and building collapse
Tornadoes	_____
_____	Riots, civil disturbances, and stampedes
Tsunamis	_____
_____	Sniper, shooter, and hostage situations
Landslides, avalanches, mudslides	_____
_____	Information technology (cyber) disruptions
Volcanic eruptions	_____
_____	Hazardous materials incidents
Sandstorms and dust storms	
_____	
Drought	
_____	
Meteors and space debris	
_____	

Crime Scene Awareness

Matching

Match each of the items in the right column to the appropriate definition in the left column.

_____ **1.** Any other means of egress, including windows and rear doors.

_____ **2.** The main means of escape should violence erupt. This is usually the door you used to enter the building.

_____ **3.** A gunman who has begun to fire on people and is still at large.

_____ **4.** The evidence that ties a suspect or victim to a crime. It may include body materials, objects, and impressions.

_____ **5.** Protection from being seen.

_____ **6.** Locations where illegal drugs, such as methamphetamine, lysergic acid diethylamide (LSD), ecstasy, and phencyclidine hydrochloride (PCP), are manufactured.

_____ **7.** A situation in which a paramedic becomes so completely involved with patient care that he or she fails to see the possibility of physical harm to the patient or other care providers.

_____ **8.** The oral documentation by a witness of his or her perceived facts of a criminal act.

_____ **9.** Knowing your surroundings, the people and groups in your environment, and the climate of violence or strife.

_____ **10.** A technique that involves one paramedic making contact with the patient to provide care while the second paramedic obtains patient information, gauges the level of tension, and warns his or her partner at the first sign of trouble.

_____ **11.** Obstacles that are difficult or impossible for bullets to penetrate.

_____ **12.** Specially trained paramedics who provide medical care for special weapons and tactics (SWAT) team members conducting operations, barricaded patients, patients being held hostage, and other special operations.

A. Active shooter

B. Clandestine drug laboratories

C. Concealment

D. Contact and cover

E. Cover

F. Physical evidence

G. Primary exit

H. Secondary exit

I. Situational awareness

J. Tactical paramedics

K. Testimonial evidence

L. Tunnel vision

Multiple Choice

Read each item carefully, and then select the best response.

_____ **1.** For maximum safety when arriving at incidents with a single vehicle in which the potential danger is high, your vehicle should be positioned a minimum of how many feet behind the stopped vehicle?

    A. 50

    B. 15

    C. 21

    D. 10

2. When approaching a passenger vehicle (sedan), you should stop at which column (post) of the vehicle to look in the rear and side windows?

   A. A

   B. B

   C. C

   D. D

3. When announcing your arrival at the front door of a residence, where should you stand?

   A. To the doorknob side of the door

   B. To the hinged side of the door

   C. In front of the door

   D. Ten to 15 feet back from the door

4. When you enter a structure, the door you use to enter the building is referred to as the _____ exit.

   A. tertiary

   B. secondary

   C. primary

   D. general

5. Which of the following is considered concealment when you are confronted by violence?

   A. Curb

   B. Depression in the ground

   C. Utility pole

   D. Shrubbery

6. You are dispatched to a residence for a possible sick person. En route to the call, the dispatcher informs you that the caller hung up before all the information could be collected. When you are suspicious that something is not right, prior to announcing your arrival at the door, you should do all the following, EXCEPT:

   A. listen for loud noises.

   B. look for neighbors to talk with.

   C. glance through a window for signs of a struggle.

   D. listen for threatening voices.

7. You have entered a residence that you initially thought was safe, but once inside, you and your partner are suspicious that there might be trouble. You approach the patient to start the assessment, and your partner starts to look around to see if there is any immediate danger and gather information relevant to providing care. What is this technique called?

   A. Assess and act

   B. Contact and cover

   C. Respond and react

   D. Link and look

8. In a hostage situation, you should assume all of the following, EXCEPT:

   A. other hostages may look to you for guidance.

   B. your captors could kill you at any moment.

   C. your captors will be lenient on you because your uniform is an image of authority.

   D. removing pieces of your uniform may make you less threatening to the captors.

9. In all potentially violent situations, the paramedic's best (and often only) defense is:

   A. a hidden weapon.

   B. police backup.

   C. the portable radio.

   D. situational awareness.

_____ **10.** You respond to a stabbing. While treating the patient and packaging for transport, you observe some footprints in the patient's blood, and you try to work quickly with minimal disruption to the evidence. The footprints are considered _____ evidence.

    A. physical

    B. testimonial

    C. circumstantial

    D. substantiated

Fill in the Blank

Read each item carefully, and then complete the statement by filling in the missing word(s).

1. Becoming completely involved with patient care and failing to see possible physical harm is called _____ _____.

2. For maximum safety when arriving at an incident with a single vehicle in which the potential for danger is high, position your vehicle at least _____ feet behind the stopped vehicle at a(n) _____-degree angle.

3. When there are two or more paramedics in the unit and you come to the scene of a motor vehicle crash, the person riding in the right front seat of the ambulance is the _____ _____.

4. When you approach a van in a situation where safety is a concern, move 10 to 15 feet away from the passenger side, and then belly-in and walk parallel until you are approximately 45° forward of the _____ post.

5. When you enter a structure, pick a(n) _____ exit and a(n) _____ exit to keep one means of escape accessible at all times.

6. To enter a scene where violence is suspected, one technique is for one paramedic to start providing patient care and the other to obtain information and warn the partner at the first sign of trouble. This technique is called _____ and _____.

Identify

Read the following case study, and then list the possible errors in handling scene safety, warning signs of danger, and potential evidence.

You are assigned to respond to a call for an injured person in a residence in a middle-class neighborhood. You are provided no additional information by the dispatcher because the caller hung up before more questions could be asked. You approach the house and hear a loud conversation inside, and without announcing yourself, you stand in front of the door and knock. You enter through the front door (primary exit), and without looking around, you ask what is happening. You find a woman on the couch, with bruising to the face, holding her right arm. She appears to be in considerable pain. Both you and your partner go to the patient and do not pay much attention to the person on the other side of the room, who is still arguing with the patient. You see a ceramic object in pieces on the floor and brush it out of the way with your foot as you approach the patient. You start to assess the patient, and your partner cuts and rips through the bloody shirt sleeve to examine the arm. You decide the person standing on the other side of the room is a potential threat and realize that he is between you and the front door. You notice there are a number of tables with drawers and a fire poker in a stand next to the fireplace. Just as you and your partner become anxious about the potential threats, two police officers come through the front door.

1. Errors in handling scene safety:

_____

_____

_____

_____

2. Warning signs of danger:

_____

_____

_____

_____

3. Potential evidence:

_____

_____

_____

_____

Ambulance Calls

The following case scenarios provide an opportunity to explore the concerns associated with patient management and paramedic care. Read each scenario, and then answer each question.

1. You respond to a residence that has previously had calls for domestic violence, but the dispatcher informs you that the information provided was for a medical problem including severe difficulty breathing, and no information indicated danger or that responders would be at risk. You are told the police will not arrive for another 5 minutes after you are on the scene. When you arrive at the residence, you are suspicious. What precautions might you take to help ensure that there is no immediate violence that would place you at risk?

_____

_____

_____

2. You and your paramedic partner, who is driving the ambulance, are the first emergency personnel to arrive at the scene where a car ran off the road into a guardrail. When you arrive on the scene, you see no activity around the vehicle, and you see only one person in the driver's seat of the car. You are initially suspicious.

a. How should you park and approach the scene?

_____

_____

b. What precautions should you take to identify the car?

_____

_____

c. Who should be the incident commander, and how should that person proceed?

_____

_____

3. You receive a call for a sick child. You arrive on the scene of the call, and someone is outside waiting for you. You are led into the house to find a wheezing pediatric patient who, you are told, is 7 years old. She is an asthmatic, and her family members report that they can't find her inhaler. You and your partner signal each other to use "contact and cover." You start to treat the patient, and your partner obtains information from the person who met the ambulance. Your partner's observations lead her to believe this residence is a clandestine drug laboratory.

a. What does "contact and cover" mean?

_____

_____

b. What actions should you and your partner take?

_____

_____

c. What are your concerns?

_____

_____

4. Upon arrival at the scene of a shooting, you find a young patient shot in the leg and lying in a pool of blood. You and your partner do a rapid assessment and provide care quickly. The patient is prepared for transport, placed on the stretcher, and loaded into the ambulance. What are your primary concerns when trying to preserve evidence?

_____

_____

_____

_____

True/False

If you believe the statement to be more true than false, write the letter "T" in the space provided. If you believe the statement to be more false than true, write the letter "F."

_____   **1.** Physical evidence is oral documentation by witnesses of facts.

_____   **2.** The most popular substance manufactured in clandestine labs is methamphetamine.

_____   **3.** The secondary exit is the door that you use to enter the building.

_____   **4.** When standing at the door to a residence, you should stand on the hinged side of the door.

_____   **5.** When there are two paramedics in an ambulance and you arrive on the scene where a vehicle needs to be checked out, the incident commander is the driver of the ambulance.

_____   **6.** Some agencies have developed standard operating procedures that guide how to handle potentially violent situations.

_____   **7.** When checking out a vehicle where the back seat is occupied, do not pass the C column/post until you are sure that it is safe to do so.

_____   **8.** When you arrive at the scene of a single-vehicle crash with potential danger, the ambulance should be parked at least 10 feet behind the vehicle.

_____   **9.** Many gangs use graffiti to mark off their territories.

_____   **10.** Clandestine drug laboratories are not hazardous and present no danger to emergency medical services personnel.

Short Answer

Complete this section with short written answers using the space provided.

1. You are on the scene of a call that, because of unsafe circumstances, dictates your retreat to a safe area. After you have backed away from the danger zone and are in a safe area, you supply the dispatcher with your unit identifier, your location, and the location of the injured. What additional information would you want to provide to the dispatcher?

   a. _____

   b. _____

   c. _____

   d. _____

   e. _____

2. What three immediate hazards present dangers to emergency responders in regard to a clandestine drug laboratory?

   a. _____

   b. _____

   c. _____

3. When approaching a motor vehicle, a paramedic should always be attentive to impending danger. In which locations in a vehicle could a weapon be concealed?

   a. _____

   b. _____

   c. _____

   d. _____

   e. _____

   f. _____

   g. _____

4. When you enter a structure, the primary exit is usually the door you used to enter. What is a secondary exit, and why should it be identified?

   _____

   _____

5. What is the difference between *cover* and *concealment*?

   _____

   _____

6. Give three examples each of cover and concealment that you can use when there is danger from a shooter.

   a. Cover

     (1)_____

     (2)_____

     (3)_____

   b. Concealment

     (1)_____

     (2)_____

     (3)_____

7. If you are taken hostage by a subject with a gun, what should you assume during the capture stage?

_____

_____

8. There are two general classifications of evidence. Name and provide a brief description of each.

   a._____

   b._____

CAREER DEVELOPMENT

Career Development

We didn't cover ballroom dancing...

Neither did we.

Each sport has common mechanisms of injury...

© Jones & Bartlett Learning.

Matching

Match each of the items in the right column to the appropriate definition in the left column.

_____ **1.** Paramedics who may work in military combat settings or civilian settings as part of special response teams such as special weapons and tactics (SWAT) teams.

_____ **2.** Paramedics who provide trauma care and other emergency services in remote and frontier areas.

_____ **3.** Paramedics who work as part of an air rescue team that provides either on-scene care in remote field settings or interfacility transports from one clinical setting to another.

_____ **4.** Paramedics whose primary role is to assist patients, such as those who frequently use the emergency medical services (EMS) system for health care needs that can be managed outside the emergency department, in managing their health care needs more effectively.

_____ **5.** A specialty role for paramedics, in which the paramedic is trained to provide advanced care and transport for critically injured or ill patients; also called a critical care transport professional (CCTP).

A. Critical care paramedic (CCP)

B. Flight paramedics

C. Mobile integrated health care providers/community paramedics (MIHPs/CPs)

D. Tactical paramedics

E. Wilderness paramedics

Multiple Choice

Read each item carefully, and then select the best response.

_____ **1.** According to the US Bureau of Labor Statistics, which occupation will be the fastest growing in the next 10 years?

   A. Accountants

   B. Registered nurses

   C. Emergency medical technician (EMT) and paramedic

   D. Auto mechanics

_____ **2.** Ultimately, the primary goal of an MIHP/CP is to get the right patient to the:

   A. right resource.

   B. right treatment.

   C. right tools.

   D. All of the above

_____   **3.** The training program for the MIHP/CP focuses primarily on pathophysiology, public health, prevention, and:
  A. transport ventilators.
  B. tactical weapons.
  C. social assessment needs.
  D. hemodynamic monitoring.

_____   **4.** The International Board of Specialty Certification or other local regulatory bodies often administer certification exams for:
  A. MIHP/CPs.
  B. CCTPs.
  C. tactical paramedics.
  D. bicycle response teams.

_____   **5.** A career as a flight paramedic may require any of the following skills, EXCEPT:
  A. trauma management.
  B. neurologic emergency management.
  C. cycling fundamentals for all terrains.
  D. advanced airway management.

_____   **6.** Paramedics who are specially trained to provide medical care within the "hot zone" are usually referred to as:
  A. bicycle emergency response.
  B. flight paramedics.
  C. critical care paramedics.
  D. tactical paramedics.

_____   **7.** Responsibilities of the wilderness paramedic may include any of the following, EXCEPT:
  A. general environmental medicine.
  B. providing wellness checks.
  C. improvised medicine.
  D. expedition medicine.

_____   **8.** An EMT or paramedic with experience in patient transportation and EMS care is an ideal candidate to serve as a(n):
  A. transportation coordinator.
  B. emergency management coordinator.
  C. hospital EMS coordinator.
  D. tactical paramedic.

_____   **9.** One of the best ways to maintain interest in your profession is to train and educate others to:
  A. be tactical paramedics in your community.
  B. provide the same level of care you provide.
  C. be EMS researchers in academic settings.
  D. be mobile integrated health care providers.

_____   **10.** If you were searching for an organization that can provide you with help in your interest in becoming a flight paramedic it would make sense to check the website:
  A. http://wms.org.
  B. nemsma.org.
  C. www.nasemso.org.
  D. www.iafccp.org.

Fill in the Blank

Read each item carefully, and then complete the statement by filling in the missing word(s).

1. Tactical paramedics may also serve as training instructors for the law enforcement agency in areas such as _____ and _____.

2. The wilderness paramedic role may not only be _____ demanding due to extended length of time between injury and illness and _____ care, but could also be _____ demanding.

3. Emergency _____ _____ assist hospitals with disaster planning, drills, and training on the concepts of a hospital _____ command system.

4. Visualize and _____ your career _____ in EMS.

5. When doing home visits the MIHP/CP may be trained to provide: _____ checks, obtain patient _____ inventory and determine _____ to recommended guidelines.

6. A _____ paramedic must be in _____ physical condition and able to _____ long-term fitness.

Ambulance Calls

The following case scenarios provide an opportunity to explore the concerns associated with patient management and paramedic care. Read each scenario, and then answer each question.

1. You respond to a shopping mall for a fight in which at least two individuals have been injured. On your arrival, there are shoppers who are running out the mall door stating, "Someone has a gun and is shooting people." What should you do right away, and which type of specialty training would have been helpful for you as a paramedic?

   _____

   _____

   _____

   _____

2. You and your paramedic partner just worked a 70-year-old male who was in cardiac arrest. The patient had return of spontaneous circulation (ROSC), and you transported him to a community hospital because he was not stable. The emergency department (ED) physician has decided it would be appropriate to transport the patient to the regional cardiac care center because he is a candidate for percutaneous coronary intervention (PCI).
   a. What type of specialty training would be helpful for the transport of this critical patient?

   _____

   _____

   b. The patient is on multiple IV drips to maintain his blood pressure (BP). What specific skills would be helpful for those paramedics doing this transport?

   _____

   _____

3. You receive a call for a diabetic patient who has an altered level of mental status. You have been to this location at least three times this week, and it seems the patient and family could use some help with monitoring the patient's diabetes.

    a. What type of specialty training could be helpful on calls like this as well as to prevent these calls from occurring in the first place?

_____

_____

    b. What specific responsibilities are included in this specialty training that would be helpful in this situation?

_____

_____

True/False

If you believe the statement to be more true than false, write the letter "T" in the space provided. If you believe the statement to be more false than true, write the letter "F."

_____ 1. The rise in violent crime is a reason for needing more EMS providers in the next decade.

_____ 2. Career development begins with your self-assessment.

_____ 3. The stabilization and evacuation of patients in hostile and austere environments are a key component of the MIHP/CP.

_____ 4. When the career options for paramedics increase, the opportunities for EMS educators will decrease.

_____ 5. There are roles for EMS providers in developing community programs to help prevent injury and illness.

_____ 6. The CCP is focused on functioning in nontraditional settings and providing nonemergency care with a preventive and long-term focus.

_____ 7. Learning how to use sonography and medical diagnostic tools may be a part of the training of a CCP.

_____ 8. Field sanitation, hygiene, and preventive medicine are often components of the training of the wilderness paramedic.

Short Answer

Complete this section with short written answers using the space provided.

1. List five examples of the factors influencing the need for paramedics in the next decade.

    a. _____

    b. _____

    c. _____

    d. _____

    e. _____

2. List five examples of organizations for EMS providers for career development.

    a. _____

    b. _____

    c. _____

    d. _____

    e. _____

3. When completing your training as a paramedic, it is advisable to have some short- and long-term career goals. Becoming a paramedic may be an achievement of one of your goals already! Take the time to think about and write down your short- and long-term goals. Next, discuss these goals with your instructor(s) and mentors, and obtain some advice on an action plan to help achieve your goals.

a. Short-term goal: _____

_____

_____

b. Short-term goal: _____

_____

_____

c. Short-term goal: _____

_____

_____

d. Short-term goal: _____

_____

_____

e. Short-term goal: _____

_____

_____

f. Long-term goal: _____

_____

_____

g. Long-term goal: _____

_____

_____

h. Long-term goal: _____

_____

_____

i. Long-term goal: _____

_____

_____

j. Long-term goal: _____

_____

_____

Instructor/Mentor Comments and Advice:

_____

_____

_____

Case Studies

Case Studies

Case Study 1

It is 0900 hours, and you have been dispatched to a Priority 1 (Charlie response) call for a serious injury. As you arrive at 0908 hours, the police have just arrived and are calling you to come to the side of the house right away. The scene is safe, although there is a blood trail from a basement window to the spot where the patient is lying, holding his right leg and screaming out in pain. His airway is obviously open! You don appropriate personal protective equipment (PPE) and approach the patient to find a 20-year-old man who states he tried to kick open the basement window and managed to cut the back of his knee. He said it has continued to spurt bright red blood all over the place. Quickly, you open the trauma kit and apply direct pressure with gauze to the large laceration to the artery behind the right knee. Meanwhile, your partner determines that the patient, who is screaming that he is in a lot of pain (10/10), is alert and restless. The patient reports no other injuries. His vital signs are taken and are found to be as follows: respirations of 26 breaths/min, deep and full; pulse of 100 beats/min, thready and weak at the wrist. His blood oxygen saturation (SpO_2) is 94%. His skin is pale, cool, and clammy. The patient denies any other injuries and states he feels thirsty, weak, and dizzy at this point. You are busy trying to control the bleeding, following all the appropriate methods you learned in your paramedic training. Meanwhile, your partner applies a nonrebreathing mask with 100% oxygen to the patient as you prepare to load him on the stretcher. You both decide to do the secondary assessment en route to the hospital because the patient's condition is serious. As you load him into the ambulance, you note that the time is now 0916 hours.

1. What is the appropriate order of initial management of this patient?

_____

_____

_____

_____

_____

_____

2. How will you manage the continued bleeding from the patient's injury?

_____

_____

_____

_____

_____

_____

3. What is the appropriate intravenous (IV) fluid resuscitation regimen for this patient?

_____

_____

_____

_____

_____

_____

4. What is the difference between a crystalloid and a colloid solution?

_____

_____

_____

_____

_____

5. What is the purpose of performing a secondary assessment?

_____

_____

_____

_____

_____

6. Complete the PCR.

EMS Patient Care Report (PCR)					
Date:	**Incident No.:**	**Nature of Call:**		**Location:**	
Dispatched:	**En Route:**	**At Scene:**	**Transport:**	**At Hospital:**	**In Service:**
Patient Information					
Age: **Sex:** **Weight (in kg [lb]):**			**Allergies:** **Medications:** **Past Medical History:** **Chief Complaint:**		
Vital Signs					
Time:	**BP:**	**Pulse:**		**Respirations:**	**SpO$_2$:**
Time:	**BP:**	**Pulse:**		**Respirations:**	**SpO$_2$:**
Time:	**BP:**	**Pulse:**		**Respirations:**	**SpO$_2$:**
EMS Treatment **(circle all that apply)**					
Oxygen @ _____ L/min via (circle one): **NC NRM Bag-mask device**		**Assisted Ventilation**	**Airway Adjunct**		**CPR**
Defibrillation	**Bleeding Control**	**Bandaging**	**Splinting**		**Other:**
Narrative					

Case Study 2

It is 1700 hours, and you have been dispatched to a Priority 1 (Charlie response) call for an elderly woman with breathing difficulty. As you arrive, at 1707 hours, the fire department is just pulling up in front of the house. There is a family member, most likely the patient's daughter, who meets you at the front door of the residence. The scene is safe, and you have enough help. You don your PPE as you enter the bedroom in the rear of the second floor. The patient is sitting in bed, propped with about four pillows, and is in obvious respiratory distress. She is pale with blue lips, and her skin is warm and clammy to touch. She is confused but tries to talk to you in two-word sentences. Her level of consciousness (LOC), which is altered, is a V on the AVPU scale. Her daughter begins to fill you in as your partner determines that her airway is open and clear and tries to assess her respirations. The daughter states that her mother, Millie, is 72 years old and has a long history of smoking two packs a day until she was diagnosed with emphysema a few years ago. Now she only smokes one pack a day. She is on a long list of medications, which do not seem to be working today, and she has had a fever of 101.5°F all day. She called you because Millie's breathing has continued to get worse, and now she is acting very confused. The last time she was this bad, she spent 2 weeks in a critical care unit on a respirator. Your partner reports that Millie's respirations are 28 breaths/min, labored, and shallow; her pulse is about 120 beats/min and irregular; her blood pressure (BP) is 130/90 mmHg and her SpO$_2$ is 88%; and she does feel like she is burning up.

As you begin to set up for a nebulizer treatment, you ask the daughter whether Millie has any allergies. Your partner applies the electrodes for an electrocardiogram (ECG), which reveals an atrial rhythm that is irregularly irregular. Next, her breath sounds are found to be wheezes on expiration in all lung fields. She looks like she is tiring out, so you decide to assist her breathing and "bag in the treatment" with a bag-mask device as your partner starts an IV line. Once the IV line is in place and the first treatment is on board, the next decision will likely involve a nasal intubation, or better yet, perhaps continuous positive airway pressure (CPAP) and transportation. You both decide to do the rest of the secondary assessment en route to the hospital because the patient's condition is serious. The daughter hands you a long list of medications to take along to the hospital, which includes albuterol (Ventolin), digoxin (Lanoxin), methyldopa (Aldomet), and warfarin (Coumadin). As you load Millie into the ambulance, you note that the time is now 1720.

1. What initial management is indicated for this patient?

_____

_____

_____

_____

_____

_____

2. What is your interpretation of this cardiac rhythm?

_____

_____

_____

_____

_____

_____

3. What is your field impression of this patient?

_____

_____

_____

_____

_____

4. Are the patient's vital signs and SAMPLE history consistent with your field impression?

_____

_____

_____

_____

_____

_____

5. What specific treatment is required for this patient's condition?

_____

_____

_____

_____

_____

_____

6. Is further treatment required for this patient?

_____

_____

_____

_____

_____

_____

7. Are there any special considerations for this patient?

_____

_____

_____

_____

_____

_____

8. Complete the PCR.

EMS Patient Care Report (PCR)					
Date:	**Incident No.:**	**Nature of Call:**		**Location:**	
Dispatched:	**En Route:**	**At Scene:**	**Transport:**	**At Hospital:**	**In Service:**
Patient Information					
Age: **Sex:** **Weight (in kg [lb]):**		**Allergies:** **Medications:** **Past Medical History:** **Chief Complaint:**			
Vital Signs					
Time:	**BP:**	**Pulse:**	**Respirations:**	**SpO$_2$:**	
Time:	**BP:**	**Pulse:**	**Respirations:**	**SpO$_2$:**	
Time:	**BP:**	**Pulse:**	**Respirations:**	**SpO$_2$:**	
EMS Treatment **(circle all that apply)**					
Oxygen @ _____ L/min via (circle one): NC NRM Bag-mask device		**Assisted Ventilation**	**Airway Adjunct**	**CPR**	
Defibrillation	**Bleeding Control**	**Bandaging**	**Splinting**	**Other:**	
Narrative					

Case Study 3

It is 1900 hours, and you have been dispatched to a Priority 1 (Charlie response) call for an elderly woman who fell in the hallway of the nursing home. As you arrive at 1908, an aide meets you to escort you to the location where the patient was found. Apparently, Mrs. Smith wandered out of her room and was found on the floor in the hallway near the dining room. A family member has been called and will be meeting you at the local hospital's emergency department (ED). The scene is safe, and you have enough help. You don your PPE as you approach the patient, who is lying on her back on the floor and looking very uncomfortable. The patient's right leg seems to be twisted laterally, which leads you to suspect she may have injured her hip when she fell. She is a bit confused but glad that help has arrived at her side. According to the aide, Mrs. Smith is 68 years old and has a history of diabetes and osteoarthritis. She takes medications for both conditions and has no known allergies. You ask her a few questions and determine that she is verbally responsive, and you note that she has an open airway and is breathing adequately. She is pale and clammy, and her radial pulse is fast and irregular. Your partner provides manual stabilization of the cervical spine as you do a quick head-to-toe exam on the patient. Moments later, your supervisor arrives on the scene and assists in placing the cervical collar and then securing the patient on the scoop stretcher.

Vital signs reveal the following: Respirations are 24 breaths/min and regular, her pulse is about 100 beats/min and irregular, BP is 110/70 mm Hg, and her SpO_2 is 98%. You decide to place a board between the legs to secure the possible fractured hip, then do a quick test of her blood glucose because the aide says she is usually alert and very talkative. Your partner places ECG electrodes and confirms sinus tachycardia with occasional premature ventricular contractions (PVCs) as well as a blood glucose of 70 mg/dL. You have decided that she should be moved to the stretcher and kept in a supine position, which has been a bit difficult due to the kyphosis of her spine, so giving sugar by mouth might be difficult. You therefore start an IV line and quickly administer 10% dextrose (D_{10}). Once you document another set of vital signs and note that her mental status is now alert, you decide that hypoglycemia was part of the cause of the fall. Now it is time to get rolling to the hospital because there is a potential for internal bleeding from the hip fracture, which you realize older patients do not compensate for very well. You will be reassessing the blood glucose, monitoring vital signs, listening to her lungs, carefully administering fluid, and acquiring a 12-lead ECG on the way to the hospital. As you load Mrs. Smith into the ambulance, you note that the time is now 1920.

1. What are common contributing factors to falls in the geriatric population?

_____

_____

_____

_____

_____

_____

2. What are some common causes of altered mental status in the geriatric population?

_____

_____

_____

_____

_____

_____

3. What is kyphosis? How will you immobilize this patient's spine and hip?

_____

_____

_____

_____

_____

_____

4. How does aging affect the body's ability to compensate for shock?

_____

_____

_____

_____

_____

_____

5. Complete the PCR.

EMS Patient Care Report (PCR)					
Date:	Incident No.:	Nature of Call:		Location:	
Dispatched:	En Route:	At Scene:	Transport:	At Hospital:	In Service:
Patient Information					
Age:		Allergies:			
Sex:		Medications:			
Weight (in kg [lb]):		Past Medical History:			
		Chief Complaint:			
Vital Signs					
Time:	BP:	Pulse:	Respirations:		SpO$_2$:
Time:	BP:	Pulse:	Respirations:		SpO$_2$:
Time:	BP:	Pulse:	Respirations:		SpO$_2$:
EMS Treatment (circle all that apply)					
Oxygen @ _____ L/min via (circle one): NC NRM Bag-mask device		Assisted Ventilation	Airway Adjunct		CPR
Defibrillation	Bleeding Control	Bandaging	Splinting		Other:
Narrative					

Case Study 4

It is 2200 hours, and you have been dispatched to a Priority 1 (Charlie response) call for a serious injury from a bar fight. The police are already on the scene, and they are looking for you to respond directly to the alleyway behind the tavern. As you arrive at 2206, the police are assisting a 23-year-old man to your ambulance. You barely open the doors to get your equipment out when the patient is already passing out on the ground just behind the ambulance. A firefighter begins to hold the head and neck while you note that the patient has a slash wound to his face and lots of blood on the front of his shirt. You note that the airway is patent, but he is having difficulty breathing. You assign a rescuer to control the bleeding to the face while you remove the patient's shirt and listen to his lungs. He has equal breath sounds, but you note a stab wound in the anterior chest on the left side, way too close to the heart. You seal the wound with an occlusive dressing and note that he has jugular venous distention (JVD). Your partner states that he has a barely palpable radial pulse, so the decision is to put him on a scoop stretcher, begin assisting his ventilations, and do the rest while en route to the trauma center.

Once in the ambulance, a full set of vital signs reveals the following: weak pulse of 108 beats/min, respirations of 26 breaths/min and shallow, BP of 90/60 mm Hg, and SpO_2 of 94%. You are assisting his ventilations with a bag-mask device and 100% oxygen while a large-bore IV line is inserted. A reassessment of vital signs shows a barely palpable radial pulse, and the BP is now 78/64 mm Hg. You make a quick call to the ED and tell them you suspect his heart was nicked by the knife because his pulse pressure is narrowing, his neck veins are distended, and the location of the wound is close to the heart. There is too much noise with the siren blaring to listen for muffled heart sounds. The ED appreciates the early warning so they can be prepared to crack his chest upon your arrival. As you pull up at the ED, you note that the time is now 2222.

1. What immediate care is required for this patient?

_____

_____

_____

_____

_____

_____

2. What does JVD in this patient suggest?

_____

_____

_____

_____

_____

_____

3. What additional signs may accompany JVD in a patient with penetrating chest trauma?

_____

_____

_____

_____

_____

_____

4. What specific treatment is required to treat this patient's condition?

_____

_____

_____

_____

_____

_____

5. Complete the PCR.

EMS Patient Care Report (PCR)					
Date:	Incident No.:	Nature of Call:		Location:	
Dispatched:	En Route:	At Scene:	Transport:	At Hospital:	In Service:
Patient Information					
Age: Sex: Weight (in kg [lb]):			Allergies: Medications: Past Medical History: Chief Complaint:		
Vital Signs					
Time:	BP:	Pulse:	Respirations:	SpO$_2$:	
Time:	BP:	Pulse:	Respirations:	SpO$_2$:	
Time:	BP:	Pulse:	Respirations:	SpO$_2$:	
EMS Treatment **(circle all that apply)**					
Oxygen @ _____ L/min via (circle one): NC NRM Bag-mask device		Assisted Ventilation	Airway Adjunct	CPR	
Defibrillation	Bleeding Control	Bandaging	Splinting	Other:	
Narrative					

Case Study 5

It is 0630 hours, and you have been dispatched to a Priority 2 (Bravo response) call for a sick child. As you arrive at 0640, the father is waiting at the front door of the residence. He leads you to the nursery where the 18-month-old daughter sleeps. She has not been sleeping all night, and the father states that her mom has been up with her because she was so irritable and crying. The scene is safe, and you decide to don PPE upon entering the room because the mother states her daughter is running a fever and has been vomiting. She believes she has a headache and a neck ache, and she has never seen her so irritable before. You decide that because there is no obvious immediate life threat, the child can stay in her mom's lap during your assessment.

The airway is open and clear. The breathing is slightly elevated, but skin color is good, and the tidal volume seems adequate. It is obvious that the child, whose name is Jessica, has a fever, and you decide that masks and eye shields are appropriate in addition to the gloves. As you examine the child, you see some petechiae on the extremities, but no purpura is present, and there is no obvious trauma. Jessica is alert according to the mom but still very irritable. You decide that oxygen would be helpful but do not want to get the child any more agitated than she is already, so you let Mom administer blow-by with a pediatric nonrebreathing mask. Your partner gets a full set of vital signs, and you compare them to the vital signs in the pocket guide in your pediatric kit. The pulse is fast, BP is slightly low, and respirations are on the high side of the normal range. After talking with the mother, you find this is a normally healthy child who has been sick for the last day and unable to keep any food down. The child takes no medications and has no allergies.

After consulting with your partner and the family, the plan is to wrap the child up so that she is warm and transport to the local pediatric ED. If the respirations become depressed, you will switch to bag-mask ventilations, and if the mental status changes or pulse further increases, you will consider venous access by IV or intraosseous (IO) line and then administer 20-mg/kg boluses to improve the perfusion. As you load Jessica into the ambulance, you note that the time is now 0650.

1. What is your initial treatment for this child?

_____

_____

_____

_____

_____

_____

2. What is your field impression of this child?

_____

_____

_____

_____

_____

_____

3. What are petechiae and purpura? What do they indicate?

_____

_____

_____

_____

_____

_____

4. What treatment will you provide to this child en route to the hospital?

_____

_____

_____

_____

_____

_____

5. Complete the PCR.

EMS Patient Care Report (PCR)

Date:	Incident No.:	Nature of Call:		Location:	
Dispatched:	En Route:	At Scene:	Transport:	At Hospital:	In Service:

Patient Information

Age:	Allergies:
Sex:	Medications:
Weight (in kg [lb]):	Past Medical History:
	Chief Complaint:

Vital Signs

Time:	BP:	Pulse:	Respirations:	SpO2:
Time:	BP:	Pulse:	Respirations:	SpO2:
Time:	BP:	Pulse:	Respirations:	SpO2:

EMS Treatment
(circle all that apply)

Oxygen @ _____ L/min via (circle one): NC NRM Bag-mask device	Assisted Ventilation	Airway Adjunct	CPR
Defibrillation	Bleeding Control	Bandaging	Splinting	Other:

Narrative

Skill Review

Note: Not every chapter includes skills. Skills are listed in order of chapter sequence.

Chapter 11

Skill Drill 11-1 Performing a Rapid Full-Body Scan

Step 1 Inspect and palpate head for open/closed findings and crepitus.

Step 2 Inspect and palpate neck for open/closed findings, jugular venous distention (JVD), tracheal deviation, and crepitus. In trauma patients, consider applying a cervical spinal immobilization device. Assess neck *before* covering it with a cervical collar.

Step 3 Inspect and palpate chest for open/closed findings, paradoxical motion, and crepitus. Listen to breath sounds on both sides of chest.

Step 4 Inspect and palpate abdomen for open/closed findings, rigidity (firm or soft), and distention.

Step 5 Inspect and palpate pelvis for open/closed findings. If there is no pain, gently compress pelvis downward and inward to look for tenderness and instability.

Step 6 Inspect and palpate four extremities for open/closed findings. Assess bilaterally for distal pulses and motor and sensory functions.

Step 7 Inspect and palpate back and buttocks for open/closed findings. In all trauma patients, maintain in-line stabilization of spine while rolling patient on his or her uninjured side in one smooth motion. If you place patient on a backboard, check back before you finish log rolling patient onto board. If you use a scoop stretcher, you won't be able to inspect or palpate lower thoracic and lumbar spine.

Skill Drill 11-2 Performing Percussion

Step 1 Place your hand lightly against surface to be examined.

Step 2 Hyperextend your middle finger, and apply firm pressure to surface to be percussed.

Step 3 Directly strike middle phalanx of your middle finger with one or two fingertips of your other hand. Apply same force over each area of body to accurately compare sounds produced by percussion.

Skill Drill 11-3 Performing the Full-Body Exam

Step 1   Examine face for obvious lacerations, bruises, fluids, and deformities.

Step 2   Inspect area around eyes and eyelids.

Step 3   Examine eyes for redness and for contact lenses. Use a penlight to assess pupils.

Step 4   Look behind ears for bruising (Battle sign).

Step 5   Use penlight to look for drainage of spinal fluid or blood in ears.

Step 6   Examine head for bruising and lacerations. Palpate for tenderness, skull depressions, and deformities.

Step 7   Palpate zygomas for tenderness, symmetry, and instability.

Step 8   Palpate maxillae.

Step 9   Check nose for blood and drainage.

Step 10   Palpate mandible.

Step 11   Assess mouth and nose for cyanosis, foreign bodies (eg, loose or broken teeth or dentures), bleeding, lacerations, and deformities.

Step 12   Check for unusual odors on patient's breath.

Step 13   Inspect neck for obvious lacerations, bruises, and deformities. Observe for jugular venous distention and/or tracheal deviation.

Step 14   Palpate front and back of neck for tenderness and deformity.

Step 15   Inspect chest for obvious signs of injury before you begin palpation. Watch for movement of chest with respiration. Assess work of breathing.

Step 16   Gently palpate over ribs to assess structural integrity and elicit tenderness. Avoid pressing over obvious bruises and fractures.

Step 17   Listen for breath sounds over midaxillary and midclavicular lines—a minimum of four fields if you check anterior chest, six fields if you are assessing posterior chest.

Step 18   Assess lungs including bases and apexes of lungs. At this point, also assess back for tenderness and deformities, so you log roll patient only once. Remember, if you suspect a spinal cord injury, use spinal precautions as you log roll patient.

Step 19   Look for obvious lacerations, bruising, and deformity of abdomen and pelvis. Gently palpate abdomen for tenderness. Begin by palpating quadrant diagonal from where any pain is located. If patient indicates his or her pain is localized to one quadrant, palpate that area last. Contraction of abdominal muscles in response to palpation is seen with underlying conditions such as appendicitis and is described as "guarding." When contraction persists throughout abdominal musculature, abdomen is described as "rigid," a condition seen with severe abdominal inflammation such as peritonitis.

Step 20   Gently compress pelvis from sides to assess for tenderness.

Step 21   Gently press iliac crests to elicit instability, tenderness, and/or crepitus.

Step 22   Inspect all four extremities for any lacerations, bruises, swelling, deformities, or medical alert jewelry. Also, assess distal pulses and motor and sensory functions in all extremities. Compare right and left sides whenever possible.

Skill Drill 11-4 Using a Glucometer to Assess Blood Glucose Level

Step 1 Identify need to obtain a blood glucose level, normal parameters for blood glucose level, contraindications, and possible complications. Take standard precautions. Clearly explain procedure to patient. Select, check, and assemble equipment (glucometer, test strip, needle or spring-loaded puncture device, alcohol prep pads). Turn on glucometer and insert a test strip. Cleanse fingertip with an alcohol prep pad.

Step 2 Puncture prepped site with lancet needle or puncture device, drawing capillary blood.

Step 3 Dispose of lancet needle in a sharps container.

Step 4 Express a blood sample and transfer it to test strip. Insert test strip into glucometer and activate device per manufacturer's instructions.

Step 5 Dress fingertip wound with pressure and an alcohol prep pad, and place a bandage over puncture site. Record reading from glucometer and document appropriately.

Skill Drill 11-5 Assessing the Head

Step 1 Visually inspect and palpate head for open/closed findings and crepitus.

Step 2 Palpate top and back of head to locate any subtle abnormalities. Use a systematic approach, going from front to back, to ensure nothing is missed.

Step 3 Part hair in several places to examine condition of scalp. Identify any lesions beneath hair.

Step 4 Palpate structure of face, note any open/closed findings and crepitus. Pay attention to condition of skin, hair distribution, and shape of face.

Skill Drill 11-6 Examining the Eye

Step 1 Examine exterior portion of eye. Carefully inspect and palpate upper and lower orbits, starting at nose and working toward lateral edge. Look for any obvious trauma or deformity. Ask about general problems (eg, any pain or redness, altered vision, vision loss, diplopia, photophobia, blurring, discharge, sensitivity to light, and corrective lens use). Note periorbital ecchymosis (raccoon eyes).

Step 2 Measure visual acuity by having patient count number of fingers you are holding up at varying distances (usually 6 feet [2 m], 3 feet [1 m], and 1 foot [0.3 m] away from patient). Perform this exam on each eye independently. If corrective lenses are normally worn, check visual acuity with correction in place.

Step 3 Examine pupils for size (in millimeters), shape, and symmetry. They should be equal. Test pupils for reactivity to light in as dark an environment as possible. Both pupils should constrict when exposed to light, and they should be equal in response.

Step 4 Test for cranial nerve function by asking patient to follow your fingers in a "Z" or "H" pattern. Eyes should move smoothly and symmetrically, tracking your finger movement. Evaluate whether eyes move in sync (conjugate gaze) and whether they can track in all fields (up, down, left, right). Note any abnormal movement of eyes. A visual field exam assesses retina's ability to perceive light. This is done by checking patient's peripheral vision, examining each eye separately.

Step 5 Inspect eyelids, lashes, and tear ducts for evidence of trauma, or discharge. Turn up lids to look for foreign bodies, and inspect conjunctivae and sclera. Sclera ought to be white, not jaundiced or injected (red). Painless subconjunctival hemorrhage is a common but benign presentation. Conjunctivae should be pink—not cyanotic, pale, or overly reddened. Cornea and lens will be difficult to examine without additional assessment tools, although in a trauma situation, you should note whether globe is patent. Next, examine anterior chamber and iris for clarity, noting any cloudiness or bleeding.

Skill Drill 11-7 Examining the Neck

Step 1 If spinal trauma is suspected, take precautions to protect cervical spine in accordance with your protocol. Assess for usage of accessory muscles during respiration.

Step 2 Palpate neck to find any structural abnormalities or subcutaneous air and to ensure trachea is midline. Begin at suprasternal notch and work your way toward head. Be careful when applying pressure to area of carotid arteries because doing so may stimulate a vagal response.

Step 3 Assess lymph nodes and note any swelling, which may indicate infection.

Step 4 Assess jugular veins for distention, which may indicate a problem with venous return to heart.

Skill Drill 11-8 Examining the Chest

Step 1 Ensure patient's privacy as best you can. Assess chest, inspecting and palpating for open/closed findings, paradoxical motion, and crepitus. Observe chest wall for respiratory effort, and document respiratory rate, depth, and rhythm. If you find any open wounds, dress them appropriately.

Step 2 Compare two sides of chest for symmetry. Note shape of chest—it can give you clues to many underlying medical conditions, such as emphysema. Look for any surgical scars (eg, midline "zipper" scar, which may be result of pacemaker implantation or a previous cardiac surgery). Palpate chest to reveal any air under skin (as occurs in subcutaneous emphysema).

Step 3 Auscultate lung fields. Note any abnormal lung sounds. Auscultate for heart tones. Always auscultate directly to patient's skin, not through his or her clothing. Listening over fabric will result in breath sounds being muted by clothing. With each stethoscope placement, listen to at least one full inhalation and exhalation. If patient is able to cooperate, have him or her breathe through an open mouth to help emphasize lung sounds.

Step 4 Percuss chest to detect any abnormalities. Repeat appropriate portions of exam for posterior aspect of thorax.

Skill Drill 11-9 Examining the Abdomen

Step 1 Inspect and palpate abdomen for open/closed findings, rigidity (firmness), tenderness, distention, swelling, or bruising. Look at skin as well as contour and overall appearance of abdominal wall. Note any surgical scars because they may be clues to an underlying illness, previous trauma, or surgeries. Look for symmetry and distention. Look for a rash or other signs of an allergic reaction. Finally, note any wounds, striae, dilated veins, or generalized distention or localized masses.

Step 2 Auscultate abdomen for bowel sounds (if time and noise level permit). Note presence or absence of bowel sounds. Note frequency and character of any hyperactive sounds.

Step 3 Before palpating abdomen, ask patient to point to area of greatest discomfort. Avoid touching that area until last. Systematically palpate four quadrants of abdomen, beginning with quadrant farthest from patient's complaint. Work slowly, and avoid quick movements. Perform percussion as appropriate. Pay special attention to patient's expressions because they may yield valuable information.

Skill Drill 11-10 Examining the Musculoskeletal System

Step 1 Beginning with upper extremities, inspect skin overlying muscles, bones, and joints for soft-tissue damage. Note any deformities or abnormal structures.

Step 2 Inspect and palpate hands and wrists. Note any open/closed findings and crepitus.

Step 3 Inspect and palpate elbows. Ask patient to flex and extend elbow to establish range of motion. Note any abnormalities.

Step 4 Check for adequate distal pulse, motor function, and sensation in each extremity.

Step 5 Ask patient to flex and extend joints of fingers, hands, and wrist to establish range of motion. If patient experiences any discomfort, immediately stop that portion of exam.

Step 6 Ask patient to turn his or her hand from palm-down position to palm-up position and back again.

Step 7 Inspect and palpate shoulders. Ask patient to shrug shoulders and raise and extend both arms.

Step 8 Inspect and palpate bony structures to establish range of motion. Ask patient to point and bend his or her toes.

Step 9 Ask patient to rotate ankle to check for pain or restricted range of motion.

Step 10 Inspect and palpate knee joints and patella to establish range of motion. Ask patient to bend and straighten both knees.

Step 11 Check for structural integrity of pelvis by applying gentle pressure to iliac crests, pushing in and then down.

Step 12 Ask patient to lift both legs, bend at hip, and turn legs inward and outward. Note any abnormalities.

Skill Drill 11-11 Examining the Peripheral Vascular System

Step 1 As you examine upper extremities, note any abnormalities in radial pulse, skin color, temperature, or condition.

Step 2 If you note abnormalities in distal pulse, work your way proximally, check those pulse points, and note your findings.

Step 3 Palpate epitrochlear and brachial nodes of lymphatic system. Note any swelling or tenderness.

Step 4 Examine lower extremities, noting any abnormalities in size and symmetry of legs. Evaluate temperature of each leg relative to rest of body and to each other.

Step 5 Inspect skin color and condition, noting any abnormal venous patterns or enlargement.

Step 6 Check distal pulses, noting any abnormalities.

Step 7 Palpate inguinal nodes for swelling or tenderness.

Step 8 Evaluate for pitting edema in legs and feet.

Skill Drill 11-12 Examining the Spine

Step 1 Inspect cervical, thoracic, and lumbar curves for any abnormalities.

Step 2 Evaluate height of shoulders and iliac crests. Differences between one side and other may indicate abnormal spinal curvature.

Step 3 Palpate posterior portion of cervical spine, noting any point tenderness or structural abnormalities.

Step 4 In nontrauma patient, and in absence of reported pain, ask patient to move his or her head forward, backward, and from side to side.

Step 5 Palpate each vertebra with thumbs.

Step 6 In absence of pain or trauma, ask patient to bend at waist in each direction to establish range of motion.

Skill Drill 11-13 Examining the Nervous System

Step 1 Use AVPU scale to assess patient's mental status. Note patient's posture. Evaluate cranial nerve function.

Step 2 Evaluate patient's coordination by performing finger-to-nose test using alternating hands.

Step 3 If appropriate, test patient's gait and balance by having him or her walk heel-to-toe or take a heel-to-shin stance.

Step 4 Perform pronator drift test by asking patient to close his or her eyes and hold both arms out in front of body. There should not be a difference in movement on either side.

Step 5 Evaluate patient's sensory function by checking his or her responses to both gross and light touch. If appropriate, check for deep tendon reflexes.

Chapter 14

Skill Drill 11-14 Evaluating Deep Tendon Reflexes

Step 1 Place patient in a sitting position.

Step 2 Flex patient's arm at elbow to a 45° angle. Locate biceps tendon in antecubital fossa. Place your thumb over tendon, with your fingers behind elbow. Strike your thumb with reflex hammer, note flexion of elbow.

Step 3 With patient's arm remaining at a 45° angle, rest patient's forearm on your arm, with hand slightly pronated. Strike patient's brachioradialis tendon proximal to wrist, note flexion of elbow.

Step 4 Flex patient's arm at elbow to a 90° angle, and rest his or her hand against body. Locate and strike triceps tendon, noting contraction of triceps or extension of elbow.

Step 5 Flex patient's knee to a 90° angle, allowing leg to dangle. Support upper leg with your hand, and strike patellar tendon just below patella. Note contraction of quadriceps and extension of lower leg.

Step 6 With patient's leg in same position, hold heel of patient's foot in your hand. Strike Achilles tendon, noting plantar flexion of foot.

Skill Drill 14-1 Spiking the Bag

Step 1 Take standard precautions. Ensure you've chosen correct administration set (primary or piggyback), tubing is not tangled, and protective covers are in place. Ensure you have proper solution, that it is clear and has not expired, and that protective tail port covers are in place. Move roller clamp to off position.

Step 2 Remove protective covering found on end of IV bag. Bag is still sealed and will not leak until piercing spike punctures this port. Remove protective cover from piercing spike (remember, this spike is sterile and sharp!), and slide spike into IV bag port until it is seated against bag.

Step 3 Squeeze drip chamber to fill to line marking chamber, then run fluid into line to flush air out of tubing.

Step 4 Twist protective cover of opposite end of IV tubing to allow air to escape. Do not remove this cover yet because cover keeps tubing end sterile until it is needed. Let fluid flow until air bubbles are removed from line before turning roller clamp wheel to stop flow or setting drip rate per required dose.

Step 5 Next, go back and check drip chamber; it should be only half-filled. Fluid level must be visible to calculate drip rates. If fluid level is too low, then squeeze chamber until it fills; if chamber is too full, with roller clamp in off position, invert bag and chamber and squeeze chamber to empty fluid back into bag. Hang bag in an appropriate location with end of IV tubing easily accessible.

Skill Drill 14-2 Obtaining Vascular Access

Step 1   Choose appropriate fluid, and examine bag for clarity and expiration date. Ensure no particles are floating in fluid and that fluid is appropriate for patient's condition and not expired. Choose appropriate drip set, and attach it to fluid. A macrodrip set (eg, 10 gtt/mL) should be used for a patient who needs volume replacement; a microdrip set (eg, 60 gtt/mL) should be used for a patient who needs a medication infusion. If an IV extension set is available, then attach it to end of tubing to assist hospital staff in manipulating IV tubing at hospital. Fill drip chamber by squeezing it.

Step 2   Flush or "bleed" tubing to remove any air bubbles by opening roller clamp. Ensure no errant bubbles are floating in tubing.

Step 3   Before venipuncture, tear tape needed to secure site and collect and open antiseptic swabs, gauze pads, and anything else needed for vascular access per local practice.

Step 4   Take standard precautions before making contact with patient. Palpate a suitable vein. Veins should be "springy" when palpated. Avoid areas that are hard when palpated.

Step 5   Apply constricting band above intended IV site. It should be placed approximately 4 to 8 inches (10 to 20 cm) above intended site.

Step 6   Clean area using aseptic technique. Use an alcohol pad to cleanse in a circular motion from inside out. Use a second alcohol pad to wipe straight down center.

Step 7   Choose appropriately sized catheter, and twist catheter to break seal. Do not advance catheter upward because this may cause needle to shear catheter. Examine catheter, and discard it if you discover any imperfections. Occasionally you will find "burrs" on edge of catheter. Loosen catheter hub.

Step 8   Advise patient to expect a needlestick. While applying distal traction at site with one hand, insert catheter at an angle of approximately 45° with bevel up.

Step 9   Feel for a "pop" as stylet enters vein and observe for "flashback" as blood enters catheter. Clear chamber at top of catheter should fill with blood when catheter enters vein. If you note only a drop or two, then you should gently advance catheter farther into vein, approximately ⅛ to ¼ inches (0.3 to 0.6 cm). Apply pressure to site to occlude catheter and prevent blood from leaking while removing stylet. Hold hub while withdrawing needle so as not to pull catheter out of vein.

Step 10   Immediately dispose of all sharps in proper container.

Step 11   Attach prepared IV line. Hold hub of catheter while connecting IV line.

Step 12   Remove constricting band.

Step 13   Open IV line to ensure fluid is flowing and IV is patent. Observe for any swelling or infiltration around IV site. If fluid does not flow, then check whether constriction band has been released. If infiltration is noted, then immediately stop infusion and remove catheter while holding pressure over site with a piece of gauze to prevent bleeding.

Step 14   Secure catheter with tape or a commercial device.

Step 15   Secure IV tubing and adjust flow rate while monitoring patient.

Skill Drill 14-3 Gaining Intraosseous Access with an EZ-IO Device

Step 1 Check selected IV fluid for proper fluid, clarity, and expiration date. Look for discoloration and for particles floating in fluid. If particles are found in fluid, then discard bag and choose another bag of fluid.

Select appropriate equipment (ie, intraosseous [IO] needle, syringe, saline, extension set, antiseptic swabs, and gauze pads).

A three-way stopcock may also be used to facilitate easier fluid administration.

Select proper administration set. Connect administration set to bag. Prepare administration set. Fill drip chamber and flush tubing. Ensure all air bubbles are removed from tubing.

Prepare syringe and extension tubing. Ensure tubing is not tangled.

Cut or tear tape and prepare bulky dressings. This can be done at any time before IO puncture.

Step 2 Take standard precautions. This must be done before IO puncture.

Step 3 Identify proper anatomic site for IO puncture. Palpate landmarks and then prepare site.

- **Tibia placement.** This site is reserved for EZ-IO and BIG.
- **Humerus placement.** Humeral placement is typically reserved for adults when using EZ-IO or BIG.

Step 4 Cleanse site appropriately. Follow aseptic technique by cleansing in a circular manner from inside out.

Step 5 Attach needle to EZ-IO gun, and remove protective cover. Examine needle. If you find any imperfections, then discard needle and select another one.

Step 6 Perform IO puncture by first stabilizing tibia, then placing a folded towel under knee, and finally holding extremity in a manner to keep your fingers away from site of puncture. For humeral placement, continue to apply pressure on anterior and inferior aspects of humerus.

Insert needle at a 90° angle to insertion site. Advance needle with a twisting motion until a "pop" is felt. Unscrew cap, and remove stylet from needle.

Step 7 Remove stylet from catheter.

Step 8 Attach syringe and extension set to IO needle. Pull back on syringe to aspirate blood and particles of bone marrow to ensure proper placement. Absence of marrow does not mean access failed. Check site for other signs of extravasation.

Slowly inject saline to ensure proper placement of needle. Responsive patients should receive 1% lidocaine prior to infusion of fluids. Watch for extravasation, and stop infusion immediately if it is noted. It is possible to fracture bone during insertion of IO needle. If this happens, then remove IO needle and switch insertion site.

Connect administration set and adjust flow rate as appropriate. Fluid does not flow as rapidly through an IO catheter as through an IV line; crystalloid boluses should be given with a syringe in children and a pressure infuser device in adults.

Secure needle with tape, and support it with a bulky dressing. Stabilize in place in same manner that an impaled object is stabilized. Use bulky dressings around catheter, and tape securely in place. Be careful not to tape around entire circumference of leg because this could impair circulation and potentially result in compartment syndrome.

Dispose of needle in proper container.

Skill Drill 14-4 Administering Medication via a Nasogastric Tube

Step 1 Take standard precautions. Confirm proper gastric tube placement. Attach a 60-mL cone-tipped syringe to gastric tube, and slowly inject air as you or your partner auscultates over epigastrium. To further confirm proper placement, withdraw plunger of syringe, and observe for return of gastric contents in tube. Leave gastric tube open to air.

Step 2 Draw up 30 to 60 mL of normal saline into syringe, and irrigate gastric tube. If you meet resistance, ensure tube is not kinked.

Step 3 Draw up appropriate amount of medication, ensure it is correct medication and amount, and slowly inject medication into gastric tube.

Step 4 Inject 30 to 60 mL of normal saline into gastric tube following administration of medication. This will ensure tube is flushed and patient has received entire dose of medication.

Step 5 Clamp off proximal end of gastric tube. Do not attach gastric tube to suction because this will result in removal of medication from stomach. Monitor patient for adverse reactions. Document: medication given, route, dose, administration time, and patient condition and response. Repeat medication dose if indicated.

Skill Drill 14-5 Drawing Medication from an Ampule

Step 1 Check medication, ensuring expiration date has not passed and that it is correct drug and concentration.

Shake medication into base of ampule. If some of drug is stuck in neck, then gently thump or tap stem.

Step 2 Using a 4-inch × 4-inch (10-cm × 10-cm) gauze pad, an alcohol prep, or an ampule breaker, grip neck of ampule and snap it off where ampule is scored. If ampule is not scored and an attempt is made to break it, some sharp edges may be present. Drop stem in sharps container.

Step 3 Insert a filtered needle into ampule without touching outer sides of ampule. Draw solution into syringe, and dispose of ampule in sharps container.

Step 4 Hold syringe with needle pointing up, and gently tap barrel to loosen air trapped inside and cause it to rise.

Step 5 Press gently on plunger to dispel any air bubbles. Recap needle using one-handed method. Dispose of needle in sharps container, and attach a standard hypodermic needle to syringe if necessary to administer medication.

Skill Drill 14-6 Drawing Medication from a Vial

Step 1 Check medication, ensuring expiration date has not passed and that it is correct drug and concentration.

Remove sterile cover, or clean top with alcohol if vial was previously opened.

Step 2 Determine amount of medication that you will need, and draw that amount of air into syringe. Allow a little extra room to expel some air while removing air bubbles.

Step 3 Invert vial, clean rubber stopper with an alcohol prep, and insert needle through rubber stopper into medication. Expel air in syringe into vial, and then withdraw amount of medication needed.

Step 4 Once you have correct amount of medication in syringe, withdraw needle from vial, and expel any air in syringe.

Step 5 Recap needle using one-handed method. Label syringe if it is not immediately given to patient.

Skill Drill 14-7 Administering Medication via the Subcutaneous Route

Step 1 Take standard precautions. Determine need for medication based on patient presentation. Obtain a history, including any drug allergies and vital signs. Follow standing orders, or contact medical control for permission. Check medication to ensure that it is correct, that it is not cloudy or discolored, and that expiration date has not passed, and determine appropriate amount and concentration for correct dose.

Step 2 Advise patient of potential discomfort while explaining procedure.

Assemble and check equipment needed: alcohol preps and a 3-mL syringe with a 24- to 26-gauge needle. Draw up correct dose of medication and dispel air while maintaining sterility.

Step 3 Cleanse area for administration (usually upper arm or thigh) using aseptic technique.

Step 4 Pinch skin surrounding area, advise patient of a stick, and insert needle at a 45° angle. Inject medication and remove needle. Immediately dispose of needle and syringe in sharps container.

Step 5 To disperse medication through tissue, rub area in a circular motion with your gloved hand (unless contraindicated for medication). Properly store any unused medication. Monitor patient's condition, and document medication given, route, administration time, and patient response.

Skill Drill 14-8 Administering Medication via the Intramuscular Route

Step 1   Take standard precautions. Determine need for medication based on patient presentation. Obtain a history, including any drug allergies and vital signs. Follow standing orders, or contact medical control for permission.

Check medication to ensure that it is correct, that it is not cloudy or discolored, and that expiration date has not passed, and determine appropriate amount and concentration for correct dose.

Advise patient of potential discomfort while explaining procedure.

Assemble and check equipment needed (eg, alcohol preps and a 3- to 5-mL syringe with a 21-gauge, 1-inch or 2-inch [4-cm or 5-cm] needle). Draw up correct dose of medication, and dispel air while maintaining sterility.

Step 2   Cleanse area for administration (usually upper arm or hip) using aseptic technique.

Step 3   Stretch skin over cleansed area, advise patient of a stick, and insert needle at a 90° angle.

Pull back on plunger to aspirate for blood (presence of blood in syringe indicates you may have entered a blood vessel). In such a case, remove needle, and hold pressure over site. Discard syringe and needle in sharps container. Prepare a new syringe and needle, and select another site.

If there is no blood in syringe, then inject medication and remove needle.

Step 4   Immediately dispose of needle and syringe in sharps container. Store any unused medication properly. Monitor patient's condition, and document: medication given, route, administration time, and response of patient.

Skill Drill 14-9 Administering Medication via the Intravenous Bolus Route

Step 1   Take standard precautions. Determine need for medication based on patient presentation. Obtain a history, including any drug allergies and vital signs.

Follow standing orders, or contact medical control for permission.

Check medication to ensure that it is correct, that it is not cloudy or discolored, and that expiration date has not passed, and determine appropriate amount and concentration for correct dose.

Explain procedure to patient and need for medication. Assemble needed equipment, and draw up medication. Expel any air in syringe. Draw up 20 mL of normal saline to use as a flush for medication.

Cleanse injection port with alcohol, or remove protective cap if using needleless system.

Step 2   Insert needle into port, and pinch off IV tubing proximal to administration port. Failure to shut off line will result in medication taking pathway of least resistance and flowing into bag instead of into patient.

Administer correct dose of medication at appropriate rate. Some medications must be administered quickly, whereas others must be pushed slowly to prevent adverse effects.

Step 3   Place needle and syringe into sharps container.

Unclamp IV line to flush medication into vein. Allow it to run briefly wide open, or flush with a 20-mL bolus of normal saline.

Readjust IV flow rate to original setting.

Properly store and label any unused medication.

Monitor patient's condition, and document medication given, route, time of administration, and patient response.

Skill Drill 14-10 Administering a Medication via Intravenous Piggyback Infusion

Step 1 Take standard precautions. Ensure established IV line is patent.

Step 2 Determine need for medication based on patient presentation. Obtain a history, including any drug allergies and vital signs. Follow standing orders, or contact medical control for permission. Identify concentration, then determine appropriate dose and rate of infusion. Check medication to ensure that it is correct, that it is not cloudy or discolored, and that expiration date has not passed, and determine appropriate amount and concentration for correct dose. Explain procedure to patient and/or parent and need for medication.

Step 3 Assemble needed equipment. Check medication clarity and expiration date. Ensure you have proper IV solution and that it is clear, sterile, and not expired. Ensure you have correct administration set and correct drip rating. Check for tangling and that protective covers are on ends. Flow clamp should be closed.

Step 4 Cleanse injection port of secondary IV bag (into which medication will be infused) with alcohol. Inject medication into second IV bag, and then place syringe into sharps container. Gently swirl IV bag to mix injected medication into solution. Note: Drawing up medications may not be necessary if manufacturer attaches medication to second IV bag (IV antibiotics, some antidysrhythmics, etc).

Step 5 Remove protective cover on secondary IV bag. Insert tubing spike into second IV bag tail port. Turn bag with medication upright. Squeeze drip chamber until it is half full. Maintain sterility.

Step 6 Unclamp line from secondary IV bag to dispel air from it, or utilize infusion pump to accomplish this step. Maintain sterility. While removing air, try to minimize loss of fluid. Clamp line after all air bubbles have been removed.

Step 7 If applicable, program IV infusion pump with appropriate dose and rate. Place cartridge from secondary IV bag in pump.

Step 8 Cleanse a port on primary IV line. Attach distal end of secondary IV line to a port on primary IV line. Begin flow and ensure that rate is appropriate. Maintain sterility.

Step 9 Label secondary IV bag. Monitor patient's condition, and document: medication given, route, concentration, dose, date time, and your initials. Document patient's response to medication.

Skill Drill 14-11 Administering Medication via the Intraosseous Route

Step 1 Take standard precautions. Determine need for medication based on patient presentation. Obtain a history, including any drug allergies and vital signs. Follow standing orders, or contact medical control for permission. Check medication to ensure that it is correct, that it is not cloudy or discolored, and that expiration date has not passed, and determine appropriate amount and concentration for correct dose.

Explain procedure to patient and/or parent and need for medication.

Assemble needed equipment, and draw up medication. Also draw up 20 mL of normal saline for a flush.

Step 2 Cleanse injection port of extension tubing with alcohol, or remove protective cap if using needleless system.

Step 3 Insert needle into port, and clamp off IV tubing proximal to administration port. This is usually managed with a three-way stopcock. Failure to shut off line will result in medication taking pathway of least resistance and flowing into bag instead of into patient.

Administer correct dose of medication at proper push rate. Some medications must be administered quickly, whereas others must be pushed slowly to prevent adverse effects.

Step 4 Place needle and syringe into sharps container. Unclamp IV line to flush medication into site. Flush with at least a 20-mL bolus of normal saline. Readjust IV flow rate to original setting. Store any unused medication properly.

Monitor patient's condition, and document: medication given, route, time of administration, and response of patient.

Skill Drill 14-12 Administering Medication via the Sublingual Route

Step 1 Take standard precautions. Determine need for medication based on patient presentation. Obtain a history, including any drug allergies and vital signs. Follow standing orders, or contact medical control for permission. Check medication to ensure that it is correct and that its expiration date has not passed, and determine appropriate amount for correct dose.

Step 2 Ask patient to rinse his or her mouth with a little water if mucous membranes are dry. Explain procedure, and ask patient to lift his or her tongue.

Place tablet or spray dose under tongue, or ask patient to do so. Advise patient not to chew or swallow tablet but to let it dissolve slowly.

Monitor patient's condition, and document: medication given, route, administration time, and patient's response.

Skill Drill 14-13 Administering Medication via the Intranasal Route

Step 1 Take standard precautions. Determine need for medication based on patient presentation. Obtain a history, including any drug allergies and vital signs. Follow standing orders, or contact medical control for permission. Check medication to ensure it is correct and its expiration date has not passed, and determine appropriate amount for correct dose.

Step 2 Ask patient to rinse mouth with a little water if mucous membranes are dry. Explain procedure, and ask patient to lift his or her tongue.

Place tablet or spray dose under tongue, or ask patient to do so. Advise patient not to chew or swallow tablet but to let it dissolve slowly.

Monitor patient's condition, and document: medication given, route, administration time, and patient's response.

Step 3 Attach mucosal atomizer device to syringe, maintaining sterility.

Step 4 Explain procedure to patient (or to a relative if patient is unresponsive) and need for medication. Stop ventilation of patient if necessary; remove any mask. Insert mucosal atomizer device into larger and less deviated or less obstructed nostril.

Step 5 Quickly spray half of medication dose into a nostril.

Step 6 Dispose of atomizer device and syringe in appropriate container.

Step 7 Monitor patient's condition. Document medication given, route, time of administration, and patient response.

Skill Drill 14-14 Assisting a Patient With a Metered-Dose Inhaler

Step 1 Take standard precautions. Obtain an order from medical control, or follow local protocol. Assemble needed equipment.

Ensure you have right medication, right patient, right dose, right route, and that medication is not expired.

Ensure patient is alert enough to use inhaler. Check to see whether patient has already taken any doses. Obtain baseline breath sounds for comparison after a few minutes of inhaler use. Ensure inhaler is at room temperature or warmer.

Step 2 Shake inhaler vigorously several times. Stop administering supplemental oxygen, and remove any mask from patient's face. Ask patient to exhale deeply and, before inhaling, to put his or her lips around opening of inhaler.

Step 3 If patient has a spacer, then attach it to allow more effective use of medication.

Have patient depress handheld inhaler as he or she begins to inhale deeply.

Instruct patient to hold his or her breath for as long as he or she comfortably can to help lungs absorb medication.

Step 4 Continue administering supplemental oxygen.

Allow patient to breathe a few times, then give second dose per direction from medical control or according to local protocol. Monitor patient's condition, and document: medication given, route, administration time, and patient response.

Skill Drill 14-15 Administering a Medication via a Small-Volume Nebulizer

Step 1 Take standard precautions. Determine need for an inhaled bronchodilator based on patient presentation. Obtain a history, including any drug allergies and vital signs.

Follow standing orders, or contact medical control for permission. Check medication and its expiration date. Make sure that you have right medication and that it is not cloudy or discolored. Assemble and check needed equipment.

Step 2 If medication is in a premixed package, then add it to bowl of nebulizer. If it is not premixed, then add medication to bowl and mix with specified amount of normal saline, usually 2.5 to 3 mL.

Step 3 Connect "T" piece with mouthpiece to top of bowl, or mask to bowl, and connect it to oxygen tubing.

Set flowmeter at 6 L/min to produce a steady mist. Remove oxygen mask from patient if oxygen is being administered.

Step 4 With metered-dose inhaler (MDI) or handheld nebulizer in position, instruct patient on proper way to breathe. Have patient breathe as deeply as possible and hold his or her breath for 3 to 5 seconds before exhaling. Continue to coach patient as needed.

Monitor patient's condition, and document medication given, route, time of administration, and response of patient to medication.

Cardiac monitoring is essential when administering a beta agonist. If cardiac dysrhythmias are noted, then stop administering medication, manage in accordance with current resuscitation guidelines, and contact medical control.

Skill Drill 14-16 Accessing a Tunneling Device

Step 1 Use aseptic technique. Prepare all appropriate equipment: empty 10- to 20-mL syringe (nothing less than a 10-mL syringe should be used), 10-mL normal saline flush, sterile gloves, alcohol prep, 10-gtt administration set, 500 mL normal saline.

Ensure all lumens are clamped. Air embolism is a serious risk with these patients because many of these devices go directly into vena cava. That is why central lines must be clamped whenever they are not in use.

Use an alcohol prep to prepare lumen that will be used.

Step 2 Attach empty syringe, and withdraw a minimum of 10 mL of blood from lumen. Discard this immediately into sharps container. Do not withdraw too forcefully. If you meet some resistance, then gently flush and withdraw. Ask patient to turn his or her head in opposite direction of central line.

Step 3 After you have withdrawn 10 mL of blood, attach 10-mL syringe filled with normal saline and slowly administer it.

Step 4 Attach prepared IV drip set and set it up for at least 10 mL/h. Depending on size of catheter, you can infuse at a rate of 125 to 250 mL/h. The line must be running continuously because heparin is not available.

Administer IV medications through attached IV drip set.

Monitor patient's condition, and document: medication given, route, administration time, and patient response.

Chapter 15

Skill Drill 15-1 Removing an Upper Airway Obstruction With Magill Forceps

Step 1   With patient's head in sniffing position, open patient's mouth and insert laryngoscope blade.

Step 2   Visualize obstruction and retrieve object with Magill forceps.

Step 3   Remove object with Magill forceps.

Step 4   Attempt to ventilate patient.

Skill Drill 15-2 Using CPAP

Step 1   Take standard precautions. Assess patient for indications and contraindications of continuous positive airway pressure (CPAP). Confirm patient's BP, and explain procedure to him or her. Check your equipment, then connect circuit to CPAP device.

Step 2   Connect face mask to circuit tubing. After system is connected, look for an on/off button or switch. Some models have this feature. Confirm device is powered on and working before you apply CPAP to patient.

Step 3   Connect tubing to oxygen tank.

Step 4   Place mask over patient's mouth and nose, creating as much of an airtight seal as possible. Place patient in a high Fowler position to facilitate breathing, and coach him or her through initial application of mask. To reduce some of stress and anxiety associated with application of CPAP, it may be beneficial to initially allow patient to hold mask to his or her face. Allow patient to get used to mask.

Step 5   After mask is placed on face and patient adjusts to it, use strapping mechanism to secure it to patient's head. Ensure seal between mask and face remains intact. Consult manufacturer's guidelines for specific strapping instructions.

Step 6   Adjust positive end-expiratory pressure (PEEP) valve and FIO_2 level according to manufacturer's recommendations to maintain adequate oxygenation and ventilation. With CPAP in place, patient's oxygenation saturation level should improve, work of breathing should decrease, ease of speaking should increase, and breath sounds should improve. Constantly reassess patient for signs of clinical deterioration and/or complications (ie, pneumothorax).

Skill Drill 15-3 Inserting a Nasogastric Tube in a Responsive Patient

Step 1 Explain procedure to patient, and oxygenate him or her if necessary and possible. Ensure patient's head is in a neutral or slightly flexed position. Suppress gag reflex with a topical anesthetic spray.

Step 2 Constrict blood vessels in nares with a topical alpha-agonist, if available.

Step 3 Measure tube for correct depth of insertion (nose to ear to xiphoid process).

Step 4 Lubricate tube with a water-soluble gel.

Step 5 Advance tube gently along nasal floor.

Step 6 Encourage patient to swallow or drink to facilitate passage of tube into esophagus.

Step 7 Advance tube into stomach.

Step 8 Confirm proper placement: Auscultate over epigastrium while injecting 20 to 30 mL of air into tube, and/or observe for gastric contents in tube. There should be no reflux around tube.

Step 9 Apply suction to tube to aspirate stomach contents, and secure tube in place. Blue extension of gastric tube should remain open to air.

Skill Drill 15-4 Inserting an Orogastric Tube in an Unresponsive Patient

Step 1 Position patient's head in a neutral or slightly flexed position. Measure tube for correct depth of insertion (mouth to ear to xiphoid process).

Step 2 Lubricate tube with a water-soluble gel.

Step 3 Introduce tube at midline, and advance it gently into oropharynx. Advance tube into stomach.

Step 4 Confirm proper placement: Auscultate over epigastrium while injecting 20 to 30 mL of air and/or observe for gastric contents in tube. There should be no reflux around tube. Afterwards, auscultate over lung fields to confirm ET tube has not been dislodged.

Step 5 Apply suction to tube to aspirate stomach contents.

Step 6 Secure tube in place.

Skill Drill 15-5 Suctioning of a Stoma

Step 1 Take standard precautions.

Step 2 Inject 3 mL of sterile saline through stoma and into trachea.

Step 3 Instruct patient to exhale (if he or she is responsive), and insert catheter without providing suction until resistance is felt (no more than 12 cm).

Step 4 Suction while withdrawing catheter.

Skill Drill 15-6 Ventilating Through a Stoma Using a Resuscitation Mask

Step 1 Position patient's head in a neutral position with shoulders slightly elevated.

Step 2 Locate and expose stoma site.

Step 3 Place resuscitation mask over stoma, and ensure an adequate seal. For best results, use a pediatric mask.

Step 4 Maintain patient's neutral head position, and ventilate patient by exhaling directly into resuscitation mask. Assess patient for adequate ventilation by observing his or her chest rise and feeling for air leaks around mask.

Step 5 If air leakage is evident, then seal patient's mouth and nose and ventilate.

Skill Drill 15-7 Ventilating a Stoma With a Bag-Mask Device

Step 1 With patient's head in a neutral position, locate and expose stoma.

Step 2 Place bag-mask device (with a pediatric mask) over stoma, and ensure an adequate seal. Ventilate patient by squeezing bag-mask device, and assess for adequate ventilation by observing chest rise and feeling for air leaks when using a mask. Seal mouth and nose if an air leak is evident from upper airway.

Step 3 Auscultate over lungs to confirm adequate ventilation.

Skill Drill 15-8 Replacing a Dislodged Tracheostomy Tube With a Temporary Endotracheal Tube

Step 1 Take standard precautions. Assemble equipment.

Step 2 Lubricate same-sized tracheostomy tube or an ET tube (at least 5.0 mm) with a water-soluble gel.

Step 3 Instruct patient to exhale, and gently insert tube approximately 0.5 to 0.75 inches (1 to 2 cm) beyond balloon cuff.

Step 4 Inflate balloon cuff.

Step 5 Ensure patient is comfortable, and confirm patency and proper placement of tube by listening for air movement from tube and noting patient's clinical status. Ensure that a false lumen (placement of tube into soft tissue of neck, rather than in trachea) was not created.

Step 6 Auscultate lungs to confirm correct tube placement.

Skill Drill 15-9 Performing Orotracheal Intubation Using Direct Laryngoscopy

Step 1   Take standard precautions. If you suspect trauma, then maintain manual in-line stabilization of head.

Step 2   Measure for proper size, and insert an oropharyngeal airway (OPA).

Step 3   Ventilate patient with a bag-mask device at a rate of 10 to 12 breaths/min with sufficient volume to produce chest rise. Preoxygenate for 2 to 3 minutes with 100% oxygen.

Step 4   Check, prepare, and assemble your equipment.

Step 5   Place patient's head in sniffing position.

Step 6   Remove OPA, then insert blade into right side of patient's mouth, and displace tongue to left.

Step 7   Gently lift long axis of laryngoscope handle until you can visualize glottic opening and vocal cords.

Step 8   Insert ET tube through right corner of mouth.

Step 9   Visualize entry of ET tube between vocal cords.

Step 10   Remove laryngoscope from patient's mouth.

Step 11   Note depth of ET tube (in centimeters) at patient's teeth, and remove stylet from ET tube.

Step 12   Inflate distal cuff of ET tube with 5 to 10 mL of air, and immediately detach syringe from inflation port.

Step 13   Attach ETCO$_2$ detector (waveform capnography preferred) to ET tube.

Step 14   Attach ETCO$_2$ detector to cardiac monitor/ defibrillator and observe for a capnographic waveform and numeric CO$_2$ reading.

Step 15   Attach ventilation device and ventilate. Listen over epigastrium and over both lungs.

Step 16   Secure ET tube with a commercial device or tape. Ventilate patient at proper rate while monitoring capnography and pulse oximetry.

Skill Drill 15-10 Performing Orotracheal Intubation Using Video Laryngoscopy

Step 1   Take standard precautions. If you suspect trauma, then maintain manual in-line stabilization of head.

Step 2   Measure for proper size, and insert an OPA.

Step 3   Ventilate patient with a bag-mask device at a rate of 10 to 12 breaths/min with sufficient volume to produce chest rise. Preoxygenate for 2 to 3 minutes with 100% oxygen.

Step 4   Check, prepare, and assemble your equipment. Turn on video laryngoscope, and ensure light and camera are functioning.

Step 5   Remove OPA and place patient's head in sniffing position.

Step 6   Insert video laryngoscope blade into right side of patient's mouth. Sweep tongue to left (displacing laryngoscope) or midline of mouth (nondisplacing laryngoscope). Visualize epiglottis, vocal cords, and arytenoid cartilage.

Step 7   Visualize entry of ET tube between vocal cords on video monitor.

Step 8   Remove laryngoscope from patient's mouth.

Step 9   Remove stylet from ET tube (if used).

Step 10   Inflate distal cuff of ET tube with 5 to 10 mL of air, and immediately detach syringe from inflation port.

Step 11   Attach ETCO$_2$ detector (waveform capnography preferred) to ET tube.

Step 12   Attach ETCO$_2$ detector to cardiac monitor/ defibrillator and observe for a capnographic waveform and numeric CO$_2$ reading.

Step 13   Attach ventilation device and ventilate. Auscultate over epigastrium and over both lungs.

Step 14   Secure ET tube with a commercial device or tape.

Step 15   Ventilate patient at proper rate while monitoring capnography and pulse oximetry.

Skill Drill 15-11 Performing Nasotracheal Intubation

Step 1   Take standard precautions.

Step 2   Preoxygenate whenever possible with a bag-mask device and 100% oxygen. Auscultate patient's breath sounds to confirm adequate ventilation.

Step 3   Check, prepare, and assemble your equipment.

Step 4   Place patient's head in a neutral position.

Step 5   Preform nasotracheal tube by bending it in a circle.

Step 6   Administer nasal spray to cause vasoconstriction of nasal mucosa

Step 7   Lubricate tip of nasotracheal tube with a water-soluble gel.

Step 8   Gently insert nasotracheal tube into more compliant nostril, with bevel facing toward nasal septum, and advance tube along nasal floor. Pause to ensure that tip of tube is positioned just superior to vocal cords. Observe for condensation in tube, and note audible breath sounds from proximal end of tube.

Step 9   Advance nasotracheal tube through vocal cords as patient inhales. BAAM® device can be helpful in this step. Ensure that patient is aphonic (unable to speak).

Step 10   Inflate distal cuff with 5 to 10 mL of air, and immediately detach syringe.

Step 11   Attach ETCO$_2$ detector (waveform capnography preferred) to nasotracheal tube.

Step 12   Attach ETCO$_2$ detector to cardiac monitor/defibrillator.

Step 13   Attach bag-mask device, ventilate, and auscultate over epigastrium and over both lungs. Ensure proper tube placement with waveform capnography. Secure nasotracheal tube. Ventilate patient at appropriate rate while monitoring capnography and pulse oximetry.

Skill Drill 15-12 Performing Transillumination Intubation

Step 1   Take standard precautions.

Step 2   Preoxygenate for 2 to 3 minutes with a bag-mask device and 100% oxygen.

Step 3   Check, prepare, and assemble your equipment.

Step 4   Insert lighted stylet into ET tube.

Step 5   Bend ET tube by placing a slight curve at its distal end (like a hockey stick), and turn on lighted stylet.

Step 6   Lift patient's tongue and mandible anteriorly.

Step 7   Insert ET tube into midline of patient's mouth and slowly advance toward larynx, but stop before passing through vocal cords.

Step 8   Observe for a tightly circumscribed light at midline of neck, and advance ET tube approximately 1 to 1.5 inches (2 to 4 cm) farther.

Step 9   Remove stylet from ET tube.

Step 10   Inflate distal cuff of ET tube with 5 to 10 mL of air, and immediately detach syringe.

Step 11   Attach ETCO$_2$ detector (waveform capnography preferred) to ET tube.

Step 12   Attach ventilation device, ventilate, and auscultate over apices and bases of both lungs and over epigastrium. Ensure proper tube placement with waveform capnography.

Step 13   Secure ET tube, and recheck breath sounds.

Skill Drill 15-13 Performing Retrograde Intubation

Step 1 Take standard precautions. Place patient supine. Ventilate patient with 100% oxygen via appropriate device while preparing equipment and patient. Cleanse anterior part of neck from laryngeal prominence to just below cricoid ring, and position a fenestrated drape. A fenestrated drape is a sheet with a round or slit-like opening in center that is positioned over site where incision will be made.

Step 2 If patient is responsive, then consider numbing area over cricothyroid membrane using a local anesthetic.

Step 3 Puncture cricothyroid membrane using a large needle aligned with airway and pointed approximately 30° cephalad (toward head), perpendicular at level of cricothyroid membrane.

Step 4 Identify tracheal lumen by aspirating air into syringe attached to needle.

Step 5 Pass 28-inch (70-cm) guide wire through catheter until it appears in oropharynx.

Step 6 Grasp guide wire with a clamp/Magill forceps, and pull wire partially out of mouth, ensuring that distal end is still emerging from neck and wire is pulled taut.

Step 7 Insert guide wire, emerging from mouth, through lumen of ET tube.

Step 8 Advance ET tube into trachea.

Step 9 Verify tube placement by auscultating lungs bilaterally and over epigastrium. Attach an ETCO$_2$ detector (waveform capnography preferred) to ensure proper tube placement.

Step 10 After tube placement is confirmed, remove guide wire by pulling on distal end emerging from neck, then advance tube approximately 1 inch (2 to 3 cm) further.

Step 11 If tube placement is incorrect, then remove tube and attempt to ventilate. If ventilating adequately, then continue to ventilate with high-flow oxygen and reassess. Determine whether additional attempts at retrograde intubation are warranted or whether another means of securing airway is necessary (such as cricothyrotomy).

Step 12 Secure ET tube in place, and continue to ventilate.

Skill Drill 15-14 Performing Tracheobronchial Suctioning

Step 1 Check, prepare, and assemble your equipment.

Step 2 Lubricate suction catheter.

Step 3 Preoxygenate patient.

Step 4 Detach ventilation device and inject 3 to 5 mL of sterile water down ET tube.

Step 5 Gently insert catheter into ET tube until you feel resistance.

Step 6 Suction in a rotating motion while withdrawing catheter. Monitor cardiac rhythm and oxygen saturation level during procedure.

Step 7 Reattach ventilation device and resume ventilation and oxygenation.

Skill Drill 15-15 Inserting a King LT Airway

Step 1 Take standard precautions.

Step 2 Preoxygenate with a bag-mask device and 100% oxygen.

Step 3 Gather your equipment. Choose proper size of King LT airway for patient. Test cuffs for proper inflation. Ensure all air is removed from cuffs before insertion. Lubricate tip of device with a water-soluble gel for easy insertion and minimal airway damage.

Step 4 Place patient's head in a neutral position, unless contraindicated (use jaw-thrust maneuver if trauma suspected). In your dominant hand, hold King LT at connector. With your other hand, hold patient's mouth open while positioning head. Insert tip of King LT airway into midline of mouth.

Step 5 Advance tip beyond base of tongue. If you meet resistance, then rotate device slightly, change your angle, and advance it again. Continue to gently advance device until base of connector is aligned with patient's teeth or gums. Do not use excessive force. Inflate cuffs with recommended amount of air or just enough to seal device.

Step 6 Attach tube to ventilation device, and confirm tube placement by auscultating lungs and epigastrium and attaching waveform capnography. Add additional air to cuffs to maximize airway seal, if needed; however, avoid exceeding manufacturer's recommended maximum amount of air. After placement is confirmed, continue to ventilate patient.

Skill Drill 15-16 Inserting an LMA

Step 1 Take standard precautions. Check cuff of LMA by inflating it with 50% more air than is required for size of airway to be used.

Step 2 Deflate cuff completely so that no folds appear near tip. Deflation is best accomplished by pressing device, cuff facing down, on a flat surface to remove all wrinkles from cuff.

Step 3 Lubricate outer rim of device.

Step 4 Preoxygenate before insertion. Do not interrupt ventilation for more than 30 seconds to accomplish airway placement. Place patient in sniffing position.

Step 5 Proper insertion of LMA depends on holding device properly. Insert your finger between cuff and tube. Place index finger of your dominant hand in notch between tube and cuff. Open patient's mouth. Lift jaw with one hand, and begin to insert device with other hand.

Step 6 Insert LMA along roof of mouth. The key to proper insertion is to slide convex surface of airway along roof of mouth. Use your finger to push airway against hard palate. After it slides past tongue, LMA will move easily into position.

Step 7 Inflate cuff with amount of air indicated for airway being used. If LMA is properly positioned, then it will move out of airway slightly 0.5 to 0.75 inches (1 to 2 cm) as it moves into position (a good indication that LMA is in correct position).

Step 8 Begin to ventilate patient. Confirm chest rise and presence of breath sounds. Ensure proper tube placement with waveform capnography. Continuously and carefully monitor patient's condition.

Skill Drill 15-17 Inserting an i-gel Supraglottic Airway

Step 1 Take standard precautions.

Step 2 Lubricate back, sides, and front of cuff with a thin layer of water-soluble gel.

Step 3 Preoxygenate before insertion. Do not interrupt ventilation for more than 30 seconds to accomplish airway placement. Place patient in sniffing position.

Step 4 Open airway with tongue-jaw lift maneuver, and position i-gel so that cuff outlet is facing toward patient's chin.

Step 5 Introduce leading soft tip of i-gel into patient's mouth, directing it toward hard palate.

Step 6 Glide i-gel downward and backward along hard palate with a continuous but gentle push until a definitive resistance is felt.

Step 7 Begin to ventilate patient. Confirm chest rise and presence of breath sounds. Ensure proper tube placement with waveform capnography. Continuously and carefully monitor patient's condition.

Step 8 Secure i-gel in place with provided strap.

Skill Drill 15-18 Performing an Open Cricothyrotomy

Step 1 Take standard precautions.

Step 2 Check, assemble, and prepare equipment. Place a 90° bend in a 6.0-mm ET tube (with a stylet inserted), just proximal to cuff.

Step 3 With patient's head in a neutral position, palpate for and locate cricothyroid membrane.

Step 4 Cleanse area with an iodine-or chlorhexidine-containing solution.

Step 5 Stabilize larynx, and make a vertical incision (approximately 0.5 to 0.75 inch [1 to 2 cm]) over cricothyroid membrane.

Step 6 Puncture cricothyroid membrane.

Step 7 Make a horizontal incision (approximately 0.5 inch [1 cm]) in each direction from midline. Insert scalpel handle into opening and rotate it.

Step 8 Insert tube into trachea as you remove scalpel handle.

Step 9 Manually stabilize ET tube between your thumb and index finger, carefully remove stylet, and inflate distal cuff.

Step 10 Attach an ETCO$_2$ detector between tube and ventilation device.

Step 11 Ensure proper tube placement with waveform capnography. Attach ETCO$_2$ detector to monitor. Ventilate patient.

Step 12 Confirm correct tube placement by auscultating apices and bases of both lungs and over epigastrium.

Step 13 Secure tube with a commercial device or tape. Reconfirm correct tube placement, and resume ventilations at appropriate rate.

Chapter 17

Skill Drill 15-19 Performing Needle Cricothyrotomy and Translaryngeal Catheter Ventilation

Step 1 Take standard precautions.

Step 2 Attach a 14- to 16-gauge IV catheter to a 10-mL syringe containing approximately 3 mL of sterile saline or water.

Step 3 With patient's head in a neutral position, palpate for and locate cricothyroid membrane.

Step 4 Cleanse area with an iodine-containing solution.

Step 5 Stabilize larynx, and insert needle into cricothyroid membrane at a 45° angle toward feet.

Step 6 Aspirate with syringe to determine correct catheter placement.

Step 7 Slide catheter off of needle until hub of catheter is flush with patient's skin.

Step 8 Place syringe and needle in a puncture-proof container.

Step 9 Connect one end of oxygen tubing to catheter and other end to jet ventilator. Maintain manual stabilization of catheter until it has been secured in place to avoid dislodgment with jet ventilation.

Step 10 Press or occlude ventilation valve on jet ventilator for 1 second while observing for chest rise. Release ventilation valve for 2 to 3 seconds to allow for exhalation.

Step 11 Auscultate apices and bases of both lungs and over epigastrium to confirm correct catheter placement.

Step 12 Secure catheter with a 4-inch × 4-inch (10-cm × 10-cm) gauze pad and tape. Continue ventilations while frequently reassessing for adequate ventilations and potential complications.

Skill Drill 17-1 Performing Cardiac Monitoring

Step 1 Take standard precautions. Check your equipment. Ensure there are no loose pins in end of ECG cable and that cable/lead wires are intact. Ensure monitor has an adequate paper supply. Connect ECG cable to machine. Connect lead wires to ECG cable (if not already connected). Turn on power to monitor. Adjust screen contrast if necessary.

Step 2 Explain procedure to patient. To minimize distortion of ECG tracing, prepare skin for electrode placement by briskly rubbing it with a dry gauze pad to remove skin oils and improve impulse transmission. If you are applying electrodes to patient's chest, rather than to his or her limbs, then ensure good contact by shaving small amounts of chest hair if needed.

Step 3 Attach electrodes to lead wires before placing them on patient.

Step 4 One at a time, remove backing from each electrode and apply it to patient.

Step 5 If you plan to obtain a 12-lead tracing as well, then place limb leads. Limb-lead electrodes are usually placed on wrists and ankles but may be positioned anywhere on appropriate limb. To reduce muscle tension, ensure patient's limbs are resting on a supportive surface. Do not apply electrodes over bony areas, broken skin, joints, skin creases, scar tissue, or rashes.

Step 6 Turn on monitor and select desired lead, which is typically lead II. Adjust ECG size if necessary to ensure machine detects patient's QRS complexes. Feel patient's pulse, and compare it with heart rate indicator on monitor. If not already preset, then set heart rate alarms on monitor according to your agency's policy.

Step 7 Record tracings.

Step 8 Label each strip.

Skill Drill 17-2 Performing Transcutaneous Pacing

Step 1 Select, check, and assemble all necessary equipment, including a monitor/defibrillator with pacing capability, ECG electrodes, pacing pads, medication for pain or sedation (to be used if necessary), oxygen, and an appropriate oxygen administration device. Take standard precautions. Apply ECG electrodes, and assess patient's vital signs. Ensure patient is oxygenated adequately, and establish a patent IV line.

Step 2 Identify rhythm and confirm transcutaneous pacing (TCP) is warranted. Obtain a baseline rhythm strip.

Step 3 Ensure scene and environment are safe; evaluate risk of sparks, combustibles, oxygen-rich atmosphere. Explain need for procedure to patient and family. Apply pacing pads to patient according to manufacturer's recommendations. Sedation or analgesia may be needed to minimize discomfort associated with this procedure. Ask patient about any medication allergies before administering medications.

Step 4 Switch on power to pacer.

Step 5 Set pacing rate to desired number of paced pulses per minute (ppm). A rate between 60 and 80 beats/min is usually selected.

Step 6 Set current (milliamps) to be delivered to minimum setting. While watching monitor screen, slowly but steadily increase current until you achieve electrical capture (each pacer spike is followed by a wide QRS complex).

Step 7 Evaluate mechanical capture by assessing patient's pulse and BP. Reassess patient's mental status, SpO_2, color, and level of discomfort.

Step 8 Obtain rhythm strips for documentation, and continuously monitor patient's condition.

Skill Drill 17-3 Performing Synchronized Cardioversion

Step 1 Select, check, and assemble all necessary equipment, including a monitor/defibrillator with defibrillation pads, ECG electrodes, medication for pain or sedation (to be used if necessary), oxygen, and an appropriate oxygen administration device. Take standard precautions. Assess patient's vital signs. Ensure patient is oxygenated adequately, and establish a patent IV line.

Step 2 Place ECG electrodes in same position as you would when performing cardiac monitoring. Obtain a baseline rhythm strip. Identify rhythm and confirm that cardioversion is warranted. If patient is responsive, you should consider appropriate medication to sedate patient. Ask about medication allergies before administering sedation.

Step 3 Ensure environment is safe (evaluate risk of sparks, combustibles, oxygen-rich atmosphere). Explain need for procedure to patient and family. Apply defibrillation pads to patient according to manufacturer's recommendations. Turn on power to defibrillator.

Step 4 Connect pads to monitor.

Step 5 Select appropriate energy setting. Turn synchronize switch on machine to on position.

Step 6 Observe ECG rhythm. Confirm that a sense marker appears near middle of each QRS complex. If sense markers are not visible or appear in wrong location (eg, on T wave), adjust ECG size or select another lead until machine reads QRS complexes appropriately. Clear area by announcing, "All clear!"; ensure everyone is clear of patient.

Step 7 Depress *Shock* buttons. Keep them depressed until defibrillator discharges.

Step 8 Reassess ECG rhythm and patient (pulse and BP). If tachycardia persists, ensure machine is in sync mode before delivering another shock. If rhythm changes to ventricular fibrillation (VF), ensure patient has no pulse. If no pulse is present, ensure sync control is off, and proceed with defibrillation.

Skill Drill 17-4 Performing Manual Defibrillation

Step 1   Select, check, and assemble all necessary equipment, including a monitor/defibrillator with defibrillation pads, oxygen, and an appropriate oxygen administration device. Take standard precautions, and ensure scene and environment are safe (evaluate risk of sparks, combustibles, oxygen-rich atmosphere).

Step 2   If available (and possible without interrupting care), ask bystanders about events surrounding arrest. Check responsiveness. Request additional help, if needed.

Step 3   Assess patient for breathing while simultaneously checking for a carotid pulse.

Step 4   Begin chest compressions if patient is not breathing or is only gasping and has no pulse. Ensure an adequate depth and rate, use correct compression-to-ventilation ratio, allow chest to recoil completely, deliver an adequate volume for each breath, and keep interruption of chest compressions to 10 seconds or less throughout resuscitation effort.

Step 5   Turn on power to defibrillator. If EMS providers have been using machine in AED mode before your arrival, switch machine to manual mode.

Step 6   Remove clothing from patient's upper body. With gloves, remove any medication paste or patches from patient's chest, and wipe away any residue.

Step 7   If using standard paddles, place pre-gelled defibrillator pads on patient's chest (or apply defibrillator gel to electrode surface of paddles). If using adhesive electrodes, place one electrode just to right of sternum just below clavicle, and place other on left lower chest area with top of pad 2 to 3 inches below armpit (or position electrodes according to manufacturer's instructions). Do not place electrodes on top of breast tissue. If necessary, lift breast out of way and place electrode underneath.

Step 8   Stop CPR, identify rhythm, and confirm that defibrillation is warranted. After verifying that a shockable rhythm is present, set defibrillator to proper energy setting.

Step 9   Charge defibrillator.

Step 10   Clear area. Announce, "All clear!"; ensure no one is touching patient. Press *Shock* button on machine if using a hands-free system. If using paddles, depress *Shock* button on each paddle at same time, and hold until defibrillator discharges. Resume CPR immediately.

Skill Drill 17-5 Performing Defibrillation with an AED

Step 1 Select, check, and assemble all necessary equipment, including AED, AED pads, oxygen, and an appropriate oxygen administration device. Take standard precautions, and ensure scene and environment are safe (evaluate risk of sparks, combustibles, oxygen-rich atmosphere).

Step 2 If available (and possible without interrupting care), ask bystanders about events surrounding arrest. Check responsiveness. Request additional help, if needed.

Step 3 Assess patient for breathing while simultaneously checking for a carotid pulse.

Step 4 If CPR is already in progress, then assess effectiveness of chest compressions. If patient is not breathing or is only gasping and has no pulse, and CPR has not been started, then begin chest compressions and rescue breaths. Ensure an adequate depth and rate, use correct compression-to-ventilation ratio, allow chest to recoil completely, deliver an adequate volume for each breath, and keep interruption of chest compressions to 10 seconds or less throughout resuscitation effort. Continue until an AED arrives and is ready for use.

Step 5 Turn on AED. Remove clothing from patient's upper body. With gloves, remove medication paste or patches from patient's chest, if present, and wipe away any residue.

Step 6 Follow machine's prompts; apply AED pads to patient's bare chest according to manufacturer's recommendations. Attach pads to AED.

Step 7 Stop CPR and press *Analyze* button (some AEDs will begin analyzing patient's rhythm automatically). Ensure everyone is clear of patient. Wait for AED to analyze cardiac rhythm. If no shock is advised, then resume CPR, starting with chest compressions. Perform five cycles (about 2 minutes) of CPR, and then reanalyze cardiac rhythm. If a shock is advised, then recheck that all are clear, and press *Shock* button.

Step 8 After shock is delivered, immediately resume CPR, beginning with chest compressions. Do not interrupt chest compressions for more than 10 seconds. Do not turn off AED during CPR. Continue to follow AED prompts. To reduce likelihood of rescuer fatigue, rotate position of chest compressor and ventilator during AED's analysis phase.

Skill Drill 17-6 Acquiring a 12-lead ECG

Step 1 Take standard precautions. Check your equipment. Ensure end of ECG cable has no loose pins and that cable or lead wires are intact. Ensure monitor has an adequate paper supply. Connect ECG cable to machine. Connect lead wires to ECG cable (if not already connected).

Step 2 Explain procedure to patient. Prepare patient's skin for electrode placement; shave and cleanse patient's skin as needed before placing monitoring electrodes.

Step 3 Attach electrodes to leads before you place them on patient.

Step 4 Position electrodes on patient. Connect four limb electrodes. Place them on arms and legs. Do not place electrodes on trunk of body, as is sometimes done for ECG monitoring. Double-check to confirm correct electrode has been positioned on each limb (LA electrode on left arm, RA electrode on right arm, and so on). Once limb electrodes have been secured, connect and apply electrodes for precordial leads:

- V_1—Fourth intercostal space (ICS) to right of sternum
- V_2—Fourth ICS to left of sternum
- V_3—Directly between leads V_2 and V_4
- V_4—Fifth ICS at left midclavicular line
- V_5—At level of lead V_4 at left anterior axillary line
- V_6—At level of lead V_4 at left midaxillary line

Step 5 Connect cables to monitor. Ensure patient is sitting or lying still, extremities are not crossed, and he or she is breathing normally and is not talking. Turn on power to monitor, and adjust screen contrast if necessary. Ensure all electrodes and cables are still connected and that no error message is displayed.

Step 6 Press *12-Lead Analyze* button.

Step 7 Obtain 12-lead ECG recording.

Step 8 Examine tracing for acceptable quality. Interpret 12-lead ECG, label it, and determine whether additional views of right and posterior walls (15- or 18-lead tracings) are needed. Obtain a 12-lead ECG every 5 to 10 minutes in high-risk patients and post-treatment.

Chapter 19

Skill Drill 19-1 Examining the Eye with an Ophthalmoscope

Step 1 Darken environment as much as possible. Ask patient to look straight ahead and focus on a distant object.

Step 2 Set light on ophthalmoscope to a setting no brighter than necessary and lens to 0, unless another setting works better for your eyes. Use your right hand and eye to examine patient's right eye; use your left hand and eye to examine patient's left eye.

Step 3 Place scope to your eye, and look into patient's pupil from 10 to 20 inches (25 to 51 cm) away at a 45° angle to eye. You should see retina as a "red reflex" or a bright orange glow. Slowly move toward patient to appreciate structures of fundus. Adjust lens as needed to improve focus. Locate a blood vessel, and follow it back to disk. Use this blood vessel as a point of reference.

Step 4 Inspect for size, color, and clarity of disk. Note integrity of blood vessels and any lesions present on retina. Move nasally to observe macula. Repeat process with other eye.

Skill Drill 19-2 Examining the Ear with an Otoscope

Step 1 Select an appropriately sized speculum. Dim lights as much as possible. Ensure ear is free of foreign bodies. Place your hand firmly against patient's head, and gently grasp auricle. Move ear to best visualize canal, usually upward and backward in an adult patient.

Step 2 To avoid damaging ear, instruct patient not to move during exam. Turn on otoscope, and insert speculum into ear. Do not insert speculum deeply into canal.

Step 3 Inspect canal for any lesions or discharge. A small amount of cerumen (earwax) is normal. Visualize tympanic membrane (eardrum), and inspect it for integrity and color. It should be translucent or a pearly gray color. Note any signs of inflammation, including swelling or discoloration (a pink-tinged or red ear canal or tympanic membrane).

Chapter 28

Skill Drill 28-1 Restraining a Patient

Step 1   Law enforcement officers should bring down patient into prone position. Then, acting at same time, secure patient in supine or left lateral position with wrist and ankle restraints. Some services require use of backboard for restraint so that a patient who becomes unconscious or who vomits can be turned onto his or her side quickly to manage airway.

Step 2   Use stretcher straps or sheets to secure legs.

Step 3   Fasten remaining stretcher straps.

Step 4   Continue to verbally reassure and calm patient following chemical/physical restraint. Regularly check circulation to extremities.

Skill Drill 30-2 Applying a Commercial Tourniquet (Combat Application Tourniquet)

Step 1   Hold direct pressure over bleeding site, and place tourniquet proximal to injury, preferably at groin or axilla. Wrap band around limb, and fasten it to buckle.

Step 2   Pull band tightly, and secure band back on itself. Ensure that tips of three fingers cannot fit between band and limb.

Step 3   Tighten rod (windlass) until bleeding stops.

Step 4   Secure rod inside clip. Ensure bleeding is still controlled, and assess for a distal pulse.

Step 5   Wrap rest of band through clips. Secure rod with strap labeled *TIME:*, and document time.

Chapter 30

Skill Drill 30-1 Managing External Hemorrhage

Step 1   Take standard precautions. Maintain airway with cervical spine immobilization if mechanism of injury (MOI) suggests possibility of spinal injury. Apply direct, even pressure over wound with a dry, sterile dressing.

Step 2   If bleeding stops, apply a pressure dressing and/or splint. Hold pressure dressing in place using gauze.

Step 3   If direct pressure does not rapidly control bleeding on an extremity injury, apply a tourniquet above level of bleeding.

Step 4   Tighten tourniquet until bleeding stops. Position patient supine unless contraindicated. Apply oxygen as necessary. Keep patient warm, transport promptly, monitor serial vital signs, and watch diligently for developing shock.

Skill Drill 30-3 Managing Internal Hemorrhage

Step 1   Take standard precautions. Maintain airway with cervical spine immobilization if mechanism of injury (MOI) suggests possibility of spinal injury. Administer supplemental oxygen as needed, and assist ventilation if necessary.

Step 2   Control all obvious external bleeding, and treat suspected internal bleeding using a splint if possible. Apply a tourniquet for severe bleeding from an extremity that cannot be controlled with direct pressure.

Step 3   Depending on local protocols, if a pelvic fracture is suspected, use a pelvic binder or sheets to bind pelvic area.

Step 4   Monitor and record vital signs at least every 5 minutes.

Chapter 34

Skill Drill 34-1 Performing Spinal Immobilization of a Supine Adult Patient

Step 1   Take standard precautions, and then begin manual in-line stabilization from a kneeling position at patient's head. Hold head firmly with both hands. The provider at head directs all patient movement.

Support lower jaw with your index and middle fingers, and support head with your palms. If patient's head is not facing forward, gently move it until patient's eyes are looking straight ahead and head and torso are in alignment (neutral alignment). Never twist, flex, or extend head or neck excessively. Do not remove your hands from patient's head until patient is properly secured to a backboard and head is immobilized.

Evaluate patient's reliability in giving a history.

Step 2   Assess distal pulses and motor and sensory function in each extremity.

Step 3   Apply a well-fitting cervical collar as previously discussed.

Step 4   Other team members should position immobilization device (backboard) beside patient and place their hands on patient's far side to increase their leverage while kneeling. Instruct them to use their body weight, shoulders, and back muscles to ensure a smooth, coordinated pull. The pull should concentrate on heavier portions of body.

Step 5   On count/command from paramedic at patient's head, rescuers should roll patient toward themselves until patient is balanced on his or her side. This prevents patient from twisting as he or she is pulled down by gravity and up by provider. One rescuer should then quickly examine back while patient is rolled on side, and then slide backboard behind and under patient. The team should then roll patient back onto board, avoiding rotation of head, shoulders, and pelvis.

Step 6   Ensure patient is centered on board. Alternatively, patient may be moved onto board as follows: board is placed beside patient with foot end at level of patient's hips. The patient is log rolled, then patient is pulled onto board along axis of spine to a centered position. This alternative method results in only moving patient twice (one roll and one slide).

Step 7   Apply padding as necessary to fill voids between patient and device. When possible, prepare blanket rolls ahead of time, and have them ready to go. When you have blankets prepared, you need only seconds to place them. Use of blanket rolls has been shown to dramatically improve effectiveness of immobilization.

Step 8   Center patient on backboard.

Step 9   Secure upper torso to board after patient has been centered on backboard.

Step 10 Secure pelvis and upper legs, using padding as needed. For pelvis, use straps over iliac crests and/or groin loops (leg straps).

Step 11 Pad behind patient's head and neck as needed to maintain a neutral in-line position.

Step 12 Immobilize head to board with a commercial immobilization device per manufacturer's instructions. Secure head to board only after entire torso has been secured. If head is secured first and body shifts, spine may be compromised. Securing most of body weight first creates better protection.

Step 13 Secure patient's lower legs to board.

Step 14 Secure patient's arms with a single strap.

Step 15 Check and readjust straps as needed to ensure that entire body is snugly secured and will not slide during movement of board or during patient transport. Reassess distal pulse, motor function, and sensation (PMS) function in each extremity and repeat periodically.

Skill Drill 34-2 Using a Scoop Stretcher

Step 1   With scoop stretcher separated, measure length of scoop and adjust to proper length.

Step 2   Position stretcher, one side at a time. Lift patient's side slightly by pulling on far hip and upper arm while your partner slides stretcher into place.

Step 3   Lock stretcher ends together by engaging their locking mechanisms one at a time, and continue to lift patient slightly as needed to avoid pinching patient or your fingers.

Step 4   Apply and tighten straps to secure patient to scoop stretcher before transferring to stretcher.

Skill Drill 34-3 Performing Spinal Immobilization of a Seated Adult Patient

Step 1   Take standard precautions, and direct your assistant to place and maintain head in a neutral in-line position. Stabilize head and neck with manual in-line stabilization until patient is secured to long backboard. Evaluate patient's reliability as a historian. Assess distal pulse and motor and sensory function in each extremity.

Apply a well-fitting cervical collar. Because cervical collar does not completely stabilize cervical spine, continue manual stabilization of head and neck until patient is fully immobilized on a backboard.

Step 2   Insert immobilization device between patient's upper back and seat back.

Step 3   Open board's side flaps (if present), and position them around patient's torso, snug to armpits.

Step 4   When device is properly positioned, secure upper torso straps.

Step 5   Position and fasten both groin/leg straps. Pad groin as needed. Check all torso straps, and make sure they are secure. Make any necessary adjustments without excessively moving patient.

Step 6   Pad any space between patient's head and device. Secure forehead strap or tape head securely, and then fasten lower head strap around rigid cervical collar. Reevaluate patient to assure that he or she is adequately immobilized. Reassess distal pulses and motor and sensory function in each extremity.

Step 7   Place long backboard next to patient's buttocks, perpendicular to trunk.

Step 8   Turn patient parallel to long board, and slowly lower him or her onto it. Lift patient and vest-type board together as a unit (without rotating patient), and slip long backboard under patient and device. Slide patient onto backboard as a unit using any handles that may be built into device. Release leg straps and loosen chest strap to allow legs to straighten and give chest room to fully expand.

Step 9   Secure short board and long backboard together. Do not remove vest-type board from patient. Reassess distal pulse and motor and sensory function in all four extremities. Note your findings on PCR and prepare for transport.

Chapter 35

Skill Drill 35-1 Needle Decompression (Thoracentesis) of a Tension Pneumothorax

Step 1   Assess patient to ensure that presentation matches that of a tension pneumothorax. Look for difficult ventilation despite an open airway, jugular venous distention (JVD; may not be present with associated hemorrhage), absent or decreased breath sounds on affected side, hyperresonance to percussion on affected side, tracheal deviation away from affected side (late sign, not always present), pulsus paradoxus, and tachycardia.

Step 2   Prepare and assemble all necessary equipment, including a large-bore IV catheter, preferably 14- to 16-gauge and at least 3.25 inches (8 cm) long (this ensures ability of needle to reach intended depth to relieve pressure); alcohol or povidone iodine (Betadine) preps; a flutter valve (cut off one finger of a glove to use as a substitute if you do not have a commercial device available); and adhesive tape. A two-way or three-way stopcock can also be used to seal or relieve pressure should it begin to build within thoracic cavity. Obtain medical control if required by regional protocols.

Step 3   Locate appropriate site. Find second or third rib. Insert needle just above third rib into intercostal space at midclavicular line on affected side. If there is significant trauma to anterior portion of chest, or chest wall is too deep, use intercostal space between fourth and fifth ribs at midaxillary line on affected side.

Step 4   Cleanse appropriate area using aseptic technique.

Step 5   Make a one-way valve, or flutter valve, by inserting catheter through end of finger of a medical glove, cut off from glove. Alternatively, use a commercially prepared device.

Step 6   Insert needle at a 90° angle, and listen for release of air. Insert needle just superior to third rib, midclavicular line, or just above sixth rib, midaxillary line. (To avoid nerves, arteries, and veins, run along inferior borders of each rib.)

Step 7   Remove needle, and properly dispose of needle in sharps container.

Step 8   Secure catheter in place in same manner you would use to secure an impaled object. Monitor patient closely for recurrence of tension pneumothorax. This procedure may need to be repeated several times before arrival at ED.

Chapter 37

Skill Drill 37-1 Performing a Motor Function and Sensory Exam

Step 1 Have patient flex his or her arms at elbow to test musculocutaneous nerve motor function.

Step 2 Have patient extend arms at elbow to test radial nerve motor function.

Step 3 Have patient extend thumbs (thumbs up) to test radial nerve motor function.

Step 4 Have patient make an "okay" sign to test median nerve motor function.

Step 5 Have patient spread his or her fingers apart to test ulnar nerve motor function.

Step 6 Instruct patient to extend his or her legs at knee to test femoral nerve motor function.

Step 7 Have patient flex his or her feet and ankles downward (plantarflex) to test tibial nerve motor function.

Step 8 Instruct patient to flex feet and ankles upward (dorsiflex) to test deep peroneal nerve motor function.

Step 9 Lightly touch lateral surface of shoulder (over deltoid) to test axillary nerve sensory function using corner of a bandage or tissue to make contact with skin.

Step 10 Lightly touch anterolateral surface of forearm to test musculocutaneous nerve sensory function.

Step 11 Lightly touch dorsal surface of web space of thumb to test radial nerve sensory function.

Step 12 Lightly touch volar surface of distal thumb, index, and middle fingers to test median nerve sensory function.

Step 13 Lightly touch distal volar surface of small finger to test ulnar nerve sensory function.

Step 14 Lightly touch anteromedial surface of thigh to test femoral nerve sensory function.

Step 15 Lightly touch plantar surface of toes to test tibial nerve sensory function.

Step 16 Lightly touch web space between great toe and second toe to test peroneal nerve sensory function.

Chapter 39

Skill Drill 39-1 Performing Two-Rescuer Adult CPR

Step 1 Take standard precautions, and ensure scene safety. Move to patient's head and establish unresponsiveness while your partner moves to patient's side to be ready to deliver chest compressions.

Step 2 If patient is unresponsive, then simultaneously check for breathing and palpate for a carotid pulse; take no more than 10 seconds to do this. If patient has no pulse and is either not breathing or only gasping, then apply an AED if available.

Step 3 If an AED is unavailable, begin chest compressions at a ratio of 30:2. After an advanced airway is inserted, rescuers should switch from cycles of CPR to continuously delivered compressions at a rate of 100 to 120/min.

Step 4 If patient has a pulse, position patient to open airway according to your suspicion of spinal injury. If breathing is adequate, then place patient in recovery position, and monitor breathing and pulse.

Step 5 If patient has a pulse but is not breathing adequately, then deliver rescue breaths at a rate of 10 breaths/min (1 breath every 6 s).

Step 6 If CPR was started, then compressor and ventilator should switch positions after 2 min. Switch time should take no longer than 5 s. If a third rescuer is available, then position him or her at chest opposite compressor. If only two rescuers are available, then switch mid-cycle during compressions.

Step 7 Reassess patient every few minutes. Each assessment should last no more than 10 s. Depending on patient's condition, continue CPR, continue rescue breathing only, or place patient in recovery position, monitoring breathing and pulse.

Note: After an advanced airway has been inserted, compressions and ventilations are no longer performed in cycles. Instead, they are performed individually, are not timed, and do not require waiting for other rescuer to pause (asynchronous). Compressor provides between 100 and 120 compressions/min without pausing for breaths, and ventilator gives 10 breaths/min (1 breath every 6 s). Because compressor will inevitably get tired, switch compressors every 2 min, but minimize break in compression cycle to approximately 5 s.

Skill Drill 39-2 Performing CPR on a Child

Step 1   Take standard precautions, and ensure scene safety. Move to child's head and establish unresponsiveness while your partner moves to patient's side to be ready to deliver chest compressions. If patient is unresponsive, then simultaneously check for breathing and palpate for a pulse; take no more than 10 seconds to do this. If patient has no pulse and is either not breathing or only gasping, then apply an AED if available.

Step 2   Place child on a firm surface. Prepare to place heel of one or both hands in center of chest, in between nipples, avoiding xiphoid process.

Step 3   Compress chest one-third anterior-posterior diameter of chest (approximately 2 in. [5 cm] in most children) at a rate of 100 to 120/min. In between compressions, allow chest to fully recoil; do not lean on chest. Compression and relaxation time should be same duration. Use smooth movements. Hold your fingers off child's ribs, and keep heel of your hand(s) on sternum.

Step 4   Coordinate compressions and ventilations in a 30:2 ratio for one rescuer and 15:2 for two rescuers, making sure chest rises with each ventilation. At end of each cycle, pause for two ventilations.

Step 5   Continue cycles of compressions and ventilations until an AED becomes available or patient shows signs of spontaneous breathing. If child resumes effective breathing, then place him or her in a position that allows for frequent reassessment of airway and vital signs during transport.

Step 6   If child remains in cardiac arrest, continue CPR. Rotate compressors every 2 minutes of CPR.

Note: After an advanced airway has been inserted, compressions and ventilations are no longer performed in cycles. Instead, they are performed continuously at a rate of at least 100 breaths/min, without pauses for ventilation. Ventilations should be delivered at breath every 6 to 8 s (8 to 10 breaths/min). Because compressor will inevitably get tired, switch compressors every 2 min but limit break in compressions to approximately 5 s.

Skill Drill 39-3 Infant CPR

Step 1   Take standard precautions, and ensure scene safety. Move to infant's head and establish unresponsiveness while your partner moves to patient's side to be ready to deliver chest compressions. If patient is unresponsive, then simultaneously check for breathing and palpate for a brachial pulse; take no more than 10 seconds to do this. If patient has no pulse and is either not breathing or only gasping, then apply an AED if available.

Step 2   Place infant on a firm surface, using one hand to keep head in an open airway position. You can also use a pad or wedge under shoulders and upper body to keep head from tilting forward.

Step 3   Imagine a line drawn between nipples. Place two fingers in middle of sternum, about 0.5 in. (1 cm) below level of imaginary line (one finger width). Using two fingers, compress sternum at least one-third anterior-posterior diameter of chest (approximately 1.5 in. [4 cm] in most infants). Compress chest at a rate of 100 to 120/min. After each compression, allow sternum to return briefly to its normal position. Allow equal time for compression and relaxation of chest. Do not remove your fingers from sternum, and avoid jerky movements.

Step 4   Coordinate compressions and ventilations in a 30:2 ratio for one rescuer and 15:2 for two rescuers, making sure chest rises with each ventilation. At end of each cycle, pause for two ventilations. Continue cycles of compressions and ventilations until an AED becomes available or infant shows signs of spontaneous breathing. If infant resumes effective breathing, place him or her in a position that allows for frequent reassessment of airway and vital signs during transport.

Chapter 42

Skill Drill 42-1 Intubating a Newborn

Step 1 Pre-oxygenate newborn by bag-mask ventilation to an oxygen saturation greater than 95%. Administering 100% oxygen is not needed and can have deleterious effects in preterm infants.

Step 2 Suction oropharynx if there are copious secretions that prevent adequate ventilation. This can be a vagal stimulus, so pay close attention to pulse rate, and avoid repeated or vigorous suctioning. Provide bag-mask ventilation if bradycardia results.

Step 3 Place laryngoscope blade in oropharynx. Visualize vocal cords. Avoid applying torque to blade because it increases risk of trauma. Place ET tube between vocal cords until black line on ET tube is at level of cords. For full-term newborns, ET tube is usually advanced until it is at 9 cm at lip. For a premature newborn, you may need to advance ET tube to only 6.5 to 7 cm at lip. Limit intubation attempt to 20 seconds, and initiate bag-mask ventilation if it is unsuccessful or if significant bradycardia develops.

Step 4 Confirm ET tube placement. Observe chest rise, auscultate laterally in epigastric region and high on chest, note mist in ET tube (seen when patient exhales through tube from condensation of humidified air leaving lungs), note equal breath sounds on both sides, and observe for clinical improvement. Monitor ETCO$_2$ via waveform capnography, and consider using pulse oximetry. This is often earliest indicator of return of spontaneous circulation (ROSC). Pulse oximetry monitoring provides peripheral oxygen saturation and reflects response to adequate oxygenation and ventilation.

Step 5 Tape ET tube in place on face to minimize risk of tube dislodging. Monitor newborn closely for complications such as tube dislodgement, tube occlusion by mucous plug or meconium, or pneumothorax.

Skill Drill 42-2 Inserting an Orogastric Tube in the Newborn

Step 1 Measure for correct depth. Use an 8F feeding tube, and measure length from bottom of earlobe to tip of nose to halfway between xiphoid process (lower tip of sternum) and umbilicus.

Step 2 Insert tube through mouth to appropriate depth. Leave nose open to allow for ventilation.

Step 3 Attach a 10-mL syringe and suction stomach contents. Tape tube to newborn's cheek. Remove syringe from feeding tube to allow venting of air from stomach. Intermittently suction feeding tube.

Chapter 43

Skill Drill 43-1 Inserting an Oropharyngeal Airway in a Pediatric Patient

Step 1 Determine appropriately sized airway by measuring from corner of mouth to angle of jaw or by using a length-based resuscitation tape to measure patient. Place airway next to face, with flange at level of central incisors and bite block segment parallel to hard palate. The tip of airway should reach angle of jaw.

Step 2 Position patient's airway. For medical patients, use head tilt–chin lift maneuver, avoiding hyperextension. If patient has a traumatic injury, use jaw-thrust maneuver and provide in-line spinal stabilization.

Step 3 Open mouth by applying pressure on chin with your thumb. Insert airway by depressing tongue with a tongue blade on base of tongue and inserting airway directly over tongue blade. If a tongue blade is not available, point airway tip toward roof of mouth to depress tongue. Gently rotate airway into position as it passes through mouth toward curve of tongue. Insert airway until flange rests against lips. Reassess airway after insertion.

Skill Drill 43-2 Inserting a Nasopharyngeal Airway in a Pediatric Patient

Step 1 Determine appropriately sized airway. External diameter of airway should not be larger than diameter of naris, and there should be no blanching (turning white) of naris after insertion. Place airway next to patient's face to make sure length is correct. Airway should extend from tip of nose to tragus of ear (ie, small cartilaginous projection in front of opening of ear). Position patient's airway, using techniques described for oropharyngeal airway (OPA).

Step 2 Lubricate airway with a water-soluble lubricant. Insert tip into right naris with bevel pointing toward septum.

Step 3 Carefully move tip forward, following curvature of nose, until flange rests against outside of nostril. If you are inserting airway on left side, insert tip into left naris upside down, with bevel pointing toward septum. Move airway forward slowly until you feel a slight resistance, and then rotate airway 180°. Reassess airway after insertion.

Skill Drill 43-3 Performing One-Person Bag-Mask Ventilation on a Pediatric Patient

Step 1   Open airway and insert appropriate airway adjunct.

Step 2   Hold mask on patient's face by using one-handed head tilt–chin lift technique (E-C grip) method. To use E-C method, form a C with your thumb and index finger along mask while your other three fingers form an E along mandible. With infants and toddlers, support jaw with only your third finger. Do not compress area under chin because you may push tongue into back of mouth and block airway. Keep your fingers on mandible. Ensure mask forms an airtight seal on face. Maintain seal while checking that airway is open.

Step 3   Squeeze bag, using correct ventilation rate: 12 to 20 breaths/min for infants and children (1 breath every 3 to 5 seconds). Allow 1 second per ventilation, providing adequate time for exhalation.

Step 4   Assess effectiveness of ventilation by watching bilateral rise and fall of chest.

Skill Drill 43-4 Performing Pediatric Endotracheal Intubation

Step 1   Take standard precautions (gloves and face shield).

Step 2   Check, prepare, and assemble your equipment.

Step 3   Measure length of child using a length-based resuscitation tape to aid in determining needed equipment sizes.

Step 4   Manually open child's airway.

Step 5   Measure for proper size, and then insert oropharyngeal airway (OPA) or nasopharyngeal airway (NPA).

Step 6   Ventilate patient with a bag-mask device at a rate of 12 to 20 breaths/min with sufficient volume to produce visible chest rise. Attach pulse oximeter, and note child's oxygen saturation level. Preoxygenate child for at least 2 to 3 minutes with 100% oxygen.

Step 7   Place patient's head in a neutral or sniffing position; add padding as needed to achieve proper positioning. Remove airway adjunct, then insert laryngoscope into right side of mouth, and sweep tongue to left. Lift tongue with firm, gentle pressure. Avoid using teeth or gums as a fulcrum.

Step 8   Identify vocal cords. If cords are not yet visible, instruct your partner to perform BURP maneuver (also called external laryngeal manipulation) if possible.

Step 9   Introduce ET tube in right corner of child's mouth.

Step 10   Pass ET tube through vocal cords to approximately 2 to 3 cm below vocal cords. Remove laryngoscope from patient's mouth. Inflate cuff to proper pressure, and immediately remove syringe if a cuffed tube is used.

Step 11   Attach an end-tidal carbon dioxide detector (waveform capnography preferred). Attach bag-mask device, and auscultate for equal breath sounds over each lateral chest wall high in axillae. Ensure absence of breath sounds over epigastrium. Assess for hypoxia during intubation attempt.

Step 12   Secure ET tube with a commercial device or tape, noting placement of distance marker at child's teeth or gums. Ventilate patient at proper rate and volume while monitoring capnography and pulse oximetry.

Skill Drill 43-5 Performing Pediatric IO Infusion

Step 1   Check selected IV fluid for proper fluid, clarity, and expiration date. Look for any discoloration or particles floating in fluid. If any are found, discard fluid and choose another bag of fluid. Select appropriate equipment, including an intraosseous (IO) needle, syringe, saline, and extension set. A three-way stopcock may also be used to facilitate easier fluid administration.

Step 2   Select proper administration set. Connect administration set to bag. Prepare administration set. Fill drip chamber, and flush tubing. Ensure no air bubbles remain in tubing. Prepare syringe and extension tubing.

Step 3   At any time before IO puncture, cut or tear tape and prepare bulky dressings. Before IO puncture, take standard precautions. Identify proper anatomic site for IO puncture. To miss epiphyseal (growth) plate, you should measure two fingerbreadths below knee on medial side of leg.

Step 4   Cleanse site using aseptic technique (ie, in a circular manner from inside out). Stabilize tibia. Place a folded towel under knee, and hold it so that you keep your fingers away from puncture site. Insert needle at a 90° angle to leg. Advance needle with a twisting motion until you feel a "pop."

Step 5   Unscrew cap, and remove stylet from needle.

Step 6   Remove stylet from catheter. Attach syringe and extension set to IO needle. Pull back on syringe to aspirate blood and particles of bone marrow to ensure placement. If you are not able to aspirate marrow but IO flushes easily, with no signs of infiltration (swelling around insertion site), then continue to flush. Slowly inject saline to ensure proper placement of needle. Watch for infiltration, and stop infusion immediately if any is noted. It is possible to fracture bone during insertion of IO needle; if this happens, you should remove IO needle and switch to other leg. Connect administration set, and adjust flow rate as appropriate. Fluid does not flow well through an IO needle, and boluses are given by administering fluid using syringe and three-way stopcock.

Step 7   Secure needle with tape, and support it with a bulky dressing. Be careful not to tape around entire circumference of leg because doing so could impair circulation and create compartment syndrome. Dispose of needle in proper container.

Skill Drill 43-6 Immobilizing a Child

Step 1 Use a towel under shoulders of a child to maintain head in a neutral position.

Step 2 Apply an appropriately sized cervical collar.

Step 3 Carefully log roll child onto immobilization device.

Step 4 Secure child's torso to immobilization device first.

Step 5 Secure child's head to immobilization device.

Step 6 Complete immobilization by ensuring that child is strapped in properly.

Skill Drill 43-7 Immobilizing an Infant

Step 1 Carefully stabilize infant's head in a neutral position, and lay seat down into a reclined position on a hard surface.

Step 2 Position a pediatric board or a similar device between infant and surface on which infant is resting.

Step 3 Slide infant onto board.

Step 4 Make sure infant's head is in a neutral position by placing a towel under infant's shoulders.

Step 5 Secure torso first, and place padding to fill any voids.

Step 6 Secure infant's head to backboard.

Chapter 45

Skill Drill 45-1 Cleaning a Tracheostomy Tube

Step 1 Wash your hands and apply a mask, goggles, and clean nonlatex gloves. Suctioning a home care patient is a clean procedure, not a sterile one. Open supplies may be used. For cost reasons, home care patients often reuse their suction catheters. If catheters do not have visible contamination and have been stored in a clean manner, they are acceptable for use. Remove inner cannula, and check with your patient's caregiver, if available, regarding appropriate solution for soaking device, then place device to soak in recommended solution. If caregiver is not available, use a mixture of hydrogen peroxide and water. Placing cannula in plain water is acceptable in short-term situations. With one-piece tracheostomy tubes, this step is unnecessary. If patient is dependent on a ventilator, have a replacement cannula immediately available.

Step 2 Attach catheter to negative pressure. Check suction and clear catheter by drawing up a small amount of saline.

Step 3 Have patient take a deep breath, or preoxygenate patient using ventilator.

Step 4 Insert catheter into trachea without suction. Apply intermittent suction while removing catheter. Repeat as necessary. Keep patient well oxygenated during procedure.

Step 5 Clean inner cannula with tracheostomy brush, rinse, and replace and lock into place. Omit this step for a one-piece tracheostomy tube. Remove your gloves and wash your hands. Document procedure and assessment on PCR.

Skill Drill 45-2 Replacing an Ostomy Device

Step 1 Help position patient in a comfortable area in which to change appliance and easily dispose of contaminated articles. Wash your hands and apply a mask, goggles, and clean nonlatex gloves. Open supplies. Ostomy equipment includes a skin barrier called a wafer and one of several styles of drainage bags. Some bags can be opened along bottom and emptied at regular intervals; others are sealed around a system similar to a urine drainage bag. Empty/remove current appliance, and dispose of it appropriately.

Step 2 Wash area around stoma with soap and water. Cleanse stoma with water only, being careful not to rub or irritate area.

Step 3 Place a clean gauze pad over stoma to prevent contamination of clean skin with stool or urine.

Step 4 Cut wafer to correct size using patient's measurement or tracing. Home care patients usually have stoma already sized or have a tracing to cut a hole in wafer large enough for stoma but keeping exposed skin to a minimum.

Step 5 Attach appliance to wafer. Be sure distal end is closed.

Step 6 Remove gauze.

Step 7 Remove paper backing from wafer.

Step 8 Apply appliance with stoma centered in wafer cutout. Remove your gloves and wash your hands. Document procedure and assessment on PCR.

Skill Drill 45-3 Catheterizing an Adult Male Patient

Step 1 Help position patient supine with legs slightly spread apart. Maintain privacy as much as possible. Wash your hands and apply a mask, goggles, and sterile nonlatex gloves.

Open supplies, including urinary catheter and placement kit. Home care patients may reuse their catheters provided that they have been stored in a clean manner. Place necessary supplies onto a clean area within reach. If placing an indwelling catheter, use sterile technique throughout. Do not allow catheter that will be inserted to come into contact with anything that is not also sterile. If you are inserting an indwelling catheter, connect a syringe filled with saline to balloon port. Also, connect indwelling catheter to drainage system. There are no connecting ports for either a balloon or a drainage bag on a straight catheter.

Wash penis with solution included in kit. Make sure foreskin has been retracted. Use great caution throughout to avoid breaks in sterile technique.

Coat end of catheter with a water-soluble gel. Hold penis at a 90° angle to body and insert catheter.

Step 2 When urine is evident in tubing, insert catheter until Y between drainage port and balloon port is at tip of penis. For a straight catheter, insert approximately 1 inch (2.5 cm) more.

Inflate balloon, and gently pull back on catheter until you feel resistance, which indicates that balloon is snug against neck of bladder. This step is unnecessary for a straight catheter. Never inflate balloon if you do not see any urine in tubing or if you meet resistance to inflation, as doing so may indicate that balloon is in urethra instead of bladder, and inflation would therefore cause urethral injury.

Step 3 Allow urine to drain. Note amount and color.

To remove a catheter, remove saline in balloon port and pull back gently until catheter is free of tip of penis. Never remove an indwelling catheter without using a syringe to remove saline from balloon because it may damage urinary sphincter. For a straight catheter, simply pull back gently to remove catheter. Wash according to home care instructions. Remove your gloves and wash your hands, following standard precautions. If catheter is to remain in place, secure it to patient's leg according to home care instructions. Document procedure and assessment on PCR.

Skill Drill 45-4 Catheterizing an Adult Female Patient

Step 1 Help position patient supine with legs spread apart or side lying with top knee flexed. Maintain privacy as much as possible. Wash your hands and apply nonlatex gloves.

Open supplies including urinary catheter and placement kit. Home care patients may reuse their catheters provided that they have been stored in a clean manner. Place necessary supplies onto a clean area within reach. If placing an indwelling catheter, use sterile technique throughout. Do not allow catheter that will be inserted to come into contact with anything that is not also sterile. If you are inserting an indwelling catheter, connect a syringe filled with saline to balloon port. Also, connect indwelling catheter to drainage system. There are no connecting ports for either a balloon or a drainage bag on a straight catheter.

Wash perineal area with solution included in kit. First cleanse outer area of perineum, and then spread labia minora and thoroughly wash mucosa surrounding vagina and urinary meatus. Dry with a clean towel. Coat end of catheter with a water-soluble gel. Locate urinary meatus anterior to vagina and insert catheter. Depending on age of patient, integrity of her pelvic musculature, and other factors, locating urinary meatus can be difficult.

Step 2 When urine is evident in tubing, insert catheter another 1 to 3 inches (2.5 to 8 cm).

Step 3 Inflate balloon and gently pull back on catheter until you feel resistance, which indicates that balloon is snug against neck of bladder. This step is unnecessary for a straight catheter. Allow urine to drain. Note amount and color.

To remove a catheter, remove saline in balloon port and pull back gently until catheter is free of tip of meatus. Never remove an indwelling catheter without using a syringe to remove saline from balloon because it may damage urinary sphincter. For a straight catheter, simply pull back gently to remove catheter. If catheter is to be reused, it should be cleaned. Remove your gloves and wash your hands.

If catheter is to remain in place, secure it to patient's leg or abdomen according to patient's needs. Document procedure and assessment on PCR.

Chapter 48

Skill Drill 48-1 Breaking Tempered Glass Using a Spring-Loaded Center Punch

Step 1   Take standard precautions and don appropriate PPE. Ensure that scene is safe and vehicle is stable. Using window farthest from patient, place palm of your hand facedown against lower corner of window and frame, with your index finger and thumb facing upward. Position and rest body of spring-loaded center punch in ridge section of your palm (V-section of your hand) between your index finger and thumb.

Step 2   Ensure that patient is protected from flying glass. Warn personnel verbally, "Breaking glass!" With point of tool directly on glass, apply pressure until spring is activated and glass breaks.

Step 3   Use a piece of cribbing to remove remaining fragments of tempered glass from around window frame.

Skill Drill 48-2 Stabilizing a Suspected Spinal Injury in the Water

Step 1   Turn patient supine by rotating entire upper half of patient's body as a single unit. Twisting only head, for example, may aggravate any injury to cervical spine. Two rescuers are usually required to turn patient safely, although one may suffice.

Step 2   As soon as patient is turned, have other rescuer support head and trunk as a unit while you open airway and begin artificial ventilation using mouth-to-mouth method or a pocket mask. Immediate ventilation is primary treatment of all submersion patients as soon as patient is faceup in water.

Step 3   Float a buoyant backboard under patient as you continue ventilation.

Step 4   Secure trunk and head of patient to backboard to eliminate motion of cervical spine. Do not remove patient from water until this is done.

Step 5   Remove patient from water, on backboard.

Step 6   Remove patient's wet clothes and cover him or her with a blanket. Administer supplemental oxygen if patient is breathing adequately; give positive-pressure ventilation if he or she is apneic or breathing inadequately. Begin CPR if breathing and pulse are absent.

Chapter 49

Skill Drill 49-1 Using the *ERG* to Research Materials

Step 1   Identify chemical name and/or chemical ID number for suspect material.

Step 2   Look up material name in appropriate section. Use yellow section to obtain information based on chemical ID number. Use blue section to obtain information based on alphabetical chemical name. *Note any listing that has been highlighted because this should lead you to evacuation distance section of* ERG.

Step 3   Determine correct emergency action guide to use for chemical identified.

Step 4   Identify potential fire and explosion and/or health hazards of chemical identified.

Step 5   Identify isolation distance and protective actions required for chemical identified.

Step 6   Identify emergency response actions for chemical identified.